NUTRIENT REQUIREMENTS OF SMALL RUMINANTS

NUTRIENT REQUIREMENTS OF SMALL RUMINANTS

SHEEP, GOATS, CERVIDS, AND NEW WORLD CAMELIDS

Committee on Nutrient Requirements of Small Ruminants

Board on Agriculture and Natural Resources

Division on Earth and Life Studies

NATIONAL RESEARCH COUNCIL
OF THE NATIONAL ACADEMIES

THE NATIONAL ACADEMIES PRESS
Washington, D.C.
www.nap.edu

THE NATIONAL ACADEMIES PRESS • 500 Fifth Street, N.W. • Washington, DC 20001

NOTICE: The project that is the subject of this report was approved by the Governing Board of the National Research Council, whose members are drawn from the councils of the National Academy of Sciences, the National Academy of Engineering, and the Institute of Medicine. The members of the committee responsible for the report were chosen for their special competences and with regard for appropriate balance.

This study was supported by grants from the National Sheep Industry Improvement Center (U.S. Department of Agriculture), the Joe Skeen Institute for Rangeland Restoration (Montana State University, New Mexico State University, and Texas A&M University), the American Sheep Industry Association, the Montana Sheep Institute, internal National Research Council funds, and general support of the Animal Nutrition series provided by the Department of Health and Human Services (U.S. Food and Drug Administration) under Award No. 223-01-01-2460. Any opinions, findings, conclusions, or recommendations expressed in this publication are those of the author(s) and do not necessarily reflect the views of the organizations or agencies that provided support for the project.

Library of Congress Cataloging-in-Publication Data

Nutrient requirements of small ruminants : sheep, goats, cervids, and New World camelids / Committee on Nutrient Requirements of Small Ruminants, Board on Agriculture and Natural Resources, Division on Earth and Life Studies, The National Research Council.

p. cm.

Includes bibliographical references and index.

ISBN 0-309-10213-8 (cloth) — 978-0-309-10213-1 (cloth) 1. Ruminants—Feeding and feeds. 2. Ruminants—Nutrition—Requirements. I. National Research Council (U.S.). Committee on Nutrient Requirements of Smal Ruminants.

SF95.N78 2006

636.3′0852—dc22

2006028306

Additional copies of this report are available from the National Academies Press, 500 Fifth Street, N.W., Lockbox 285, Washington, DC 20055; (800) 624-6242 or (202) 334-3313 (in the Washington metropolitan area); Internet, http://www.nap.edu

Printed in the United States of America

THE NATIONAL ACADEMIES

Advisers to the Nation on Science, Engineering, and Medicine

The **National Academy of Sciences** is a private, nonprofit, self-perpetuating society of distinguished scholars engaged in scientific and engineering research, dedicated to the furtherance of science and technology and to their use for the general welfare. Upon the authority of the charter granted to it by the Congress in 1863, the Academy has a mandate that requires it to advise the federal government on scientific and technical matters. Dr. Ralph J. Cicerone is president of the National Academy of Sciences.

The **National Academy of Engineering** was established in 1964, under the charter of the National Academy of Sciences, as a parallel organization of outstanding engineers. It is autonomous in its administration and in the selection of its members, sharing with the National Academy of Sciences the responsibility for advising the federal government. The National Academy of Engineering also sponsors engineering programs aimed at meeting national needs, encourages education and research, and recognizes the superior achievements of engineers. Dr. Wm. A. Wulf is president of the National Academy of Engineering.

The **Institute of Medicine** was established in 1970 by the National Academy of Sciences to secure the services of eminent members of appropriate professions in the examination of policy matters pertaining to the health of the public. The Institute acts under the responsibility given to the National Academy of Sciences by its congressional charter to be an adviser to the federal government and, upon its own initiative, to identify issues of medical care, research, and education. Dr. Harvey V. Fineberg is president of the Institute of Medicine.

The **National Research Council** was organized by the National Academy of Sciences in 1916 to associate the broad community of science and technology with the Academy's purposes of furthering knowledge and advising the federal government. Functioning in accordance with general policies determined by the Academy, the Council has become the principal operating agency of both the National Academy of Sciences and the National Academy of Engineering in providing services to the government, the public, and the scientific and engineering communities. The Council is administered jointly by both Academies and the Institute of Medicine. Dr. Ralph J. Cicerone and Dr. Wm. A. Wulf are chair and vice chair, respectively, of the National Research Council.

www.national-academies.org

COMMITTEE ON NUTRIENT REQUIREMENTS OF SMALL RUMINANTS

JAMES E. (ED) HUSTON, *Chair,* Texas A&M University, San Angelo
ROBERT G. WHITE, *Vice-Chair,* University of Alaska, Fairbanks
BRIAN J. BEQUETTE, University of Maryland, College Park
HUGH DOVE, Commonwealth Scientific and Industrial Research Organisation, Canberra, Australia
ARTHUR L. GOETSCH, Langston University, Langston, Oklahoma
BRET W. HESS, University of Wyoming, Laramie
MAXIMINO HUERTA BRAVO, Universidad Autónoma Chapingo, Texcoco, Mexico
DAVID G. PUGH, Fort Dodge Animal Health, Waverly, Alabama
SANDRA G. SOLAIMAN, Tuskegee University, Alabama

Staff

AUSTIN J. LEWIS, *Study Director*
JAMIE S. JONKER, *Study Director**
DONNA LEE JAMEISON, *Senior Project Assistant***
RUTH S. ARIETI, *Project Assistant*
PEGGY TSAI, *Research Associate*

External Support

PAULA T. WHITACRE, *Editor*

*Through June 2004
**Through January 2006

Preface

Small ruminants, especially sheep and goats, are an important part of the economic and social life of many nations throughout the world. Numerous other species of small ruminants range the Earth in undomesticated herds, some of which are managed and others which are not. Information about the dietary habits and nutrient requirements of these animals is crucial in managing their wellbeing and in contributing to the livelihoods of people who depend on them. Proper nutrition and management of small ruminants is also essential for the maintenance of various natural ecosystems from the Arctic Circle to the Sahara Desert.

The National Research Council has published reports on the *Nutrient Requirements of Sheep* (6th edition, 1985) and the *Nutrient Requirements of Goats* (1st edition, 1981), but a large amount of new information has accumulated during the last 25 years. Other small ruminants have not been addressed in the *Nutrient Requirements* series. This new publication updates the sheep and goat publications and adds information about other small ruminant species. In addition, information about New World camelids (alpacas and llamas) is included to the extent that it is available.

The committee appointed to write this report faced two important decisions at the outset. The first decision was which species to include as "small ruminants." After considering various factors such as body size, amount of scientific research data, absence of alternative sources of information, and general interest of potential users, the committee decided to include the following species: sheep (*Ovis aries*), goats (*Capra hircus*), cervids (white-tailed deer [*Odocoileus virginianus*], red deer [*Cervus elaphus*], wapiti/American elk [*Cervus elaphus*], and caribou/reindeer [*Rangifer tarandus*]), and New World camelids (alpacas [*Lama glama*] and llamas [*Vicugna pacos*]). The second important decision was how to organize the publication—by species or by topic, such as individual nutrients. Ultimately, the committee decided that to organize the report by species would result in a large amount of repetition and redundancy. Therefore, the report is organized by topic. Thus, for example, there are chapters on individual nutrients, and the species are covered within each chapter. The committee recognized that this makes the publication somewhat less convenient for readers interested in one species only. To address this, tables of nutrient requirements are organized by species, and one chapter discusses practical feeding and nutrition on a species-by-species basis.

This report represents the concerted efforts of all committee members. The committee was appointed in April 2004 and held its first meeting in May 2004. After two more in-person meetings and several teleconferences, an initial draft was sent to reviewers in November 2005. The committee hopes the publication will serve as an important reference for all concerned with the nutrition, feeding, health, and welfare of small ruminants and that it will also serve to stimulate more research on this important group of animals.

ED HUSTON
Chair, Committee on
Nutrient Requirements of
Small Ruminants

Acknowledgments

This report has been reviewed in draft form by persons chosen for their diverse perspectives and technical expertise in accordance with procedures approved by the National Research Council's Report Review Committee. The purpose of this independent review is to provide candid and critical comments that will assist the institution in making its published report as sound as possible and to ensure that the report meets institutional standards of objectivity, evidence, and responsiveness to the study charge. The review comments and draft manuscript remain confidential to protect the integrity of the deliberative process. We wish to thank the following individuals for their review of this report:

Antonello Cannas, University of Sassari, Sardinia, Italy
George F. W. Haenlein, University of Delaware, Newark, DE (retired)
Patrick G. Hatfield, Montana State University, Bozeman, MT
Robert J. Hudson, University of Alberta, Edmonton, Alberta, Canada
Lyndon N. Irwin, Southwest Missouri State University, Springfield, MO
Woody Lane, Lane Livestock Services, Roseburg, OR
Jean-Marie Luginbuhl, North Carolina State University, Raleigh, NC
Daniel G. Morrical, Iowa State University, Ames, IA
John V. Nolan, University of New England, Armidale, NSW, Australia
Fredric N. Owens, Pioneer Hi-Bred International, West Des Moines, IA
Rodney L. Preston, Texas Tech University, Lubbock, TX (retired)
Duane E. Ullrey, Michigan State University, East Lansing, MI (retired)
Larry W. Varner, Purina Mills Inc, Seguin, TX

Although the reviewers listed above have provided constructive comments and suggestions, they were not asked to endorse the conclusions or recommendations, nor did they see the final draft of the report before its release. The review of this report was overseen by Michael L. Galyean, Texas Tech University. Appointed by the National Research Council, he was responsible for making certain that an independent examination of this report was carried out in accordance with institutional procedures and that all review comments were carefully considered. Responsibility for the final content of this report rests entirely with the author committee and the institution.

We are grateful for contributions of Larry Miller, CSREES-USDA, who has been a good friend to the industries that will be served by this report. Larry is an ever-present entity whenever the animal industries, the scientific community, and U.S. governmental agencies interact and always a facilitator, a role that he fulfilled in the production of this document.

Members of the author committee express appreciation to the National Research Council and parent agency, The National Academies, for entrusting us to prepare this greatly anticipated and respected document. Special thanks are given to Charlotte Kirk Baer, former Director of the Board on Agriculture and Natural Resources, for her initiation of this project and early guidance, and to Robin Schoen, current Director, for her administrative oversight of this process and continued encouragement. A deeply felt thank you goes to Donna Lee Jameison, Senior Project Assistant, and to Ruthie Arieti, Project Assistant, for their technical contributions in monitoring, formatting, editing, posting, and other responsibilities, and for their extremely good nature while performing these vital services. Finally, the committee wishes to thank Austin Lewis, Study Director, who led us on a daily basis by giving us information, feedback, critique, and encouragement and brought us to successful completion.

Contents

Tables and Figures

TABLES

FIGURES

Summary

Publications in the National Research Council's series on nutrient requirements of domestic animals support proper animal feeding practices for the production of meat, milk, and fiber, and give advice on feeding animals that provide companionship and recreation to world societies. Requirements for energy, protein, minerals, vitamins, and water are defined, based on scientific evidence published in peer-reviewed technical sources. Feeding standards, developed from nutrient requirements of the animals and nutrient composition of feedstuffs, provide readers with the knowledge and means to adopt proper feeding practices. Periodic updating of these publications is needed as new research information accumulates and new needs surface.

This report combines revisions of *The Nutrient Requirements of Sheep* (1985) and *The Nutrient Requirements of Goats* (1981), with considerations of other small ruminants and ruminant-like species addressed for the first time. Inclusion of the new species (e.g., cervids) required an expanded view of products to include antlers and aesthetic value. The sheep series began publication in 1945, and it was revised periodically until the sixth edition in 1985. The first edition of the goat series, published in 1981, remains the most recent. Implicit in the charge given to the committee (Appendix A) was that other small ruminants and ruminant-like species be identified and included if justified by anatomical, physiological, behavioral, and/or socioeconomic similarities. The species listed below were identified for inclusion in this publication.

Sheep (*Ovis aries*)
Goats (*Capra hircus*)
Cervids
– White-tailed deer (*Odocoileus virginianus*)
– Red deer (*Cervus elaphus*)
– Wapiti/American elk (*Cervus elaphus*)
– Caribou/reindeer (*Rangifer tarandus*)
New World Camelids
– Llamas (*Lama glama*)
– Alpacas (*Vicugna pacos*)

This edition updates the requirements of sheep based on recent research and a need to consider higher levels of productivity by larger and improved genotypes. It also represents a major revision of the first edition of the goat requirements, which was prepared from the scant research data available at that time. During the last 25 years, voluminous research results on goat nutrition, especially on energy and protein, have accumulated. Similar to those considered in the first edition of the goat publication, data used in estimating requirements of cervids and New World camelids are limited, but estimates derived from those data and extrapolated from data from similar species are presented as the current standards.

The audience for this report is varied, as evidenced by the nature of the many sponsors. The U.S. Department of Agriculture (USDA) Multistate Research Committee concerned with efficiency of sheep production issued a resolution stating the urgent need to revise the existing nutrient requirement publications for sheep and goats. Sponsors that were forthcoming included the USDA Cooperative State Research, Education, and Extension Service (USDA-CSREES; www.csrees.usda.gov) and the Joe Skeen Institute for Rangeland Restoration (http://www.animalrangeextension.montana.edu/joe_skeen/contact.htm; Montana State University, New Mexico State University, and Texas A&M University System); American Sheep Industry Association (www.sheepusa.org); National Sheep Industry Improvement Center (www.nsiic.org); the Montana Sheep Institute (www.sheepinstitute.montana.edu/index.htm), and general support of the Animal Nutrition Series provided by the Department of Health and Human Services (U.S. Food and Drug Administration; www.fda.gov/cvm/). These agencies and organizations are interested in the current and potential socioeconomic roles of small ruminants and in the impact of small ruminants (both domestic and wild) on sustaining environmental quality. Appreciation for this diverse audience guided the structure of this report to address multilayers of users from biologists, ecologists, and environmental scientists to practical nutritionists and flock or herd managers. Some portions of the report will be too technical for readers with less advanced training, while some readers may consider other sections too elementary. Attempts were made to ease these difficulties by providing topical chapters for selective reading.

The publication begins with a brief introduction in Chapter 1. Then, Chapter 2 describes commonalities among the animal species in anatomical and physiological characteristics, as well as some subtle differences. Similarities and differences in size, shape, and location of the components of the gastrointestinal tracts of the animal species are considered. This explanation aids the reader in understanding the sites, rates, and partitioning that occur during the ingestion and processing of food as it flows through the digestive tract. Terms relating to nutrients are defined and illustrated so the reader is not confused by too many abbreviations. Nitrogen recycling is also described in this chapter. Finally, Chapter 2 summarizes the roles of minerals and vitamins as body components and in the various metabolic pathways.

Small ruminants are important in their association with vegetation, both in their reliance for diet and in their impact on renewable resources. Chapter 3 addresses the feeding behavior of small ruminants, including differences in diet selection and intake and how they are affected by the characteristics and availabilities of various diet sources.

Chapters 4, 5, 7, 8, and 9 provide discussions on requirements for energy, protein, minerals, vitamins, and water, respectively. The methods and equations used in calculating or estimating requirements are described in detail, and pertinent references to data used are cited. Except in a few instances when data were unavailable, the factorial method for calculating requirements was used. That is, separate estimates for requirements for the different physiological processes, including maintenance, pregnancy, lactation, body weight gain, and fiber production, are given. These separate estimates are used to construct the requirements tables presented at the end of the publication, but are available to the reader to customize requirements to fit unique circumstances. In some cases, requirements are estimated using data from other species of animals. This occurs most frequently when requirements for various minerals and vitamins for cervids and New World camelids are extrapolated from sheep, goat, or cattle data. Less frequently, goat requirements are calculated from sheep or cattle data.

Lipids and essential fatty acids are covered in Chapter 6. Although some fatty acids are metabolically essential, seldom are they of concern in small ruminants. However, dietary lipids for animals providing sources for human food are topics of discussion and scientific study as they may relate to human nutrition and health. This chapter gives a thorough overview of the state of knowledge of lipids in small ruminant diets.

Chapter 10 describes the physical and chemical nature of plants in respect to the content and availability of required nutrients. The practical aspects of evaluating feedstuffs and plant communities as sources of nutrients for small ruminants and designing management strategies are topics of Chapter 11. Chapter 12 discusses the various possibilities of negative environmental impacts of small ruminants and how these can be avoided. Also, opportunities for positive influences on the environment, mainly through the suppression of noxious weeds by selective grazing, are discussed.

Chapter 13 identifies nutrition-related diseases and deficiency symptoms and describes strategies for prevention and treatment. Some maladies are recognized problems among all species, whereas others are considered unique or more common to one or more species.

A guide for the practical use of this publication is provided in Chapter 14, and this chapter is recommended as primary reading for some users. Although other chapters are cited, all essential information is provided for determining the needs for the different nutrients and for using the requirements tables in formulating diets or supplements.

The final section of the publication contains requirements tables for sheep, goats, cervids, and New World camelids and composition tables for both common and novel feedstuffs. Regrettably, some nutrients were not available for some of the ingredients listed. Assistance in interpreting and using these tables is included in Chapter 14.

This publication was a challenge to prepare because it addressed multiple species for a diverse audience. Although conciseness was an ever-present goal, completeness was never sacrificed. The sheep portions update the 1985 edition in that a greater range in body size, litter size, and milk production were considered. The quality and accuracy in the goat considerations greatly exceed those contained in the first edition because of the large amount of research efforts invested since that document was published in 1981. However, many requirement issues in minerals and vitamins have not been resolved for goats. Rather, requirements were estimated from values derived in sheep and cattle studies. Considerable data are available for cervids, but estimates for requirements for nutrients are somewhat sketchy and variable. Similarly for New World camelids, some data are available, but many have not been validated by multiple independent studies. To produce adequately complete requirements tables for cervids and camelids, it was necessary to extrapolate from data generated from experiments with similar species. After enhanced efforts to generate definitive information in mineral and vitamin requirements for goats and all nutrients for camelids, the next edition of the *Nutrient Requirements of Small Ruminants* will be much more complete. However, the discussions, expressions, and values presented in this current edition are considered valid to the level of present knowledge.

1

Introduction

Small ruminants are important to world agriculture and natural resource management. This publication addresses the nutrient requirements of this subset of animal species within the larger population of ruminating animals. Separation of the class of ungulates into "small ruminants" and "large ruminants" is arbitrary, although there is general recognition of the differences between small and large domestic ruminant species. The separation was more difficult for undomesticated species. Including a subset of camelids (llamas and alpacas), which technically are not ruminants, complicated the grouping further. In the final analysis, practical considerations drove the decisions on which species to include. Considering various factors such as body size, availability of sufficient scientific documentation, absence of alternative sources of information, and general interest of potential users, a decision was made to include the following species in this report:

Sheep (*Ovis aries*)
Goats (*Capra hircus*)
Cervids[1]
– White-tailed deer (*Odocoileus virginianus*)
– Red deer (*Cervus elaphus*)
– Wapiti/American elk (*Cervus elaphus*)
– Caribou/reindeer (*Rangifer tarandus*)
New World Camelids
– Llamas (*Lama glama*)
– Alpacas (*Vicugna pacos*)

Although red deer and wapiti/American elk are classified as a single species, they are considered separately in this publication because they behave as separate biotypes, have different body weights, occupy different niches, and attract different clientele of interest. Furthermore, managers of these biotypes have different expectations in terms of levels of production.

[1]Certain other wild species will be considered through data extrapolation.

This first edition of the series devoted to small ruminants includes an update of a longstanding series (sheep), a major revision of a first edition (goats), and a first step in reporting nutrient requirements of the remaining species. The first and latest (sixth) editions of the sheep series were published in 1945 and 1985, respectively. This edition on small ruminants includes the first revision of the series on goats since its initial publication in 1981. The requirements of the other small ruminants and camelids have not been reported by the National Research Council (NRC). This publication includes updated materials for sheep pertaining mainly to genetic changes in size and productivity. Data provide for larger mature size, greater lamb numbers (litters), and higher milk production. Major revisions in the information on goats include updated equations based on more recent and sound information and a greater understanding of modern goat types and differences. Unlike previous editions, this edition accommodates users of nutritional information to support commercial sized sheep or goat dairies and modern, heavier weight sheep and goat flocks. For the species addressed for the first time, recommendations are derived from the scientific base available. These recommendations offer an acceptable level of confidence, but with the understanding that additional data that accumulate hereafter will lead to greater accuracy and precision in future editions. For all the species covered, an effort was made to review research data published throughout the world. However, because of the number of species and complexity of the task, it was not possible to complete an exhaustive international review.

This edition presented a challenge to the committee charged with its writing to properly serve the needs of the individual users of the product. The authors chose the approach of addressing species of small ruminants both as a distinct group and as individuals. The first three chapters of this edition describe behavioral, anatomical, and physiological characteristics of small ruminants that set them apart as a group. Discussions under chapters 4–9 apply generally to all small ruminants, although specific references are made when necessary and when citing sources of information. Similarly, much of the material in chapters 10–14 also applies to all small ruminants. However, Chapter 14, entitled *Providing Required Nutrients to Small Ruminants*, contains individual considerations of (1) sheep, (2) goats, (3) cervids (white-tailed deer, red deer, reindeer/caribou, and elk/wapiti), and (4) New World camelids (llamas and alpacas). In this chapter, information was drawn from previous sections and used in concert with information contained in applicable tables for practical application. Users who want to identify nutritional needs and develop feeding strategies will find this chapter an abridged and user-friendly tool. Those interested in the details of requirements, nutrient uses, and deficiencies will find pertinent information provided in the previous chapters.

Small ruminants provide food, fiber, recreation, and natural resource enhancement for human populations throughout the world, often from marginal and limited resources. Their ability to utilize poor-quality materials or seek out marginally accessible nutrient rich materials allows them to thrive in arid environments and on non-cultivatable terrain. Although the 2005 U.S. inventory of sheep (6.14 million) and goats (2.5 million) and their products are more than twofold lower than in the mid-1980s (USDA NASS, 2005), with numbers also lower in some other developed countries, their importance on the world stage has never been greater (FAOSTAT, 2005). Interest in small ruminant wildlife species and in New World camelids for recreation and alternative economic development is high and increasing. Differences between small ruminants and their larger counterparts in food selection and gastrointestinal physiology determine their special niches in the natural distribution of animal species. These unique characteristics identify these species as a separate group with valuable roles in the different socioeconomic circumstances in various regions of the world.

REFERENCES

FAOSTAT (Food and Agriculture Organization of the United Nations, FAO Statistical Databases). 2005. Agricultural Data. Available at faostat.fao.org/faostat/collections?version=ext&hasbulk=0&subset=agriculture/. Accessed October 25, 2005.

USDA NASS (U.S. Department of Agriculture, National Agricultural Statistics Service). 2005. Agricultural Statistics Board, Sheep and Goats. Available at usda.mannlib.cornell.edu/reports/nassr/livestock/pgg-bb/. Accessed October 25, 2005.

2

Anatomy, Digestive Physiology, and Nutrient Utilization

INTRODUCTION

An understanding of the digestive system of small ruminants is essential for the proper application of nutrient requirements. Ruminants are cud-chewing, even-toed ungulates that form a suborder (Ruminantia) of the mammal order Artiodactyla. Ruminants possess a unique "stomach" with four compartments (reticulum, rumen, omasum, and abomasum), which supports fermentation before digesta reach the small and large intestines. This publication also includes two species (llamas and alpacas) of another suborder of Artiodactyla known as Tylopoda (camelids). Llamas and alpacas are sometimes described as New World camelids (NWC) or South American camelids. Camelids also possess a multi-compartmented stomach, but they have three compartments (C1, C2, and C3), rather than four. Ruminants and NWC are found in diverse and extreme climates, and therefore diets, feed resources, and behavioral preferences for plant growth forms that differ in compositional chemistry and fiber type and content vary widely. The anatomy and physiological function of the gastrointestinal tract (GIT) has adapted to a wide range of feed resources and the fermentation capacity of the forestomachs (rumen-reticulum and omasum and C1–C2) enables utilization of cellulosic materials. Publications by Church (1988), Hofmann (1989), and Van Soest (1994) contain extensive discussions on GIT anatomy and comparisons among species.

ANATOMY

Morphological Feeding Type

Although all ruminants have the characteristic four-compartmented stomach, differences in GIT functioning are evident even among the species discussed in this document and are largely based on adaptation to feed resources. Ruminants can be classified according to their morphological feeding type into three groups: concentrate selector (CS), intermediate type (IM), and grass/roughage eater (GR) (Hofmann and Stewart, 1972; Hofmann, 1989). Concentrate selectors are animals that select diets of plants that are highly digestible, and high in starch, proteins, and lipids, depending on plant growth stage. Diets are low in fiber, and CS species have a limited ability to ferment cellulosic fractions of cell walls. In contrast, GR species have a highly developed fermentation system that enables them to digest cellulosic fractions of plant cell walls that characterize the high fiber content of graminoid diets. Forages consumed by GR include most of the agriculturally important pasture species found in improved and native pastures and ranges. The IM group consumes mixed diets and forages based on season and opportunity. These animals prefer diets based on the concentrate components of plant material and will select shrubs and browse, but also possess the ability to digest cellulosic materials. All three ecophysiological feeding types (CS, IM, and GR) deal with seasonal changes in plant development and nutritional quality of preferred forage types. In winter, or the dry season, depending on the biome or ecosystem, the fiber component increases for both grass-based and browser specialists. However, adaptation for dealing with mature grasses and browse is as equally specialized as processing the more nutrient-rich summer vegetation. Of the five ruminant species covered in this document, the white-tailed deer is a CS; the goat, wapiti, and caribou/reindeer are IM; and the sheep is a GR (Hofmann, 1989).

Anatomy of the Gastrointestinal Tract

The GIT is a complex system that begins with the prehensile organs of the mouth and ends with the rectum and anus. In between are components of a long digestive tract through which all ingested feeds are exposed to mastication, microbial fermentation, and enzyme digestion. For most ingested feeds, chemical modifications in the forestomachs and abomasum must occur before the nutrients or nutrient precursors can be absorbed and utilized by the animal. The GIT of the sheep and llama are illustrated in Figure 2-1.

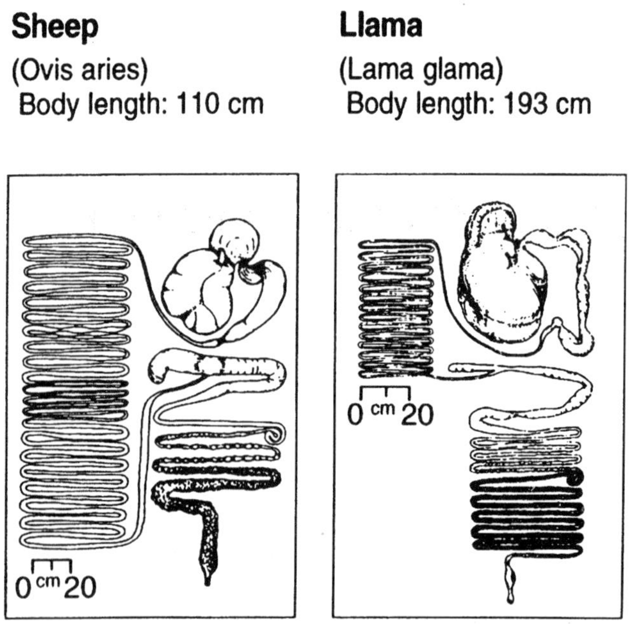

FIGURE 2-1 Drawings of the gastrointestinal tracts of the sheep (a grass/roughage eater morphological feeding type) and the llama. Adapted from Stevens and Hume (1998). Reprinted with the permission of the American Physiological Society.

Mouth

The act of prehension, which is the ingestion of feedstuffs, differs among ruminants and is affected by anatomical diversity. In general, GR species have short lips and broad mouths, whereas CS species have narrow but deep mouth openings to facilitate the intake of specific plant parts and fruit (Hofmann, 1989). In CS species, lips that are well developed with small papillae and narrow but deep mouths allow selective harvesting of soft leafy tissue of spiny and woody shrubs. The deep mouth allows stripping of leaves and effective harvesting of the highest quality current annual growth of woody browse (Bunnell and Gillingham, 1985; Cooper and Owen-Smith, 1985). These selection processes are aided by a relatively long freely mobile part of the tongue and short torus component of the thick part of the tongue. The wide, flat mouth of GR species maximizes intake of grasses and sedges at low biomass, and the long torus of GR species is associated with a more cornified tip of the tongue, which is thought to aid in tearing of grasses and sedges of high biomass (Hofmann, 1989). Morphology of the tongue and hard palate also allow processing in the mouth that assists in preferential retention and rejection of plant parts based on taste. The dental pad and hard palate make up the roof of the oral cavity. With the absence of upper incisors, this pad aids the tongue in grasping feed during the ingestion process. In ruminant species selecting for cell contents (forbs, fruit-eating species), the number of palatine ridges on the hard palate are fewer, but they have more and longer papillae associated with the ridges (Hofmann, 1989).

Dentition of ruminant species also varies and is correlated with preferred feed types. In all ruminants, incisors are absent from the upper jaw. Canines are also absent in most ruminants with the exception of wapiti and red deer. The lateral chewing action characteristic of ruminants is required to cut plant tissues because rows of molars and premolars are wider on the maxillary jaw than on the mandibular jaw.

The salivary glands in ruminants consist of both paired and unpaired glands that serve several important functions during ingestive and digestive processes. Saliva is also an important route of nitrogen recycling to the rumen, which is discussed in more detail later in this chapter. In most ruminants, the paired parotid glands (located at the base of each ear and extending to the posterior end of the mandible) are major contributors of saliva produced. Buccal and pharyngeal glands are also important contributors and secrete mucous type saliva. Parotid gland secretions are of the serous (thin, watery) type, and secretion is on a continuous basis, although flow will increase during eating and rumination. A more complete discussion on salivary glands and their production, functions, and composition of their secretions can be found in Church (1988) and Stevens (1988).

Compartments of the Ruminant Stomach

Ingested feed reaches the stomach via the esophagus, which is a tube that connects the mouth to the reticulum. The esophagus also serves an important role in the rumination process. It transports previously ingested feed back to the mouth during regurgitation followed by reswallowing of ingesta back to the rumen.

The esophagus opens into an upper part of the reticulum known as the cardia. At this point there is a groove known as the ventricular groove (formerly incorrectly termed the "esophageal groove"). The ventricular groove consists of two sections, a reticular portion and a short omasal portion. Normally the groove is open and digesta arrive in the reticulum. However, the two lips of the groove can close, diverting digesta to the abomasum. This occurs in suckling ruminants and channels milk directly to the abomasum. Closure of the groove can also be stimulated by certain chemical substances in adults, and may be an important means of bypassing slurries of plant juice past the rumen in some adult ruminants.

The four compartments of the stomach (reticulum, rumen, omasum, and abomasum) fit compactly into the abdominal cavity (Figure 2-2).

The ruminant stomach showing the arrangement of the four compartments is illustrated in Figure 2-3.

Actual and relative sizes and capacities of these compartments differ among species. Figure 2-4 shows the four compartments of a young white-tail deer. Each of the four compartments has unique and specialized functions.

The reticulum is the region where feed boluses enter upon swallowing and passage through the esophagus. This compartment is characterized by a honeycomb pattern ep-

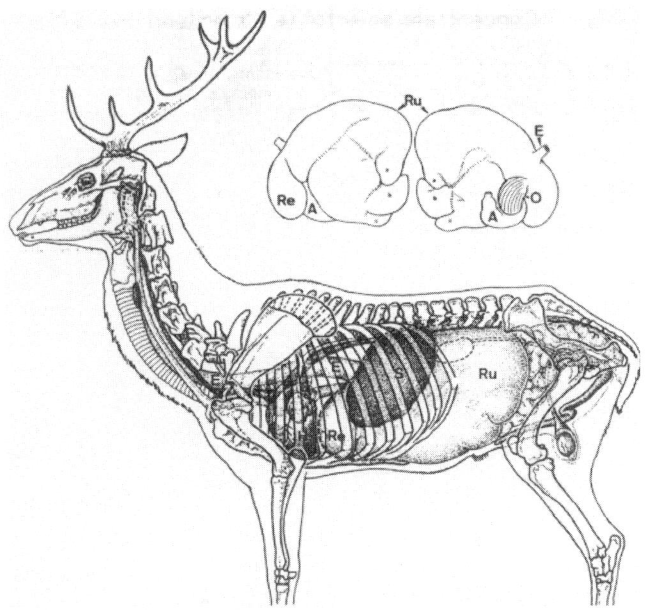

FIGURE 2-2 A drawing of the red deer (an intermediate morphological feeding type) showing the stomach in situ and isolated. A = abomasum, E = esophagus, H = heart, O = omasum, Re = reticulum, Ru = rumen, and S = spleen. From Hofmann (1989). Reprinted with the permission of Oecologia.

ithelial lining (Figure 2-5). It has the ability to contract to a fraction of its resting size. This contraction enables the mixing and movement of feeds into and throughout the rumen, regurgitation of digesta from the rumen to the mouth, expulsion of contents to the omasum, and expiration of fermentation gases.

The rumen is the largest of the four compartments. It serves as a storage site and fermentation vat and houses a large and diverse microbial population. The rumen provides a holding area for feed that is consumed quickly and later regurgitated and ruminated. As in the reticulum, motor activity that facilitates continuous mixing and movement of contents is an essential part of rumen function. In GR species, there are thick pillars between the rumen and reticulum. This affects rumination and mixing and can result in stratification of grass-based diets and formation of a "fiber raft" that characterizes the reticulum-rumen contents of some GR species (Clauss et al., 2003). The rumen epithelium is lined with papillae that are the sites of absorption of fermentation acids produced within this compartment (Figure 2-5). Papillae cover the entire lining of the rumen, but size and density vary with developmental stage, and in response to diet, season, and the ruminal environment (Hofmann, 1989; Forsyth and Fraser, 1999; Mathiesen et al., 2000; Knott et al., 2004).

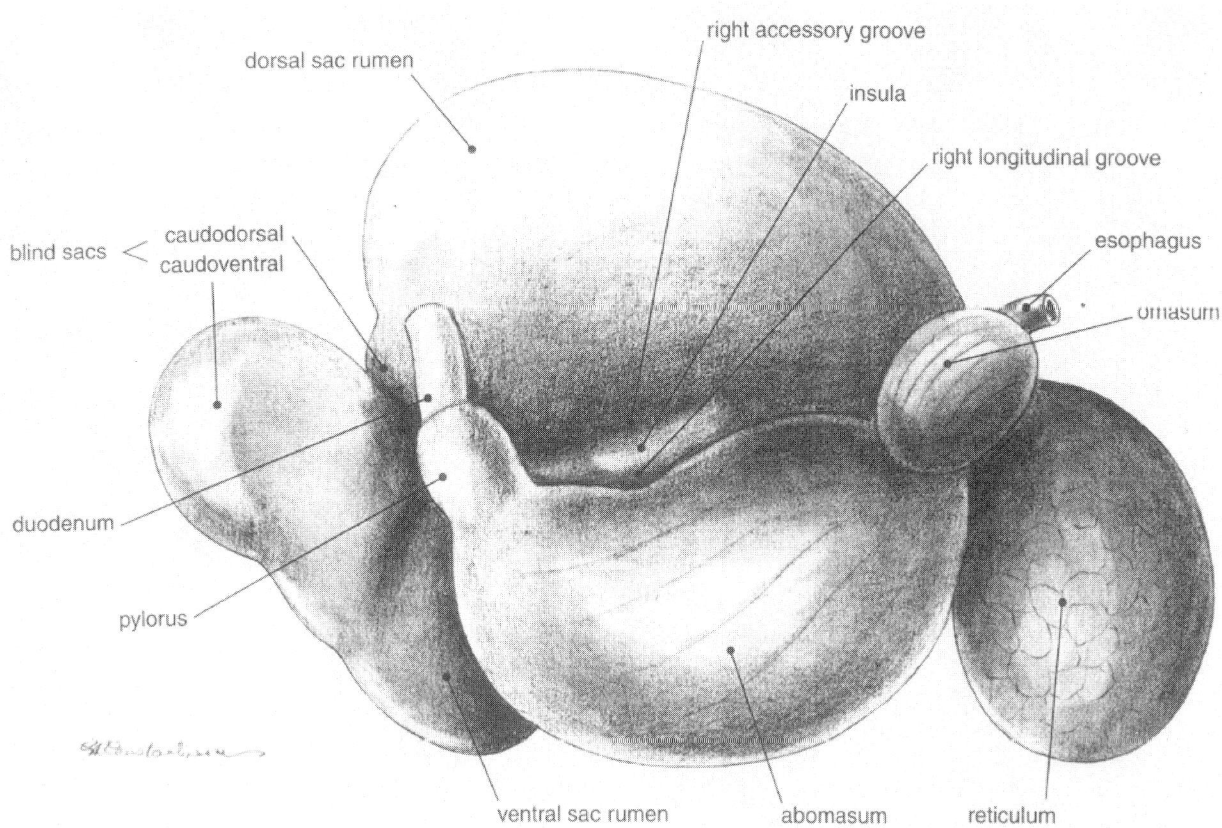

FIGURE 2-3 A drawing of the right aspect of the stomach of the goat (an intermediate morphological feeding type). From Constantinescu (2001). Reprinted with the permission of Iowa State University Press and Blackwell Publishing.

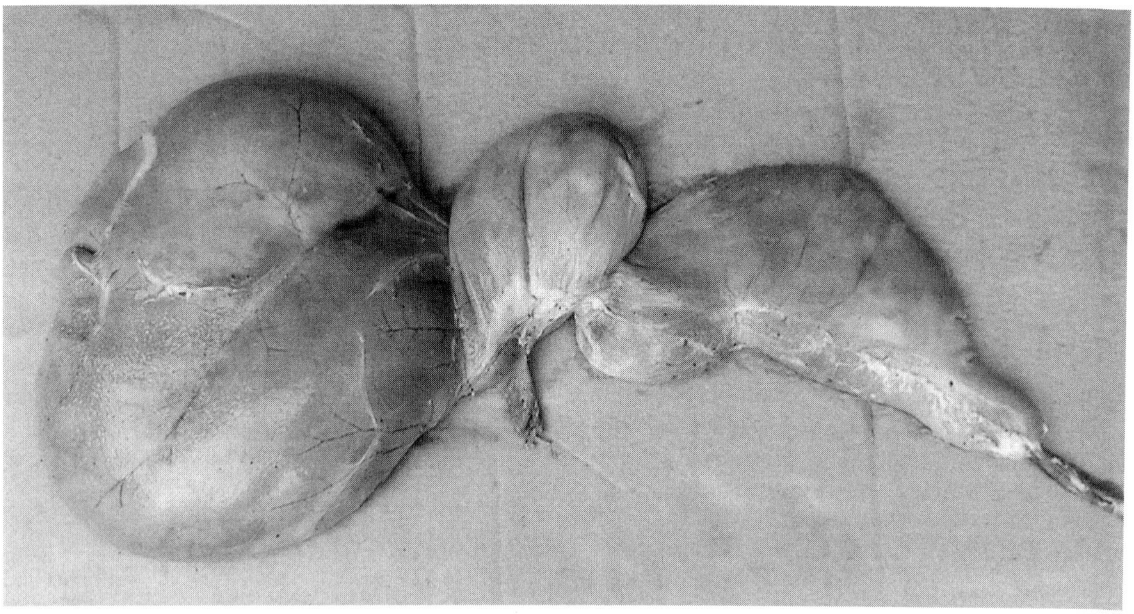

FIGURE 2-4 Photograph of the four stomach compartments of a yearling white-tailed deer (a concentrate selector morphological feeding type). From left to right, the rumen, the reticulum, the omasum, and the abomasum. Photo courtesy of G. F. W. Haenlein, Emeritus Professor, University of Delaware.

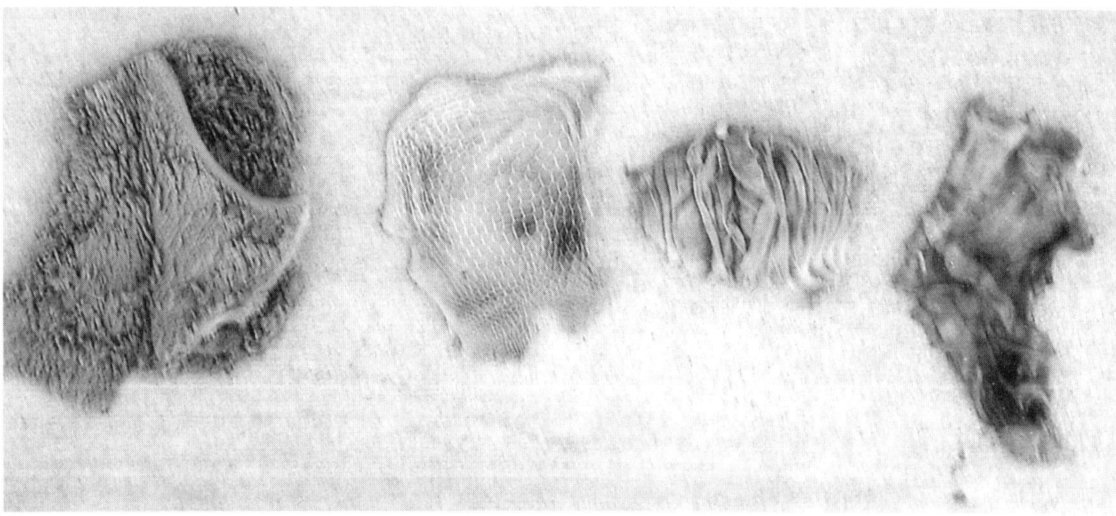

FIGURE 2-5 The inside structure of the four stomach compartments of a white-tailed deer (a concentrate selector morphological feeding type). From left to right, the papillae and muscular structures of the rumen, the honeycomb netting of the reticulum, the manyply leaves of the omasum, and the irregular folds of the abomasum. Photo courtesy of G. F. W. Haenlein, Emeritus Professor, University of Delaware.

Because of their physically close proximity to each other and the continuous mixing and movement between these two compartments, the reticulum and rumen are often discussed as a single compartment.

In general, total fermentation volume increases with body weight (Van Soest, 1994). The volume of the reticulum-rumen (in liters) can be estimated as: $0.77 \times$ body weight (kg)$^{0.57} - 3.49$ (Bunnell and Gillingham, 1985). The GR species have a larger reticulum-rumen per unit of body weight than do CS species, which compensate with an increase in omasum size. In IM species, the relative size of the reticulum-rumen is seasonally adaptive, being largest in summer and smallest in winter, when forage availability is limiting. Within species, reticulum-rumen size is associated with voluntary feed intake, and particularly with digestible dry matter (DM) intake. Because of a narrow opening to the omasum in GR species, retention of fiber in the reticulum-rumen maximizes fiber digestion. In contrast, passage of larger particles by CS species consuming woody browse allows them to maintain intake of woody fiber of low potential digestibility. The same effect allows for rapid processing of cell contents of high-quality forbs and leafy browse by CS species. Higher rates of passage of liquid and particulates found in CS species are associated with more daily feeding events than in GR species (Hofmann, 1989).

The omasum is composed of many layers of tissue all with an absorptive epithelial lining (Figure 2-5). Relatively little if any digestive activity occurs in this compartment, although water and minerals are removed from the ingesta before passage to the abomasum. Omasum size and number of lamina increase from CS to IM species and are largest in GR species (Hofmann, 1989). The reticulum-omasal opening is responsible for control of rate of reticulum-rumen emptying, which is relatively greater in species that have a smaller omasum.

The abomasum is similar in function to the stomach of a nonruminant animal (Figure 2-5). Secretions into the abomasum make the digesta leaving this compartment for passage to the small intestine high in water content. The abomasum of CS and IM species is relatively larger than that of GR species, mainly due to a thicker wall, and is capable of more copious parietal gland secretions. Presumably the morphology is associated with a greater production of pepsin-HCl by CS and IM species, and therefore a presumed relatively greater dependence on post-reticulum-rumen digestion, compared with GR species (Hofmann, 1989).

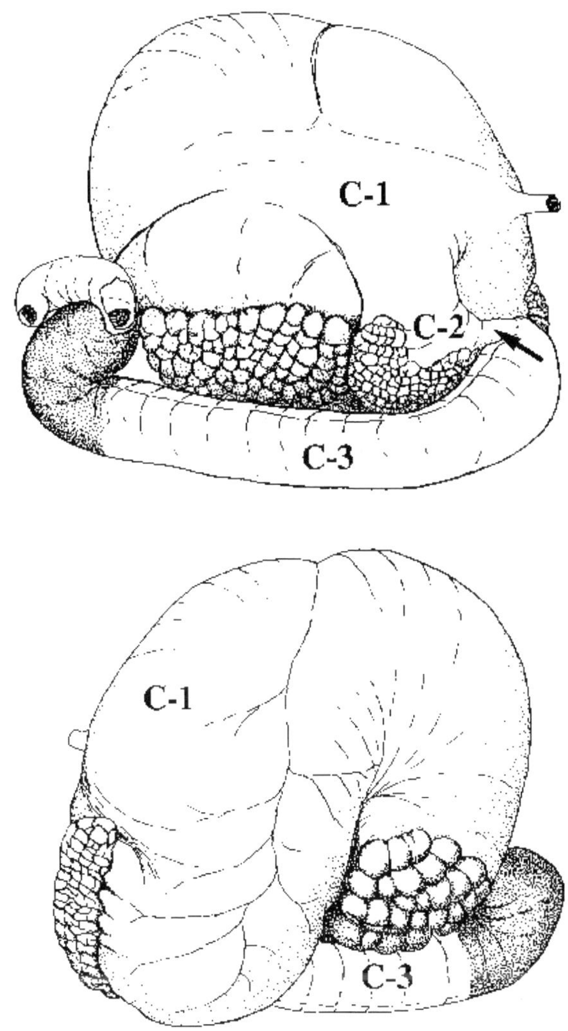

FIGURE 2-6 Drawings of the three stomach compartments of the llama. Illustration courtesy of K. I. Timm, Emeritus Associate Professor, Oregon State University.

Compartments of the Camelid Stomach

In contrast to ruminants, NWC have forestomachs with three compartments (C1, C2, and C3). An illustration of the camelid stomach appears in Figure 2-6. Compartments 1 and 2 contain 85 to 90 percent of the total stomach volume and function as fermentation vats, similar to the reticulum-rumen of true ruminants (Vallenas et al., 1971). Unlike ruminants, the C1 contains saccules that are lined by glandular epithelium (Vallenas et al., 1971; Rubsamen and Engelhardt, 1979). NWC seem to have increased volatile fatty acid (VFA) absorption and have a higher fermentation chamber pH than the rumen of ruminants (Eckerlin and Stevens, 1973; Vallenas et al., 1973; Lemosquet et al., 1996; Van Saun, 2003). The cranial portion of C3 functions as a fermentation vat, while the caudal one-fifth of the compartment is "abomasum-like" (Johnson, 1989; San Martin and Bryant, 1989; Van Saun, 2003). The forestomach motility of NWC is also different than that of true ruminants. NWC have greater forestomach activity, three to four eructations per motile cycle, a more homogenous mixture of ingesta than that of true ruminants, and a more rapid forestomach fluid passage rate (Clemens and Stevens, 1980; San Martin and Bryant, 1989; Van Saun, 2003). The microbial populations found in the foregut of NWC compartments are similar to those found in ruminants (Navarre et al., 1999). The remainder of the GIT is anatomically and physiologically similar to that of ruminants, with the possible exception that the rate of ingesta passage is slightly slower in llamas (San Martin and Bryant, 1989). This slowed rate of passage results in better degradation of ingested feed, particularly the cell wall fraction of poor-quality forages that are low in protein (Hintz et al., 1973; San Martin and Bryant, 1989; Warmington et al., 1989; Cordesse et al., 1992; Fraser and Baker, 1998; Genin et al., 1994; Lopez et al., 1998).

Small and Large Intestines

The small and large intestines, including the cecum and colon and the rectum, complete the distal portions of the GIT. There is considerable variation among species in the relative proportions of the small and large intestines. Figure 2-1 shows the major differences between the sheep and the llama.

The small intestine, a long and convoluted tube, is the primary site of remaining digestive activities. Villi lining the small intestine are a primary site of absorption of nutrients for distribution throughout the body. Secretions added to intestinal contents that aid in the digestive processes come from the pancreas, gall bladder, and intestinal cells. These secretions work to break down protein, fat, and starch components of the intestinal contents. End products of digestion, including amino acids, fatty acids, and sugars, are absorbed from the small intestine and enter the blood or lymph for distribution. Contents of the small intestine that are not broken down sufficiently for absorption from the tract pass on to the large intestine. Absorption from the intestines is controlled by flow into the small intestine (Kay and Pfeffer, 1970), intestine length, surface area enlargement by mucosa villi (Snipes, 1994), and epithelial transporters, which are differentially affected by developmental changes associated with ontogeny of the nutritional niche (Knott et al., 2004), seasonality, and diet (Hofmann, 1989). The GR species have a long intestinal length relative to their body length (BL) (25–30 × BL), with 80–82 percent as small intestine. In contrast, the intestine length of CS species is shorter (12–15 × BL), and a smaller proportion (65–73 percent) is associated with the small intestines (Hofmann, 1989).

Most digestion and absorption of energy and protein by ruminants is completed before the contents reach the large intestine. However, the absorption of water and inorganic ions by the large intestine is essential to the water and mineral balance of the animal (White et al., 1984; Staaland et al., 1986; Stevens, 1988), and absorption of many vitamins also occurs in the large intestine (Stevens, 1988). The storage capacity and size of the cecum varies by species. The CS species have relatively large ceca to rumen volume ratios (1:6–10) compared to the GR species (1:15–30) (Hofmann, 1989). The IM species are intermediate in cecum volume, with a ratio of 1:9–24. Digesta remaining in the tract postcecum are likely to be excreted from the body as feces. Feces contain undigested feed residue, microbial cells, and cells sloughed from the GIT itself. The fecal pellet formation of some ruminant species occurs in the spiral colon portion of the large intestine and is the result of a series of specific contractions in this region (Stevens, 1988). Although small ruminants do not routinely practice coprophagy, sheep fed high-concentrate diets are occasionally observed eating feces, and deer fed a low-protein diet will eat feces of animals fed a high-protein diet if they have the opportunity. Goats avoid feed contaminated with feces.

FERMENTATIVE AND DIGESTIVE PROCESSES OF RUMINANTS

Rumination

Rumination, or cud-chewing, begins with regurgitation of a bolus (consisting of previously ingested feed) back to the mouth via the esophagus. This is accomplished by a series of reticular contractions and antiperistaltic movements through the esophagus (Grovum, 1986; Stevens, 1988). In the mouth the bolus is re-chewed, additional saliva is added to the mix, and it is re-swallowed. This rumination process is important as a means of reducing the size of feed particles and volume in the rumen, allowing more feed to be consumed. By reducing particle size and increasing surface area, the likelihood of degradation during fermentation and digestion is enhanced (Faichney, 1986).

Fermentation

The symbiotic relationship between the host animal and the diverse resident microbial population accomplishes three functions of importance to the nutritional wellbeing of ruminants: (1) fermentation of structural carbohydrates (e.g., cellulose and hemicellulose) into readily absorbable and utilizable sources of energy, (2) conversion of nonprotein nitrogen into utilizable protein sources, and (3) synthesis of vitamin K and the B vitamins. These processes have been described in detail by Van Soest (1994).

The end products of fermentation provide the primary means by which ruminants are supplied with nutrients from the consumed feeds. Within the rumen, complex and diverse microbial populations are maintained in a specialized anaerobic environment with conditions normally in the following ranges: pH, 5.5 to 7.2; temperature, 38 to 42°C; and oxidation-reduction potential (Eh), –250 to –450 mV (Clarke, 1977). The contents of the rumen continually change as ingested feed, salivary secretions, and products of the rumination process are added; gaseous products of microbial fermentation are removed; and particulates pass to the lower tract. Copious amounts of saliva containing bicarbonate and phosphate buffers maintain a relatively constant pH (Kay, 1966).

Microbial fermentation is the mechanism by which ruminants benefit from the consumption of fibrous feeds. The microorganisms can ferment fiber, which is not susceptible to degradation by mammalian enzymes. The microbes use the nutrients extracted from the fiber and other sources to synthesize microbial proteins that subsequently become an available protein source for the host ruminant. End products of microbial activity include the production of large quantities of gases—mainly carbon dioxide and methane. The gases are removed from the animal via the esophagus and mouth through the processes of respiration and eructation (Stevens and Sellers, 1968). These gases must be expelled from the animal on a continuous basis, or bloat, ending in death, can occur quickly.

Volatile Fatty Acid Production and Use

Complete degradation of feeds to carbon dioxide and water does not occur in the anaerobic conditions of the rumen environment. Most of the energy contained in feedstuffs is converted to the byproducts of microbial fermentation (van Houtert, 1993). For the host animal the most are important byproducts are VFAs, predominantly acetate, propionate, and butyrate. Other fermentation byproducts found in smaller concentrations in the rumen include formate, lactate, succinate, ethanol, and hydrogen. A complete review of the production and metabolism of VFAs and their association with the nutritional status of forage-fed ruminants is provided by van Houtert (1993).

VFAs are produced primarily from dietary carbohydrates, although proteins and lipids also contribute to the pool. Plant carbohydrates, including monosaccharides, storage carbohydrates (primarily starch), and structural carbohydrates (primarily cellulose, hemicellulose, and pectin) produce VFAs through a variety of metabolic pathways that have been well described (Baldwin, 1965; Hungate, 1966; Demeyer, 1981; Wolin and Miller, 1983; Bergman, 1990).

Profiles of VFA production and resulting molar ratios found in the rumen will vary in response to diet. For example, diet type (high forage vs. high concentrate) is a major determinant of the microbial population that will be resident and will affect the VFA profile accordingly. In the case of a high-forage diet, a relatively high ruminal pH will favor fiber-digesting bacteria and acetate production will predominate. In contrast, a high-concentrate diet will produce an environment that is lower in pH, thereby selecting against fiber-digesting microbes in favor of more acid-tolerant starch-digesting organisms and, as a result, propionate fermentation pathways will increase.

As early as 1942, Phillipson and McAnally reported that VFAs were absorbed directly from the rumen of sheep and entered the blood stream. More recently the mechanism for absorption of VFAs across the epithelial cell in the rumen has been defined (Stevens et al., 1980). Nearly all acetate and propionate are removed from the GIT at the rumen or omasum and are transported to the liver via the hepatic portal vein. A small portion of acetate is oxidized to carbon dioxide within the ruminal epithelium. As with acetate, propionate is largely unaltered at the rumen epithelium. Butyrate is extensively metabolized (up to 90 percent) within the rumen and omasum epithelial cells to form acetoacetate and β-hydroxy butyrate (Bergman, 1990; van Houtert, 1993).

After absorption from the rumen, the fates of VFAs differ, as does their role in contributing to the energy status of the ruminant. Of the three major VFAs, only acetate is found circulating in the peripheral blood to any great extent. A small amount of acetate is removed from the portal blood by the liver, but most passes through to the periphery. The acetate that is removed is used primarily for the de novo synthesis of long-chain fatty acids and cholesterol (van Houtert, 1993). Circulating acetate is primarily used by muscle, portal drained viscera, and adipose tissue, where it is oxidized or used for fatty acid synthesis. The mammary gland is an important user of acetate for milk fat synthesis in the lactating ruminant.

Propionate is extensively metabolized in the liver (Bergman and Wolff, 1971), and the primary pathway for propionate metabolism is gluconeogenesis (Judson et al., 1968; Steel and Leng, 1973). With little direct absorption of glucose occurring in the ruminant GIT, glucose synthesis is a vital step in cellular metabolism for many of the body systems. Propionate is the primary precursor for glucose synthesis with lesser contributions originating from amino acids, lactate, and glycerol (van Houtert, 1993). Ruminants consuming forage-based diets may have small amounts of propionate that exit the liver and circulate to the periphery. When available, the mammary gland and other tissue will readily absorb this VFA and the primary metabolic pathway is oxidation.

Similar to acetate, though present in much smaller quantities, any butyrate in the peripheral circulation is either oxidized or contributes to fatty acid synthesis.

ENERGY AND NUTRIENT UTILIZATION

Energy

Energy is defined as the potential to do work and can be measured only in its transformation from one form to another. Feedstuffs contain variable amounts of energy that fuel the body upon consumption and transformation within the animal body during the digestive processes. Energy requirements vary among and within animals and depend on many factors including: species, age, sex, climate, physiological stage of production, and amount of activity. The joule (J) is the accepted unit for expressing energy in most countries, although the calorie (cal) is still used extensively in the United States. One calorie is defined as 4.184 J, and is equal to the amount of energy required to increase the temperature of 1 g of water from 16.5 to 17.5°C. Both the joule and calorie are small, and larger units are typically used in nutrition (i.e., kJ = 1,000 J; MJ = 1,000,000 J; kcal = 1,000 cal; Mcal = 1,000,000 cal).

As energy flows through the animal, energetic inefficiencies occur, and there are losses at various stages. The nutritional energetics of domestic animals have been discussed in detail (NRC, 1981a), and so only the key points are described here.

Gross Energy

Gross energy (GE) represents the total energy content of a feedstuff or diet and is determined by oxidation in a bomb calorimeter. During this process, the feed resource is completely oxidized to carbon dioxide and water and the resulting amount of heat produced is measured. This measurement has little or no value in predicting animal performance or describing energy requirements because it does not take into account the availability of that energy to the animal. The GE content of feedstuffs depends on concentrations of carbohydrate, protein, and fat, with average heats of combustion of 3.7 (glucose) to 4.2 (starch), 5.6, and 9.4 kcal/g, respectively.

Digestible Energy

Apparent digestible energy (DE) is the difference between GE intake and energy voided in feces (FE). It is termed "apparent" because some of the fecal energy is of nondietary origin, such as secretions of the GIT, sloughed epithelial cells, and microbial cells. For sheep, FE is typically 40–50 percent and 20–30 percent of GE with consumption of forage and high-concentrate diets, respectively. In general, FE increases and DE decreases as feed intake increases, because of decreased ruminal residence time of digesta and factors influencing capacity and motility of the GIT. However, this is not true for all diets and feed ingredients.

Total Digestible Nutrients

Total digestible nutrients (TDN) also allows for energy lost in feces, but in addition it accounts for the higher energy concentration in lipids (TDN is the sum of digestible carbohydrates, digestible crude protein (CP), and 2.25 times digestible crude fat). In most cases today, the TDN content of feedstuffs is predicted from established empirical equations based on concentrations of chemical constituents such as CP, and neutral and/or acid detergent fiber. Frequently, TDN is related to DE by assuming 1 kg TDN = 4.4 Mcal DE (NRC, 1985a, 2000). Many reported TDN values are misleading and overestimate the energetic value of feedstuffs, especially when fed above maintenance intakes and when high-fiber diets and diets with low-quality roughages are compared to low-fiber diets and mixed diets (Moore et al., 1953; NRC 1981a).

Metabolizable Energy

Although DE and TDN are frequently used to evaluate feedstuffs and to express energy requirements, the use of apparent metabolizable energy (ME) instead of DE or TDN has important advantages for ruminants. To calculate ME, energy losses in urine (UE) and combustible gases (GasE) are subtracted from DE (i.e., ME = DE – UE – GasE). Thus, ME represents the portion of GE that is captured as a useful product (in tissue, milk, wool, conceptus) or is lost as heat. Urine energy accounts for a higher proportion of GE in ruminants (4–5 percent) than in nonruminants (2–3 percent of GE). This is because of the presence of more nonurea nitrogenous compounds, such as hippuric acid (Robbins, 1993). Major factors influencing UE are diet protein levels, diet roughage levels, and essential oil content (Robbins, 1993). Gaseous energy losses are a consequence of digestive processes—primarily fermentation. As feedstuffs are exposed to microorganisms in the rumen, a significant part of the GE in the feedstuff is metabolized to combustible gases, primarily methane, that escapes from the rumen as eructated or expired gas. A small amount of combustible gas is also produced from hindgut fermentation. In ruminants GasE is normally 5–8 percent of GE intake, although in cattle it has been noted to range from 2–12 percent (Johnson and Johnson, 1995). Gaseous energy increases with increasing dietary forage content. It is also affected by level of feed intake, decreasing as a percentage of GE with increasing level of intake. Hence, methane loss as a percentage of GE is lowest with ad libitum intakes of high-concentrate diets (Johnson and Johnson, 1995), or when browse is an important dietary component (Schwartz et al., 1987; Galbraith et al., 1998; Robbins 1993; Woodward et al., 2001; White and Lawler, 2002). Because of increasing FE and decreasing GasE as level of feed intake increases, feed intake generally has a lesser effect on ME than DE concentration (NRC, 2001).

Energy losses from urine and combustible gases are highly predictable, and, therefore, DE and ME are highly correlated. For most forages and mixtures of forages and cereal grains, the conversion of DE to ME can be expressed as ME = DE × 0.82, except for high-grain and high-browse diets where higher ratios have been reported (Johnson, 1972; Robbins, 1993). Although this "standard" conversion from DE to ME is useful for many purposes, it is important to recognize its limitations and the wide variability because of the factors just discussed.

Net Energy

Net energy (NE) is the most refined expression of the value of energy in a feedstuff or an animal's energy requirement, although it is not as commonly used in evaluating feedstuffs and expressing requirements of small ruminants as ME primarily because of insufficient data. Net energy is the amount of energy available to the animal for maintenance and productive functions. Determination of NE requires one measurement in addition to those required for calculating ME. This is the heat increment (HiE), which is defined as the increase in heat produced following the consumption of feed by an animal in a thermoneutral environment (NRC, 1981a). HiE is the inefficiency of ME use for any given function. Thus, NE = ME – HiE. Net energy represents energy that is completely used by the animal body after accounting for all energetic losses and inefficiencies. This assumes that HiE includes both the heat from fermentations in the digestive tract and the heat liberated during nutrient metabolism. Under most conditions, HiE is of no value to the animal and frequently is a burden, because additional energy is required for dissipation. However, when ruminants are exposed to low environmental temperatures, HiE may be useful in maintaining body temperature. Heat increment usually ranges from 25–40 percent of GE, with the percentage increasing with increasing dietary forage content, decreasing forage quality, increasing level of intake, and increasing energy used for tissue gain vs. maintenance and splanchnic tissue metabolism (Hudson and Christopherson, 1985; Burrin et al., 1989; Goetsch, 1998). Because NE is the only energy expression to account for HiE, the other systems (DE, TDN, and ME) overestimate the energetic value of forage relative to concentrate feedstuffs, with the overestimate increasing with level of intake and with the proportion of nutrient use for tissue gain.

Net energy for maintenance (NEm) includes the NE for basal metabolism that relates to muscular activity, tissue repair and replacement, and involuntary metabolic processes such as maintenance of ionic gradients. Also included as NEm is the minimal voluntary activity necessary to sustain life. The amount of energy needed to satisfy voluntary activity needs (activity increment) varies widely depending on the availability of feed, water, and shade and the topography of the environment. Extreme examples of management systems—confinement vs. arid range—may cause the activity increment to be a major factor in determining NEm. During hot or cold weather, the animal uses ME to cool or heat its body; the energy required for this is also part of NEm and is widely variable depending on environmental factors.

Net energy available to an animal in excess of that required for maintenance is used in a variety of productive processes. These include the net energy for growth, lactation, reproductive processes, and production of wool or hair. Where applicable, NE for physical work, in addition to that required by the activity increment, may also be included.

Energy Needs for Growth, Gestation, Lactation, and Fiber Production

Energy required to support tissue gain depends on the energy composition of the gain. Water, lipid, and protein contents of gain vary with the growth stage of an animal. For example, each kilogram of empty body gain requires between 1.2 Mcal (when composition is mainly protein and water) and 8.0 Mcal (when the composition is mainly lipid and water) (NRC, 1985a). Within species, energy density of gain is also known to be affected by genotype, sex, body weight, level of intake, rate of gain, and energy concentration of the diet.

The efficiency with which energy is used for pregnancy (which includes the gravid uterus plus mammary gland development) is affected by stage of gestation, number of fetuses, and diet (Rattray et al., 1974a,b). As fetal development progresses from early through late gestation, additional energy is needed because fetal growth accelerates. The number of fetuses in utero can range from one to greater than five in some breeds of sheep, and as these numbers increase, energy demands increase, especially in late gestation. To date there are relatively few studies that define energy requirements during gestation, especially for genotypes that have been selected over time to produce larger animals and support higher levels of production (prolificacy, growth rate, milk production).

Defining the requirements and energetic efficiency in lactation is confounded by energy contributions from the mobilization of body energy reserves in addition to dietary intakes. Furthermore, deposition of energy in the body of a lactating animal is also a consideration. In general, it is assumed that the energetic efficiency from mobilizing body reserves for lactation is 0.84 (ARC, 1980), although it is recognized that the efficiency is lower under some circumstances (e.g., protein deficiency). The average lactational efficiency of metabolizable energy use for ruminants is estimated to be 0.62 and varies with metabolizability of the diet (ARC, 1980). Defining energy needs for lactating ruminants requires an assessment of the relationship between body energy retention and milk secretion.

Energy is also required to support fiber growth of some ruminants. Current requirement recommendations for fiber production are based on fiber growth, an assumed energy concentration in fiber, and direct estimates of the efficiency of ME use for fiber growth. Although Angora goats seem to be more efficient in fiber production (g/kg BW; Gallagher and Shelton, 1972), the ME requirement and efficiency of ME use for mohair fiber growth are similar to those for wool growth by sheep (as discussed in Chapter 4).

Carbohydrates

Carbohydrates are the main source of dietary energy in ruminant diets. Carbohydrates found in feed resources include a large and diverse group of compounds that are generally classified as monosaccharides (simple sugars such as aldopentoses and aldohexoses), oligosaccharides (containing 2 to 10 sugar units linked by glycosidic bonds), and polysaccharides (long chain, high molecular weight units such as cellulose, hemicellulose, starch, and pectin). Polysaccharides are the primary contributors of energy in most ruminant diets.

Functions and Sources of Carbohydrates

The primary role of dietary carbohydrates is to provide energy—first to the rumen microbial populations and second to the host ruminant. Another, less obvious role of carbohydrates in the ruminant system is to help maintain a stable GIT environment, which is aided by the consumption of fibrous feedstuffs. Rumen microbes readily attack all carbohydrates presented to them and can adapt to dietary shifts in type and amount of carbohydrate. Adequate energy for the resident microbial population is an important factor in determining level of production that can be attained by the host animal. End products of microbial fermentation include the primary source of energy for the host animal—the VFA. Energy used in the process of ruminal fermentation also subsequently supports rumen microbial protein and vitamin synthesis. Nonstructural polysaccharides, primarily starch, that escape ruminal fermentation and appear at the small intestine can directly supply energy to the animal after enzymatic hydrolysis and absorption, although some may escape digestion and appear in the feces.

Structural polysaccharides make up the bulk of the dietary carbohydrates in small ruminants consuming forage- or browse-based diets. However, in more intensive production settings, high-concentrate diets are frequently used, and in these diets the starch in cereal grains provides the majority of the dietary energy. Ruminants consuming fruits and plants high in cell contents and low in structural carbohydrates will have a dietary carbohydrate profile that is higher in monosaccharides and starch. Dietary differences such as these result in a range of ruminal fermentation patterns and fermentation end products and a range in dietary energy uses and efficiencies.

Carbohydrate Digestion and Metabolism in the Rumen

A key factor influencing the rate and pattern of ruminal fermentation is the nature of the feed carbohydrates, because they form the most important source of energy for rumen microbes and thus, ultimately, for the host animal. The carbohydrate composition of the feed also affects the extent of formation of "rafts" of grass particles (Sutherland, 1988) by grazers or "homogeneous" mixes by browsers (Clauss et al., 2003).

The soluble carbohydrate components of plant material, especially the simple sugars, are very rapidly metabolized in the rumen and usually result in a propionate-dominant fermentation. At the other extreme, the structural carbohydrates of plants are much more slowly fermented, with acetate fermentation being dominant. Starch is digested rapidly in the rumen, though less rapidly than simple sugars. The rate of fermentation of plant carbohydrate in relation to the rate of rumen protein degradation to ammonia is a major determinant of microbial protein production. However, the balance between the rates of fermentation of the different plant carbohydrate pools is also crucial. Increased soluble carbohydrate supply can result in an increased rate of fermentation, increased propionate supply, and increased incorporation of rumen ammonia into microbial protein (Dove and Milne, 1994; Trevaskis et al., 2001). However, the rapid fermentation of soluble carbohydrate can also reduce rumen pH to the point that the rate of fermentation of structural carbohydrate is decreased.

Regardless of the type of carbohydrate, the ultimate fate of plant carbohydrate in the rumen is to be degraded to its constituent sugars and then fermented to VFAs via pyruvate (Annison and Bryden, 1998). VFAs (mainly acetate, propionate, and butyrate) account for 50–70 percent of DE intake. Increases in acetate:propionate ratio in the rumen may reduce the efficiency of utilization of ME and microbial protein production (SCA, 1990; Dove and Milne, 1994), and Corbett (1987) suggested that when this ratio exceeds 3:1, the supply of readily available energy can be regarded as limiting microbial protein synthesis. Stated more directly, rumen microbial protein production can be directly related to rumen propionate concentration (Dove and Milne, 1994; Trevaskis et al., 2001). Further details of the fate of plant carbohydrate during rumen and postruminal digestion are discussed by Annison et al. (2002) and Mackie et al. (2002).

Postruminal Carbohydrate Digestion and Metabolism

Although ruminal fermentation provides the primary opportunity for the degradation and utilization of cellulose and hemicellulose, which are not subject to mammalian enzyme breakdown, fermentation is an energetically inefficient process for the breakdown of starch. Ruminal fermentation losses are estimated to be 13–18 percent of GE (Harmon and McLeod, 2001). In a review of factors affecting intestinal starch digestion in ruminants, Harmon et al. (2004) estimated that approximately 75–80 percent of starch intake is digested in the rumen. Of the starch that escapes ruminal fermentation and reaches the small intestine, 35–60 percent is digested there by enzymatic hydrolysis. Starch still present in the GIT and presented to the large intestine is then subject to hindgut fermentation, and approximately 35–50 percent of that starch is digested. Energetic efficiencies can be increased by increasing the proportion of starch that is digested and glucose absorbed directly from the small intestine.

Many factors are known to affect starch availability and use in the small intestine. These factors include diet type and feed processing, energy intake, adequate pancreatic amylase, and glucose transport mechanisms (Harmon et al., 2004).

Lipids

Lipids are hydrophobic, organic substances that are soluble in organic solvents. The terms "fats" and "lipids" are often used interchangeably because all fats are lipids; however, not all lipids are fats. Whereas fats consist of one or more fatty acids esterified with glycerol, lipids include both glycerol-based and nonglycerol-based compounds (e.g., sterols and waxes). The principal lipids of importance in animal nutrition are fatty acids. Therefore, determination of total fatty acid concentration would be a preferred method of lipid analysis (Palmquist and Jenkins, 2003).

The lipid components of small ruminant tissues are generally similar to those of other mammals, although fatty acids are generally more saturated and there are differences among the CS, IM, and GR morphological types (Meyer et al., 1998). Animal tissues are composed of both simple lipids (acylglycerols), compound lipids (phospholipids, glycolipids, and lipoproteins), and derived lipids (sterols and fatty acids). Simple lipids or true fats are the major storage form of body lipids. The principal role of compound lipids involves structure and function, and the fatty acids contained within the compound lipids contribute to a specific tissue's fatty acid composition. Lipids derived from tissue metabolism also contribute to a tissue's fatty acid composition. Fatty acids actually represent the greatest fraction of lipids because they are components of all three classes of lipids. Unique aspects of lipid digestion by ruminant animals have been thoroughly reviewed by authors in the monographs edited by Christie (1981) and Wiseman (1984).

Functions and Sources of Lipids

Lipids serve three basic functions in the animal body: structural, regulatory, and nutritional. Structurally, lipids are components of cell membranes. Regulatory functions are related to hormone and eicosanoid actions. Nutritionally, lipids have greater energetic value than any of the other nutrients and are also the most important energy storage reservoir in the animal. The main purpose of dietary lipids is to provide a concentrated source of energy. Nutritional manipulation via dietary lipids is also emerging as a means to alter fatty acid composition of ruminant-derived food products.

Ruminants obtain fatty acids from the diet and through de novo synthesis. In feeds, fatty acids are present primarily as triacylglycerols or part of compound lipids, such as phospholipids or glycolipids. Forage lipids, predominantly phospholipids and glycolipids, typically contain < 50 percent fatty acid, whereas lipids of seeds contain from 70–80 percent fatty acid for grains to 90 percent fatty acid for oilseeds (Palmquist, 1988). Adipose tissue of the nonlactating animal is the principal site of synthesis of fatty acids from acetate, whereas the predominant site of de novo fatty acid synthesis shifts to the mammary gland in the lactating animal. Fatty acid synthesis de novo may be altered by plane of nutrition (Andersen et al., 1996), physiological stage of production (McNamara and Hillers, 1986; Smith and Walsh, 1988), and through provision of a dietary fat (Chilliard, 1993; McNamara et al., 1995; Ahnadi et al., 2002) or specific fatty acids (Bauman et al., 2003). Direct use of long-chain fatty acids for milk fat secretion or body fat deposition is more energetically efficient than de novo synthesis from acetate and glucose (Chilliard, 1993; Palmquist, 1994).

Lipid Digestion and Metabolism in the Rumen

Lipids of feeds consumed by small ruminants are altered in the rumen before they are available for metabolism by the animal. The initial step in the ruminal transformation of dietary acyl lipids is hydrolysis of ester linkages by microbial lipolytic enzymes to liberate glycerol and free fatty acids (Jenkins, 1993). Glycerol may then be metabolized by the ruminal microorganisms to produce VFAs (Nagaraja et al., 1997). Once liberated as free fatty acids, unsaturated fatty acids are subject to biohydrogenation by the ruminal bacteria. The presence of a free carboxyl group of an unesterified fatty acid is absolutely required for hydrogenation to proceed (Kepler et al., 1970; Hazelwood et al., 1976). The end product of complete biohydrogenation of 18-carbon fatty acids is stearic acid; however, incomplete hydrogenation results in formation of conjugated isomers of linolenic and linoleic acids as well as various isomeric forms of oleic acid.

The stepwise process of ruminal biohydrogenation was described by Harfoot and Hazelwood (1997). The present consensus is that the bacteria are largely responsible for biohydrogenation in the rumen. This is accomplished with a range of bacteria having various capacities to biohydrogenated unsaturated fatty acids (Kemp and Lander, 1984). Several factors related to the diet influence biohydrogenation in the rumen. Forage maturity (Gerson et al., 1985, 1986), forage species, harvesting and processing methods (Dewhurst et al., 2003), dietary forage-to-concentrate ratio (Kucuk et al., 2001), dietary nitrogen content (Gerson et al., 1982, 1983), and some ionophores (Van Nevel and Demeyer, 1995; Wang et al., 2005) affect the degree with which dietary fatty acids are metabolized in the rumen. Supplementing the diet with fats in the form of whole oilseeds has provided protection of unsaturated fatty acids from ruminal biohydrogenation (Baldwin and Allison, 1983). Lipid composition of supplemental feeds also affects the extent of biohydrogenation in the rumen. Protein-formaldehyde treatments have been used to protect lipids from ruminal biohydrogenation (Scott and Cook, 1975). Because a free carboxyl group is an absolute requirement for biohydrogenation, fatty acyl amides (Fotouhi and Jenkins, 1992; Jenkins, 1995) and insoluble calcium soaps of fatty acids (Enjalbert et al., 1994) provide partial protection against ruminal biohydrogenation. Dietary supplements containing fatty acids with relatively high concentrations of polyunsaturated fatty acids, such as linoleic acid (Scholljegerdes et al., 2004), or those with > 20 carbons (Khanal and Olson, 2004) may not be completely hydrogenated due to irreversible inhibition (Harfoot et al., 1973) of select bacteria growth or through inhibition of their hydrogenases (Griinari and Bauman, 1999). Less extensive ruminal biohydrogenation resulted in greater flow of linoleic and linolenic acids to the duodenum as dietary level of soybean oil increased (Kucuk et al., 2004). Increased duodenal flow of linoleic acid that occurred from increased dietary oil could be accounted for by increased flow of esterified linoleic acid (Atkinson et al., 2005), which may be associated with intracellular lipid inclusion by the ruminal bacteria (Bauchart et al., 1990) or by contamination of the bacterial fraction with feed particles (Harfoot and Hazelwood, 1997). Accumulation of lipid in the bacteria accompanied a reduction in the extent of biohydrogenation (O'Kelly and Spiers, 1991).

The nature of the ruminal microorganism lipids is of importance because of microbial contributions to the composition of the lipid component available to the host animal in postruminal digesta. Chikunya et al. (2004) estimated that about 30 percent of the fatty acids reaching the proximal duodenum were of microbial origin. De novo synthesis of lipids by the microbial population occurs in the rumen, and free acids may be incorporated into microorganisms in the course of cell synthesis (Harfoot and Hazelwood, 1997). However, the rate of de novo synthesis tends to diminish as the amount of exogenous lipid increases (Demeyer et al., 1978) because incorporation of dietary fatty acids into cellular lipids inhibits microbial de novo fatty acid synthesis (Byers and Schelling, 1988). Estimates of incorporation of dietary lipids into microbial cells have ranged from 8 percent (Jenkins, 1993) to approximately 30 percent (Wu et al., 1991).

Postruminal Lipid Digestion and Metabolism

The aforementioned factors that influence lipid composition available to the host animal are important because the digestibility of lipids is dependent on its fatty acid composition. Although Doreau and Ferlay (1994) suggested that ruminal absorption of free fatty acids is possible if large amounts of fatty acids are available in the rumen, it is generally accepted that there is negligible disappearance of long-chain fatty acids from the rumen either by absorption across the ruminal epithelium (Moore and Christie, 1984) or by ruminal catabolism (Jenkins, 1993). The small intestine is therefore the primary absorptive site for fatty acids. For absorption to occur, the fatty acids must be transferred from the insoluble particulate phase and emulsified into micelles, a process that is aided by bile salts and pancreatic secretions (Byers and Schelling, 1988; Palmquist, 1988). Unsaturated fatty acids are absorbed somewhat more efficiently than saturated fatty acids (Lennox and Garton, 1968). A linear decrease in intestinal disappearance of total fatty acids was attributed to reduced disappearance of saturated fatty acids (primarily stearic acid) in sheep fed increasing levels of soybean oil (Kucuk et al., 2004).

Energetic Value of Dietary Lipids

The energy available for metabolism when lipids are added to the diet is 85–90 percent of theoretical estimates (Chilliard, 1993). In addition to the expected discount in energy value associated with reduced intestinal digestibility of fatty acids as the level of supplemental lipid increases, fat additions to the diet can exert antimicrobial actions (Jenkins, 1993) and adversely affect ruminal fermentation and diet digestibility (Palmquist and Jenkins, 1980). Total tract digestibility of structural carbohydrates decreased about 25 percent in sheep fed diets with 6 percent added fat (Ikwuegbu and Sutton, 1982; Nelson et al., 2001). Decreased digestibility of structural carbohydrates may be largely attributed to reduced ruminal digestion. Ikwuegbu and Sutton (1982) reported a 68 percent decrease in ruminal disappearance of structural carbohydrates in sheep fed fat at approximately 6 percent of the diet. Although Jenkins (1995) reported that adding fat at 5 percent of the diet decreased total tract fiber digestibility by 15 percent, Ludden et al. (1995) found that adding fat at 5 percent of diet DM had no effect on the digestibility of the DM of the total diet. Thus, the negative effects of lipid supplements on diet digestibility can be avoided by limiting the level of added fat to 5 percent or less. In an experiment in which lambs were limit fed (Kucuk et al., 2004), there were no negative effects on digestibility when soybean oil levels as high as 9.4 percent of DM were added.

Despite the potential adverse effects of added lipid on fiber digestibility, energy digestibility may not be affected (Jenkins, 1995, 1997; Ludden et al., 1995) because digestibility of fatty acids is typically greater than that of the nonlipid fraction of the basal diet (Chilliard, 1993). In a summary of results from 11 experiments, Chilliard (1993) demonstrated that the energy values of diets supplemented with 3.9 percent lipids were 9 percent greater than those of control diets, and observations were not linked clearly to the nature of lipid supplements. This increase is remarkably close to the 8.8 percent increase in the ME content of diets containing 4 percent added fat (Nelson et al., 2001). Likewise, DE content increased by 10.5 percent in wethers fed 5 percent added dietary fat (Ludden et al., 1995). Metabolizable energy content increased by 14.7 percent with 6 percent added fat and reached a plateau at an increase of 17.6 percent for diets with 8 and 10 percent added fat (Nelson et al., 2001). These observations are consistent with the conclusions of Palmquist (1994), who surmised that effects imposed by high amounts of dietary fat limit its incorporation in ruminant diets to 16–20 percent of ME. Nevertheless, the energy provided by supplemental lipids affords feed managers the opportunity to increase energy density of the diet.

Protein

Protein and Amino Acid Supplies

The ability of ruminants to synthesize microbial protein in the rumen from nonprotein nitrogen sources as well as from dietary protein sources complicates their protein and nitrogen metabolism. The goal in meeting the protein needs of ruminants is to optimize the contributions of both microbial protein and dietary protein that escape ruminal degradation to the supply of amino acids available for absorption. Historically, the CP and digestible protein (DP) systems were used to express protein requirements of small ruminants. Now, the metabolizable protein (MP) system is viewed as the most appropriate method of defining protein requirements.

Metabolizable Protein

Metabolizable protein is defined as the true protein, derived from a combination of dietary and microbial protein, that is digested postruminally and from which the constituent amino acids are absorbed from the intestine. Minor contributions from endogenous proteins (e.g., sloughed epithelial cells) are also present within the digestive tract, but these are not usually directly considered in MP systems. Metabolizable protein is based on the quantity of protein absorbed from the small intestine, which is largely determined by factors influencing microbial protein synthesis and ruminal outflow of intact feed proteins. The MP system is preferred over the DP system for a number of reasons. Primarily, fecal CP excretion, the basis for DP, is appreciably influenced by factors unrelated to amino acid absorption.

The evaluation or prediction of MP intake requires information on the factors that influence microbial protein synthesis and the extent of ruminal outflow of intact feed protein. The most important factor affecting microbial protein synthesis is the quantity of ruminally fermented energy or organic matter. Hence, the MP system predicts microbial protein synthesis based on some measure of energy that is derived from ruminal fermentation and is available to support microbial cell growth. A variety of methods have been used to estimate microbial protein synthesis (SCA, 1990; Sniffen et al., 1992; AFRC, 1993, 1998; NRC, 2001; Luo et al., 2004a,b; Nsahlai et al., 2004).

Microbial Protein Synthesis

Many factors determine microbial protein synthesis. The most important of these is the adequacy of ruminal availability of nitrogenous compounds to meet microbial growth requirements. Other factors include feed intake and the supply and sources of fermentable energy. Rumen microbes differ in preferences for nitrogen sources, with ammonia being the preferred source of many bacteria. For example, fibrololytic bacteria prefer ammonia. In contrast, many amylolytic bacteria prefer amino acids and/or peptides, and ruminal protozoa derive their nitrogen from degradation of bacterial, feed, and fungal proteins. When quantities of ruminally available nitrogen are limited, microbial protein synthesis is restricted. However, the concentration of rumi nal ammonia at which microbial protein synthesis is limited under different dietary and animal feeding conditions has not been well established.

The rate that digesta fractions pass from the rumen to the intestines also affects both microbial protein synthesis and flow to the small intestine. In general, microbial protein synthesis and ruminal outflow increase with increasing passage rate because of a decreasing proportion of ruminally fermented energy used for microbial cell maintenance, concomitant with an increased rate of replication to maintain cell numbers. Short ruminal digesta residence time selects for more efficient microbes with relatively high rates of replication. However, the extent of organic matter digestion in the rumen decreases with increasing digesta passage rate. Therefore, the net effect of change in passage rate depends on magnitudes of change in efficiency of microbial growth and ruminally fermented energy.

Typically, digesta passage from the rumen is addressed by consideration of both fluid and particulate fractions. Although both generally change together, an increase in fluid passage rate is thought to have relatively greater effect on microbial cell outflow. Ruminal outflow of protozoa is very slow relative to their contribution to microbial mass in the rumen. The inability to predict accurately both fluid and particulate passage rates under various feeding conditions has led some nutrient requirement systems to use only one general digesta passage rate term (e.g., AFRC, 1992).

To determine the contribution of microbial CP to MP, true protein concentration and digestibility in the small intestine must be addressed. Assumed values differ only slightly among most MP systems, such as a true protein concentration of 75 and 80 percent and digestibility of 85 and 75 percent for NRC (2000, 2001) and AFRC (1993, 1998), respectively, resulting in microbial MP estimates of 64 and 60 percent of microbial CP.

Ruminal Outflow of Intact Feed Protein

The approaches to predict ruminal outflow of intact feed protein are similar among various MP systems, with some differences in how dietary CP is fractionated. The NRC (2001) divides CP into three fractions based on rate of degradation in the rumen. The Cornell Net Carbohydrate and Protein System (CNCPS) Level II approach (Sniffen et al., 1992) entails a greater degree of fractionation, but is still based on rate of ruminal degradation. Other systems (AFRC, 1993, 1998; Luo et al., 2004a,b; Nsahlai et al., 2004) define additional insoluble and indigestible fractions and assign rates of passage to them.

Passage rate has an appreciable effect on degraded intake protein and undegraded intake protein and is known to be affected by DM intake, forage type, and diet composition (NRC, 2001). An equation developed with cattle (Ngwa et al., 2001) was used to estimate fluid passage rate from particulate passage rate, which was used to estimate flow of soluble true protein. Cannas et al. (2004) used equations developed mainly from cattle data to predict passage rate in sheep based on neutral detergent fiber intake and dietary CP concentration.

Small intestinal absorption rate of amino acids from feed protein escaping the rumen intact seems to be more variable than that of amino acids from microbial protein. Presently there are insufficient data available for accurately predicting amino acids absorbed. The AFRC (1993) assumed a small intestinal digestion coefficient for feed protein of 85 percent. The NRC (2000) assumed 80 percent intestinal digestibility of undegraded intake protein, which apparently includes acid detergent fiber nitrogen.

Nitrogen Recycling and Conservation in Small Ruminants

The ability of ruminants to recycle urea synthesized in the liver to the rumen for microbial protein synthesis is a significant aspect of ruminant nitrogen metabolism. Urea recycling, also known as the "protein regeneration cycle," has long been recognized as a major mechanism to improve the quality of protein supply (Houpt, 1959; Cocimano and Leng, 1967; Robbins et al., 1974). Recycling also allows ruminants to conserve nitrogen when dietary intake of nitrogen is low (Schmidt-Nielsen et al., 1957; Houpt, 1959). For example, urea recycling is important for survival of wild deer, North American elk (wapiti), and reindeer/caribou when forage availability and quality are low in the fall and winter months. For sheep and goats in semi-arid and arid environments, urea recycling enables them to meet maintenance protein requirements when forage quality is low.

As in recent NRC reports (2000, 2001), the present report does not explicitly represent urea nitrogen recycling in the prediction of available MP from diets. This decision was based on the following. First, despite the large number of studies where urea recycling has been measured in domesticated and wild ruminants, there continues to be insufficient information related to animal and diet effects to predict accurately the amount of urea that is transferred to the rumen and the extent to which this urea nitrogen is incorporated into microbial protein. Second, at present, there are no generalized empirical equations to predict bacterial CP synthesis and efficiency, particularly at the low intakes of TDN of many wild and grazing ruminants. In consequence, it is not possible to predict accurately the contribution of recycled urea nitrogen to rumen microbial protein outflow. Whole tract and rumen models have been developed that include some representation of the contribution of recycled urea nitrogen to protein nutrition of ruminants (Nolan and Leng, 1972; Dijkstra et al., 1992; Model Level II NRC, 2000). However, none of these models has been comprehensively evaluated for practical application, and for two of the models detailed descriptions of feed composition are required. And, lastly, the Beef report (NRC, 2000) made the assumption that the requirement for nitrogen (ruminally degraded protein, recycled urea, other nonprotein nitrogen sources) by rumen microbes equals microbial protein synthesis and, therefore, that losses of ammonia from the rumen equate to the amount of urea nitrogen recycled (i.e., net urea recycling equal to zero). Stated another way, excess rumen ammonia results in ammonia absorption, whereas a deficiency of rumen ammonia encourages urea recycling, and so long as ruminally degraded protein intake is in close balance with microbial protein synthesis, the need to account for urea recycling is minimal.

In the previous Sheep (NRC, 1985a) and Goat (NRC, 1981b) reports and in the recent Dairy (NRC, 2001) report, the lack of sufficient information on urea recycling and use led to the decision not to incorporate it explicitly into the prediction equations. In contrast, the Beef report (NRC, 2000) accepted the recommendation of the Ruminant Nitrogen Usage report (NRC, 1985b) and in Level I employed an iterative equation with nitrogen recycled being a function of dietary CP and TDN content. This equation was acknowledged as unsuitable for diets below 8 percent CP, and no validations have been conducted. Given the magnitude and potential that recycling of urea to the rumen has on overall nitrogen economy in all ruminants, it is clear that further efforts will need to be made to define feeding conditions when the partition of blood urea to the rumen (urea recycling) has major impact on the protein supply for maintenance and productive functions.

The amount of urea produced by the liver exceeded the amount of urea excreted into the urine by 74 percent in sheep (Ford and Milligan, 1970), 93 percent in beef bulls, 107 percent in caribou in summer, and 139 percent in caribou in winter (Wales et al., 1975). Urea not excreted into the urine has two potential fates: (1) partition to the rumen where it is rapidly hydrolyzed to ammonia and then either used by microbes for protein synthesis or absorbed into blood, and (2) partition to the lower GIT (cecum, large intestines), where it is ultimately excreted in feces as microbial protein-nitrogen.

The proportion of urea transferred to the GIT (10–80 percent) is often of critical importance to the overall nitrogen economy in ruminants compared to other species (Table 2-1). To appreciate the importance of this process in ruminants, consider that the ratio of liver urea synthesis to digestible nitrogen intake averages 0.87 for dairy cows, 1.07 for steers, 1.15 for bulls, 1.42 for sheep fed forage diets, 2.34 for sheep fed hay/barley diets, 1.05–1.21 for growing goats, 2.83–4.86 for wapiti, 0.54–1.32 for white-tailed deer, and 0.82–1.79 for reindeer/caribou. In cases where urea synthesis exceeds digestible nitrogen intake, urea must be recycled to the rumen for microbial protein synthesis and to meet the maintenance and growth needs of the animal. Therefore, the ability of reindeer/caribou to meet maintenance requirements in winter and the ability of the other species to meet requirements for maintenance plus gain as tissue protein (meat, wool) or milk protein depends on these animals recycling a significant portion of urea to the rumen.

Fates of Urea Recycled to the Ruminant Gastrointestinal Tract

Urea is water soluble and distributed throughout all body fluids. Thus, urea has the potential to enter all compartments of the GIT through normal GIT secretions (i.e., saliva, gastric juice, bile, and pancreatic juice) and by diffusion from blood (Kennedy and Milligan, 1980; Egan et al., 1986). However, depending on diet characteristics that may shift fermentative activity throughout the GIT, urea transfer to the rumen can be variable.

Estimates in sheep, goats, and elk are that 18–85 percent of blood urea is directed to the rumen either via saliva or diffusion from blood (Nolan and Leng, 1972; Kennedy and Milligan, 1978; Harmeyer and Martens, 1980; Obara and Shimbayashi, 1980; Mould and Robbins, 1981; Koenig et al., 2000), with the remainder entering the hindgut. Most

TABLE 2-1 Digestible Nitrogen (N) Intake and Urea Synthesis and Recycling in Different Animal Species (g N/day)

Species	N Intake	Digestible N	Urea-N Synthesis	Urea-N Recycled to GIT	Urea Recycled: Urea Synthesis
Dairy cows[a]	450	301	262	171	0.65
Steers[b]	64	33.1	35.4	28.1	0.79
Yearling bulls[c]	70	(42)	48.2	23.2	0.48
Sheep—forage diet[d]	17.1	11.5	16.3	9.9	0.61
Sheep—hay/barley diet[e]	12.9	(8.7)	20.4	8.7	0.42
Goats—hay/grain diet, 7.8% CP[f]	9.3	3.7	3.9	2.7	0.69
Goats—hay/grain diet, 11.2% CP[f]	14.5	8	9.7	4.1	0.42
Elk/wapiti[g]	41/51	15/36	73/102	63/30	0.85/0.29
White-tailed deer[h]	15/84	13.2/76	17.4/41	15.4/17	0.89/0.41
Reindeer/caribou					
Summer[i]	77	56	46	23.8	0.52
Winter[i]	36	24	43	25	0.58
Cats[j]	1.7	1.5	1.1	0.2	0.18
Pigs[k]	28.1	18.8	21	9.7	0.46

[a]Lapierre and Lobley (2001), [b]Archibeque et al. (2000b), [c]Wales et al. (1975), [d]Lobley et al. (2000), [e]Ford and Milligan 1970, [f]Obara and Shimbayashi (1980), [g]*Cervus elaphus nelsoni*, fed a 7.6% vs. 17.6% CP diet to maintenance energy, Mould and Robbins (1981), [h]*Odoceilius virginianus*, fed a 5.1% vs. 26% CP diet to ad libitum intake, Robbins et al. (1974), [i]*Rangifer tarandus*, fed a 12% CP diet in summer and a 8% CP lichen/pellet diet in winter, Wales et al. (1975), [j]Russell et al. (2000), [k]Mosenthin et al. (1992).

of the urea entering the GIT is hydrolyzed to ammonia by the action of bacterial urease at the luminal surfaces of the rumen, small intestines, cecum, and large intestines (Wallace et al., 1979). The released ammonia is either reabsorbed into blood or is used as a nitrogen source for microbial protein synthesis, some of which may be excreted into the feces (approximately 10 percent; Lapierre and Lobley, 2001). Thus, if bacterial synthesis from the hydrolyzed urea occurs in either the cecum or large intestines, sites where amino acid absorption does not occur, then the urea recycled to these compartments will be lost to the feces.

Saliva can be a significant route (15–100 percent) of urea nitrogen transfer to the rumen, the extent of which depends on the type (e.g., concentrate vs. forage; Huntington, 1989) and processing (e.g., dried vs. ensiled grass; Siddons et al., 1985) of the diet. Forage has most influence on saliva flow rate and rumination activity, as well as level of feed intake (Egan et al., 1986). For example, a diet high in fiber or a dried-forage diet stimulates rumination activity, and in turn increases saliva flow to the rumen. Obara and Shimbayashi (1980) observed an increase in salivary transfer of urea by goats when switched from a low (7.8 percent CP) to a high (11.2 percent CP) diet. Generally, salivary transfer of urea dominates in ruminants fed forage diets (approximately 70 percent), but when higher concentrate diets are fed most (67 percent) of urea transfer is via the blood (Lapierre and Lobley, 2001). Size of salivary glands also may influence saliva production and hence urea transfers to the rumen (Kay, 1966). The large submaxillary and parotid glands of CS and IM species (1.2–1.8 g/kg BW [body weight]) greatly exceed that for grazer species (approximately 0.6 g/kg BW), suggesting a greater saliva production (Kay et al., 1980; Hofmann 1989), and urea transfer through saliva in CS species (white-tailed deer) and IM species (goats, elk/wapiti, reindeer/caribou) compared with GR species (sheep). Ammonia not captured by bacteria is absorbed from the rumen, removed by the liver, and again converted to urea (Sarraseca et al., 1998; Milano et al., 2000), and the cycle continues. General trends are that urea transferred to the rumen in animals (sheep, beef) fed low-protein diets is utilized more efficiently (approximately 85–90 percent capture) for microbial protein synthesis compared to urea transferred in animals fed higher (> 14 percent) CP diets (< 50 percent capture; Marini and Van Amburgh, 2003; Sunny et al., 2004).

Contributions of recycled urea nitrogen toward rumen microbes, feces, and urine depend on feed intake (Sarraseca et al., 1998) and the conditions in the rumen (pH, ammonia:ammonium concentration, fermentable carbohydrates), which themselves are determined by dietary factors such as protein content (Marini and Van Amburgh, 2003), nitrogen solubility, the concentrate:forage ratio of the diet (Lobley et al., 2000), available or fermentable energy (Norton et al., 1982), and others. Because lichens represent a highly fermentable resource for deer and reindeer/caribou in winter, access and intake of lichens should support the capture of the high rates of urea recycled to the rumen in winter compared with summer (0.65 vs. 0.37 g per $kg^{-0.75}$ per day; Wales et al., 1975).

Dietary Factors Affecting Urea Recycling and Utilization in Ruminants

The proportion of recycled urea that is used for bacterial protein synthesis within the rumen can range from 5 to 95 percent, depending on animal species, the level of intake, type of diet, and fermentable energy intake (Schmidt-Nielsen et al., 1957; Sarraseca et al., 1998; Lobley et al., 2000; Archibeque et al., 2000a,b). In general, at low-protein intakes and when low-quality roughage diets are fed, ruminants tend to have lower blood concentrations of urea, lower urinary urea excretion, and increased transfer of urea to the GIT (Robbins et al., 1974; Wales et al., 1975; Harmeyer and Martens, 1980; Bunting et al., 1987; Huntington, 1989; Marini and Van Amburgh, 2003). In sheep fed low-quality hay, urea recycled to the GIT accounted for 80–90 percent of blood urea and a higher proportion of absorbed nitrogen was retained (Bunting et al., 1987). In red deer, Mould and Robbins (1981) reported greater urea recycling when deer were fed timothy hay compared to feeding fresh wheat herbage.

Increasing the fermentable carbohydrate fraction of the diet increases urea recycling to the rumen but urea transfer to hindgut tissues is reduced (Kennedy, 1980; Kennedy and Milligan, 1980; Norton et al., 1982; Reynolds and Huntington, 1988; Huntington, 1989). Thus, supplemental grain, starch, dried pulp, and sucrose provided as energy sources significantly increase urea nitrogen capture in the rumen. By contrast, when fermentable carbohydrates reach the cecum, the higher fermentation increases the proportion of urea nitrogen reaching the hindgut (70 percent) and being excreted in the feces (10–25 percent; Thornton et al., 1970; Reynolds and Huntington, 1988). This probably explains why feeding large amounts of resistant starch results in high fecal nitrogen losses in feedlot animals.

Feed processing also influences urea recycling through effects on fermentation activity. Theurer et al. (2002) observed an increase in urea nitrogen recycling to the GIT and a reduction in urinary urea nitrogen output in growing beef steers fed steam-flaked sorghum compared to dry-rolled sorghum. They also observed greater transfer of urea to the rumen (77 percent) vs. to the small intestines (23 percent). The same researchers (Alio et al., 2000) fed steam-flaked sorghum to the steers at decreasing flake densities (437, 360, and 283 g/L) and also observed increasing rates of urea nitrogen transfer to the GIT of beef steers. This processing technique increases starch and CP digestibility, which may result in rapid capture and lowering of rumen ammonia to allow greater diffusion of blood urea through the GIT wall (Huntington, 1997).

Minerals

Minerals are required for an array of important functions in the animal body (Underwood and Suttle, 1999). Primary functions include roles as structural components of organs and tissues, including bone and teeth, and as constituents of body fluids and tissues. Within body fluids and tissues, minerals have important physiological roles as electrolytes, maintaining osmotic pressure, acid-base balance, membrane permeability, and nervous transmission. They also function in the regulation of cell replication and differentiation (Underwood and Suttle, 1999). Important functions of some minerals are as coenzymes, cofactors, and metaloenzymes, participating in many metabolic activities in the body. Some minerals are components of hormones. Recent reviews of minerals in animal nutrition were published by McDowell (2003) and NRC (2005).

Classification of Minerals

Minerals that are required in gram quantities per day are classified as the macroelements, whereas those found in very low concentrations in the body (parts per million or less), and are required in small quantities, are classified as the microelements. Macroelements include calcium, phosphorus, magnesium, sodium, chlorine, potassium, and sulfur. Essential microelements include copper, zinc, selenium, iodine, manganese, cobalt, and iron. There are 13 other elements that are considered essential under certain conditions and for certain species of animals. These are chromium, molybdenum, nickel, fluorine, vanadium, tin, silicon, arsenic, boron, aluminum, lead, lithium, and rubidium (Underwood and Suttle, 1999). Excessive intakes of fluorine, molybdenum, lead, arsenic, aluminum, cadmium, and mercury may exert toxic effects.

Mineral Requirements

Many of the essential elements are found in sufficient quantities in diets typically consumed by small ruminants. Other elements are often deficient in the diets consumed and, when possible, should be supplemented to optimize animal performance and health. Toxicity is a potential problem with some minerals. Therefore, in addition to identifying requirements for the elements, maximum tolerable levels (the dietary level that, when fed for a defined period of time, will not impair animal performance; NRC, 2005) may also need to be considered.

The concentrations of minerals within feed resources vary greatly. In addition to differences among feed type and plant species, mineral content can be affected by production and management practices. Soil type and pH will affect mineral content, as will fertilization practices and application rates. Climatic conditions affecting plant growth rate and plant maturity can alter mineral content. Bioavailability of minerals contained in feed resources is an important consideration in evaluating dietary adequacy (Ammerman et al., 1995).

Vitamins

Vitamins are a group of complex organic compounds that are essential in trace amounts for normal metabolism and physiological processes. Vitamins have diverse functions including involvement in many metabolic processes, immune cell function, and gene regulation. A deficiency of a single vitamin will produce specific clinical signs and symptoms. Subclinical deficiencies may occur in which clinical signs are not evident but animal productivity or overall health is less than optimal. A comprehensive review of vitamins in animal nutrition was published by McDowell (2000).

Classification of Vitamins

The traditional classification of vitamins depends on their solubility in fat or water. Fat-soluble vitamins are A, D, E, and K, whereas vitamins of the B complex (thiamin, riboflavin, niacin, vitamin B_6, pantothenic acid, biotin, folacin, vitamin B_{12}, choline), C, and other vitamin-like compounds are classified as water soluble. Fat-soluble vitamins are found associated with lipids in feedstuffs. The fat-soluble vitamins are absorbed in the small intestine by mechanisms similar to those involved in long-chain fatty acid absorption. Unlike the fat-soluble vitamins, water-soluble vitamins are not associated with fats and alterations in fat absorption do not affect their absorption. Fat-soluble vitamins are stored in appreciable amounts in the animal body. Most water-soluble vitamins, with the exception of vitamin B_{12}, are not stored in significant amounts and excesses are rapidly excreted. Thus, a continuous supply of water-soluble vitamins is needed to avoid deficiencies. Water-soluble vitamins are relatively nontoxic, but excesses of vitamins A and D can cause serious problems.

Vitamin Requirements

Although small ruminants have a physiological requirement for the vitamins, not all vitamins are required in the diet. Some vitamins are considered metabolic essentials, but not dietary essentials, because they can be synthesized in amounts sufficient to satisfy physiological requirements. Vitamins A and E are the only vitamins with an absolute dietary requirement, although even this requirement can be met with injectable forms of these vitamins. Many natural feedstuffs contain vitamin A precursors and vitamin E, and these vitamins need not be supplemented in many situations. Vitamin D is synthesized by ultraviolet radiation of plant material and an animal's skin. However, management systems in which animals are maintained in confinement with less exposure to sunlight and fresh forage may increase the need to add supplemental sources of vitamins A, D, and E. Except during specific conditions, small ruminants with a fully functioning rumen satisfy their needs for vitamin K and the B vitamins from these vitamins naturally present in their feed plus those synthesized by symbiotic microorganisms. Vitamin C, or ascorbic acid, is synthesized from L-gulonic acid within the cells of the small ruminant's body. The neonatal small ruminant, however, relies on dietary intake of the vitamins to fulfill their requirement. The ruminal flora may contribute significant amounts of the B vitamins as early as 8 days with self-sufficiency occurring once the rumen becomes fully functional (Smith, 1970), whereas vitamin C may not be synthesized in sufficient amounts until about 3 weeks of age (Cummins and Brunner, 1991).

REFERENCES

AFRC (Agriculture and Food Research Council). 1992. Nutritive Requirements of Ruminant Animals: Protein. Technical Committee on Responses to Nutrients, Report No. 8. Wallingford, UK: CAB International.

AFRC. 1993. Energy and Protein Requirements of Ruminants. An Advisory Manual Prepared by the AFRC Technical Committee on Responses to Nutrients. Wallingford, UK: CAB International.

AFRC. 1998. The Nutrition of Goats. New York: CAB International.

Ahnadi, C. E., N. Beswick, L. Delbecchi, J. J. Kennelly, and P. Lacasse. 2002. Addition of fish oil to diets for dairy cows. II. Effects on milk fat and gene expression of mammary lipogenic enzymes. J. Dairy Res. 69:521–531.

Alio, A., C. B. Theurer, O. Lozano, J. T. Huber, R. S. Swingle, A. Delgado-Elorduy, P. Cuneo, D. DeYoung, and K. E. Webb, Jr. 2000. Splanchnic nitrogen metabolism by growing beef steers fed diets containing sorghum grain flaked at different densities. J. Anim. Sci. 78:1355–1363.

Ammerman, C. B., D. H. Baker, and A. J. Lewis, eds. 1995. Bioavailability of Nutrients for Animals: Amino Acids, Minerals and Vitamins. San Diego, CA: Academic Press.

Andersen, M. K., J. W. Bailey, C. Wilken, and D. C. Rule. 1996. Lipoprotein lipase and glycerolphosphate acyltransferase in ovine tissues are influenced by growth and energy intake regimen. Nutr. Biochem. 7:610–616.

Annison, E. F., and W. L. Bryden. 1998. Perspectives on ruminant nutrition and metabolism. I. Metabolism in the rumen. Nutr. Res. Rev. 11: 173–198.

Annison, E. F., D. B. Lindsay, and J. V. Nolan. 2002. Digestion and metabolism. Pp. 95–118 in Sheep Nutrition, M. Freer and H. Dove, eds. Wallingford, UK: CAB International.

ARC (Agricultural Research Council). 1980. The Nutrient Requirements of Ruminant Livestock. Slough, UK: Commonwealth Agricultural Bureaux.

Archibeque, S. L., J. C. Burns, and G. B. Huntington. 2000a. Urea flux in beef steers: Effects of forage species and fertilization. J. Anim. Sci. 78(Suppl. 1):282(Abstr.).

Archibeque, S. L., J. C. Burns, and G. B. Huntington. 2000b. Nitrogen metabolism of beef steers fed endophyte-free fescue hay: Effects of rumen protected methionine supplementation. J. Anim. Sci. 78(Suppl. 1):302(Abstr.).

Atkinson, R. L., E. J. Scholljegerdes, S. L. Lake, V. Nayigihugu, B. W. Hess, and D. C. Rule. 2005. Site and extent of digestion, duodenal flow, and intestinal disappearance of total and esterified fatty acids in sheep fed a high-concentrate diet supplemented with high-linoleate safflower oil. J. Anim. Sci. 84:287–296.

Baldwin, R. L. 1965. Pathways of carbohydrate metabolism in the rumen. Pp. 379–389 in Physiology of Digestion in the Ruminant, R. W. Dougherty, ed. Washington, DC: Butterworths.

Baldwin, R. L., and M. J. Allison. 1983. Rumen metabolism. J. Anim. Sci. 57(Suppl. 2):461–477.

Bauchart, D., F. Legay-Carmier, M. Doreau, and B. Gaillard. 1990. Lipid metabolism of liquid-associated and solid-adherent bacteria in the rumen of dairy cows. Reprod. Nutr. Dev. 28:139–140.

Bauman, D. E., B. A. Corl, and D. G. Peterson. 2003. The biology of conjugated linoleic acid in ruminants. Pp. 146–173 in Advances in Conjugated Linoleic Acid Research, Vol. 2, J. L. Sebedio, W. W. Christie, and R. Adlof, eds. Champaign, IL: AOCS Press.

Bergman, E. N. 1990. Energy contributions of volatile fatty acids from the gastrointestinal tract in various species. Physiol. Rev. 70:567–590.

Bergman, E. N., and J. E. Wolff. 1971. Metabolism of volatile fatty acids by liver and portal drained viscera in sheep. Am. J. Physiol. 221: 586–592.

Bunnell, F. L., and M. P. Gillingham. 1985. Foraging behavior: Dynamics of dining out. Chapter 3. Pp. 53–79 in Bioenergetics of Wild Herbivores, R. J. Hudson and R. G. White, eds. Boca Raton, FL: CRC Press.

Bunting, L. D., J. A. Boling, C. T. MacKown, and R. B. Muntifering. 1987. Effect of dietary protein level on nitrogen metabolism in lambs: Studies using ^{15}N-nitrogen. J. Anim. Sci. 64:855–867.

Burrin, D. G., C. L. Ferrell, J. H. Eisemann, R. A. Britton, and J. A. Nienaber. 1989. Effect of level of nutrition on splanchnic blood flow and oxygen consumption in sheep. Br. J. Nutr. 62:23–34.

Byers, F. M., and G. T. Schelling. 1988. Lipids in ruminant nutrition. Pp. 298–312 in The Ruminant Animal: Digestive Physiology and Nutrition, DC. Church, ed. Prospect Heights, IL: Waveland Press.

Cannas, A., L. O. Tedeschi, D. G. Fox, A. N. Pell, and P. J. Van Soest. 2004. A mechanistic model for predicting the nutrient requirements and feed biological values for sheep. J. Anim. Sci. 82:149–169.

Chikunya, S., G. Demirel, M. Enser, J. D. Wood, R. G. Wilkinson, and L. A. Sinclair. 2004. Biohydrogenation of dietary *n*-3 PUFA and stability of ingested vitamin E in the rumen, and their effects on microbial activity in sheep. Br. J. Nutr. 91:539–550.

Chilliard, Y. 1993. Dietary fat and adipose tissue metabolism in ruminants, pigs, and rodents: A review. J. Dairy Sci. 76:3897–3931.

Christie, W. W. 1981. Lipid Metabolism in Ruminant Animals. Oxford, UK: Pergamon Press.

Church, D. C., ed. 1988. The Ruminant Animal: Digestive Physiology and Nutrition. Prospect Heights, IL: Waveland Press.

Clarke, R. T. J. 1977. Methods for studying gut microbes. Pp. 1–33 in Microbial Ecology of the Gut, R. T. J. Clarke and T. Bauchop, eds. New York: Academic Press.

Clauss, M., M. Lechner-Doll, and W. J. Streich. 2003. Ruminant diversification as an adaptation to the physicomechanical characteristics of forage. A reevaluation of an old debate and a new hypothesis. Oikos 102: 253–262.

Clemens, E. T., and C. E. Stevens. 1980. A comparison of gastrointestinal transit time in ten species of mammal. J. Agric. Sci. 94:735–737.

Cocimano, M. R., and R. A. Leng. 1967. Metabolism of urea in sheep. Br. J. Nutr. 21:353–371.

Constantinescu, G. M. 2001. Guide to Regional Ruminant Anatomy Based on the Dissection of the Goat. Ames: Iowa State University Press.

Cooper, S. M., and N. Owen-Smith. 1985. Condensed tannins deter feeding by browsing ruminants in a South African savanna. Oecologia 67:142–146.

Corbett, J. L. 1987. Energy and protein utilization by grazing animals. Pp. 341–355 in Temperate Pastures, J. L. Wheeler, C. J. Pearson, and G. E. Robards, eds. Melbourne, Australia: Australian Wool Corporation/ CSIRO.

Cordesse, R., M. Inesta, and J. Gaubert. 1992. Intake and digestibility of four forages by llamas and sheep. Ann. Zootech. 41:70.

Cummins, K. A., and C. J. Brunner. 1991. Effect of calf housing on plasma ascorbate and endocrine and immune function. J. Dairy Sci. 74: 1582–1588.

Demeyer, D. I. 1981. Rumen microbes and digestion of plant cell walls. Agric. Environ. 6:295–337.

Demeyer, D. I., C. Henderson, and R. A. Prins. 1978. Relative significance of exogenous and *de novo* synthesised fatty acids in the formation of rumen microbial lipids *in vitro*. Appl. Environ. Microbiol. 35:24–31.

Dewhurst, R. J., N. D. Scollan, M. R. F. Lee, H. J. Ougham, and M. O. Humphreys. 2003. Forage breeding and management to increase the beneficial fatty acid content of ruminant products. Proc. Nutr. Soc. 62:329–336.

Dijkstra, J., H. D. Neal, D. E. Beever, and J. France. 1992. Simulation of nutrient digestion, absorption and outflow in the rumen: Model description. J. Nutr. 122:2239–2256.

Doreau, M., and A. Ferlay. 1994. Digestion and utilisation of fatty acids by ruminants. Anim. Feed Sci. Technol. 45:379–396.

Dove, H., and J. A. Milne. 1994. Digesta flow and rumen microbial protein production in ewes grazing perennial ryegrass. Aust. J. Agric. Res. 45:1229–1245.

Eckerlin, R. H., and C. E. Stevens. 1973. Bicarbonate secretion by the glandular saccules of the llama stomach. Cornell Vet. 63:436–445.

Egan, A. R., K. Boda, and J. Varady. 1986. Regulation of nitrogen metabolism and recycling. Pp. 386–402 in Control of Digestion and Metabolism in Ruminants, L. P. Milligan, W. L. Grovum, and A. Dobson, eds. Englewood Cliffs, NJ: Prentice-Hall.

Enjalbert, F., M. C. Nicot, M. Vernay, R. Monocoulon, and D. Griess. 1994. Effect of different forms of polyunsaturated fatty acids on duodenal and serum fatty acid profiles in sheep. Can. J. Anim. Sci. 74:595–600.

Faichney, G. J. 1986. The kinetics of particulate matter in the rumen. Pp. 173–195 in Digestion and Metabolism in the Ruminant, I. W. McDonald and A. C. I. Warner, eds. Armidale, Australia: The University of New England Publishing Unit.

Ford, A. L., and L. P. Milligan. 1970. Tracer studies of urea recycling in sheep. Can. J. Anim. Sci. 50:129–135.

Forsyth, D. M., and K. W. Fraser. 1999. Seasonal changes in the rumen morphology of Himalayan tahr (Hemitragus jemlahicus) in the Two Thumb Range, South Island, New Zealand. J. Zool. (Lond.) 249: 241–248.

Fotouhi, N., and T. C. Jenkins. 1992. Ruminal biohydrogenation of linoleyl methionine and calcium linoleate in sheep. J. Anim. Sci. 70:2574–2580.

Fraser, M. D., and D. H. Baker. 1998. A comparison of voluntary intake and in vivo digestion in guanacos (*Lama guanicoe*) and sheep given fresh grass. J. Anim. Sci. 67:567–572.

Galbraith, J. K., G. W. Mathison, R. J. Hudson, T. A. McAllister, and K. J. Cheng. 1998. Intake, digestibility, methane and heat production in bison, wapiti, and white-tailed deer. Can. J. Anim. Sci. 78:681–691.

Gallagher, J. R., and M. Shelton. 1972. Relative efficiencies of conversion of feed to fiber of Angora goats and Rambouillet sheep. J. Anim. Sci. 34:319–324.

Genin, D., Z. Villea, and P. Obasto. 1994. Diet selection and utilization by llamas and sheep in a high altitude arid rangeland of Bolivia. J. Range Manage. 47:245–248.

Gerson, T., A. John, and A. S. D. King. 1985. The effects of dietary starch and fiber on the in vitro rates of lipolysis and hydrogenation by sheep rumen digesta. J. Agric. Sci. 105:27–30.

Gerson, T., A. John, and A. S. D. King. 1986. Effects of feeding ryegrass of varying maturity on the metabolism and composition of lipid in the rumen of sheep. J. Agric. Sci. 106:445–448.

Gerson, T., A. John, I. D. Shelton, and B. R. Sinclair. 1982. Effects of dietary N on lipids of rumen digesta, plasma, liver, muscle and perirenal fat in sheep. J. Agric. Sci. 99:71–78.

Gerson T., A. John, and B. R. Sinclair. 1983. The effect of dietary N on *in vitro* lipolysis and fatty acid hydrogenation in rumen digesta from sheep fed diets high in starch. J. Agric. Sci. 101:97–101.

Goetsch, A. L. 1998. Splanchnic tissue energy use in ruminants that consume forage-based diets ad libitum. J. Anim. Sci. 76:2737–2746.

Griinari, J. M., and D. E. Bauman. 1999. Biosynthesis of conjugated linoleic acid and its incorporation into meat and milk in ruminants. Pp. 180–200 in Advances in Conjugated Linoleic Acid Research, Vol. I, M. P. Yurzwecz, M. M. Mossoba, J. K. G. Kramer, M. W. Pariza, and G. J. Nelson, eds. Champaign, IL: AOCS Press.

Grovum, W. L. 1986. The control of motility of the ruminoreticulum. Pp. 18–40 in Digestion and Metabolism in the Ruminant, I. W. Mc-

Donald and A. C. I. Warner, eds. Armidale, Australia: The University of New England Publishing Unit.

Harfoot, C. G., and G. P. Hazelwood. 1997. Lipid metabolism in the rumen. Pp. 382–426 in The Rumen Microbial Ecosystem, P. N. Hobson, and C. S. Stewart, eds. London: Blackie Academic and Prof., an imprint of Chapman and Hall.

Harfoot, C. G., R. C. Noble, and J. H. Moore. 1973. Factors influencing the extent of biohydrogenation of linoleic acid by rumen micro-organisms *in vitro*. J. Sci. Food Agric. 24:961–970.

Harmeyer, J., and H. Martens. 1980. Aspects of urea metabolism in ruminants with reference to the goat. J. Dairy Sci. 63:1707–1728.

Harmon, D. L., and K. R. McLeod. 2001. Glucose uptake and regulation by intestinal tissues: Implications and whole-body energetics. J. Anim. Sci. 79:E59–E72.

Harmon, D. L., R. M. Yamka, and N. A. Elam. 2004. Factors affecting intestinal starch digestion in ruminants: A review. Can. J. Anim. Sci. 84:309–318.

Hazelwood, G. P., P. Kemp, D. Lander, and R. M. C. Dawson. 1976. C_{18} unsaturated fatty acid hydrogenation patterns of some rumen bacteria and their ability to hydrolyse exogenous phospholipid. Br. J. Nutr. 35: 293–297.

Hintz, H. F., H. F. Schryver, and M. Halbert. 1973. A note on the comparison of digestion by new world camelids, sheep, and ponies. Anim. Prod. 16:303–305.

Hofmann, R. R. 1989. Evolutionary steps of ecophysiological adaptation and diversification of ruminants: A comparative view of their digestive system. Oecologia 78:443–457.

Hofmann, R. R., and D. R. M. Stewart. 1972. Grazer or browser: A classification based on the stomach structure and feeding habits of East African ruminants. Mammalia 36:226–240.

Houpt, T. R. 1959. Utilization of blood urea in ruminants. Am. J. Physiol. 197:115–120.

Hudson, R. J., and R. J. Christopherson. 1985. Maintenance metabolism. Chapter 6. Pp. 121–142 in Bioenergetics of Wild Herbivores, R. J. Hudson and R. G. White, eds. Boca Raton, FL: CRC Press.

Hungate, R. E. 1966. The Rumen and Its Microbes. London: Academic Press.

Huntington, G. B. 1989. Hepatic urea synthesis and site and rate of urea removal from blood of beef steers fed alfalfa hay or a high concentrate diet. Can. J. Anim. Sci. 69:215–223.

Huntington, G. B. 1997. Starch utilization by ruminants: From basics to the bunk. J. Anim. Sci. 75:852–867.

Ikwuegbu, O. A., and J. D. Sutton. 1982. The effect of varying the amount of linseed oil supplementation on rumen metabolism in sheep. Br. J. Nutr. 48:365–375.

Jenkins, T. C. 1993. Lipid metabolism in the rumen. J. Dairy Sci. 76: 3851–3863.

Jenkins, T. C. 1995. Butylsoyamide protects soybean oil from ruminal biohydrogenation: Effects of butylsoamide on plasma fatty acids and nutrient digestion in sheep. J. Anim. Sci. 73:818–823.

Jenkins, T. C. 1997. Ruminal fermentation and nutrient digestion in sheep fed hydroxyethylsoyamide. J. Anim. Sci. 75:2277–2283.

Johnson, D. E. 1972. Heat increment of acetate and corn and effects of casein infusions with growing lambs. J. Nutr. 102:1093–1100.

Johnson, K. A., and D. E. Johnson. 1995. Methane emissions from cattle. J. Anim. Sci. 73:2483–2492.

Johnson, L. W. 1989. Nutrition. Vet. Clin. North Am. Food Anim. Pract. 5:37–54.

Judson, G. J., E. Anderson, J. R. Luick, and R. A. Leng. 1968. The contribution of propionate to glucose synthesis in sheep given diets of different grain content. Br. J. Nutr. 22:69–75.

Kay, R. N. B. 1966. The influence of saliva on digestion in ruminants. World Rev. Nutr. Diet. 6:292–325.

Kay, R. N. B., and E. Pfeffer. 1970. Movements of water and electrolytes into and from the intestine of sheep. Pp. 390–402 in Physiology of Digestion and Metabolism in the Ruminant, A. T. Phillipson, ed. Newcastle upon Tyne, UK: Oriel Press.

Kay, R. N. B., W. V. Engelhardt, and R. G. White. 1980. The digestive physiology of wild ruminants. Pp. 743–761 in Digestive Physiology and Metabolism in Ruminants, Y. Ruckebusch and P. Thivend, eds. Lancaster, UK: MTP Press Ltd., International Medical Publishers.

Kemp, P., and D. J. Lander. 1984. Hydrogenation *in vitro* of α-linolenic acid to stearic acid by mixed cultures of pure strains of rumen bacteria. J. Gen. Microbiol. 130:527–533.

Kennedy, P. M. 1980. The effects of dietary sucrose and concentrations of plasma urea and rumen ammonia on the degradation of urea in the gastrointestinal tract of cattle. Br. J. Nutr. 43:125–140.

Kennedy, P. M., and L. P. Milligan. 1978. Transfer of urea from the blood to the rumen of sheep. Br. J. Nutr. 40:149–154.

Kennedy, P. M., and L. P. Milligan. 1980. The degradation and utilization of endogenous urea in the gastrointestinal tract of ruminants: A review. Can. J. Anim. Sci. 60:205–221.

Kepler, C. R., W. P. Tucker, and S. B. Tove. 1970. Biohydrogenation of unsaturated fatty acids. IV. Substrate specificity and inhibition of linoleate Δ^{12}-*cis*, Δ^{11}-*trans* isomerase from *Butyrivibrio fibrisolvens*. J. Biol. Chem. 245:3612–3620.

Khanal, R. C., and K. C. Olson. 2004. Factors affecting conjugated linoleic acid (CLA) content in milk, meat, and egg: A review. Pak. J. Nutr. 3:82–98.

Knott, K. K., P. S. Barboza, R. T. Bowyer, and J. E. Blake. 2004. Nutritional development of feeding strategies in arctic ruminants: Digestive morphometry of reindeer, *Rangifer tarandus*, and muskoxen, *Ovibos moschatus*. Zoology 107:315–333.

Koenig, K. M., C. J. Newbold, F. M. McIntosh, and L. M. Rode. 2000. Effects of protozoa on bacterial nitrogen recycling in the rumen. J. Anim. Sci. 78:2431–2445.

Kucuk, O., B. W. Hess, P. A. Ludden, and D. C. Rule. 2001. Effect of forage:concentrate ratio on ruminal digestion and duodenal flow of fatty acids in ewes. J. Anim. Sci. 79:2233–2240.

Kucuk, O., B. W. Hess, and D. C. Rule. 2004 Soybean oil supplementation of a high-concentrate diet does not affect site and extent of organic matter, starch, neutral detergent fiber, or nitrogen digestion, but influences both ruminal metabolism and intestinal flow of fatty acids in limit-fed lambs J. Anim. Sci. 82:2985–2994.

Lapierre, H., and G. E. Lobley. 2001. Nitrogen recycling in the ruminant: A review. J. Dairy Sci. 84(E. Suppl.):E223–E236.

Lemosquet, S., C. Dardillant, M. Jailler, and J. P. Dulphy. 1996. Voluntary intake and gastric digestion of two hays by llamas and sheep: Influence of concentrate supplementation. J. Agric. Sci. 127:539–548.

Lennox, A. M., and G. A. Garton. 1968. The absorption of long-chain fatty acids from the small intestine of the sheep. Br. J. Nutr. 22:247–253.

Lobley, G. E., D. M. Bremner, and G. Zuur. 2000. Effects of diet quality on urea fates in sheep as assessed by refined, non-invasive [$^{15}N^{15}N$]urea kinetics. Br. J. Nutr. 84:459–468.

Lopez, A., J. Maiztegui, and R. Cabrera. 1998. Voluntary intake and digestibility of forages with different nutritional quality in alpacas. Small Ruminant Res. 29:295–301.

Ludden, P. A., M. J. Cecava, and K. S. Hendrix. 1995. The value of soybean hulls as a replacement for corn in beef cattle diets formulated with or without added fat. J. Anim. Sci. 73:2706–2711.

Luo, J., A. L. Goetsch, I. V. Nsahlai, T. Sahlu, C. L. Ferrell, F. N. Owens, M. L. Galyean, J. E. Moore, and Z. B. Johnson. 2004a. Metabolizable protein requirements for maintenance and gain of growing goats. Small Ruminant Res. 53:309–326.

Luo, J., A. L. Goetsch, I. V. Nsahlai, T. Sahlu, C. L. Ferrell, F. N. Owens, M. L. Galyean, J. E. Moore, and Z. B. Johnson. 2004b. Prediction of metabolizable energy and protein requirements for maintenance, gain and fiber growth of Angora goats. Small Ruminant Res. 53:339–356.

Mackie, R. I., C. S. McSweeney, and A. V. Klieve. 2002. Microbial ecology of the ovine rumen. Pp. 71–94 in Sheep Nutrition, M. Freer and H. Dove, eds. Wallingford, UK: CAB International.

Marini, J. C., and M. E. Van Amburgh. 2003. Nitrogen metabolism and recycling in Holstein heifers. J. Anim. Sci. 81:545–552.

Mathiesen, S. D., Ø. E. Haga, T. Kaino, and N. J. C. Tyler. 2000. Diet composition, rumen papillation and maintenance of carcass mass in female Norwegian reindeer (*Rangifer tarandus tarandus*) in winter. J. Zool. (Lond.) 251:129–138.

McDowell, L. R. 2000. Vitamins in Animal and Human Nutrition. Ames: Iowa State University Press.

McDowell, L. R. 2003. Minerals in Animal and Human Nutrition. Amsterdam: Elsevier.

McNamara, J. P., and J. K. Hillers. 1986. Adaptations in lipid metabolism of bovine adipose tissue in lactogenesis and lactation. J. Lipid Res. 27:150–154.

McNamara, J. P., J. H. Harrison, R. L. Kincaid, and S. S. Waltner. 1995. Lipid metabolism in adipose tissue of cows fed high fat diets during lactation. J. Dairy Sci. 78:2782–2796.

Meyer, H. H. D., A. Rowell, W. J. Streich, B. Stoffel, and R. R. Hofmann. 1998. Accumulation of polyunsaturated fatty acids by concentrate selecting ruminants. Comp. Biochem. Physiol. A120:263–268.

Milano, G. D., A. Hotston-Moore, and G. E. Lobley. 2000. Influence of hepatic ammonia removal on ureagenesis, amino acid utilization and energy metabolism in the ovine liver. Br. J. Nutr. 83:307–315.

Moore, J. H., and W. W. Christie. 1984. Digestion, absorption and transport of fats in ruminant animals. Pp. 123–149 in Fats in Animal Nutrition, J. Wiseman, ed. London: Butterworths.

Moore, L. A., H. M. Irvin, and J. C. Shaw. 1953. Relationships between TDN and energy value of feeds. J. Dairy Sci. 36:93–99.

Mosenthin, R., W. C. Sauer, and C. F. M. de Lange. 1992. Tracer studies of urea kinetics in growing pigs: I. The effect of intravenous infusion of urea on urea recycling and site of urea secretion into gastrointestinal tract. J. Anim. Sci. 70:3458–3466.

Mould, F. D., and C. T. Robbins. 1981. Nitrogen metabolism in elk. J. Wildl. Manage. 45:323–334.

Nagaraja, T. G., C. J. Newbold, C. J. Van Nevel, and D. I. Demeyer. 1997. Manipulation of ruminal fermentation. Pp. 523–632 in The Rumen Microbial Ecosystem, P. N. Hobson and C. S. Stewart, eds. London: Blackie Academic and Prof., an imprint of Chapman and Hall.

Navarre, C. B., D. G. Pugh, A. M. Heath, and A. Simpkins. 1999. Analysis of first gastric compartment fluid collected via percutaneous paracentesis from healthy llamas. J. Am. Vet. Med. Assoc. 214:812–815.

Nelson, M. L., H. H. Westberg, and S. M. Parish. 2001. Effects of tallow on the energy metabolism of wethers fed barley finishing diets. J. Anim. Sci. 79:1892–1904.

Ngwa, A. T., I. V. Nsahlai, and M. L. K. Bonsi. 2001. The effect of feeding pods of multipurpose trees (MPTs) on the degradability of dry matter and cell wall constituents of maize stover and alfalfa in the rumen of sheep. J. Sci. Food Agric. 81:1235–1243.

Nolan, J. V., and R. A. Leng. 1972. Dynamic aspects of ammonia and urea metabolism in sheep. Br. J. Nutr. 27:177–192.

Norton, B. W., J. B. MacKintosh, and D. G. Armstrong. 1982. Urea synthesis and degradation in sheep given pelleted-grass diets containing flaked barley. Br. J. Nutr. 48:249–264.

NRC (National Research Council). 1981a. Nutritional Energetics of Domestic Animals and Glossary of Energy Terms. Washington, DC: National Academy Press.

NRC. 1981b. Nutrient Requirements of Goats: Angora, Dairy, and Meat Goats in Temperate and Tropical Countries. Washington, DC: National Academy Press.

NRC. 1985a. Nutrient Requirements of Sheep, 6th rev. ed. Washington, DC: National Academy Press.

NRC. 1985b. Ruminant Nitrogen Usage. Washington, DC: National Academy Press.

NRC. 2000. Nutrient Requirements of Beef Cattle (Update 2000). Washington, DC: National Academy Press.

NRC. 2001. Nutrient Requirements of Dairy Cattle, 7th rev. ed. Washington, DC: National Academy Press.

NRC. 2005. Mineral Tolerance of Animals, 2nd rev. ed. Washington, DC: The National Academies Press.

Nsahlai, I. V., A. L. Goetsch, J. Luo, Z. B. Johnson, J. E. Moore, T. Sahlu, C. L. Ferrell, M. L. Galyean, and F. N. Owens. 2004. Metabolizable protein requirements of lactating goats. Small Ruminant Res. 53:327–338.

Obara, Y., and K. Shimbayashi. 1980. The appearance of recycled urea in the digestive tract of goats during the final third of a once daily feeding of a low-protein diet. Br. J. Nutr. 44:295–305.

O'Kelly, J. C., and W. G. Spiers. 1991. Influence of host diet on the concentrations of fatty acids in rumen bacteria from cattle. Aust. J. Agric. Res. 42:243–252.

Palmquist, D. L. 1988. The feeding value of fats. Pp. 293–311 in Feed Science, E. R. Orskov, ed. Amsterdam: Elsevier.

Palmquist, D. L. 1994. The role of dietary fats in efficiency of ruminants. J. Nutr. 124:1377S–1382S.

Palmquist, D. L., and T. C. Jenkins. 1980. Fat in lactation rations. Review. J. Dairy Sci. 63:1–14.

Palmquist, D. L., and T. C. Jenkins. 2003. Challenges with fats and fatty acid methods. J. Anim Sci. 81:3250–3254.

Phillipson, A. T., and R. A. McAnally. 1942. Studies on the fate of carbohydrates in the rumen of the sheep. J. Exp. Biol. 19:199–214.

Rattray, P. V., W. N. Garrett, N. E. East, and N. Hinman. 1974a. Efficiency of utilization of metabolizable energy during pregnancy and the energy requirements for pregnancy in sheep. J. Anim. Sci. 38:383–393.

Rattray, P. V., W. N. Garrett, N. E. East, and N. Hinman. 1974b. Growth, development and composition of the ovine conceptus and mammary gland during pregnancy. J. Anim. Sci. 38:613–626.

Reynolds, C. K, and G. B. Huntington. 1988. Partition of portal-drained visceral net flux in beef steers. 1. Blood flow and net flux of oxygen, glucose and nitrogenous compounds across stomach and post-stomach tissues. Br. J. Nutr. 60:539–551.

Robbins, C. T. 1993. Wildlife Feeding and Nutrition, 2nd ed. San Diego, CA: Academic Press.

Robbins, C. T., R. L. Prior, A. N. Moen, and W. J. Visek. 1974. Nitrogen metabolism of white-tailed deer. J. Anim. Sci. 38:186–191.

Rubsamen, K., and W. V. Engelhardt. 1979. Morphological and functional peculiarities of the llama forestomach. Ann. Rech. Vet. 10:473–475.

Russell, K., G. E. Lobley, J. Rawlings, D. J. Millward, and E. J. Harper. 2000. Urea kinetics of a carnivore, Felix silvestris catus. Br. J. Nutr. 84:597–604.

San Martin, F. A., and F. C. Bryant. 1989. Nutrition of domesticated and South American llamas and alpacas. Small Ruminant Res. 2:191–216.

Sarraseca, A., E. Milne, M. J. Metcalf, and G. E. Lobley. 1998. Urea recycling in sheep: Effects of intake. Br. J. Nutr. 79:79–88.

SCA (Standing Committee on Agriculture). 1990. Feeding Standards for Australian Livestock. Ruminants. East Melbourne, Australia: CSIRO Publications.

Schmidt-Nielsen, B., K. Schmidt-Nielsen, T. R. Houpt, and S. A. Jarnum. 1957. Urea excretion in the camel. Am. J. Physiol. 188:477–484.

Scholljegerdes, E. J., B. W. Hess, G. E. Moss, D. L. Hixon, and D. C. Rule. 2004. Influence of supplemental cracked high-linoleate or high-oleate safflower seeds on site and extent of digestion in beef cattle. J. Anim. Sci. 82:3577–3588.

Schwartz, C. C., W. L. Regelin, A. W. Franzmann, and M. Hubbert. 1987. Nutritional energetics of moose. Swed. Wildl. Res. Viltrevy Suppl. 1:265–279.

Scott, T. W., and L. J. Cook. 1975. Effect of dietary fat on lipid metabolism in ruminants. Pp. 510–532 in Digestion and Metabolism in the Ruminant, I. W. McDonald and A. C. I. Warner, eds. Armidale, Australia: University of New England Publishing Unit.

Siddons, R. C., J. V. Nolan, D. E. Beever, and J. C. MacRae. 1985. Nitrogen digestion and metabolism in sheep consuming diets containing contrasting forms and levels of N. Br. J. Nutr. 54:175–187.

Smith, R. W., and A. Walsh. 1988. Effects of pregnancy and lactation on the metabolism of bovine adipose tissue. Res. Vet. Sci. 44:349–353.

Smith, S. E. 1970. Vitamins. Pp. 634–659 in Duke's Physiology of Domestic Animals, 8th ed., M. J. Swenson, ed. Ithaca, NY: Cornell University Press.

Sniffen, C. J., J. D. O'Connor, P. J. Van Soest, D. G. Fox, and J. B. Russell. 1992. A net carbohydrate and protein system for evaluating cattle diets: II. Carbohydrate and protein availability. J. Anim. Sci. 70:3562–3577.

Snipes, R. L. 1994. Morphometric methods for determining surface enlargement at the microscopic level in the large intestine and their application. Pp. 234–263 in The Digestive System in Mammals: Food, Form and Function, D. L. Chivers and P. Langer, eds. Cambridge, UK: Cambridge University Press.

Staaland, H., K. Hove, and R. G. White. 1986. Mineral absorption in relation to nutritional ecology of reindeer. Rangifer Special Issue No. 1: 279–287.

Steel, J. W., and R. A. Leng. 1973. Effects of plane of nutrition and pregnancy on gluconeogenesis in sheep. 2. Synthesis of glucose from ruminal propionate. Br. J. Nutr. 30:475–489.

Stevens, C. E. 1988. Comparative Physiology of the Vertebrate Digestive System. Cambridge, UK: Cambridge University Press.

Stevens, C. E., and I. D. Hume. 1998. Contributions of microbes in vertebrate gastrointestinal tract to production and conservation of nutrients. Physiol. Rev. 78:393–427.

Stevens, C. E., and A. F. Sellers. 1968. Rumination. Pp. 2699–2704 in Handbook of Physiology. Sec. 6. Alimentary Canal, Vol. 5: Bile; digestion; ruminal physiology, C. F. Code and W. Heidel, eds. Washington, DC: American Physiological Society.

Stevens, C. E., R. A. Argenzio, and E. T. Clemens. 1980. Microbial digestion: Rumen versus large intestine. Pp. 685–706 in Digestive Physiology and Metabolism in Ruminants, Y. Ruckebusch and P. Thivend, eds. Lancaster, UK: MTP Press.

Sunny, N. E., L. H. Hanus, S. W. El-Kadi, S. L. Owens, and B. J. Bequette. 2004. Regulation of urea recycling to the gastrointestinal tract and ammonia metabolism in ruminants. J. Anim. Sci. 87(Suppl. 1):127(Abstr.).

Sutherland, T. 1988. Particle separation in the forestomach of sheep. Pp. 43–73 in Aspects of Digestive Physiology in Ruminants, A. Dobson and M. J. Dobson, eds. Ithaca, NY: Cornell University Press.

Theurer, C. B., G. B. Huntington, J. T. Huber, R. S. Swingle, and J. A. Moore. 2002. Net absorption and utilization of nitrogenous compounds across ruminal, intestinal, and hepatic tissues of growing beef steers fed dry-rolled or steam-flaked sorghum grain. J. Anim. Sci. 80:525–532.

Thornton, R. F., P. R. Bird, M. Somers, and R. J. Moir. 1970. Urea excretion in ruminants III. The role of the hind-gut (caecum and colon). Aust. J. Agric. Res. 21:345–354.

Trevaskis, L. M., W. J. Fulkerson, and J. M. Gooden. 2001 Provision of certain carbohydrate-based supplements to pasture-fed sheep, as well as time of harvesting of the pasture, influences pH, ammonia concentration and microbial protein synthesis in the rumen. Aust. J. Exp. Agric. 41:21–27.

Underwood, E. J., and N. Suttle. 1999. The Mineral Nutrition of Livestock, 3rd ed. New York: CAB International.

Vallenas, A., J. A. Cummings, and J. F. Munnell. 1971. A gross study of the compartmentalized stomach of two new world camelids, the llama and guanaco. J. Morph. 134:399–423.

Vallenas A., J. Esquerre, A. Valenzuela, E. Candela, and D. Chauca. 1973. Volatile fatty acids and pH in the first two stomach compartments in the alpaca and sheep. Rev. Invest. Pecu. (IVITA) 2:115.

van Houtert, M. F. J. 1993. The production and metabolism of volatile fatty acids by ruminants fed roughages: A review. Anim. Feed Sci. Technol. 43:189–225.

Van Nevel, C. J., and D. I. Demeyer. 1995. Lipolysis and biohydrogenation of soybean oil in the rumen in vitro: Inhibition by antimicrobials. J. Dairy Sci. 78:2797–2806.

Van Saun, R. J. 2003. Feeding the Alpaca. Pp. 179–232 in The Complete Alpaca Book, E. Hoffman, ed. Santa Cruz, CA: Bonny Doon Press.

Van Soest, P. J. 1994. Nutritional Ecology of the Ruminant, 2nd ed. Ithaca, NY: Comstock.

Wales, R. A., L. P. Milligan, and E. H. McEwan. 1975. Urea recycling in caribou, cattle and sheep. Pp. 297–307 in Proc. First Int'l. Reindeer Caribou Symp., J. R. Luick, P. C. Lent, D. R. Klein, and R. G. White, eds. Biol. Papers, Univ. of Alaska, Spec. Report No. 1.

Wallace, R. J., K. J. Cheng, D. Dinsdale, and E. R. Ørskov. 1979. An independent microbial flora of the epithelium and its role in the ecomicrobiology of the rumen. Nature 279:424–426.

Wang, J. H., B. W. Zhu, M. K. Song, and Y. J. Choi. 2005. Effect of monensin, fish oil or their combination on in vitro fermentation and conjugated linoleic acid (CLA) production by ruminal bacteria. Anim. Feed Sci. Technol. 120:341–349.

Warmington, B. G., G. F. Wilson, and T. N. Bany. 1989. Voluntary intake and digestion of rye grass straw by llama/guanaco crossbreds and sheep. J. Agric. Sci. 113:87–91.

White, R. G., and J. P. Lawler. 2002. Can methane suppression during digestion of woody and leafy browse compensate for energy costs of detoxification of plant secondary compounds? A test with muskoxen fed willows and birch. Comp. Biochem. Physiol. A 133:849–859.

White, R. G., E. Jacobsen, and H. Staaland. 1984. Secretion and absorption of nutrients in the alimentary tract of reindeer fed lichens or concentrates during the winter. Can. J. Zool. 62:2364–2376.

Wiseman, J. 1984. Fats in Animal Nutrition. London: Butterworths.

Wolin, M. J., and T. L. Miller. 1983. Interactions of microbial populations in cellulose fermentation. Fed. Proc. 42:109–113.

Woodward, S. L., G. C. Waghorn, M. Ulyatt, and K. R. Lassey. 2001. Early indications that Lotus will reduce methane emissions from ruminants. Proc. N. Z. Soc. Anim. Prod. 61:23–26.

Wu, Z., O. A. Ohajuruka, and D. L. Palmquist. 1991. Ruminal synthesis, biohydrogenation, and digestibility of fatty acids by dairy cows. J. Dairy Sci. 74:3025–3034.

3

Ingestive Behavior and Feed Intake

INTRODUCTION

When animals are managed under housed conditions or in feedlots (and perhaps under zoo conditions), the degree of control that can be exerted over their diet is such that rations can be formulated based on requirements, and the nutrient intake of individual animals can be related to their requirements. However, a feature of many of the animals for which requirements are given in this publication is that they may obtain much of their nutrients from grazing or browsing. This means that their feeding environment is highly variable in both time and space, and the manager can exert less control over the nutrient intake of individual animals. Although nutritional management would usually be expected to start with knowledge of nutrient intake, for free-ranging animals the estimation of both diet composition and total intake is fraught with difficulty (Cornelis et al., 1999; Mayes and Dove, 2000). This is especially the case for wild cervids, and also for camelids under some management systems, because of the difficulty of capture/recapture required to make such estimates in wild animals. While some estimates of diet composition might be obtained in such animals from the analysis, for example, of plant fragments in feces or the stomach contents of slaughtered animals (Cornelis et al., 1999), estimates of total intake are very difficult. Nevertheless, unless some estimate of nutrient intake can be obtained or predicted, it will be difficult to apply the nutrient requirements listed in this publication, no matter how accurately they are estimated. It is possible to predict intake, by using current live weight and a measure of animal performance (e.g., milk yield), together with known requirements, to infer what intake must have been (Reeves et al., 1996). However, as Corbett and Freer (2003) have pointed out, this severely constrains nutritional management of grazing/browsing animals, in which the reverse procedure is wanted—the prediction of the intake of nutrients and then, by comparing these with nutrient requirements, the prediction of the resultant production. Both NRC (1996) and the Cornell Net Carbohydrate and Protein System (Tedeschi et al., 2000; Cannas et al., 2004) attempt the prediction of intake from live weight and the net energy (NE) content of a defined diet, while Tedeschi et al., (2000) extend this to include the rumen-degradable nitrogen content of a defined diet. However, the only nutrient requirement system that explicitly attempts to predict intake and the digestibility and protein content of the consumed diet, in relation to the characteristics of the forage resource and of the animals that graze it, is that in use in Australia (SCA, 1990; Freer et al., 1997). Details of that system relating to the prediction of intake are discussed in more detail below, but it should be noted that the estimates of intake in SCA (1990) are based on temperate pastures. In particular, they do not apply to browse forages nor tropical pastures.

Although "domesticated" plants of agricultural-pastoral importance, both monocotyledons and dicotyledons, may contain harmful secondary compounds, in general they contain fewer chemical or physical (spines and thorns) defenses than the plants consumed in natural systems. As a result, much understanding of the processes of prehension, digestion, and metabolism is limited to plants of agricultural importance. This report differs from previous sheep and goat reports (NRC, 1981, 1985) in that nonagricultural plants are given greater consideration because the particular ruminant and ruminant-like species can utilize a wide range of plant species.

FACTORS INFLUENCING DIET SELECTION

Free-ranging ruminants are selective when choosing what to consume and, in general, will select a diet of better quality (higher digestibility and protein content, fewer secondary compounds) than the average of the plant biomass on offer. The factors that influence selection and intake can be viewed as relating to the nature of the animals themselves, the nature of the plant resource, and the extent to which the management/feeding system permits the processes of diet selection/intake to proceed.

An extensive literature discusses the effects of both plant and animal characteristics on diet selection and intake. The process of harvesting nutrients has repercussions both for the animal (nutrient intake) and for the plant resource that is harvested (preferential utilization of parts of the biomass). The harvesting process can itself range from controlled grazing of sown pastures by domestic ruminants, through bipedal browsing (e.g., by goats) to situations as extreme as tree-climbing by goats to obtain leaf tissue, as has been observed in Morocco. A further consideration is the question of scale, both in a spatial sense (single bite, patch, landscape) and a temporal sense (bite time, day, lifetime). This has resulted in a wide range of approaches to and even terminologies for discussing diet selection and intake by herbivores. The following publications present a more detailed discussion: The relationships between the processes of foraging and natural selection in natural systems are discussed in detail by Belovsky et al. (1999), while Illius and Gordon (1999) discuss the processes of diet selection and intake in relation to the physiological ecology of herbivores. The spatial distribution of harvestable plant material is a major issue, especially for ruminants in diverse habitats; at varying scales, these aspects are discussed by Laca and Demment (1996), Ungar (1996), and Hobbs (1999). Aspects of diet choice in relation to plant defense mechanisms, especially the content of secondary compounds, have been extensively reviewed by Launchbaugh (1996), Foley et al. (1999), Duncan and Gordon (1999), and Iason (2005). The influence of plant secondary compounds on the ultimate provision of nutrients from the animals' feed resource is also discussed in Chapter 10 of this volume. Finally, diet selection in New World camelids (NWC) has been discussed by Bas and Bonacic (2003).

Association of plant selection behaviors with morpho-physiological adaptations of the digestive tracts of ruminants (Hofmann, 1989) has been a useful construct (though not universally accepted) in discussions of diet selection and intake. Shrub-eating foregut fermenters evolved to process plant cell contents and have been termed concentrate selectors (CS; they select diets of at least 75 percent tree/shrub stem and foliage, fruit, or dicotyledonous leaf). By contrast, "grazer species" (which select diets of < 25 percent browse) co-evolved with the later arrival of grasses and sedges. Another component of this radiation in the Eocene is a group of species that present as intermediate or mixed foragers (IM), mixing foraging on monocotyledons and dicotyledons depending on season or on opportunity (Hofmann and Stewart, 1972; Hofmann, 1989; Shipley, 1999).

In the suite of small ruminants in this publication, sheep represent a typical grazer (GR), with white-tailed deer, the CS. Goat, red deer, and reindeer/caribou represent an intermediate (IM) group of mixed foragers that frequently exhibit seasonal changes in diet choice. In this system, GR species are considered "monocotyledon specialists," but opportunistically take dicotyledons. Likewise CS species are "dicotyledon specialists," but will opportunistically forage on nondicotyledon species. The system is thus one of flexibility in function, and somewhat in form (anatomy).

In general, woody browse plants have a greater content of cell contents, lignin, secondary compounds, and nitrogen than do grasses, though the protein of browse can be rendered less available for digestion through binding with secondary compounds during chewing. Conversely, cell wall constitutes a greater proportion of the total dry matter (DM) of grasses, but it is generally more digestible than the cell wall of browse (Shipley, 1999; Gordon, 2003). In terms of digestibility and protein content, the tissues of browse can also be less uniform than grasses (e.g., leaf vs. woody stem) and may be processed differently by CS and GR herbivores (Clauss et al., 2002). As discussed above, attempts have been made to relate these categories of diet choice to the features of browse vs. grasses and to features of the animals, such as dental and buccal architecture, salivary gland size, and gut morphology (Hofmann, 1989; Shipley, 1999). Such attempts have been criticized as only reflecting the overarching importance of body size (Gordon and Illius, 1994; Robbins et al., 1995; Illius and Gordon, 1999; Gordon, 2003), which results in larger animals being better able to process roughage such as grass (because the size of body components scales to weight$^{1.0}$ whereas increasing energy requirements only scale to weight$^{0.75}$). Gordon (2003) suggested that there was ". . . little substantive evidence for differences in morphology and physiology . . ." between these categories, after allowing for differences in phylogenetic relationships and in body size. Equally, he suggested that until it had been better tested within controlled experiments, the hypothesis ". . . linking food, form and function should not be dismissed out-of-hand." On this basis, the classification into grazers, browsers/concentrate selectors, and intermediate feeders is adopted in this publication.

There are many reports of the species composition of the diet consumed by individual species of small ruminants, but fewer studies in which diet composition of sheep, goats, cervids, and NWC are compared. A selection of published comparisons is summarized in Table 3-1. A consistent result in comparative studies of sheep and goats is that goats consume a diet containing a higher proportion of browse when such species are available and appear to digest fiber better, due to their more efficient particle size reduction and greater nitrogen recycling to the rumen (Domingue et al., 1990, 1991). However, the actual preference rankings for individual species often depend upon what other species are present (Walker et al., 1994). When only grass species are present, the species composition of the diet consumed by sheep and goats tends to be similar (Hadjigeorgiou et al., 2003).

Comparisons of sheep and NWC again show a tendency for llamas to consume more browse or coarse grass species than either sheep (Genin et al., 1994) or alpacas (Wackwitz et al., 1999), though this tendency appears less marked than for goats vs. sheep.

TABLE 3-1 Selected Comparisons of Diet Compositions of Small Ruminants

Comparison	Source	Results
Sheep vs. goats	Clark et al. (1982)	"Scrub-pasture" association in New Zealand. Grass-predominant diet component for both species. Goats ate less white clover (*Trifolium repens*) than in sward and more gorse (*Ulex* spp.). Sheep ate very little gorse.
	Walker et al. (1994)	Goats preferred leafy spurge (*Euphorbia esula*) compared with sheep, though diet preferences influenced by which other plant species present.
	Gong et al. (1996)	Turves of grass/legume pasture offered to housed sheep, goats. Sheep grazed leaf components of tall swards, goats less selective and consumed more stem.
	Penning et al. (1997)	Higher preference for white clover cf. perennial ryegrass (*Lolium perenne*) in sheep.
	Hart (2001)	Review publication indicating goats consume more browse than either cattle or sheep.
	Pande et al. (2002)	Under mixed browse/pasture conditions, the three most-preferred species were the same for sheep and goats, but goats browsed more than three times as much as sheep.
	Hadjigeorgiou et al. (2003)	When offered a range of graminaceous forages, sheep and goats had similar preferences.
	Holst et al. (2004a,b)	Pasture dominated by the grass *Microlaena stipoides*, together with either Scotch broom (*Cytisus scoparius*) or nodding thistle (*Carduus nutans*). Goats had higher preference for these weed species.
Camelid vs. sheep	Genin et al. (1994) (llama)	Higher proportion of "coarse bunchgrasses" in llama diet. Higher proportion of herbs and "soft grasses" in sheep diet.
	Fraser and Baker (1998) (guanaco)	Guanaco selected for emerging inflorescence of grass, tolerated mature inflorescence. Sheep tolerated former, avoided latter.
	Pinares-Pitaño et al. (2003) (alpaca)	Sheep consumed higher-quality diet both indoors and while grazing grass/legume or legume pastures.
Alpaca vs. llama	Wackwitz et al. (1999)	Compared with alpacas, llamas consumed more shrubs during dry season, more forbs during rainy season.
Feral goat; fallow, red, white-tailed deer	Forsyth et al. (2002)	Provides preference rankings among these animal species for the indigenous forest plant species of New Zealand.

The species composition of cervid diets is strongly influenced by the seasonal availability of different plant species (Cornelis et al., 1999; Johnson et al., 2001; Mårell et al., 2002) and the extent to which seasonal conditions permit access to preferred plant species. For example, Bugalho et al. (2005) used plant wax alkane profiles to demonstrate that the diet composition of red deer consisted of mainly browse during summer but mainly herbage during spring. Similarly, although woodland caribou showed a preference for terrestrial lichens in the forest, they foraged on arboreal lichens when snow depth and hardness limited access to the terrestrial species (Johnson et al., 2001). Neither reindeer (Mårell et al., 2002) nor forest caribou (Johnson et al., 2001) selected feeding sites or plant species with the highest nutritional value, in contrast with what might be expected from optimal-foraging theory (Belovsky et al., 1999).

The phenological development of potential forage plants as the season progresses provides extra diet choice in terms of the production of buds, inflorescences, seed/fruits, and vegetative storage units such as tubers and roots. These plant parts are frequently consumed as part of small ruminant diets and, as in grazed pastures, represent a series of food-source pulses that are superimposed on well-documented general seasonal trends in forage biomass, characterized by declining quality from spring to winter, or wet to dry season (Crampton and Harris, 1969; Albon and Langvatn, 1992; Johnstone et al., 2002). Foraging ecology and changes in diet composition in relation to phenological events and seasonal progression in biomass and plant quality are well documented for small ruminants in the wild and under rangeland grazing conditions (Klein, 1970; Moen, 1973; Van der Wal et al., 2000; Owen-Smith, 2002). Small ruminants under rangeland or wild conditions heavily utilize new spring buds of many shrubs and forage trees. For example, goats, deer, reindeer/caribou, and wapiti all strip buds and unfurling young leaves to maximize foraging efficiencies. Similarly, flower buds and early inflorescences of tussock cotton grass are extremely important diet components contributing to milk production and survival of caribou and reindeer calves on the calving grounds in spring (Griffith et al., 2002); during summer, a progression of flowering plants, including legumes and louseworts, raise the crude protein (CP) content of grass- and sedge-based diets (White et al., 1981). In contrast to systems based on grazing livestock, a most important dietary component that contributes to the autumn fattening of deer and indirectly affects their over-winter survival is the availability of mast, particularly acorns (Moen, 1973; McCullough and Ullrey, 1985). The extent to which these plant parts or products contribute to the actual nutrient intake of small ruminants, particularly the wild species, is discussed in more detail in Chapter 10.

A degree of caution is also required in evaluating the diet composition data discussed above and presented in Table 3-1, for two reasons:

1. Estimates of diet composition can be influenced by the techniques used to obtain them (Cornelis et al., 1999; Mayes and Dove, 2000). For example, estimates based on the proportion of time spent consuming one type or species of plant compared with another (Penning et al., 1997) or comparisons of the number of bites from different plant species (Genin et al., 1994) do not directly equate to proportions of DM intake, because bite sizes can differ among plant species. Similarly, diet composition estimates based on the identification of plant cuticular fragments in either stomach contents or especially feces will be biased toward those plants that have lower digestibilities and thus remain for longer in digesta or feces (Cornelis et al., 1999; Mayes and Dove, 2000). The use of the profiles of plant cuticular wax components as chemical "fingerprints" of different plant species in the diet (Mayes and Dove, 2000; Bugalho et al., 2005) offers great promise as an alternative to these approaches, but still requires development in order to be able to identify a sufficient number of plant species in species-diverse habitats.

2. Even if the technique used does provide an accurate and unbiased estimate of diet composition, it must be remembered that what is estimated is the outcome ("diet selected") rather than the process ("diet selection") (Mayes and Dove, 2000). It is a much more difficult task to establish *why* the animal has selected a particular species or class of species, or perhaps why it has *not* so selected. In terms of the effect of unpleasant post-ingestive feedback signals, it may be easier to suggest why a particular species has not been selected, though our understanding of this area remains rudimentary (Duncan and Gordon, 1999). In terms of selection for a particular species or plant part, recent research has provided strong evidence that the influence of water-soluble carbohydrate (WSC) content of herbage may have been underestimated as a determinant of diet selection (Fisher et al., 1999; Leury et al., 1999; Ciavarella et al., 2000a). However, what the animal actually perceives as the signal coming from "water-soluble carbohydrate" and how this is integrated with other physical or physiological signals are not well understood.

Many of the above investigations of diet composition relate to either natural plant associations in which there are a wide range of plant species, or to sown or native pastures invaded by shrub or weed species. In farming systems, especially with botanically simple sown pastures, the degree of selection possible might be more restricted and involve only possible selection between green and dead herbage, or between grass and legume components of the pasture. In general, instances of preference of dead herbage over green herbage are rare (Arnold, 1981). However, if the proportion of dead material in the sward changes with pasture height or mass, grazing animals may consume substantial quantities of dead pasture simply because they cannot physically select against the dead material. For example, in swards of phalaris (*Phalaris aquatica*) and subterranean clover (*Trifolium subterraneum*) ranging in height from 1 to 10 cm, Ciavarella (2002) found that the content of green material in both the sward (SW) and the diet of sheep (DS) decreased significantly with pasture height (H) in a curvilinear fashion:

$$SW = 8.32 + 16.07H - 0.98H^2 \ (r = 0.931)$$
$$DS = 20.11 + 15.85H - 1.01H^2 \ (r = 0.610)$$

Although these relationships suggest that the diet always contained slightly more green material than was in the sward, it can be shown that the above curves do not differ significantly, indicating no active selection for green material.

The issue of whether or not grazing livestock select in favor of legume has been the subject of many studies, but the question of whether there is selection in favor of legume remains unresolved. There have been numerous studies reporting a preference for legume (Laidlaw, 1983; Ridout and Robson, 1991; Penning et al., 1997; Dove, 1998) and many reporting no preference (Grimes et al., 1966; Arnold, 1987; Ciavarella, 2002). Cosgrove et al. (1996) found that preference changed with season, while Kelman et al. (2003) found that in a mixed sward, sheep selected in favor of *Lotus* spp. but against white clover. These conflicting findings may well relate as much to the way the trials were conducted as to any underlying preference by the animals. For example, published reports on dietary preference for legume have differed in the following ways:

1. The species of legume involved has often been white clover (Penning et al., 1997), but studies have also used red clover (Laidlaw, 1983), subterranean clover (Ciavarella, 2002), or *Lotus* spp. (Kelman et al., 2003). The preference by sheep for these species may well differ, and preference

for a given legume may also differ depending on what else is in the sward (Kelman et al., 2003).

2. The physical presentation of grass and legume has ranged from alternating strips or squares of grass and legume (Clark and Harris, 1985; Penning et al., 1997) to mixed pastures (Dove, 1998; Ciavarella, 2002; Kelman et al., 2003). This is likely to alter preference (Clark and Harris, 1985). Similarly, the legume content of material on offer has ranged from < 20 percent (Ciavarella, 2002) to as much as 70–80 percent (Penning et al., 1997; Dove, 1998).

3. Preference for clover has been estimated using a wide range of techniques including grazing behavior/location (Cosgrove et al., 1996; Penning et al., 1997); changes in legume content before and after grazing (Clark and Harris, 1985); the legume content of samples collected by animals fistulated at the esophagus (Clark and Harris, 1985); or from the profiles in grass, legume, and feces of markers (alkanes, long-chain alcohols) from plant cuticular wax (Dove, 1998; Ciavarella, 2002; Kelman et al., 2003).

4. Partly because of differences in the techniques used to estimate preference, studies have also been conducted over different time scales, ranging from minutes (Clark and Harris, 1985) to hours (Newman et al., 1992) to several days to a week (Penning et al., 1997; Dove 1998). This is a real issue, since the duration of the preference measurement can influence the result (Parsons et al., 1994; Dove, 1998), as can the previous experience of the animals (Parsons et al., 1994; Ciavarella, 2002) and the grazing pressure. Variations in preference for legume vs. grass have been observed, with a lower preference for legume being observed in the afternoon (Parsons et al., 1994; Penning et al., 1997). Parsons et al. (1994) suggested that by consuming more legume than grass in the early part of the day, animals could achieve a higher intake because of the more rapid movement of the legume through the digestive tract. However, the balance between photosynthesis and respiration also results in a marked diurnal variation in WSC content in grass, with a peak in the afternoon (Orr et al., 1997; Fisher et al., 1999; Ciavarella et al., 2000a,b). Increased preference for grass later in the day may thus represent a response of diet selection to increased WSC (Ciavarella et al., 2000a).

The issue of whether small ruminants select for legume is a real one and of economic significance, since at the same digestibility, the intake of legume has been shown to be higher than that of grass, with resultant better liveweight gain (Freer and Jones, 1984). However, the question remains unresolved, and none of the published systems for expressing nutrient requirements contains algorithms representing selection for legume. For example, in the intake prediction equations, which make up part of the Australian feeding standards (SCA, 1990; Freer et al., 1997), there is no attempt to model selection in favor of legume. If the pasture contains legume, then predicted total intake will be higher (Freer and Jones, 1984; Freer et al., 1997; see below), but the proportion of legume in the intake will be the same as that in the sward.

FACTORS INFLUENCING INTAKE

Just as with diet selection, many factors influence and control intake by both grazing and browsing ruminants. In relation to the animal species described here as "small ruminants," a feature of the literature is that for animals under "natural" conditions, there are usually more estimates of diet composition than of intake. By contrast, for grazing livestock, there are more estimates of daily intake (Mayes and Dove, 2000). Applying techniques developed with domestic livestock for estimating intake in wild animals is difficult.

Most of the comments made above about the relationships between diet selection and the processes of foraging and natural selection in natural systems (Belovsky et al., 1999), the physiological ecology of herbivores (Illius and Gordon, 1999), and the spatial distribution of harvestable plant material (Laca and Demment, 1996; Ungar, 1996; Hobbs, 1999) apply equally to intake. A feature of the literature in relation to natural systems, and, to some extent, in grazing systems as well, is the issue of why the animal chooses to leave one feeding station and move to another, and the effect that this ultimately has on the components of intake (bite size, biting rate, grazing time). For discussions of the issues involved in "optimal foraging theory" or the "marginal value theorem," the reader is referred to discussions in the above reviews and in Prache and Peyraud (2001). A cornerstone of such discussions has been the so-called "functional response": that is, the relationship between intake rate by the animals and the abundance (mass/unit area) of the plant biomass (Ungar, 1996; Belovsky et al., 1999; Shipley, 1999). This is often described as a rising asymptotic curve (Spalinger and Hobbs, 1992; see Figure 3-4 below), as is frequently observed when grazers consume predominantly grass pastures (Penning et al., 1991; Ciavarella, 2002). As Gordon (2003) has discussed, the consumption of browse by browsers can give a linear relationship between intake and biomass, which has led to the view that plant biomass is a better descriptor of "food availability" for grazers than for browsers (Gordon 2003). However, it should be noted that asymptotic relationships have been found with browsers (Ginnett and Demment, 1995) and linear relationships with sown swards (Merchant and Riach, 1994). It is possible that this variability relates, at least in part, to the fact that descriptions of the functional response are typically determined as instantaneous intake rates and are hard to scale up to daily intakes simply by multiplying by grazing time (Parker, 2003). The functional response also takes little account of the quality of the plant material on offer. Moreover, as Ungar (1996) has stressed, plant biomass is a two-dimensional description of a sward, while bites are taken in three dimensions. This means that while descriptions of intake in terms of the functional response may be useful at the ecological level, they may not predict intake sufficiently well to allow its relation to nutrient requirements. Belovsky et al. (1999) go so far as to suggest, "Herbivore optimal foraging theory may not have much to offer to researchers concerned with animal husbandry and livestock production" because ". . . the intensive production schemes . . . may have created . . . production systems that bear little resemblance to those structured by natural selection and the population dynamics of an ecological steady . . . state."

In relation to published estimates of nutrient requirements, daily intake of herbage or browse is an appropriate measurement to consider. One of the consequences of there being relatively fewer estimates of daily intake in cervids or camelids offered the same plant material as either sheep or goats is that it is more difficult to establish comparative intakes. Most data exist for the comparison between sheep and goats, for which published data are inconclusive. The material reviewed by Brown and Johnson (1984) indicated that DM intake was usually higher in sheep than in goats when offered the same diet, though goats had relatively greater intakes of high-fiber diets. The results of Giger et al. (1987) and Gong et al. (1996) also indicate lower intakes by goats, but Blanchart et al. (1980) reported higher intakes by castrate goats than castrate sheep. Neither Doyle et al. (1984) nor Reid et al. (1990) found a difference in intake between these species. Because the data are equivocal, the Australian feeding standards (SCA, 1990) assume no difference in potential intake between the species and further assume that the equations presented for estimating potential intakes apply equally to both species.

Milne et al. (1978) compared the voluntary intakes of a range of diets by red deer or Scottish Blackface sheep fed at different times of the year. In winter, the sheep ate more dried grass pellets than the deer (71.3 vs. 57.3 g organic matter [OM]/kg$^{0.75}$), but intakes were similar (and higher) in summer (88.2 vs. 82.3 OM/kg$^{0.75}$). The voluntary intake of *Agrostis-Festuca* spp. and of heather (*Calluna vulgaris*) by deer was twice that of sheep (*Agrostis-Festuca*: deer 51.5 vs. sheep 22.6 g OM/kg$^{0.75}$; heather: deer 39.5 vs. sheep 19.5 g OM/kg$^{0.75}$), and marked seasonal trends in intake were observed with both animal species. Domingue et al. (1990) compared voluntary intakes of chaffed lucerne hay in red deer, sheep, and goats and found that in winter, the deer had a lower intake (46.7 g DM/kg$^{0.75}$) than either the sheep (54.8 g DM/kg$^{0.75}$) or goats (57.4 g DM/kg$^{0.75}$). In summer, intake by deer and goats increased and was comparable (62.5, 68.7 g DM/kg$^{0.75}$, respectively) and higher than sheep (52.2 g DM/kg$^{0.75}$). Latupeirissa (2002) noted that in rusa deer and Merino sheep, comparative intakes depended on diet quality. When fed lucerne hay, deer and sheep had similar intakes (74.8 and 77.7 g DM/kg$^{0.75}$), whereas deer had the higher intakes of both Rhodes grass hay (38.4 vs. 27.4 g OM/kg$^{0.75}$, respectively) and barley straw (34.9 vs. 24.9 g OM/kg$^{0.75}$, respectively). A general finding has thus been that deer tend to have higher voluntary intakes per kg$^{0.75}$ than sheep, except in those situations where intakes by deer are reduced in response to photoperiod.

In general, NWC have smaller stomach compartments and slower particulate outflow rates than true ruminants (San Martin, 1987). This might be expected to result in lower intakes in camelids vs. ruminants, but published reports are equivocal on this point. San Martin and Bryant (1987) suggested that on natural pastures, these camelids ate 26 percent less than true ruminants, which at maturity have potential intakes of about 80–90 g DM/kg$^{0.75}$ (ARC, 1980; SCA, 1990). By contrast, Fraser and Baker (1998) reported daily intakes of 44–56 g DM/kg$^{0.75}$ in grazing guanaco, whereas Warmington et al. (1989) found that relative to metabolic live weight (W), sheep and llama × guanaco crossbreds ate similar amounts (mean 37.6 g DM/kg$^{0.75}$) of a low-quality roughage (OM digestibility 0.502). Newman and Paterson (1994) noted an effect of season on voluntary intake by alpacas, with intakes 45 percent higher in summer than in winter (68 vs. 47 g DM/kg$^{0.75}$/day). On better-quality roughage (OM digestibility 0.72–0.82), Fraser and Baker (1998) reported similar intakes (43–55 g DM/kg BW$^{0.75}$) and digestibilities by guanaco and sheep. However, Lemosquet et al. (1996) reported higher OM digestibility in guanaco (0.597) vs. sheep (0.541) though intakes were similar (55 vs. 61 g DM/kg BW$^{0.75}$). Pinares-Patiño et al. (2003) reported a mean intake of 37.5 g DM/kg$^{0.75}$ in alpaca, compared with 90.6 g DM/kg$^{0.75}$ in sheep under the same conditions. Hence, there is some evidence that sheep do consume more per unit metabolic live weight than NWC, but this is not a consistent finding.

The control of feed intake in the free-ranging herbivore is exceedingly complex and has been the subject of many reviews (Forbes, 1996; Weston, 1996; Fisher, 2002). It involves factors that relate to the energy demands of the animal (Weston, 1996), the physical and physiological consequences of the processes of digestion (Forbes, 1996; Fisher, 2002), and the amount of plant material available for consumption (e.g., Penning et al., 1991). A further complication may be the seasonal change in voluntary intake that can be related to photoperiod, over and above any changes in the quality or quantity of the diet with changing season. This has been observed in a range of small ruminants, both wild and domesticated (Milne et al., 1978; Barry et al., 1991; Iason et al., 2000; Clarke, 2001). In general, the seasonality of feed intake is less in domesticated ruminants than in wild species such as cervids (Milne et al., 1978; Iason et al., 2000; Rhind et al., 2002). Nevertheless, such seasonality also has been demonstrated in sheep (Iason et al., 2000; Clarke, 2001) and is influenced by diet quality and breed (Iason et al., 2000). A detailed review of the seasonality of voluntary feed intake is beyond the scope of this volume and, for a recent discussion of the literature, the reader is referred to Rhind et al. (2002). These authors also present developments in the understanding of the mechanisms underpinning intake seasonality. An intriguing suggestion is that the response may be related to an interaction between photoperiod and intake that alters the species balance of the rumen microbial population, independent of the effect of dietary composition (McEwan et al., 2005).

Apart from such seasonal effects, the potential feed intake of an animal can be regarded as set by a combination of its demand for energy and its physical capacity for feed, both of which can be related to current body size and the expected mature weight. The current weight of the animal is not a useful predictor of body size, because it is confounded with body condition and the degree of maturity of the animal. INRA (1978), ARC (1980), SCA (1990), and Cannas et al. (2004) present equations for estimating potential intake in grazing livestock. Those given by INRA (1978) and ARC (1980) result in a linear increase in intake with live weight, but have been criticized because they make no allowance for differences in mature size of individual sheep or cattle breeds. The equations will thus predict the same intake for a fat, less mature animal and a lean mature animal of the same current weight. Moreover, predicted intakes for young animals are lower than those observed in grazing or penned sheep (see SCA [1990] for supporting discussion). The equations used by Cannas et al. (2004) are based on those developed by Pulina et al. (1996) for housed sheep. They are nonlinear, being based on metabolic live weight ($W^{0.75}$), but again make no allowance for differences in mature live weight of sheep breeds. Differences in the extent of maturity of the animals in question are accommodated by having a separate equation for animals before their first pregnancy. Moreover, the prediction of intake by lactating ewes requires knowledge of daily milk production and milk fat content. This makes the equations difficult to apply under field conditions where these are usually not known.

The approach taken by SCA (1990) has thus been adopted in this publication and forms the basis of the assessment of the intakes tabulated in the nutrient requirement tables. The intake prediction equations in SCA (1990) are taken to apply equally to goats because of the lack of unequivocal data that there is a real difference in potential intake between the species. However, it should be noted that the applicability of the equations to goats has not been explicitly tested. The potential intake of sheep consuming an all-grass pasture of nonlimiting DM digestibility (> 0.8) (I, kg DM/day) is estimated by SCA (1990) from the equation

$$I = 0.04 \times A \times Z(1.7 - Z)$$

The term A is the "standard reference weight" defined as the weight of the dry, nonpregnant animal (kg) when it reaches mature skeletal size and has a condition score in the middle of the range used. For the present purposes, this is equated with the mature weight values used in the nutrient requirement tables. The term Z is "relative size," which is the ratio of the normal weight of an immature animal at a given age (see equation 6.1, SCA, 1990) to its mature weight as defined above, again when condition score is in the middle of the range used. An immature animal that weighs 45 kg and has an expected mature weight of 75 kg would thus have a relative size of 0.60. It follows that the value of relative size cannot exceed 1.

This equation accommodates both the mature size of the animal (A) and its current normal weight (A × Z), and, for example, will generate different predicted intakes of all-grass pasture for a 60-kg dry ewe of mature size 60-kg (0.04 × 60 × 1 × (1.7 – 1) = 1.68 kg DM/day), and a 60-kg ewe of mature size 80 kg (0.04 × 80 × 0.75 × (1.7 – 0.75) = 2.28 kg DM/day). The above equation also implies that potential intake reaches a peak when the relative size of the animals is 0.85, i.e., when the actual weight of the animal in average condition score is 0.85 of its mature weight at the same condition.

As discussed by SCA (1990), the equation is empirical and based on a wide range of published data. The validation of such equations, as with many "models" of biological systems, raises some difficult points. First, there is the point that if good data had been available with which to validate the equation, they would probably have been used to build it in the first place; this is a general problem often faced in modeling. Second, the validation should relate to the grazing situation in which the equation is to be used, but this is the very situation in which estimates of actual intake with which to compare predicted intake are so technically difficult to obtain (Mayes and Dove, 2000). Moreover, the equation provides a "point estimate" of intake, whereas intake estimates are made over time courses approaching a week. Nevertheless, the above equation provides predicted intakes for mature animals that are similar to those of ARC (1980), and, for immature animals, it predicts intakes that are in accord with published results (e.g. Langlands, 1972; Allden 1979; Weston, 1980). Subsequent validations of the equation and related feed intake functions have been made with the functions operating within the decision support tool GrassGro (Moore et al., 1997). This has allowed the point estimates provided by the functions to be integrated over time. Because of the difficulty of obtaining good estimates of intake in the field, the actual validation arises from the comparison of the animal production arising from the predicted intakes with observed levels of animal production. These comparisons showed good agreement between observed and predicted animal performance under diverse grazing conditions in both the Southern and Northern Hemispheres (Stuth et al., 1999; Clark et al., 2000; Cohen et al., 2003).

Intakes of an all-grass diet (of nonlimiting digestibility; see above) predicted by this equation for sheep of mature live weight 40–140 kg and a range of relative sizes are shown in Figure 3-1, which also demonstrates the slight decline in intake for animals with relative size > 0.85. This family of curves can be generalized by dividing through each curve by the applicable mature weight and thus expressing potential intakes per kg of mature live weight, i.e.,

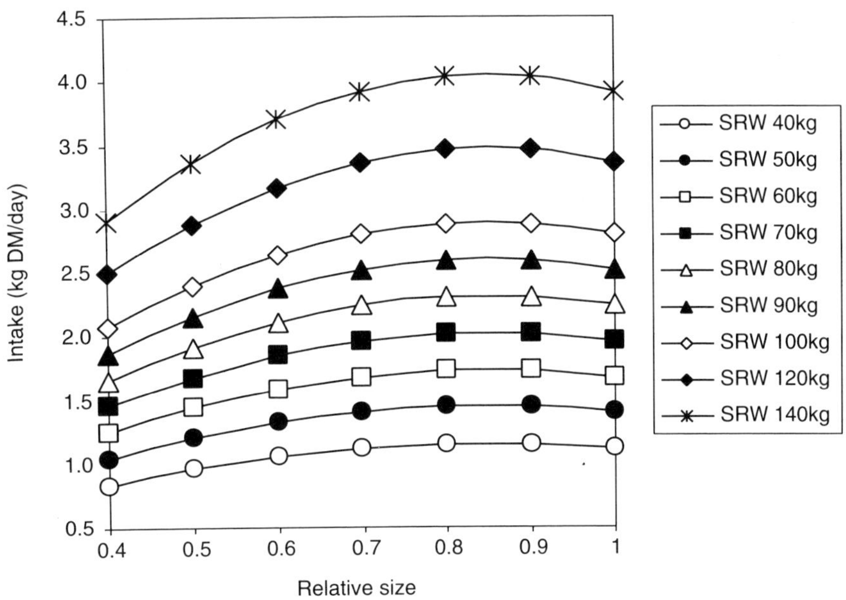

FIGURE 3-1 Influence of standard reference weight of sheep (SRW; mature size when in average condition score) and relative size (current weight as a proportion of mature weight) on predicted intakes of an all-grass diet of nonlimiting digestibility (> 0.8).

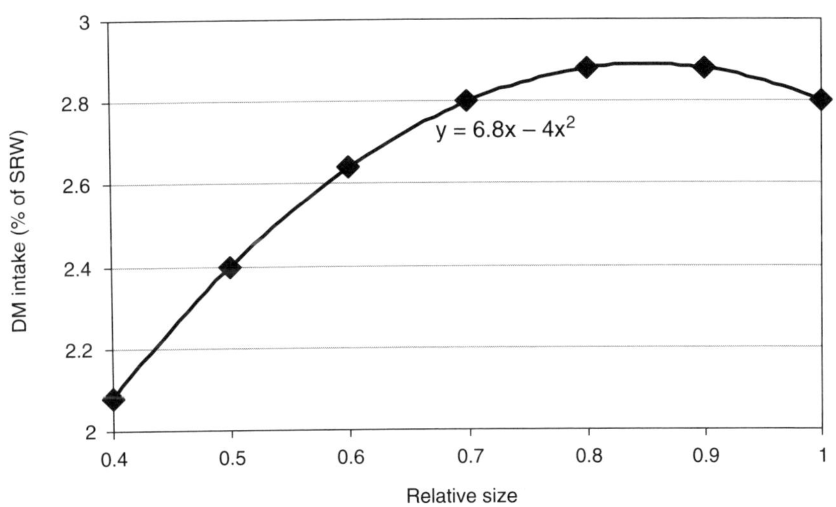

FIGURE 3-2 Influence of relative size (proportion of mature live weight) on predicted DM intakes, expressed in relation to mature size.

$$I/A = 0.068Z - 0.04Z^2$$

or, as a percentage of mature weight

$$\text{Intake (\% of mature weight)} = 6.8Z - 4Z^2 \quad \text{(x)}$$

The latter relationship is shown in Figure 3-2 and can be used to estimate the potential intake of a theoretical all-grass diet of digestibility > 0.8 for any combination of current weight and mature weight. For example, for a ewe with current live weight (at average condition score) = 68 kg and mature live weight (at average condition score) = 80 kg (i.e., relative size = 0.85), predicted intake can be calculated to be 2.89 percent of mature live weight or 2.31 (80 × 0.0289) kg DM/day.

The potential intakes calculated from equation (x) refer to the specific conditions of an all-grass diet of nonlimiting digestibility, and will alter depending on the animals' physiological state and on the amount, species composition (legume content), and quality of the plant biomass. In SCA (1990), potential intake is not increased during pregnancy, but is increased during lactation by a factor (with values in the range 1–2) that varies with time from lambing in a manner similar to published relationships for the lactation curve

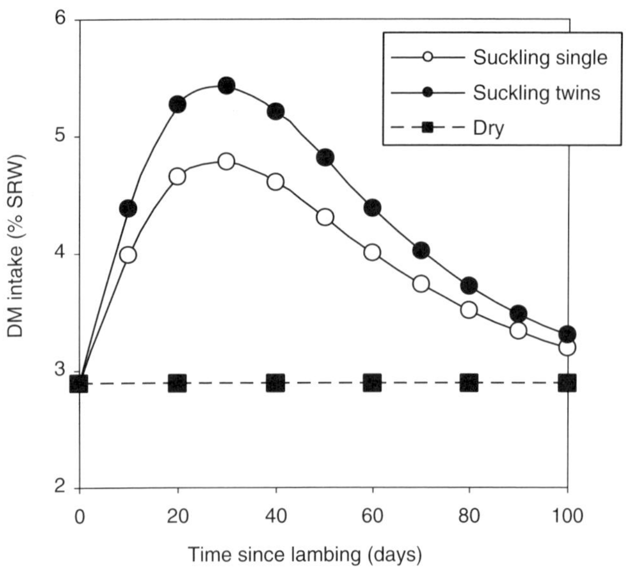

FIGURE 3-3 Influence of time since lambing on the predicted DM intake (% of standard reference weight) of ewes of relative size 0.85 consuming an all-grass diet and suckling either single or twin lambs.

(Wood, 1969) according to the following equation (equation 6.4, SCA 1990):

$$\text{Intake factor} = 1.0 + 0.025\ \text{n}\ \text{T}^{\ 1.4e(-0.05T)} \qquad \text{(y)}$$

where n has a value of 1.0 for a ewe with a single lamb and 1.35 for a ewe with twins.

This equation plus equation (x) above have been used to compute the potential intakes (percent of mature weight) of ewes suckling single or twin lambs over the first 100 days of lactation (Figure 3-3). The potential intake of dry ewes under the same conditions (2.89 percent of mature live weight; see Figure 3-2) is shown for comparison. These curves, plus equation (x) above, can be used to calculate the potential intakes of dry ewes and ewes suckling either single or twin lambs, for comparison with the intakes in the nutrient requirement tables that are required to meet energy requirements when the diet has an M/D (metabolizable energy MJ/kg DM; ARC, 1980) content of 12 MJ ME/kg DM. This will provide an indication of whether the "required" intakes are achievable.

When the digestibility (Dig) of the diet is reduced, the potential intakes implied by Figures 3-2 and 3-3 will also be reduced by a factor which can be computed from a simplification of equation 6.8 of SCA (1990), viz.:

$$\text{Quality constraint} = 1 - 1.7(0.8 - \text{Dig}) \qquad \text{(z)}$$

For diets with M/D = 10 MJ ME/kg DM (equivalent to Dig = 0.67) or 8 MJ ME/kg DM (equivalent to Dig = 0.55), the quality constraints can be computed to be 0.779 and 0.575, respectively. As an example, the effects of these constraints on the maximum likely intakes of twin-suckling ewes are shown in Table 3-2, relative to time since lambing.

TABLE 3-2 Potential Intakes (kg DM/day) of Twin-Suckling Ewes (Mature Weight 60 kg; Relative Size 0.85), when Eating Grass Diets of 8, 10, or 12 MJ ME/kg DM during Lactation[a]

Time from Lambing (Days)	60 kg Ewe, Twins M/D = 12 (kg DM/day)	60 kg Ewe, Twins M/D = 10 (kg DM/day)	60 kg Ewe, Twins M/D = 8 (kg DM/day)
0	1.73	1.35	0.99 (1.14)
10	2.63	2.05	1.51 (1.74)
20	3.16	2.46	1.82 (2.09)
30	3.26	2.54	1.87 (2.15)
40	3.12	2.43	1.79 (2.06)
50	2.88	2.24	1.66 (1.90)
60	2.63	2.05	1.51 (1.74)
70	2.41	1.88	1.39 (1.59)
80	2.23	1.74	1.28 (1.47)
90	2.09	1.63	1.20 (1.38)
100	1.98	1.54	1.14 (1.31)

[a]Calculations based on equations 6.3, 6.4, and 6.8 of SCA (1990). Values in parentheses are the intakes predicted if the legume content of the diet is 0.5.

Calculations such as those shown in Table 3-2 can be used to assess the intakes in the nutrient requirement tables required to meet energy requirements for diets of M/D = 8 or 10 MJ ME/kg DM and, as discussed above, provide an indication of when required intakes exceed potential intakes under the prevailing conditions. In these cases, the animal is unlikely to meet the suggested energy requirement unless diet quality is increased.

The proportion of legume in the diet of the animal can exert a powerful influence on intakes, because at a given digestibility, sheep are able to consume about 17 percent more legume than grass (see Freer and Jones, 1984). Equation (z) above can thus be restated:

$$\text{Quality constraint} = 1 - 1.7(0.8 - \text{Dig}) + 0.17\text{L} \qquad \text{(z)}$$

where L is the proportion of legume in the diet (following equation 6.8; SCA, 1990). If the legume proportion in the diet of the ewes consuming a diet of M/D = 8 MJ ME/kg DM in Table 3-2 were to increase from 0 to 0.5, then the predicted intakes would increase by about 15 percent and are shown in parentheses.

Under grazing conditions, actual intakes will depend on the available herbage mass and its average digestibility, and usually increase in a curvilinear fashion when related to either of these variables (Penning et al., 1991; Ciavarella, 2002). Potential intakes for a mature grazing sheep (standard reference weight 50 kg) at different herbage masses and digestibilities are shown in Figure 3-4, together with intakes calculated from the relationship given by Ciavarella (2002). It should be noted that in the latter case, herbage digestibilities were not constant.

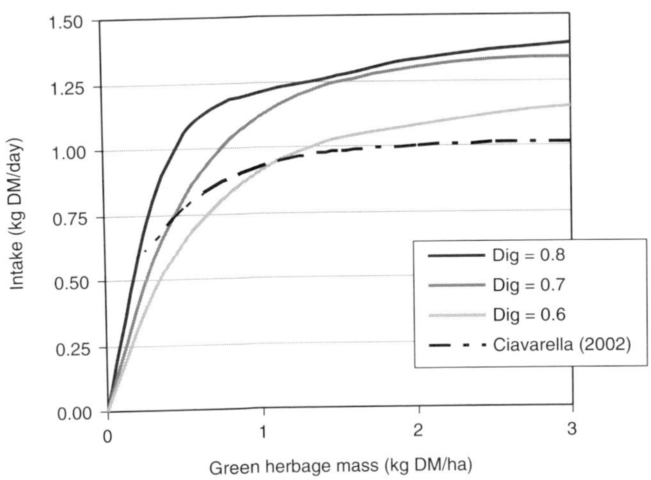

FIGURE 3-4 Pasture intakes (kg DM/day) predicted for sheep of standard reference weight 50 kg, grazing improved grass pastures differing in average digestibility (computed using the decision-support tool GrazFeed [Freer et al., 1997]). The dotted line is derived from the function fitted to actual intakes at different herbage masses (Ciavarella, 2002) for sheep grazing phalaris/subterranean clover pastures, after converting from OM to DM intake. In this case, the digestibility of the consumed diet varied with herbage mass.

It is clear that the shape of the intake response at a given average digestibility is similar to that suggested fcr the functional response in natural systems. The effect of pasture digestibility is also clear, especially as mean digestibility falls below 0.7. The predicted intakes in Figure 3-4 refer to improved grass pastures without legume. Predicted intakes would be higher for pastures containing legume (see equation 6.8, SCA, 1990, and equation (z) above), following Freer and Jones (1984).

For the sake of clarity, the effects of digestibility, legume content, and pasture mass have been discussed separately. However, in grazed systems, it is rare for only one of these to change. More usually, there will be contemporaneous changes in legume content, herbage mass, and average sward digestibility and, if there are areas of bare ground in the sward, pasture height itself may become an important variable, over and above its effect on herbage mass. Under these circumstances, it becomes exceedingly difficult to compute a predicted intake by hand, for comparison with estimates of requirements. To address these issues, computer-based decision support tools have been developed that can estimate the likely pasture intake, given a description of the animal and the pasture (see Freer et al., 1997; Freer, 2002). A further complication in relating forage intake to nutrient requirements is the provision of supplements to domestic livestock in grazing systems.

Finally, there do not appear to be sufficient data to derive similar relationships for either NWC or the cervids discussed here. In the latter case, and as discussed above, the situation is further complicated by the pronounced seasonal pattern of intake as day length varies.

THE SUPPLEMENT RESPONSE

In livestock production systems, animals are often given supplementary feed when the quantity or quality of available pasture is thought to limit nutrient intake. Supplementation may also occur in wild ruminant species, usually in relation to their utilization as game animals (Putman and Staines, 2004). At its simplest, a supplement can be defined as "something added to remedy a deficiency" (Doyle, 1987), but responses to supplements in grazing systems can be erratic, suggesting something more complex than "remedying a deficiency" is occurring. Supplement responses in grazing livestock have been reviewed elsewhere (Doyle, 1987; Dove, 2002; O'Reagain and McMeniman, 2002) and will not be revisited here. In general, if the supplement is given to overcome a known deficiency in the diet (e.g., a mineral, vitamin, or rumen-degradable nitrogen), then a common response to supplementation is for intake to increase (complementation), though it is often difficult to know by how much. If the supplement is given because the amount of forage or the energy content of the forage is too low to meet energy requirements, consumption of the supplement results in a reduction in forage intake (substitution). In some intermediate circumstances, supplementation can be additive, i.e., forage intake is not affected by feeding of supplement.

Dove (2002) discussed factors influencing the degree of substitution during supplementation of sheep on pasture. In general, the level of substitution will be greater under the following circumstances:

1. If there is more pasture available
2. If herbage quality is high
3. If supplement quality is high
4. If more supplement is fed
5. If animals do not have a high demand for nutrients; lower substitution rates have been observed in lactating animals (Dove et al., 2000)
6. If supplements are fed less frequently in a given time period.

It should be noted that exceptions to all of these have been recorded, so the prediction of the likely effect of supplementation on the net supply of nutrients to the animal is very difficult (Dove, 2002). A further point to note is that supplements that provide a readily fermented form of energy can, in fact, result in a greater supply of post-ruminal protein, due to their allowing a greater amount of rumen ammonia to be converted into microbial protein. This results in the blurring of the distinction between the common descriptions of feeds as "energy" or "protein" supplements.

CONCLUSION

Despite many years of research effort, it remains difficult to predict the likely diet composition and intake of free-ranging animals. Without doubt, part of this problem relates to the difficulty of measuring these, but even with better measurement, the confounding of the responses to such things as species composition, average quality of the material on offer, the amount of material available, and the provision of supplements make intake prediction very difficult. Stuth et al. (1999) and Freer (2002) have suggested that diet selection/intake responses are so complicated under field conditions that computer-based simulations or decision-support tools may be the only feasible approach to predicting them.

REFERENCES

Albon, S. D., and R. Langvatn. 1992. Plant phenology and the benefits of migration in a temperate ungulate. Oikos 65:502–513.

Allden, W. G. 1979. Feed intake, diet composition and wool growth. Pp. 61–78 in Physiological and Environmental Limitations to Wool Growth, J. L. Black and P. J. Reis, eds. Armidale: University of New England Publishing Unit.

ARC (Agricultural Research Council). 1980. The Nutrient Requirements of Ruminant Livestock. Slough, UK: Commonwealth Agricultural Bureaux.

Arnold, G. W. 1981. Grazing behaviour. Pp. 79–104 in Grazing Animals, F. H. W. Morley, ed. World Animal Science B1. Amsterdam: Elsevier.

Arnold, G. W. 1987. The influence of biomass, botanical composition and sward height of annual pastures on foraging behaviour of sheep. J. Appl. Ecol. 24:759–772.

Barry, T. N., J. M. Suttie, J. A. Milne, and R. N. B. Kay. 1991. Control of food intake in domesticated deer. Pp. 385–401 in Physiological Aspects of Digestion and Metabolism in Ruminants (Proc. VII Int. Symp. Rum. Physiol.). London: Academic Press.

Bas, F., and C. Bonacic. 2003. Adaptive strategies of South American camelids. Pp. 23–33 in Matching Herbivore Nutrition to Ecosystems Biodiversity, L.'t Mannetje, L. Ramírez-Avilés, C. Sandoval-Castro, and J. C. Ku-Vera, eds. Mérida, Mexico: Universidad Autónoma de Yucatán.

Belovsky, G. E., J. M. Fryxell, and O. J. Schmitz. 1999. Natural selection and herbivore nutrition: Optimal foraging theory and what it tells us about the structure of ecological communities. Pp. 1–70 in Nutritional Ecology of Herbivores, H. J. G. Jung and G. C. Fahey, eds. Savoy, IL: American Society of Animal Science.

Blanchart, G., J. Brun-Bellut, and B. Vignon. 1980. Comparison of goats and sheep with respect to the ingestion, digestibility and nutritive value of various diets. French. Reprod. Nutr. Dev. 20:1731–1737.

Brown, L. E., and W. L. Johnson. 1984. Comparative intake and digestibility of forage and by-products by goats and sheep: A review. Int. Goat Sheep. Res. 2:212–226.

Bugalho, M. N., J. A. Milne, R. W. Mayes, and F. C. Rego. 2005. Plant-wax alkanes as seasonal markers of red deer dietary components. Can. J. Zool. 83:465–473.

Cannas, A., L. O. Tedeschi, D. G. Fox, A. N. Pell, and P. J. Van Soest. 2004. A mechanistic model for predicting the nutrient requirements and feed biological values for sheep. J. Anim. Sci. 82:149–169.

Ciavarella, T. A. 2002. Attributes of pasture influencing the diet of grazing sheep. PhD thesis, University of Melbourne.

Ciavarella, T. A., H. Dove, B. J. Leury, and R. J. Simpson. 2000a. Diet selection by sheep grazing *Phalaris aquatica* L. pastures of differing water-soluble carbohydrate content. Aust. J. Agric. Res. 51:757–764.

Ciavarella, T. A., R. J. Simpson, H. Dove, B. J. Leury, and I. M. Sims. 2000b. Diurnal changes in the concentration of water-soluble carbohydrates in *Phalaris aquatica* L. pasture in spring, and the effect of short-term shading. Aust. J. Agric. Res. 51:749–756.

Clark, D. A., and P. S. Harris. 1985. Composition of the diet of sheep grazing swards of differing white clover content and spatial distribution. NZ J. Agric. Res. 28:233–240.

Clark, D. A., M. G. Lambert, M. P. Rolston, and N. Dymock. 1982. Diet selection by goats and sheep on hill country. Proc. NZ Soc. Anim. Prod. 42:155–157.

Clark, S. G., J. R. Donnelly, and A. D. Moore. 2000. The GrassGro decision support tool: Its effectiveness in simulating pasture and animal production and value in determining research priorities. Aust. J. Exp. Agric. 40:247–256.

Clarke, I. J. 2001. Sex and season are major determinants of voluntary food intake in sheep. Reprod. Fertil. Dev. 13:577–582.

Clauss, M., M. Lechner-Doll, and W. J. Streich. 2002. Faecal particle size distribution in captive wild ruminants: An approach to the browser/grazer dichotomy from the other end. Oecologia 131:343–349.

Cohen, R. D. H., J. P. Stevens, A. D. Moore, and J. R. Donnelly. 2003. Validating and using the GrassGro decision support tool for a mixed grass/alfalfa pasture in western Canada. Can. J. Anim. Sci. 83:171–182.

Corbett, J. L., and M. Freer. 2003. Past and present definitions of the energy and protein requirements of ruminants. Asian-Aust. J. Anim. Sci. 16:609–624.

Cornelis, J., J. Casaer, and M. Hermy. 1999. Impact of season, habitat and research techniques on diet composition of roe deer (*Capreolus capreolus*): A review. J. Zool. (Lond.) 248:195–207.

Cosgrove, G. P., C. B. Anderson, and R. H. Fletcher. 1996. Do cattle exhibit a preference for white clover? In Agronomy Society of New Zealand Special Publication no. 11, Grassland Research and Practice series 6:83–86.

Crampton, E. W., and L. E. Harris. 1969. Applied Animal Nutrition, 2nd ed. San Francisco: W. H. Freeman.

Domingue, B. M. F., D. W. Dellow, P. R. Wilson, and T. N. Barry. 1990. Comparative nutrition of deer and goats, goats and sheep. Proc. NZ Soc. Anim. Prod. 50:39–42.

Domingue, B. M. F., D. W. Dellow, and T. N. Barry. 1991. Voluntary intake and rumen digestion of a low-quality roughage by goats and sheep. J. Agric. Sci., Camb. 117:111–120.

Dove, H. 1998. Pastures and grazing animals—the interaction continues. (The 1998 Underwood Lecture). Anim. Prod. in Aust. 22:3–13.

Dove, H. 2002. Principles of supplementary feeding in sheep-grazing systems. Pp. 119–142 in Sheep Nutrition, M. Freer and H. Dove, eds. Wallingford, UK and Melbourne, Australia: CABI Publishing in association with CSIRO Publishing.

Dove, H., M. Freer, and J. Z. Foot. 2000. The nutrition of grazing ewes during pregnancy and lactation: A comparison of alkane-based and chromium/in vitro-based estimates of herbage intake. Aust. J. Agric. Res. 51:765–777.

Doyle, P. T. 1987. Supplements other than forages. Pp. 429–464 in The Nutrition of Herbivores, J. B. Hacker and J. H. Ternouth, eds. Sydney, Australia: Academic Press.

Doyle, P. T., J. K. Egan, and A. J. Thalen. 1984. Intake, digestion, and nitrogen and sulfur retention in Angora goats and Merino sheep fed herbage diets. Aust. J. Exp. Agric. Anim. Husb. 24:165–169.

Duncan, A. J., and I. J. Gordon. 1999. Habitat selection according to the ability of animals to eat, digest and detoxify foods. Proc. Nutr. Soc. 58:799–805.

Fisher, D. S. 2002. A review of a few key factors regulating voluntary feed intake in ruminants. Crop Sci. 42:1651–1655.

Fisher, D. S., H. F. Mayland, and J. C. Burns. 1999. Variation in ruminants' preference for tall fescue hays cut either at sundown or at sunup. J. Anim. Sci. 77:762–768.

Foley, W. J., G. R. Iason, and C. McArthur. 1999. Role of plant secondary metabolites in the nutritional ecology of mammalian herbivores: How far have we come in 25 years? Pp. 130–209 in Nutritional Ecology of Herbivores, H. J. G. Jung and G. C. Fahey, eds. Savoy, IL: American Society of Animal Science.

Forbes, J. M. 1996. Integration of regulatory signals controlling forage intake in ruminants. J. Anim. Sci. 74:3029–3035.

Forsyth, D. M., D. A. Coomes, G. Nugent, and G. M. J. Hall. 2002. Diet and diet preferences of introduced ungulates (Order: Artiodactyla) in New Zealand. NZ J. Zool. 29:323–343.

Fraser, M. D., and D. H. Baker. 1998. A comparison of voluntary intake and *in vivo* digestion in guanacos (*Lama guanacoe*) and sheep given fresh grass. Anim. Sci. 67:567–572.

Freer, M. 2002. The nutritional management of grazing sheep. Pp. 357–375 in Sheep Nutrition, M. Freer and H. Dove, eds. Wallingford, UK and Melbourne, Australia: CABI Publishing in association with CSIRO Publishing.

Freer, M., and D. B. Jones. 1984. Feeding value of subterranean clover, lucerne, phalaris and Wimmera ryegrass for lambs. Aust. J. Exp. Agric. Anim. Husb. 24:156–164.

Freer, M., A. D. Moore, and J. R. Donnelly. 1997. GRAZPLAN: Decision support systems for Australian grazing enterprises. II. The animal biology model for feed intake, production and reproduction and the GrazFeed DSS. Agric. Systems 54:77–126.

Genin, D., Z. Villca, and P. Abasto. 1994. Diet selection and utilization by llama and sheep in a high altitude-arid rangeland of Bolivia. J. Range Manage. 47:245–248.

Giger, S., D. Sauvant, J. Hervieu, and M. Dorléans. 1987. Valeur alimentaire du foin de luzerne pour la chevre. Ann. Zootech. 36:139–152.

Ginnett, T. F., and M. W. Demment. 1995. The functional response of herbivores: Analysis and test of a simple mechanistic model. Funct. Ecol. 9:376–384.

Gong, Y., J. Hodgson, M. G. Lambert, and I. L. Gordon. 1996. Short-term ingestive behaviour of sheep and goats grazing grasses and legumes 1. Comparison of bite weight, bite rate, and bite dimensions for forages at two stages of maturity. NZ J. Agric. Res. 39:63–73.

Gordon, I. J. 2003. Browsing and grazing ruminants: Are they different beasts? Forest Ecol. Manage. 181:13–21.

Gordon, I. J., and A. W. Illius. 1994. The functional significance of the browser-grazer dichotomy in African ruminants. Oecologia 98:167–175.

Griffith, B., D. C. Douglas, N. E. Walsh, D. D. Young, T. R. McCabe, D. E. Russell, R. G. White, R. D. Cameron, and K. R. Whitten. 2002. The Porcupine caribou herd. Pp. 8–37 in Arctic Refuge Coastal Plain Terrestrial Wildlife Research Summaries, D. C. Douglas, P. E. Reynolds, and E. B. Rhode, eds. U.S. Geological Survey, Biological Resources Division, Biological Science Report USGS/BRD/BSR-2002-0001.

Grimes, R. C., B. R. Watkin, and J. R. Gallagher. 1966. An evaluation of pasture quality with young grazing sheep. II. Chemical composition, botanical composition and in vitro digestibility of herbage selected by oesophageal-fistulated sheep. J. Agric. Sci., Camb. 66:113–119.

Hadjigeorgiou, I. E., I. J. Gordon, and J. A. Milne. 2003. Comparative preference by sheep and goats for *Graminaeae* forages varying in chemical composition. Small Ruminant Res. 49:147–156.

Hart, S. P. 2001. Recent perspectives in using goats for vegetation management in the USA. J. Dairy Sci. 84 (E. Suppl.):E170–E176.

Hobbs, N. T. 1999. Responses of large herbivores to spatial heterogeneity in ecosystems. Pp. 97–129 in Nutritional Ecology of Herbivores, H. G. Jung and G. C. Fahey, eds. Savoy, IL: American Society of Animal Science.

Hofmann, R. R. 1989. Evolutionary steps of ecophysiological adaptation and diversification of ruminants: A comparative review of their digestive system. Oecologia 78:443–457.

Hofmann, R. R., and D. R. M. Stewart. 1972. Grazer or browser: A classification based on the stomach structure and feeding habits of East African ruminants. Mammalia 36:226–240.

Holst, P. J., C. J. Allan, M. H. Campbell, and A. R. Gilmour. 2004a. Grazing of pasture weeds by goats and sheep. 1. Nodding thistle (*Carduus nutans*). Aust. J. Exp. Agric. 44:547–551.

Holst, P. J., C. J. Allan, M. H. Campbell, and A. R. Gilmour. 2004b. Grazing of pasture weeds by goats and sheep. 2. Scotch broom (*Cytisus scoparius*). Aust. J. Exp. Agric. 44:553–557.

Iason, G. 2005. The role of plant secondary metabolites in mammalian herbivory: Ecological perspectives. Proc. Nutr. Soc. 64:123–131.

Iason, G. R., D. A. Sim, and I. J. Gordon. 2000. Do endogenous seasonal cycles of food intake influence foraging behaviour and intake by grazing sheep? Func. Ecol. 14:614–622.

Illius, A. W., and I. J. Gordon. 1999. The physiological ecology of mammalian herbivory. Pp. 71–96 in Nutritional Ecology of Herbivores, H. J. G. Jung and G. C. Fahey, eds. Savoy, IL: American Society of Animal Science.

INRA (National Institute for Agricultural Research). 1978. Alimentation des Ruminants, R. Jarrige, ed. Versailles, France: INRA Publications.

Johnson, C. J., K. L. Parker, and D. C. Heard. 2001. Foraging across a variable landscape: Behavioral decisions made by woodland caribou at multiple spatial scales. Oecologia 127:590–602.

Johnstone, J., D. E. Russell, and G. Griffith. 2002. Variations in plant forage quality in the range of the Porcupine caribou herd. Rangifer 22:83–91.

Kelman, W. M., M. N. Bugalho, and H. Dove. 2003. Cuticular wax alkanes and alcohols used as markers to estimate the diet composition of sheep (*Ovis aries*). Biochem. Syst. Ecol. 31:919–927.

Klein, D. R. 1970. Tundra ranges north of the boreal forest. J. Range Manage. 23:8–14.

Laca, E. A., and M. W. Demment. 1996. Foraging strategies of grazing animals. Pp. 137–158 in The Ecology and Management of Grazing Systems, J. Hodgson and A. W. Illius, eds. U.K.: CABI Publishing.

Laidlaw, A. S. 1983. Grazing by sheep and the distribution of species through the canopy of a red clover-perennial ryegrass sward. Grass. Forage Sci. 38:317–321.

Langlands, J. P. 1972. Growth and herbage consumption of grazing Merino and Border Leicester lambs reared by their mothers or fostered by ewes of the other breed. Anim. Prod. 14:317–322.

Latupeirissa, C. C. E. 2002. Forage intake and digestion—a comparison of deer and sheep. M. Appl. Sci. thesis, University of Queensland, Gatton, Australia.

Launchbaugh, K. L. 1996. Biochemical aspects of grazing behaviour. Pp. 154–184 in The Ecology and Management of Grazing Systems, J. Hodgson and A. W. Illius, eds. Wallingford, UK: CAB International.

Lemosquet, S., C. Dardillat, M. Jailler, and J. P. Dulphy. 1996. Voluntary intake and gastric digestion of two hays by llamas and sheep: Influence of concentrate supplementation. J. Agric. Sci., Camb. 127:539–548.

Leury, B. J., C. Siever-Kelly, K. L. Gatford, R. J. Simpson, and H. Dove. 1999. Spray-topping annual grass pasture with glyphosate to delay loss of feeding value during summer. IV. Diet Composition, herbage intake, and performance in grazing sheep. Aust. J. Agric. Res. 50:487–495.

Mårell, A., J. P. Ball, and A. Hofgaard. 2002. Foraging and movement paths of female reindeer: Insights from fractal analysis, correlated random walks, and Lévy flights. Can. J. Zool. 80:854–865.

Mayes, R. W., and H. Dove. 2000. Measurement of dietary nutrient intake in free-ranging mammalian herbivores. Nutr. Res. Rev. 13:107–138.

McCullough, D. R., and D. E. Ullrey. 1985. Chemical composition and gross energy of deer forage plants on the George Reserve. Michigan Agricultural Experiment Station Research Report 465. 19 pp.

McEwan, N. R., L. Abecia, M. Regensbogenova, C. L. Adam, P. A. Findlay, and C. J. Newbold. 2005. Rumen microbial population dynamics in response to photoperiod. Letters Appl. Microbiol. 41:97–101.

Merchant, M., and D. J. Riach. 1994. The intake and performance of cashmere goats grazing sown swards. Grass Forage Sci. 49:429–437.

Milne, J. A., J. C. Macrae, A. M. Spence, and S. Wilson. 1978. A comparison of the voluntary intake and digestion of a range of forages at different times of the year by the sheep and the red deer (Cervus elaphus). Br. J. Nutr. 40:347–357.

Moen, A. N. 1973. Wildlife Ecology, an Analytical Approach. San Francisco: W. H. Freeman.

Moore, A. D., J. R. Donnelly, and M. Freer. 1997. GRAZPLAN: Decision support systems for Australian grazing enterprises—III. Pasture growth and soil moisture submodels and the GrassGro DSS. Agric. Syst. 55: 535–582.

Newman, J. A., A. J. Parsons, and A. Harvey. 1992. Not all sheep prefer clover: diet selection revisited. J. Agric. Sci., Camb. 119:275–283.

Newman, S. A. N., and D. J. Paterson. 1994. Effect of level of nutrition and season on fibre growth in alpacas. Proc. NZ Soc. Anim Prod. 54: 147–150.

NRC (National Research Council). 1981. Nutrient Requirements of Goats: Angora, Dairy, and Meat Goats in Temperate and Tropical Countries. Washington, DC: National Academy Press.

NRC. 1985. Nutrient Requirements of Sheep, 6th ed. Washington, DC: National Academy Press.

NRC. 1996. Nutrient Requirements of Beef Cattle, 7th ed. Washington, DC: National Academy Press.

O'Reagain, P. J., and N. P. McMeniman. 2002. Nutrition of sheep under rangeland conditions. Pp. 263–284 in Sheep Nutrition, M. Freer and H. Dove, eds. Wallingford, UK and Melbourne, Australia: CABI Publishing in association with CSIRO Publishing.

Orr, R. J., P. D. Penning, A. Harvey, and R. A. Champion. 1997. Diurnal patterns of intake rate by sheep grazing monocultures of ryegrass or white clover. Appl. Anim. Behav. Sci. 52:65–77.

Owen-Smith, R. N. 2002. Adaptive Herbivore Ecology. Cambridge, UK: Cambridge University Press.

Pande, R. S., P. D. Kemp, and J. Hodgson. 2002. Preference of goats and sheep for browse species under field conditions. NZ J. Agric. Res. 45: 97–102.

Parker, K.L. 2003. Advances in the nutritional ecology of cervids at different scales. Ecoscience 10: 395–411.

Parsons, A. J., J. A. Newman, P. D. Penning, A. Harvey, and R. J. Orr. 1994. Diet preference of sheep; Effects of recent diet, physiological state and species abundance. J. Anim. Ecol. 63:465–478.

Penning, P. D., A. J. Parsons, R. J. Orr, and T. T. Treacher. 1991. Intake and behaviour responses by sheep to changes in sward characteristics under continuous stocking. Grass Forage Sci. 46:15–28.

Penning, P. D., J. A. Newman, A. J. Parsons, A. Harvey, and R. J. Orr. 1997. Diet preferences of adult sheep and goats grazing ryegrass and white clover. Small Ruminant Res. 24:175–184.

Pinares-Patiño, C. S., M. J. Ulyatt, G. C. Waghorn, K. R. Lassey, T. N. Barry, C. W. Holmes, and D. E. Johnson. 2003. Methane emission by alpaca and sheep fed on lucerne hay or grazed on pastures of perennial ryegrass/ white clover or birdsfoot trefoil. J. Agric. Sci., Camb. 140: 215–226.

Prache, S., and J. L. Peyraud. 2001. Foraging behaviour and intake in temperate cultivated grasslands. Pp. 309–319 in Proc. XIX Int. Grassld. Cong., Sao Paolo, Brazil.

Pulina, G., T. Bettati, F. A. Serra, and A. Cannas. 1996. Razi-O: Development and validation of a software for dairy sheep feeding. Proc. XII Nat. Meeting Società Italiana de Patologia e d'Allevamento degli Ovini e dei Caprini, Varese, Italy.

Putman, R.J., and Staines, B.W. 2004. Supplementary winter feeding of wild red deer Cervus elaphus in Europe and North America: Justifications, feeding practice and effectiveness. Mammal Review 34:285–306.

Reeves, M., W. J. Fulkerson, R. C. Kellaway, and H. Dove. 1996. A comparison of three techniques to determine the herbage intake of dairy cows grazing kikuyu (*Pennisetum clandestinum*) pasture. Aust. J. Exp. Agric. 36:23–30.

Reid, R. L., G. A. Jung, J. M. Cox-Ganser, B. F. Rybeck, and E. C. Townsend. 1990. Comparative utilization of warm- and cool-season forages by cattle, sheep and goats. J. Anim. Sci. 68:2986–2994.

Rhind, S. M., Z. A. Archer, and C. L. Adam. 2002. Seasonality of food intake in ruminants: Recent developments in understanding. Nutr. Res. Rev. 15:43–65.

Ridout, M. S., and M. J. Robson. 1991. Diet composition of sheep grazing grass/white clover swards: A re-evaluation. NZ J. Agric. Res. 34:89–93.

Robbins, C. T., D. E. Spalinger, and W. Van Hoven. 1995. Adaptation of ruminants to browse and grass diets: Are anatomical-based browser-grazer interpretations valid? Oecologia 103:208–213.

San Martin, F. 1987. Comparative forage selectivity and nutrition of South American camelids and sheep, PhD thesis, Texas Technical University, Lubbock, Texas.

San Martin, F., and F. C. Bryant. 1987. Nutrición de los Camélidos Sudamericanos: Estado de nuestro conocimiento. Technical Report T–9–505. College of Agricultural Sciences, Lubbock: Texas Technical University (TTU).

SCA (Standing Committee on Agriculture). 1990. Feeding Standards for Australian Livestock: Ruminants. Standing Committee on Agriculture Ruminants Subcommittee. Melbourne, Australia: CSIRO.

Shipley, L. A. 1999. Grazers and browsers: How digestive morphology affects diet selection. Pp. 20–27 in Grazing Behavior of Livestock and Wildlife, K. L. Launchbaugh, K. D. Sanders, and J. C. Mosley, eds. Idaho Forest, Wildlife and Range Experiment Station Bulletin no. 70. Moscow, Idaho: University of Idaho.

Spalinger, D. E., and N. T. Hobbs. 1992. Mechanisms of foraging in mammalian herbivores: New models of functional response. Amer. Nat. 140:325–348.

Stuth, J. W., M. Freer, H. Dove, and R. K. Lyons. 1999. Nutritional management for free-ranging livestock. Pp. 696–751 in Nutritional Ecology of Herbivores, H. J. G. Jung and G. C. Fahey, eds. Savoy, IL: American Society of Animal Science.

Tedeschi, L. O., D. G. Fox, and J. B. Russell. 2000. Accounting for the effects of a ruminal nitrogen deficiency within the structure of the Cornell Net Carbohydrate and Protein System. J. Anim. Sci. 78:1648–1658.

Ungar, E. D. 1996. Ingestive behaviour. Pp. 185–218 in The Ecology and Management of Grazing Systems, J. Hodgson and A. W. Illius, eds. Wallingford, UK: CAB International.

Van der Wal, R., N. Madan, S. van Lieshout, C. Dormann, R. Langvatn, and S. D. Albon. 2000. Trading forage quality for quantity? Plant phenology and patch choice by Svalbard reindeer. Oecologia 123:108–115.

Wackwitz, B., G. Castellaro, H. J. Schwartz, and A. Raggi. 1999. Botanical composition of the diets of alpaca (*Lama pacos*) and llama (*Lama glama*) in the Andean rangelands of Chile. Deutscher Tropentag 1999 in Berlin, pp. 1–6.

Walker, J. W., S. L. Kronberg, S. L. Al-Rowaily, and N. E. West. 1994. Comparison of sheep and goat preferences for leafy spurge. J. Range Manage. 47:429–434.

Warmington, B. G., G. F. Wilson, and T. N. Barry. 1989. Voluntary intake and digestion of ryegrass straw by llama × guanaco crossbreds and sheep. J. Agric. Sci., Camb. 113:87–91.

Weston, R. H. 1980. Roughage intake and digestion comparisons with lambs and adult sheep. Proc. Nutr. Soc. Aust. 5:191.

Weston, R. H. 1996. Some aspects of constraint to forage consumption by ruminants. Aust. J. Agric. Res. 47:175–197.

White, R. G., F. L. Bunnell, E. Gaare, T. Skogland, and B. Hubert. 1981. Ungulates on arctic ranges. Pp. 397–483 in Tundra Ecosystems: A Comparative Analysis. IBP Vol. 25, L. C. Bliss, O. W. Heal, and J. J. Moore, eds. Cambridge, UK: Cambridge University Press.

Wood, P. D. P. 1969. Factors affecting the shape of the lactation curve in cattle. Anim. Prod. 11:307–316.

4

Energy

SPECIES

Many factors can influence energy requirements, including species. For example, NRC (1985) cited literature indicating that efficiencies of metabolizable energy (ME) use for maintenance (k_m) and gain (k_g) are similar for sheep and cattle. There do not appear available similar extensive comparisons of goats with cattle and sheep, although AFRC (1998) summarized data suggesting that the ME requirement for maintenance (ME_m) of goats, scaled by body weight $(BW)^{0.75}$, is greater than that of sheep and similar to that of cattle. Conversely, SCA (1990) assumed that ME_m of goats and sheep are similar. Regardless, given the different methods of determination of ME_m for sheep, goats, and other ruminants, as well as the varied settings in which they exist, recommended requirement expressions will be addressed separately later.

There are few direct interspecies comparisons of energy requirements, expressed as ME_m, k_m, k_g, and the efficiency of ME utilization for lactation (k_l,), either among the cervids or between cervid species and sheep or goats. Interspecies comparisons are restricted to seasonal estimates of feed intake and digestibility (Kay and Goodall, 1976; Milne et al., 1978; Fennessy et al., 1980). Estimates of ME_m for individual cervid species are reported later.

MAINTENANCE

Level of Intake

One of the most widely acknowledged effectors of ME_m is level of feed intake. At levels of intake below ME_m, fasting heat production is minimized because of decreased basal metabolic rates, for which splanchnic tissues can account for as much as 50 percent (Drouillard et al., 1991; Freetly et al., 1995a; Wester et al., 1995; Sainz and Bentley, 1997). Moreover, high levels of intake can affect ME_m, depending on the method of partitioning. That is, heat production or energy expenditure by "support" tissues, such as the splanchnic bed, increases with increasing metabolic workload associated with rising feed intake (Johnson and Johnson, 1995). The effect of metabolism by splanchnic and other support tissues is probably the basis of the higher ME_m exhibited by north temperate and Arctic cervids in summer compared with winter. The effect appears independent of basal metabolic rate because no seasonal change has been reported for a number of cervids, including reindeer, white-tailed deer, roe deer, or red deer, whereas ME_m is higher in summer than winter (Thompson et al., 1973; Holter et al., 1977; Simpson et al., 1978a; Hudson and Christopherson, 1985). This seasonal difference in ME_m reflects a complex of changes in physiology, endocrinology, and behavior that result in an increase in appetite drive and growth in summer (Hudson and Christopherson, 1985; Suttie and Simpson, 1985; Suttie and Webster, 1995, 1998; Parker et al., 1996; Tyler et al., 1999; Rhind et al., 2002). An interspecies comparison of fasting metabolic rates in winter indicates that most cervids lie above the interspecies mean of 70 kcal (293 kJ)/kg $BW^{0.75}$ (Hudson and Christopherson, 1985; Tyler and Blix, 1990; Robbins 1993), which accounts for the high ME_m of these and other cervid species compared with domestic sheep (Ullrey et al., 1970; Thompson et. al., 1973; Holter, 1977; Milne et al., 1978; Simpson et al., 1978b; Baker et al., 1979; Fennessey et al., 1981; Robbins et al., 1981; Hudson and Christopherson, 1985; Schwartz et al., 1987; Jiang and Hudson, 1992, 1994; Worden and Pekins, 1995). Because estimates of summer ME_m do not factorially remove the energy cost of summer coat growth (scurf), estimates of summer ME_m are assumed to include this cost.

Effects of level of intake on ME_m were not addressed by NRC (1985); INRA (1989) for sheep or goats; or NRC (1981b), AFRC (1998), or Drochner et al. (2003) for goats. In contrast, based on a review of pertinent beef cattle literature, NRC (2000) suggested up to a 20 percent decrease in ME_m during and following a low plane of nutrition, with impact for 2 to 3 months after the change to a higher level. A convenient means of assessing the severity of a low nutritional plane is body condition score (BCS), although it is presumed that BCS is relatively more reflective of ME_m when BCS is static rather than changing. NRC (2000) proposed a 5 percent decrease in ME_m of beef cattle for each BCS unit less than 5 (1 to 9 scale), resulting in a 20 percent lower value for a BCS of 1. Sahlu et al. (2004) proposed that the ME_m of goats be adjusted similarly for low BCS, with lower adjustments applied as time since the change from limiting to nonlimiting nutritional plane advances. SCA (1990) reviewed studies available at that time that also indicated effects of plane of nutrition on ME_m of sheep but did not recommend adjustment for BCS. Rather, in the SCA (1990) system, ME_m is varied in accordance with the degree to which ME intake (MEI) is greater or less than ME_m to account for effects of level of feed intake on energy expenditure by support tissues.

Current energy systems also vary in the means by which they adjust ME_m for effects of high levels of intake. For beef cattle, NRC (2000) recommended adjustment of ME_m for BCS above 5 (1 to 9 scale) in the same manner as when below 5. That is, ME_m is increased 5 percent for each BCS unit greater than 5, with ME_m 20 percent greater at BCS of 9. As noted earlier, the SCA (1990) system recommends an adjustment of ME_m at levels of intake both below and above ME_m to account for changes in visceral energy expenditure. Cannas et al. (2004) adopted a similar linear adjustment based on MEI and a constant k_m in the Cornell Net Carbohydrate and Protein System for sheep (CNCPS-S). Williams and Jenkins (2003) likewise have modeled heat production for support tissue metabolism in cattle when MEI is above ME_m.

Dawson and Steen (1998) discussed how such upward adjustment of ME_m for high levels of intake may be appropriate for ME_m based on fasting heat production (FHP) determined after a period of a maintenance level of intake. For ME_m assessed with producing animals (e.g., positive average daily gain [ADG] or milk or fiber production); however, such an adjustment would be inappropriate (i.e., double accounting). In this regard, since ME_m requirements for goats summarized by Sahlu et al. (2004) were determined with most animals consuming diets ad libitum, an upward adjustment of ME_m when feed intake is above maintenance was not recommended. Similarly, energy requirements of growing/finishing beef cattle of NRC (2000) are based on comparative slaughter data with levels of intake near and above maintenance rather than direct determinations of heat production while fasting. For mature animals not in the last third of gestation, lactating, or producing a significant quantity of fiber, a maintenance level of intake would be a normal occurrence other than with compensatory growth after a low nutritional plane. Therefore, there seems little need for upward adjustment of ME_m. Furthermore, for compensating animals in realimentation following a low plane of nutrition, intake is often higher than expected based on BW and diet quality, and BCS is relatively low. These factors, coupled with possibly decreased ME_m as addressed above, makes upward adjustment of ME_m for high levels of intake questionable. For energy systems in which ME_m is not increased for high feed intake or BCS, this influence is assumed to be addressed by the lower efficiencies of ME use for tissue gain (ME_g), lactation (ME_l), fiber growth (ME_f), and/or pregnancy (ME_{preg}).

For cervids, the reduction in voluntary intake in winter followed by high intake in spring and summer is associated with major protein and minor fat accretion over summer by calves, respectively 18 and 6 percent of the gain (Adamczewski et al., 1987; Gerhart et al., 1996a), whereas a major accretion of fat compared with protein occurs over summer in mature animals (Suttie et al., 1983; Adamczewski et al., 1987; Worden and Pekins, 1995). The ability to deposit fat in late summer-autumn has been associated with an increase in lipogenic activity of adipocytes (Larsen et al., 1985) combined with a low ME_m and high efficiency of gain (Worden and Pekins, 1995). This effect could be extended into winter because when pregnant reindeer consume an all-cereal grain (barley) diet ad libitum, fetal death and/or dystocia occurred in all animals and was attributable to large deposits of abdominal fat (Blanchard et al., 1984; Blanchard and Hauer, 1986).

In cervids, fiber growth occurs in summer, a time when females are lactating, and for reindeer/caribou, females produce antlers (Kelsall, 1968; Bubenik et al., 1998). Thus, for lactating reindeer/caribou, energy costs of antler growth must be added to that for maintenance, BW gain, pelage (hair coat) growth, and lactation (Moen and Pastor, 1998). Whereas antler growth commences at birth in reindeer/caribou, antler growth commences at a certain BW in fawns of other cervid species (Suttie and Kay, 1982). In adult male cervids, seasonal initiation of antler growth is under photoperiodic control (Suttie and Kay, 1982) and gonadal hormones control the termination of growth at the initiation of rut (Wislocki et al., 1947; Goss, 1963; Lincoln et al., 1972; Goss, 1995; Bubenik et al., 1997). Estimates of ME_m of male cervids in the summer invariably include some components of energy use for antlers, tissue, and pelage, which could account for high ME_m of cervids independent of any effect due to level of food intake. Determining energy requirements for antler growth is difficult (Brown, 1990; Goss, 1995) and estimates are based on theoretical cost of deposition of organic matter in the antler using a k_g of 0.4 (Moen and Pastor, 1998). During maximum antler growth rate of ~ 2 percent/d, antlers are metabolically active (Ryg, 1983a). Energy requirements increase ~ 8.5 and 1.5 percent in males and female reindeer/caribou, respectively (Moen and Pastor 1998). The ME requirements for antlers, 21 and 4.2 kcal/kg $BW^{0.75}$, for males and for female reindeer, respectively, represent 30 and 6 percent of basal metabolic rate (BMR). The major implication of antler growth for cervids is on protein, calcium, and phosphorus requirements (Ullrey, 1982; Brown, 1990; Moen and Pastor, 1998; Bubenik et al., 2000).

Genotype

The NRC (2000) summarized findings of numerous reports with beef cattle that indicated considerable variation among genotypes in ME_m. It was concluded that ME_m is positively related to genetic potential for productivity. In this regard, adjustment factors for ME_m of many beef cattle breeds were presented, and SCA (1990) also suggested adjustments for common types of Australian cattle. Conversely, Freetly et al. (1995b, 2002b) found no differences in fasting heat production (FHP) between Suffolk and Texel and between Finnsheep and Rambouillet ewes when compared at the same proportion of mature BW, in accordance with findings of Olthoff et al. (1989) with ewes of seven breeds differing in production potential. Similarly, Cannas et al. (2004) employed one ME_m requirement in the CNCPS-S for all sheep genotypes, as is also true for INRA (1989) and NRC (1985). However, there are previous reports of differences in ME_m among sheep genotypes (Blaxter et al., 1966; Graham, 1968). Comparisons do not seem available of sheep genotypes not intensively selected for production, such as local genotypes in developing countries, with genotypes that have been selected, although there have been a number of determinations with sheep breeds of developing countries. For example, Kearl (1982) suggested use of an ME_m of 92 kcal/kg $BW^{0.75}$, which was the average of values from nine reports (including one for goats: NRC, 1981b), ranging from 73 to 110 kcal/kg $BW^{0.75}$. More recently, Nsahlai et al. (1997) estimated a ME_m for Menz sheep of the Ethiopian highlands of 101 kcal/kg $BW^{0.75}$.

In measuring FHP to evaluate effects of genotype as well as other factors, perhaps it should not necessarily be assumed that differences, or lack thereof, can be directly extrapolated to ME_m. For example, differences between beef and dairy cattle in ME_m are at least partially attributable to greater energy expenditure by splanchnic tissues of dairy cattle (NRC, 2000). With FHP typically determined after 2 days of fasting, one might expect less of a difference in energy expenditure by splanchnic tissues than in a fed state. Furthermore, effects on energy expenditure of potential differences among genotypes in rates and ratios of protein anabolism and catabolism in fed states might not be fully reflected in energy expenditure from catabolism of tissue, primarily fat, on days 3 and/or 4 of fasting.

Potential impacts of genotype on ME_m of goats were not considered by NRC (1981b), INRA (1989), AFRC (1998), or Drochner et al. (2003). Many reports with estimates of FHP and ME_m for goats were recently noted by Luo et al. (2004b,d,e), and there have been few direct comparisons of different genotypes. With a compiled database of treatment mean observations from the literature, Luo et al. (2004e) were not able to address potential differences among individual genotypes because of the large number of genotypes, as well as a low number of observations for many genotypes. Hence, genotypes were categorized into different biotypes with various selection histories that potentially could affect energy and/or protein requirements (i.e., meat, ≥ 50 percent Boer; dairy; Angora; indigenous or local; all others). A greater ME_m was determined for growing dairy than for meat and indigenous goats, similar to the magnitude of difference between dairy and beef cattle breeds (NRC, 2000). These ME_m for growing goats were then extrapolated to mature goats, assuming no effect of age on the difference in ME_m between growing biotypes (NRC, 2000). The ME_m for mature Angora goats was found to be intermediate to that for dairy vs. meat and indigenous goat biotypes. Converse to grouping of genotypes into biotypes, there have been suggestions that some specific genotypes of goats have uniquely low ME_m compared with other local or indigenous types (Silanikove, 2000); however, insufficient data are presently available to describe any differences that may exist. Perhaps adequately characterizing effects on ME_m of adaptive factors such as acclimatization and nutritional plane could account for at least a portion of potential differences among goat genotypes within biotypes.

There have been few studies addressing effects of genotype on energy metabolism in cervids, although a detailed review by Suttie and Webster (1998) indicates an indirect effect due to seasonal differences in summer vs. winter growth potential in relation to latitude. In the extreme, the tropical rusa deer shows continuous annual growth, compared with a highly seasonal summer growth in north temperate and Arctic species. Therefore, the effect of latitude needs to be considered in predicting net energy requirements for growth. No studies address whether k_g varies within or among species. Given that Suttie and Webster (1998) found no effect of season on FHP in a comparison of north temperate with Arctic cervids, it is unlikely that the many genotypes of white-tailed deer, from the northern to southern ranges of distribution, would be associated with a change in FHP or ME_m, provided that appropriate account is taken of growth potential.

Mature Size

Selection history can affect energy requirements. For example, selection for milk production has yielded a greater maintenance energy requirement for dairy vs. beef cattle breeds (NRC, 2000, 2001). Similarly, some sheep breeds have been selected for size, and so mature size is now much greater than in earlier years, such as when NRC (1985) was published. Ideally, requirements can be determined based on, or evaluated with, data from the specific animals of interest. Regardless of the availability of adequate data to do so, it is useful to consider physiologically why requirements of large sheep of today may or may not differ from smaller ones of the past, with the two primary considerations being needs of maintenance and production.

Studies by Freetly et al. (1995b, 2002b), with four breeds of sheep, are pertinent for addressing requirements for maintenance. Assuming a fasted BW of 90 percent of that unshrunk (not fasted) (Freetly et al., 2002a), estimates of mature size were 78, 61, 60, and 51 kg for Suffolk, Texel, Rambouillet, and Finnsheep, respectively. Even with these different mature sizes and widely disparate selection histories, fasting heat production by mature animals relative to $BW^{0.75}$ was similar, which was also the case for younger animals when comparisons were made at the same proportions of mature size. These findings infer that, when appropriately addressed, the maintenance energy requirement of today's large sheep do not differ appreciably from smaller ones of the past.

For growth requirements, determinants are rate of gain, composition of tissue being accreted, and efficiencies of nutrient use. As noted later, efficiencies of energy and protein use for energy and protein accretion, respectively, are assumed constant regardless of mature size and growth rate in nearly all sets of recommendations of nutrient requirements of ruminants. Hence, with accurate prediction of the composition of tissue being accreted, such as through consideration of factors like the proportion of mature size, growth rate, and/or BCS, it seems unlikely that past selection for mature size has influenced requirements for growth.

Age

Fasting heat production and ME_m are thought to decrease as animals age. NRC (1985) and INRA (1989) did not address effects of age on ME_m of sheep, although Cannas et al. (2004) used the approach of SCA (1990) for the CNCPS-S, which entails an exponential decline up to 6 years. Freetly et al. (1995b, 2002a,b) reported for sheep that expressing FHP relative to $BW^{0.75}$ resulted in a curvilinear relationship with advancing age and, thus, proposed scaling for the proportion of mature BW and an exponential function to describe FHP for four breeds of sheep. However, Freetly et al. (2002a) noted that this approach was not acceptable for sheep with a restricted nutritional plane that are proportionally smaller in their mature BW. Relatedly, although a consequence of normal production practices, lower support tissue metabolism in mature animals with intake near ME_m compared with expectantly greater levels for growing animals with higher feed intake may contribute to effects of age on FHP and ME_m.

For goats, NRC (1981b), INRA (1989), AFRC (1998), and Drochner et al. (2003) did not adjust for potential effects of age on ME_m. Luo et al. (2004d,e) addressed age by categorizing goats as growing (< 1 or 1.5 years of age) or mature. For a database of dairy and indigenous goat biotypes, ME_m was less than for growing goats. Further research is needed to describe accurately how ME_m of goats changes with advancing age.

Effects of age in cervids on ME_m have not been well studied. However, similar to other neonates (Graham et al., 1974), resting metabolic rate of preweaned fawns and calves declines per unit $BW^{0.75}$ (Wesley et al., 1973; Meissner, 1976; Weiner, 1977; Parker and Robbins, 1984; Hudson and Christopherson, 1985). In maternally raised caribou, however, a decline in daily energy expenditure in the first 3 weeks is followed by a marked increase at 60 d of age (Parker et al., 1990). Most energy requirement studies have been made on calves (fawns) during their first winter or on yearlings. Under both conditions, subject animals were fed at or near maintenance requirements based on BW gain. Metabolizable energy for maintenance is lower in white-tailed deer yearlings than fawns (Ullrey et al., 1970; Thompson et al., 1973; Holter et al., 1977).

Gender

It is commonly assumed for cattle, sheep, and goats that ME_m for females and male castrates is similar (NRC, 1981b, 1985; INRA, 1989; SCA, 1990; AFRC, 1993, 1998; NRC, 2000; Drochner et al., 2003). Even though similar ME_m for females and male castrates is a common assumption, findings of Freetly et al. (1995b, 2002a,b) imply small differences at similar BW of sheep because of differences in proportion of mature BW. However, greater (e.g., 15 percent) ME_m for intact or entire males compared with females and male castrates is frequently recommended (cattle, sheep, and goats: SCA, 1990; beef cattle: NRC, 2000; sheep: Cannas et al., 2004). INRA (1989) assumed a 10 percent difference in ME_m between intact males compared with females and male castrates. Factors responsible for such differences presumably include a higher body protein concentration in intact males (Webster, 1980; Robelin and Geay, 1984; Emmans, 1994), as well as differences in stage of maturity when compared at the same BW. A comparable difference does not seem to be recommended for goats (NRC, 1981b; AFRC, 1998; Drochner et al., 2003) or sheep (NRC, 1985). In studies by Luo et al. (2004d,e), it was not possible to address directly potential gender differences in ME_m of goats because gender was not specified in many reports and treatment mean observations in some studies were averages for different genders. Hence, Sahlu et al. (2004) suggested similar ME_m for females and male castrates and a 15 percent difference between intact males vs. females and male castrates, with the difference applied to determined requirement expressions based on the proportion of genders in the data sets.

For cervids, major differences in timing and amplitude exist in seasonal body gains made by males and females. Whereas males deposit energy and protein following greenup in spring or the wet season, most females are lactating and compensatory gain does not occur until milk production declines, approximately 6 weeks after calving. During the rutting season, food intake by male cervids is very low and a weight loss ensues, whereas for females this time is part of the period of compensatory gain. In winter or the dry season, both males and females enter an endogenously controlled maintenance period. A higher resting metabolic rate has been reported for male vs. female black-tailed deer in winter (Nordan et al., 1970), whereas no differences between genders were noted in fasting metabolic rate for white-tailed deer in summer (Silver et al., 1969) or in ME_m for mule deer fawns (Baker et al., 1979) and wapiti calves in winter (Cool and Hudson, 1996). Results for red deer are mixed, with higher estimates of ME_m for males (Brockway and Maloiy, 1968; Fennessy et al., 1981; Suttie et al., 1987) and no differences between genders (Kay and Staines, 1981). Although results of the studies on fawns and yearlings could be attributable to stage of maturity, the latter findings are not easily explained (Fennessy et al., 1981). No studies attribute sex differences to the energy cost of antler growth by males; however, many studies were made outside the antler growth period. Velvet antlers are subject to injury, which limits studies involving close confinement of males in velvet.

Body Composition

There are varied opinions and findings regarding effects of body composition or degree of fatness, commonly addressed by BCS, on ME_m. More energy is required to maintain protein than fat (Webster, 1980; Emmans, 1994); hence, all other things being equal (i.e., current plane of nutrition), one would expect ME_m per unit $BW^{0.75}$ for animals at the same proportion of mature BW to decrease with increasing body fat concentration or BCS. However, as addressed by SCA (1990), this typically has not been observed in practice. Therefore, ME_m is most often based on BW regardless of BCS. In part, this may involve more than full compensation of level of support tissue metabolism for effects of body fat and protein levels. For example, for a fat animal, heat production by peripheral tissues per unit tissue mass might indeed be lower than for a lean animal, but because of a higher plane of nutrition often associated with fatness, energy expenditure by splanchnic tissues would be greater relative to whole body mass than for a lean animal on a low nutritional plane. Hence, future experimentation should address ME_m in thin animals fed to replenish body fat and possibly protein stores, as well as fat animals with restricted planes of nutrition while mobilizing tissue.

Use of Mobilized Tissue Energy

Ruminants often experience periods of BW loss as a normal part of production cycles and in response to dry seasons. Nonetheless, efficiencies of use of mobilized tissue energy for maintenance as well as other functions such as gestation, lactation, and fiber growth have received much less research attention than use of dietary energy. SCA (1990) assumed a constant efficiency of mobilized tissue energy use for maintenance (k_{mt}) of 0.80 for cattle, sheep, and goats. Cannas et al. (2004) assumed a similar k_{mt} and efficiency of use of mobilized tissue energy for lactation (k_{lt}) for sheep.

One of the most important factors influencing or at least highly related to the efficiency with which ME is used for maintenance or production is the ME concentration in the diet, possibly in regards to its impact on splanchnic tissue energy expenditure and/or the array of nutrients absorbed. In many instances, tissue is mobilized with high to moderate feed intake, such as in early lactation or with consumption of low-quality diets, suggesting that diet effects on k_{mt} or k_{lt} would not necessarily be negligible compared with times when recovered energy (RE) is zero or positive. Hence, for goats, Luo et al. (2004c) assumed k_{mt} to be the same as k_m, which varied with metabolizability as estimated by AFRC (1998). Appropriateness of such an assumption would seem strengthened by coupling of decreases in ME_m with low nutritional planes and/or BCS, as proposed by Sahlu et al. (2004) for goats. Research is needed to evaluate the accuracy of decreasing ME_m for low feed intake directly or indirectly based on BCS and also assuming very high and/or constant k_{mt}.

Tissue energy concentration is a factor that affects prediction of potential energy available from mobilized tissue for maintenance or other functions. Most systems assume energy concentration to be the same for accreted and mobilized tissue at a particular proportion of mature weight (e.g., SCA, 1990; NRC, 2000, 2001). Although this assumption may not always be valid (Aziz et al., 1994), more accurate means of prediction are not currently available. A common method to assess body energy concentration is via BCS. In this regard, Sanson et al. (1993) reported relationships between BCS (scaled 1 to 9, with 1 being emaciated and 9 extremely obese) of mature western range ewes and empty body (EB) composition, which resulted in body fat and protein concentrations at different BCS very similar to those of NRC (2000, 2001) for beef and dairy cattle. The equation for EB protein mass (percent) was: $21.14 - (0.71 \times BCS)$, and that for EB fat mass (percent) was: $0.82 + (3.66 \times BCS)$. The CNCPS-S (Cannas et al., 2004) uses an equation to predict EB fat developed by Russel et al. (1969), where BCS is scaled from 0 to 5 (EB fat, fraction = $0.0269 + (0.0869 \times BCS)$), and an equation for EB protein based on the assumption of a similar ratio of EB fat:protein for different BCS in sheep and cattle (EB protein = $0.1449 + (0.0279 \times BCS) - (0.0039 \times BCS^2)$). Body composition predictions from these equations of Sanson et al. (1993) and Cannas et al. (2004) are given for various BCS in Table 4-1. Assumed heats of combustion were 9.4 and 5.55 Mcal/kg for fat and protein, respectively. The considerable differences in composition between these equations are most likely functions of breed-specific and variable relationships between body fat and BCS and the lack of broader data sets to develop prediction equations. Although comparable data are not available for goats, several reports (Ash and Norton, 1987; Alam et al., 1991; Wuliji et al., 2003a,b) suggest a range in fat concentration similar to that reported by Sanson et al. (1993).

For cervids, BCS as an in vivo measurement of body fat has been verified in a limited number of species (Gerhart et. al., 1996a). For reindeer and caribou, a score of 1 to 5 (1 = emaciated, 5 = obese) based on palpation is made for

TABLE 4-1 Predicted Empty Body Concentrations of Fat, Protein, and Energy in Sheep from Body Condition Score (BCS) Based on Equations of Sanson et al. (1993) and Cannas et al. (2004)

Equation	BCS	% Fat	% Protein	Mcal/kg
Sanson et al. (1993)	1	4.5	20.4	1.55
	3	11.8	19.0	2.16
	5	19.1	17.6	2.77
	7	26.4	16.2	3.38
	9	33.8	14.8	3.99
Cannas et al. (2004)	0	2.7	14.5	1.06
	1	11.4	16.9	2.01
	2	20.1	18.5	2.91
	3	28.8	19.4	3.78
	4	37.5	19.4	4.60
	5	46.1	18.7	5.37

the rump, ribs, and withers and summed to give a range of 3–15, which was associated with variation of ~ 2 to > 15 percent body fat (Gerhart et al., 1996a). Although quantified for reindeer/caribou, the BCS is considered a qualitative measure giving limited precision (Parker, 2003), as are other forms of condition assessment (Hundertmark and Schwartz, 1998; Cook et al., 2001a,b; Stephenson et al., 2002). Despite its limited application in lean animals of < 4 percent body fat, but because backfat thickness is linearly related to body fat (Reimers et al., 1982; Stephenson et al., 1998; Cook et al., 2001b), back fat measurements made with ultrasound are the preferred tool for assessing body condition in cervids (Keech et. al., 1998; Stephenson et. al., 1998; Stein et. al., 2003). Use of body reserves to support energy requirements for maintenance, gestation, and lactation occurs in north temperate cervids as a product of endogenous regulation of inappetance and inanition as a product of environmental factors (Tyler et al., 1999). Isotopic studies indicate that although females catabolize dietary carbon and nitrogen in preference to endogenous fat and protein (Parker et al., 2005) during winter, most females and males lose weight, mainly as fat, but also about 30 percent of body protein can be mobilized (Reimers et al., 1982; Torbit et al., 1985; Huot, 1989; Gerhart et al., 1996b). Fat mobilization appears highest in the fattest females, and nonpregnant females mobilize more fat than those that are pregnant (Dauphiné, 1976; Mitchell et al., 1976; Ryg, 1983b; Hudson et al., 1985; Tyler, 1987; Renecker and Samuel, 1991; Cameron and White, 1996; Chan-McLeod et al., 1999). Further, most protein in fetuses is derived from maternal protein reserves (Barboza and Parker, 2006), and birth weight is related to maternal protein reserves, at least in caribou (Adamczewski et al., 1987). In general, fat content (Y, percent) of the fat + protein loss increases with the content of fat in the animal (X, percent); Y = (100 × X)/(4 + X) (Robbins, 1993). Assumed heats of combustion are 9.4 and 5.55 Mcal/kg oxidation of fat and protein, respectively; however, because of the mixed use of fat and protein and recycling of protein-N through the urea cycle, the usual range in energy content of mobilized tissue is 2–6 Mcal/kg (Robbins, 1993). Parker et al. (2005) showed that during weight loss, dietary carbon and nitrogen were catabolized in preference to endogenous body reserves, whereas maternal stores appeared a preferred source for fetal development (Barboza and Parker, 2006). For calculation purposes k_m for use of this mobilized energy is 0.82, higher than that based on metabolizable energy intake (MEI) (0.64–0.75: Hudson and Christopherson, 1985).

Activity

A factor that can have a marked effect on the energy requirement is activity (HjE). This cost is usually added to or considered part of ME_m. Perhaps because of the difficulty of study, common means of predicting the energy cost of activity for cattle, sheep, and goats do not seem to be firmly based on much data, and accuracy of predictions on a daily basis has not been thoroughly evaluated.

The NRC (1985) did not address energy expenditure due to activity (HjE) for sheep. For goats, NRC (1981b) recommended the addition of 25 percent of the suggested ME_m requirement with light activity, 50 percent with semi-arid rangeland and slightly hilly conditions, and 75 percent with sparsely vegetated rangeland or mountainous transhumace pasture. The AFRC (1998) suggested that HjE was 10 percent of FHP (10 percent of 75.3 kcal/kg $BW^{0.75}$) for stall-fed goats, with additional grazing costs based on horizontal movement (0.837 cal/(kg BW × m)), vertical movement (6.69 cal/(kg BW × m)), standing (100 cal/(kg BW × h)), and change in position (62.1 cal/(kg BW × number of changes)), and then application of k_m. These values were based primarily on reports of ARC (1980) with sheep and of Lachica et al. (1997) with goats on a treadmill placed at different slopes. Also, in the CNCPS-S, Cannas et al. (2004) proposed for grazing animals only basing HjE on flat and sloped distances traveled by sheep, with ARC (1980) costs of movement. The SCA (1990) presented a prediction equation with independent variables of dry matter (DM) digestibility, terrain score, availability of green or total forage, and BW. The NRC (2001) proposed a summative method for dairy cattle considering energy expended in three grazing functions: (1) distance walked at 454 cal/(kg BW × km) (ARC, 1980), (2) eating at 3.01 kcal/kg BW, and (3) topography or vertical ascent at 30.1 kcal/km vertical distance. Although travel should indeed affect HjE, Sahlu et al. (2004) discussed the merit of considering time spent grazing or spent grazing and walking, with the latter perhaps being more easy to assess by livestock producers. Consequently, a HjE prediction system for goats was proposed for future evaluation, with major impact of time spent grazing plus walking but also influences of herbage digestibility, distance traveled, and terrain ruggedness or topography, yielding adjustments in line with the few relevant measures available in the literature.

The activity energy cost for wild herbivores may be greater than for sheep and goats because of extensive searching for food (Robbins, 1993), predator avoidance, and daily or seasonal migration (Fancy and White, 1985a,b). Energy used for activity by cervids has been studied using a combination of summation of activity costs based on activity budgets (Fancy and White, 1985a; Robbins, 1993; Russell et al., 1993; Parker et al., 1996), combined with grazing activity, and intake based on bite-counts (Swift, 1983; Boertje, 1985; Hudson and White, 1985; Hobbs, 1989; Parker et al., 1996; Moen et al., 1997, 1998; Moen and Pastor, 1998; Russell et al., 2005). However, there have been few comparisons of estimates of energy expenditure and MEI directly to determine seasonal energy balance (Parker et al., 1996, 1999). In addition, these independent estimates should be compared with daily energy expenditure (DEE) based on doubly labeled water.

Determinations of DEE have been made for confined reindeer and caribou (Fancy et al., 1986; Parker et al., 1990; Haggarty, 2000), natural free-ranging reindeer (Gotaas et al., 2000; Haggarty, 2000), red deer (Haggarty et al., 1998), and black-tailed deer (Parker et al., 1993, 1999). Use of doubly labeled water for red deer (Haggarty et al., 1998) and reindeer (Gotaas et al., 2000; Haggarty, 2000) has indicated that HjE increases energy requirements by ~ 64 percent over confined/penned animals. Most factorial estimates of energy expenditure and HjE of the free-ranging cervid are in good agreement with those determined by doubly labeled water (Gotaas et al., 2000). Extrapolation from pen-feeding studies, and some model outputs (Boertje, 1985; Cool and Hudson, 1996), suggest that HjE for the field is 20–33 percent greater than in pens (Gotaas et al., 2000; Haggarty, 2000). This latter estimate is thought to be too low (Gotaas et al., 2000). When comparison is made of ME intake in relation to change in BW of red deer and wapiti hinds and stags held outdoors, a comparison of ME_m suggests an increase of 45–49 percent in winter and 63–72 percent in summer with a mean of 60 percent (Fennessey et al., 1981; Suttie et al., 1987; Jiang and Hudson, 1992; Wairimu et al., 1992; Haigh and Hudson, 1993). Thus, the preferred estimated increase in field cost or outdoor cost is 60–64 percent. For domestic sheep, the experimentally determined increase in ME_m requirement is 60–70 percent greater for grazing vs. housed sheep held at maintenance (Young and Corbett, 1972). Energy costs of locomotory activity of unrestrained cervids are thought to be responsible for these differences (Gotaas et al., 2000).

Season

None of the current energy requirement systems for sheep and goats recommends an adjustment of ME_m for season or photoperiod. Any such effects would therefore be assumed to be attributable to changes in other factors influencing ME_m, such as level of feed intake, acclimatization, and climatic extremes. However, NRC (2000) reviewed data showing differences among seasons in FHP and/or ME_m for cattle and also other ruminants. Although all reports cited were not in perfect agreement, the most consistent findings were lower FHP and/or ME_m in the fall and higher values in the summer. Nonetheless, observed differences were not substantial, and no adjustments were recommended. Further research in this area for seasonal breeders such as sheep and goats at different latitudes could lead to adjustment of ME_m requirements for season.

In contrast to sheep and goats, a seasonal adjustment in ME_m is recommended for north temperate cervids, including white-tailed deer, red deer, reindeer/caribou, and elk/wapiti. These adjustments possibly could be made using level of feed intake (e.g., Weber and Thompson, 1998, for fallow deer), but sufficient research has not been conducted to verify the efficacy of such adjustments. As discussed above, except for moose (Regelin et al., 1985) and muskoxen (Nilssen et al., 1994), fasting metabolic rate tends to be unaffected by season, and, therefore, a seasonal change in ME_m would be unexpected. However, a summary of estimates suggests that daily ME_m in winter is less than in summer by ~ 45 kcal/kg $BW^{0.75}$ (white-tailed deer: Thompson et al., 1973; Holter et al., 1977; red deer: Simpson et al., 1978a). A complex interaction between intrinsic changes in endocrinology, appetite, behavior, digestibility (Suttie and Webster, 1995, 1998; Tyler et al., 1999; Rhind et al., 2002), and contribution of pelage growth are potential factors that contribute to an increase in ME_m in summer and autumn. In reviewing this field, Parker (2003) stressed the requirement for more controlled studies in wildlife species.

Acclimatization

Acclimatization in the context of ME_m refers to adaptation in energy expenditure to change in climatic conditions. It is difficult to assess the need to consider potential effects of acclimatization on ME_m given the variable behavioral responses animals use to avoid extreme heat and cold conditions, such as seeking and use of shade, windbreaks, high open areas with wind on hot days, and vice versa. Furthermore, the concept of a thermoneutral "zone," rather than one particular comfort temperature, may question the logic for adjustment with actual temperature not greatly deviating from the midpoint of the thermoneutral zone. Nonetheless, some common energy requirement systems do include adjustments of ME_m for acclimatization.

Based on NRC (1981a), NRC (2000) recommended an adjustment of the net energy (NE) for maintenance (NE_m) requirement for acclimatization based on the average temperature in the previous 30 days and the midpoint thermoneutral zone temperature, which was set at 20°C. Similar adjustments were recommended for cattle, sheep, and goats by SCA (1990) and for sheep by Cannas et al. (2004). Sahlu et al. (2004) also suggested the same adjustment for goats, but stressed its optional nature and that the appropriate midpoint thermoneutral zone temperature might be different than 20°C for various types of goats and climates.

As noted before, caution should be exercised when directly extrapolating recommendations derived from data from one ruminant species to others, which seems pertinent to effects of acclimatization on ME_m of sheep and goats. In accordance, future research may lead to appropriate adjustments, or lack of a need, for various genotypes of sheep and goats in the wide array of climates in which they are reared.

An additional factor for cervids is thermal conductance, which changes seasonally. Thermal conductance is lowest when cervids are in winter coat (Scholander et al., 1950; Ryder, 1977; Parker and Robbins, 1984, 1985; Renecker and Hudson, 1986), but conductance can be increased by wetting due to rain (Parker, 1988; Cuyler and Øritsland, 2004), which could become critical to survival of the newborns of some species (Hart et al., 1961; Alexander, 1962; Markussen et al., 1985). Whole body conductance changes markedly when animals stand or become active (Gates and Hudson, 1979). Thus, estimates of lower critical temperature (T_{lc}) vary between species and in response to feeding. For reindeer/caribou, the T_{lc} is less than –30°C (Tyler and Blix, 1990); excursions to ambient temerature (T_a) < T_{lc} that occur in the Arctic could become stressful when associated with extreme wind. Although energy expenditure associated with increased feed intake, the heat increment, substitutes for thermogenic heat production and lowers T_{lc}, substitution is not complete or can be insufficient to meet thermoregulatory costs (Gates and Hudson, 1979; Jensen et al., 1999). The heat increment can, however, reduce the T_{lc} by approximately 10°C in white-tailed deer and mule deer (Moen, 1968a,b; Gates and Hudson, 1979; Parker and Robbins, 1984; Jensen et al., 1999). For young red deer, thermal conductance is not as well established as in other species, and T_{lc} is such that in northern winters, they frequently may need to mobilize both fat and protein to meet cold-induced thermogenesis (Simpson et al., 1978b).

The extent to which canopy cover contributes as a thermal cover or decreases solar radiation is complex and difficult to model to predict acclimatization effects, particularly in forest systems. Whereas dense forest cover may reduce heat loss (Moen, 1968a; Parker, 1988; Parker and Gillingham, 1990; Demarchi and Bunnell, 1993) and reduce winter mortality of deer (Armstrong et al., 1983; Ockenfels and Brooks, 1994), most studies agree that supply of adequate food is more important for responding to cold (Moen, 1968a; Swift et al., 1980; Hobbs, 1989; Gillingham et al., 1997). For elk, Cook et al. (1998) have shown negative effects of thermal cover on fat loss, and positive effects were related to an increase in solar radiation associated with low or zero thermal cover. In lieu of empirical studies, modeling and regression analysis has been used to predict effect of the thermal environment on energy requirements of cervids (Moen, 1976; Beaver et al., 1996); however, prediction of the critical thermal environment for deer is a complex challenge (Parker and Robbins, 1984, 1985; Parker, 1988; Hobbs, 1989; Parker and Gillingham, 1990; Cook et al., 1998) and modeling the effect on ME_m is not feasible except as an experimental or modeling exercise. Although studies with sheep and cattle show an increase in ME_m in response to chronic resistance to cold, winter acclimatization, or cold acclimation within the thermoneutral zone (Webster et al., 1969, 1970; Young, 1975), no equivalent response has been demonstrated for cervids.

Although the microenvironment defines the heat loss of the animal (Moen, 1968b; Parker and Gillingham, 1990; Parker and Robbins, 1984, 1985) and provisioning of shelter from wind and rain/sleet in winter is advocated, the lack of direct linkage between cover and protection from wind and winter performance (Cook et al., 1998) suggests that behavioral responses in habitat use may have more to do with hiding from predators and location of feeding sites (Swift et al., 1980; Hobbs, 1989). An exception to the lower importance of shelter to survival could involve behavioral responses of nursery groups. Although nursery pairs use other group members to seek an ameliorated microenvironment for neonates in open habitats (Moen, 1973; Gates and Hudson, 1979), an extensive review of data on barren-ground caribou by Miller and Gunn (1986) indicated that calf mortality due to adverse weather is more speculative than documented. These authors suggested, however, that calves from poorly nourished, underweight females could succumb under adverse weather. During the first hours of life, survival is assured by drying of the birthcoat by shivering and nonshivering thermogenesis, the latter supported by widely distributed brown adipose tissue (Blix and Steen, 1979; Wika and Krog, 1980; Soppela et al., 1991). Following birth and during the drying period, a high, normal, deep body temperature is established. Well-developed thermoregulation is supported by an insulative birthcoat when dry, heterothermy of the extremities, nonshivering thermogenesis, and metabolic intermediates take place (Lentz and Hart, 1960; Hart et al., 1961; Blix and Steen, 1979; Hissa et al., 1981; Nieminen et al., 1984; Timisjärvi et al., 1984; Soppela et al., 1986a,b, 1991). Newborn cervids, as exemplified by studies with reindeer and caribou, can respond with minimal thermogenic heat production to ambient temperatures as low as –10°C, and a well-established T_{lc} as low as –30°C by 3 weeks (Soppela et al., 1986a,b). Heat loss is dependent on surface area, which is highly related to BW in the young (Moen, 1973; Parker, 1987, 1989). Thus, species differences in whole body conductivity would be expected due to BW and the surface area–BW relation. Parker (1989) showed for offspring at 30 kg BW in winter, the surface area of caribou, 1.097 m^2, is 10 percent less than white-tailed deer, mule deer, and elk/wapiti at 1.209 m^2 (Moen, 1973; Parker, 1987).

Although winter cold resistance in cervids is based on low whole body conductance, a regulated hypometabolism also would conserve energy. Arnold et al. (2003) reported a nocturnal hypometabolism associated with a circadian decrease in deep body temperature in the red deer. Hypometabolism, measured as a 60 percent reduction in nadir heart rate in winter compared with that for summer, was also associated with peripheral cooling and a decrease in subcutaneous skin temperature of the side-back, to < 32°C. The effect occurred in animals both at rest and during locomotion, suggesting a sliding deep body temperature and regulation of energy metabolism more like hibernation than the current model for ruminants based on a defended body temperature that may be 1–2°C lower in winter than summer. Because no estimate of the seasonal energy savings was made by Arnold et al. (2003), the finding warrants further documentation and quantification for estimation of ME_m.

Heat and Cold Extremes

Both extreme heat and cold conditions can affect ME_m. However, because of the difficulty of study, there are no well-based prediction systems in place to address effects of heat stress apart from the general recommendation of NRC (1981a) based on the type and intensity of panting. Conversely, methods are available to address cold stress, although some include a large number of inputs that users may be unsure of, thus limiting these methods' practicality and extensiveness of use. Prediction systems of SCA (1990) for cattle, sheep, and goats, of the CNCPS-S for sheep, and of NRC (1981a) for all domesticated ruminant species consider insulation as affected by external and skin or tissue characteristics, rain, wind, solar radiation, evaporative heat loss, and lower critical and effective ambient temperatures. For goats, Sahlu et al. (2004) suggested use of the NRC (1981a) system as described for beef cattle by NRC (2000), with appropriate changes in inputs for species differences.

Unseasonable extreme heat is more of a problem for cervids in heavy winter coat than in summer. Likewise, unseasonably cold weather in early summer (see Weiner, 1977; Parker and Robbins, 1984; Mautz et al., 1992) can increase energy expenditure, and animals can visibly shiver. In the field, however, it is assumed that behavioral adjustments occur to minimize these effects (Parker, 2003). The report by Simpson et al. (1978b) suggested this might not always be possible for young cervids.

Parasitism

Because of the interrelated nature of protein and energy metabolism, internal parasitism affects energy as well as protein or amino acid requirements (Adams and Liu, 2003; Sykes and Greer, 2003). Although effects on ME_m have not yet been well quantified in regard to levels and types of parasitism, the impact of internal parasitism is thought to involve a decrease in k_m as a result of increased turnover of gastrointestinal tract protein, apart from frequent occurrences of reduced feed intake (Liu et al., 2003; Sykes and Greer, 2003). Sykes (1994) indicated that the immune responses to internal and external parasites could have nutritional costs as high as 15 percent of maintenance needs, which is supported by decreased wool growth by sheep selected for resistance to internal parasitism (Adams and Liu, 2003; Sykes and Greer, 2003). Liu et al. (2003) calculated an example cost of internal parasitism equivalent to 5 percent of ME_m, which was accompanied by a relatively greater increase in the requirement for metabolizable protein. Hence, it would seem that diet changes to increase the supply of metabolizable protein with subclinical internal parasitism, in order to meet performance targets, would be accompanied by an increase in MEI greater than the increase in ME_m from the infection. Correspondingly, the degree to which the increase in metabolizable protein requirements with subclinical internal parasitism limits performance should be greater than the change in need for ME.

Although internal parasites are thought to affect wildlife populations to the extent they influence population dynamics of the hosts (Anderson and May, 1978), possibly depressing host reproduction and survival (Gulland, 1995), few experimental studies confirm such effects (Albon et al., 2002), even though levels of infection at the end of winter and spring (Halvorsen et al., 1999) suggest the possibility of an effect on protein and energy metabolism. Since the influence of high infestation may be on both metabolism and appetite, accounting for effects of parasites on survival and productivity is confounded by climate and forage biomass and quality. Progress is being made by combining field experimentation and simulation modeling to account for effects of pasture contamination, parasite fecundity, and host density on infection (Stein et al., 2002). Cervids also are affected seasonally by external parasites such as mosquitoes (*Aedes* ssp), biting flies (*Simuliidae*), nasal bot flies (*Cephenomya trombe*), and warble flies (*Oedemagena tarandi*) that influence nutrient requirements directly through blood loss (Zhigunov, 1968), energy and protein costs of immune responses, and energy costs of responding behaviorally to minimize parasite infection rates (Reimers, 1980; White, 1983; Russell et al., 1993). Therefore, energy and protein costs of external parasites may adversely influence postnatal growth rates (Helle and Tarvainen, 1984) and compensatory growth of free-ranging adults (Cameron et al., 2005).

GROWTH

Diet

Because of the appreciable influence of diet characteristics on k_g, diet metabolizability has a larger effect on growth rate than DM intake required to satisfy ME_m. One factor that may contribute to lower k_m, and particularly k_g, for forage vs. concentrate-based diets is the higher ratio of acetate:propionate in ruminal fluid with forage diets. This can also apply to differences among forages in characteristics such as soluble carbohydrate concentration (Corbett and Freer,

2003). Propionate can increase efficiency of metabolism through conversion to glucose, thus providing NADPH for fat synthesis, and potentially sparing amino acids from use in glucose synthesis. Also, high soluble carbohydrate levels in forages may result in greater efficiency of microbial protein synthesis compared with lower levels (Corbett and Freer, 2003). However, recently there has been interest in effects of the nature of the diet on energy expenditure by the gut and liver. Relative to energy absorption, forage-based diets result in greater splanchnic tissue energy use than diets composed largely of concentrate, and this difference is likely to be less with low intakes for maintenance than with higher levels required for appreciable tissue gain (Goetsch, 1998; Williams and Jenkins, 2003). Lastly, though the nature of involved physiological processes responsible for the relationship is not well agreed upon, metabolizability influences not only k_m and k_g, but also level of intake. That is, diets of low metabolizability elicit high energy expenditure relative to MEI and limit potential MEI as well.

Diet has a major effect of growth rates in cervids, through milk production (Yates et al., 1971; Dove and Freer, 1979; Dove, 1988; White and Luick, 1984; Landete-Castillejos et al., 2001) and diet once forestomach development is completed (Knott et al., 2004, 2005). Studies to date have not determined k_g; therefore, values for sheep (ARC, 1980; NRC, 1985) have been assumed. In the first and subsequent winters, growth is minimal to negative in young and adult north temperate cervids (Wood et al., 1962; McEwan, 1968; Bandy et al., 1970; Reimers, 1972; Blaxter et al., 1974; Kay, 1979; Tyler and Blix, 1990; Worden and Pekins, 1995; Finstad and Pritchard, 2000) and the amplitude increases with age to at least 6 years in red deer (Blaxter et al., 1974). In cervids less than 6 years of age, the ratio of winter to summer growth is highly dependent on both the latitude of origin of the species, and also the current latitude, with greatest effects associated with latitude >50° north or south (Suttie and Webster, 1995, 1998).

Seasonal growth propensity is voluntary, with no apparent reduction in digestive efficiency during seasonal hyperphagia (Peltier et al., 2003). The seasonal endogenous down-regulation of BW occurs 4–7 weeks before a concurrent down-regulation in voluntary food intake (McMahon et al., 1997; Weber and Thompson, 1998). Estimates of ME_m for the autumn and winter periods of calves and summer for yearlings indicate a seasonal ranking of yearling summer > calf autumn > calf winter (Holter et al., 1977). Under some field conditions, these clearly documented changes in BW of pen-fed animals (Holter et al., 1977; Suttie, 1980; Schwartz et al., 1987; Clutton-Brock and Albon, 1989; Worden and Pekins, 1995) may be observed in the field (Tyler, 1987; Tyler and Blix, 1990; Finstad and Pritchard, 2000), but also may be dampened or less discernible (Anderson et al., 1974; Russell et al., 1996), presumably due to diet and other environmental effects.

Control of growth rate of female calves/fawns in the first winter and spring can be affected by dietary protein content (Nieminen et al., 1980; Eilertsen et al., 2001); however, this is a variable response (Nieminen et al., 1987) and is not the case for red deer stags (McMahon et al., 1997). In subsequent years, changing dietary protein level rarely increases BW gain, and very high protein in spring pastures can only be used at the expense of body fat reserves (Eilertsen et al., 2001). Most dietary effects are realized through influence on BW loss in winter. However, winter BW gains are reported for white-tailed deer (Ullrey et al., 1969), mule deer (Renecker and Samuel, 1991), and reindeer (Nilssen et al., 2000; Fauchald et al., 2004). In captive cervids, overwinter change in BW is negatively correlated with peak BW in autumn (Renecker and Samuel, 1991). The autumn BW, at which no change in overwinter BW occurs, can be considered a set point BW; thus, only those deer that enter winter with BW less than set point BW made BW gains. Those young entering winter with BW in excess of the set point lose weight in proportion to the difference from the set point. Likewise, Hudson et al. (1985) and Wairimu et al. (1992) for wapiti and Renecker and Samuel (1991) for mule deer showed that oversummer BW gain was greatest in deer with lowest BW in spring. These studies were made with captive animals consuming ad libitum on aspen parklands. Whether this compensatory growth can occur in summer probably depends on ecological conditions in the wild, as discussed for reindeer by Reimers (1983) and for red deer by Suttie (1980). Although wapiti show compensatory growth on aspen parklands (Watkins et al., 1991), for Arctic caribou, compensatory gain in summer could be documented for nonlactating females in one herd (Cameron and White, 1996), and the trend in an adjacent herd was not significant (Russell et al., 1996).

Body Composition—Stage of Maturity, Growth Rate, and Level of Intake

A key determinant of k_g and the ME requirement per unit of mass (i.e., BW change) is the composition of the tissue accreted. Energetically, it is more efficient to accrete fat than protein in part because of greater daily turnover of protein than fat, thereby necessitating greater synthesis per unit of protein accretion. However, because of the higher concentration of water in proteinaceous vs. adipose tissue, on a mass or ADG basis, gain of protein is more efficient. Therefore, on a BW mass basis, k_g declines and ME_g increases as stage of maturity rises. As growth rate and feed intake increase, the proportion of fat in accreted tissues increases while that of protein decreases. This might be expected to have effects on k_g and ME_g similar to those of increasing stage of maturity, although this may be countered by other physiological conditions responsible for decreasing efficiency of energy use as level of feed intake approaches ad libitum (Tolkamp and Ketelaars, 1992). The importance of these effects decreases as stage of maturity increases and ADG declines, and is also minimal when at a very low proportion of mature BW and physiologically there is little potential for fat deposition. With a higher plane of nutrition subsequent to a low one with limited ADG, the composition of tissue accreted may be different than that previously, the magnitude and nature of which depend on the character, length, and severity of the previous nutritional restriction (Drouillard et al., 1991; Wuliji et al., 2003a). But, though accreted tissue composition during compensatory growth may be indeed altered, this is not thought to be primarily responsible for greater than expected ADG. In general, compensatory growth seems to be a function of greater than expected feed intake given the nature of the diet and animal and/or decreased ME_m. Alterations in ME_m seem due at least partially to decreased energy expenditure by metabolically active splanchnic tissues, but reduced energy expenditure by peripheral tissues is possible as well. Although change with time has not been thoroughly characterized, the extent to which feed intake is greater than expected and ME_m is less than expected gradually decline.

For species having sufficient available data (i.e., cattle and sheep) and with use of NE, established equations are used to predict the energy concentration of BW gain based on factors such as rate of live (full or unshrunk) or empty BW gain, BCS, stage of maturity, frame score, and/or genotype classification (SCA, 1990; NRC, 2000; Cannas et al., 2004). The k_g value is assumed constant and estimated based on the ME or NE_m concentration in the diet. There are presently insufficient data available to develop means of predicting the energy concentration in tissue gain by goats. Hence, because the ME_g requirements for goats of Luo et al. (2004d,e) were determined based on BW gain and did not consider the composition of tissue gain, their accuracy should be less at extreme than typical energy or protein and fat concentrations in tissue being gained. Presently, however, the feeding of high-energy diets to goats produced for meat with harvest at high stages of maturity and degrees of fatness is not common. This suggests relatively less variation in energy concentration of accreted tissue of goats in most prevalent production systems compared with cattle and sheep.

Most estimates of ME_g requirements for cervids have been made in summer on young animals when the main proportion of gain is protein (Holter et al., 1977; Jiang and Hudson, 1992). The ME_g increases ME intake by 29–38 percent (Thompson et al., 1973; Holter et al., 1977) and ME_g is 3.8–8.8 kcal/g ADG (Jiang and Hudson, 1992; Wairimu et al., 1992). There are apparently no measurements on ME_g requirements during the seasonal BW gain or fattening period in adults. In studies on summer growth rate of fawns and calves, and of yearlings, good quality artificial diets support about the same maximum growth rates as under natural conditions. In the first summer, this growth largely reflects milk intake (Robbins et al., 1981; Loudon and Kay, 1984; White and Luick, 1984; White, 1992), which is a function of maternal condition and BW (Lenvik et al., 1988), as well as feed quality and availability (Landete-Castillejos et al., 2000). Thus, maternal body condition and BW strongly influence offspring ADG (ADG, g/d = 0.0721 × g $BW^{0.71}$: Robbins et al., 1981; Robbins, 1993), especially in relation to spring BW of females less than 5 years of age (Lenvik et al., 1988). Whether animals are gaining or losing BW, the energy content of the gain is needed to calculate feed requirements. Energy content of the gain of growing animals shows a curvilinear increase with BW to peak mature BW (Robbins, 1993). For white-tailed deer, protein content of the gain remains fairly constant, increasing from 20 percent near birth to 23 percent near maturity (Robbins, 1993). Energy content of the overwinter fat loss (Y kcal/g) is highly related to fat content of the BW loss (X, %): $Y = 1.47 + (0.07 \times X)$ (Robbins, 1993). Thus, energy content increases from 2 kcal (8.4 kJ)/g when 10 percent of the BW loss is fat to about 6 kcal (25 kJ)/g when 60 percent of the BW loss is fat. Under these conditions, the k_g used is that recommended for deer (0.50, range 0.35–0.60: Simpson et al., 1978a; Jiang and Hudson 1992, 1994) and is similar to sheep.

Gender and Genotype

Potential effects of gender on energy requirements for growth appear primarily or solely functions of differences in body composition. That is, little or no differences would exist if evaluated at the same proportion of mature BW and BCS. The same may be true for comparisons of genotypes, although contributions of potential differences in the ratio of protein anabolism:catabolism have not been extensively studied in small ruminants.

Array of Absorbed Nutrients

Diet influences k_g and the composition of tissue gain through an effect on rate of growth. However, the array of nutrients absorbed, as affected by the nature of the diet, can impact the composition of tissue gain independent of the effect of diet on ADG. For example, Wuliji et al. (2003a) noted similar ADG by growing Spanish goats, but less carcass and noncarcass fat with a dehydrated alfalfa diet compared with one having a moderate to high level of concentrate. Such findings may be most relevant to production systems not necessarily terminating in feeding of high-concentrate "finishing" diets. As noted before, currently few goats are fed high-grain diets, typically with marketing at relatively low proportions of mature BW and slow relative ADG compared with cattle and sheep in the United States.

Systems of Expression

Net energy systems for growing/finishing animals are preferred to ones based on digestible energy (DE), total digestible nutrients (TDN), or ME. However, these advantages are truly realized only with adequate data available to predict accurately energy concentration in tissue gain, k_m, and

k_g. But, as noted earlier, there are very few serial slaughter studies available with goats, and the same applies to determinations of k_m and k_g (Sahlu et al., 2004). However, Sahlu et al. (2004) proposed adjusting the estimate of DM intake necessary to achieve required levels of MEI for proportions of MEI being used for maintenance and gain based on differences among diets in k_m and k_g. This yielded intake estimates adjusted for diet effects on efficiencies of ME utilization, but that do not account for variation in energy concentration in accreted tissue.

LACTATION

Diet

Higher k_l than k_g may partially relate to the relatively lower mass of tissue contributing to RE that must be maintained by lactating vs. growing/finishing animals, thereby resulting in a relatively lower energy turnover:synthesis ratio for lactation. Another reason for differences in efficiencies relates to the complexity of biochemical transformation in tissues that are being synthesized. Moreover, the contribution of lactose to energy in milk and relatively less energy in protein in milk than in accreted tissue by growing animals in many instances may be involved in high k_l relative to k_g. Less effect of diet quality on k_l than k_g could reflect a difference in the impact of the array of nutrients absorbed on milk synthesis vs. tissue accretion.

There are differences among energy requirement systems in how k_l is addressed. The NRC (2000, 2001), for beef and dairy cattle, assumed that k_l is similar to k_m and, therefore, that one efficiency can be used for both functions. Conversely, many other systems employ k_l sufficiently less than k_m to warrant a separate accounting. For example, MAFF (1984), SCA (1990), Cannas et al. (2004), and Nsahlai et al. (2004a) assumed k_l to be constant regardless of dietary ME concentration, although INRA (1989) and AFRC (1993, 1998) varied k_l in accordance with metabolizability of the diet. However, Sahlu et al. (2004) listed adjustment factors for dietary DM required to provide the determined ME requirement of Nsahlai et al. (2004a) based on the dietary ME concentration and proportions of MEI used for maintenance and lactation, but values differed little from 1.

For cervids, no estimates of k_l have been made, and k_l is assumed to equal k_m with no adjustment for ME concentration. One study with reindeer and caribou addressed NE_g during lactation, which was only 8 percent higher than in animals that were not lactating (Chan-McLeod et al., 1994). The higher NE_g of lactating animals was associated with deposition of fat and only a slight positive deposition of lean body mass (mainly protein). Since both lactating and nonlactating reindeer were growing antlers and pelage, differences attributable to lactation should not be confounded by costs of antler and hair growth.

Level of Production and Stage of Lactation

The efficiency of energy use for lactation is normally assumed to be constant across production levels and stages of lactation both for energy systems in which ME_m is presumed constant (NRC, 1985, 2001; INRA, 1989; AFRC, 1998) and to vary with BCS (NRC, 2000) or level of intake for production relative to ME_m (SCA, 1990). Consequences of an assumed constant k_l may be relatively minor because of changes in energy expenditure by splanchnic tissues. For example, in early lactation, energy use by the liver may be greater than expected based on MEI as a result of nutrient processing associated with tissue mobilization; in late lactation, energy consumption by visceral tissues can be greater than anticipated from milk yield because of tissue energy accretion.

Under pen-feeding conditions, the lactation curve for cervids increases from parturition to 3–6 weeks postpartum, followed by an exponential decline to weaning (McEwan and Whitehead, 1971; Arman et al., 1974; Sadleir, 1980; Robbins et al., 1981; Loudon et al., 1983; Reese and Robbins, 1994). The shape and elevation of this lactation curve (Type I) resembles that proposed by Wood (1967), but it varies with species and measurement technique (Dove and Freer, 1979; Loudon and Kay, 1984; Oftedal, 1985; Parker et al., 1990; Robbins, 1993). Also, it may depend on fundamental development of cells within the mammary gland (Pulina et al., 2001). Field estimates of milk intake by young red deer, white-tailed deer, reindeer, and caribou show an exponential or linear decline from the first week (Type II curve; Loudon et al., 1983, 1984; Arman et al., 1974; White and Luick, 1984; Robbins et al., 1987; García et al., 1999) that can be changed to reflect a Type I curve by feed supplementation (Parker et al., 1990). Conversion of milk yield to energy yield requires an appropriate energy content of milk. Interspecies comparisons show variation with species and stage of lactation (Jenness and Sloan, 1970; Oftedal, 1984; Robbins, 1993). Throughout lactation, milk energy content is inversely related to milk yield (Loudon and Kay, 1984; White and Luick, 1984). Thus, differences in milk energy content and milk yield balance across species, such that for females consuming ad libitum high-quality feed and nursing one offspring, peak yield in milk energy (NE_l), whether a Type I or Type II curve, scales to maternal BW as 104 kcal/kg $BW^{0.7}$ (435 kJ/kg $BW^{0.7}$) (Oftedal, 1985). This equation slightly overestimates energy output of wapiti, but considerably underestimates energy output by the Bedouin goat. Peak milk intake for each twin-suckled deer is approximately 0.65 times that for a single deer (Sadleir, 1980, 1982). Hence, milk energy output for twins is 1.3 times that for a deer producing a single offspring. Total energy yield over the entire lactation also scales to maternal BW as 5.99 Mcal/kg $BW^{0.81}$ (25.06 MJ/kg $BW^{0.81}$) (Oftedal, 1985). Oftedal (1985) speculated that since the ratio of total lactation to peak lactation scales to maternal $BW^{0.11}$, total energy output is 80 times daily peak output for a maternal BW of 20 kg, but is 96 times daily peak output for a maternal BW of 100 kg. Within species, lactation curves are highly plastic, with a decline in peak milk production during undernutrition attributable to low maternal BW, poor body condition, and low feed availability (Loudon et al., 1983; White and Luick, 1984). Using allometric estimates of milk production, the energy requirements can be calculated using a constant k_l (0.65) across lactation. Estimated ME_l for daily peak requirement is 160 kcal/kg $BW^{0.70}$ (669 kJ/kg $BW^{0.70}$), and the total lactation requirement is 9.23 Mcal/kg $BW^{0.81}$ (38.6 MJ/kg BW $^{0.81}$: Oftedal, 1985) for cervids consuming ad libitum and raising one offspring.

Body Composition and Tissue Mobilization and Gain

Knowledge of body composition is important to assess dietary energy needs with tissue energy mobilization in early lactation and later when stores are replenished. Table 4-1 should provide reasonable approximations of tissue energy concentration for both mobilization and accretion by mature sheep. There do not seem to be available comparable data for growing sheep, such as for yearlings still increasing in proportion of mature BW. As noted before for maintenance, most energy systems assume a set k_{lt}, such as 0.80 to 0.84. Assumptions for k_g of lactating animals include 0.75 (Sahlu et al., 2004), 0.6 (SCA, 1990), and 0.95 × k_m (AFRC, 1993).

For cervids, peak feed intake may not occur until 4 weeks postpartum, after which time maternal BW increases, even for deer raising twins (Sadleir, 1982). Therefore, mobilization of nutrients to support milk synthesis is required. Costs of lactation are high, with energy expenditure of lactating females ~ 27 percent higher than nonlactating females in the first month (Mauget et al., 1997a,b). Whereas body fat and protein are mobilized for milk synthesis in the first 3 weeks, body protein seems to be protected from mobilization after 3 weeks (White et al., 1989; Russell et al., 1996; García et al., 1999), with only surplus protein not used for body tissue diverted to milk synthesis (Chan-McLeod et al., 1994). Thus, a positive correlation between maternal energy intake and maternal body protein deposition in lactating reindeer and caribou suggests that maternal protein deposition may be limited by energy availability on many diets (Chan-McLeod et al., 1994), as it is for weaned young grazing high-protein pastures (Eilertsen et al., 2001). Daily net energy requirements for lactating females are twice those for females not lactating (109 vs. 55 kcal/kg $BW^{0.75}$, 457 vs. 232 kJ/kg $BW^{0.75}$: Chan-McLeod et al., 1994). Under natural conditions the ecological energy cost to lactation in caribou over a 3.5-month period seems to be approximately 9 kg BW (Cameron et al., 2005), of which 73 percent is fat (Gerhart et al., 1996a).

Biotype or Genotype

Metabolizable energy requirements for lactation are usually deemed to be directly related to milk energy yield alone, with consideration for differences among genotypes or biotypes restricted to ME_m and FHP. Similarly, Nsahlai et al. (2004a) did not observe a difference in ME_l between dairy and other goat biotypes.

FIBER

There have been few studies concerning efficiency of ME use for fiber growth (k_f) by sheep and goats. Available estimates of k_f include 0.16–0.19 and 0.18 for clean wool fiber by Graham and Searle (1982) and Langlands and Bowles (1974), respectively. With multiple regression analysis, Herselman and Smith (1991) reported an ME_f for clean mohair fiber of 32.7 kcal/g (137 kJ/g) for South African Angora goats, which assumes 5.7 kcal/g (23.7 kJ/g) of clean mohair fiber equates to a k_f of 0.17. Similarly, with a broader database and regression analysis, Luo et al. (2004d) found an ME_f of 37.5 kcal/g (157 kJ/g) or k_f of 0.15. Other secretions such as lanolin are proportional to fiber growth, but are not retained when fiber is cleaned. Inclusion of these secretions would lower k_f. Generally, fiber requirements are expressed relative to clean fiber growth.

Some energy requirement systems for wool-producing sheep account for ME_f only with fiber growth above a threshold, such as 6 g/d (SCA, 1990), assuming the cost with lower levels is accounted for by ME_m. However, for Angoras that typically produce more fiber per unit of BW than wool-producing sheep, ME_f can be significant relative to ME_m. An alternative to considering ME_f negligible for sheep and goats with lower fiber growth would be to estimate scurf crude protein (CP) and apply a heat of combustion, such as 0.2 g CP/kg $BW^{0.6}$ (NRC, 1984) and 5.7 kcal/g (23.22 kJ/g), respectively, resulting in a scurf energy loss of 1.13 kcal/kg $BW^{0.6}$ (4.77 kJ/kg $BW^{0.6}$) or 12.0 kcal (49 kJ) for a 50 kg animal.

Low k_f may partially result from the cost of maintaining functional skin fiber follicles, since there is no turnover of protein in fiber after synthesis, as well as limiting supplies of sulfur-containing amino acids (Adams et al., 2000; Puchala et al., 2002). Effects of availability of specific amino acids on k_f have not been extensively studied, apart from the overall effect on fiber production. Seasonality may affect k_f as well. Angora goats and most wool-producing sheep grow fiber continually without an obvious period of shedding. However, there are seasonal changes in fiber growth elicited by change in photoperiod. For example, Litherland et al. (2000) noted that mohair fiber growth by yearling Angoras was greatest in summer, lowest in winter, and intermediate in fall and spring. Primary follicle activity was highly affected by season, but activity of secondary follicles was not appreciably altered. Hence, the energy cost of maintaining active secondary follicles might not have directly varied with change in fiber production.

The hair coat, or pelage, of deer varies depending on latitude, with white-tailed deer showing plasticity associated with distribution of the more than 30 subspecies (Sauer,

1984). However, for most north temperate cervids, pelage is shed twice yearly. Timing of the spring molt varies with sex, age, and pregnancy (Ryder, 1977). Pelage growth therefore occurs over summer. In most species, this thin coat (Jacobsen, 1980) is shed and a longer coat grown in late summer/autumn that is associated with growth of wool-like fibers, termed underwool, grown from secondary follicles (Sauer, 1984). Hair plus underwool, or pelage, growth is terminated in early winter. Thus, estimates of ME_m made in winter do not contain any contribution of pelage growth. Winter pelage consists of a short layer of underwool fibers surrounded by long hollow hair fibers, usually termed guard hairs. In some cases the hair fibers are of two types that grow sequentially throughout summer, with no late summer shedding, and this sequential growth accounts for changes in pelage length, thickness, coloration (e.g., a dark summer coat turns almost white by winter in Arctic caribou), and insulative properties (Scholander et al., 1950; Hammel, 1955; Jacobsen, 1980). The ME_m estimates made in summer probably contain the cost of pelage growth (Robbins, 1993). Estimates of the pelage weight have been determined for deer (Moen, 1973; Robbins, 1993) and caribou (Gerhart et al., 1996a). Hair weight in mammals is approximately 2 percent of BW and weight of hair scales at 0.035 g/g $BW^{0.92}$ (Robbins, 1993). Estimates of daily NE_f (hair fiber) for a 135-day growing period, using heat of combustion of 5.3 kcal/g (Robbins, 1993), gives 1.5–2.0 kcal/kg $BW^{0.75}$. Daily NE_f for growing white-tailed deer fawns was 35–79 kcal (Robbins et al., 1974). The daily ME_f for summer fiber and scurf loss, assuming a k_f of 0.15, is approximately 12 kcal/kg $BW^{0.75}$, which represents ~ 17 percent of BMR, and ~ 6 and 7 percent of ME_m in summer for young and mature white-tailed deer, respectively. For a 50 kg cervid, this ME_f is 226 kcal/d, which is considerably higher than the 12 kcal/d estimated for sheep and goats (above).

Wool and mohair fiber growth are influenced by physiological state, notably gestation and early lactation, which seems to be a function of increased nutrient competition with the mammary gland and gravid uterus (Adams et al., 2000) and also potential direct effects of prolactin in decreasing follicle uptake of nutrients (Puchala et al., 2003). However, how k_f might be altered in different physiological states is unclear. Similarly, effects of the nature of the diet (e.g., ME and concentrate levels) on k_f are unknown. The high priority for nutrient partitioning to follicles leads to use of mobilized tissue energy and protein for fiber growth in many instances, but possible impact of the origin of ME (diet vs. endogenous) has not been studied. Hence, Luo et al. (2004c) assumed k_f to be constant regardless of the origin of energy fueling mohair fiber growth.

PREGNANCY

Pregnancy tissues include the fetus, fetal fluids and related tissues (the sum of which is the conceptus), uterus, and mammary gland. In the final period of the last trimester of pregnancy, the majority of energy accretion is in the fetus, with relatively more energy used for development of the uterus and mammary gland earlier. The efficiency of ME use for pregnancy (k_{preg}) is low compared with k_m, k_g, and k_l, with estimates generally 0.12 to 0.16 (Rattray et al., 1974a; ARC, 1980; INRA, 1989; SCA, 1990; NRC, 2001). However, based on the data of Rattray et al. (1974a) the efficiency may be slightly less for maintenance and development of the fetus and fetal fluids and associated tissues than of the uterus and mammary gland. In 1990, SCA pointed out that k_{preg} as classically determined is low as a result of being a "gross" efficiency, pertinent to maintaining pregnancy tissue present as well as accretion. In late pregnancy, about one-half of ME use attributable to pregnancy is due to increased metabolism by nonpregnancy tissues, with one-half of that of pregnancy tissues attributable to the fetus and the other half primarily to the uteroplacenta (Ferrell and Reynolds, 1987; Freetly and Ferrell, 1997). Regarding true efficiency, Bell (1986) calculated a value for fetal growth in cattle and sheep, comparable to k_g, of 0.38, which reflects high heat production by the placenta relative to energy retained. Likewise, Hutchings (1997) used a modeling approach to suggest that the efficiency of growth of the products of conception (gravid uterus without the mammary gland) is similar to that for growth by nonpregnant animals.

The first step in estimating ME_{preg} is usually to predict mass and energy of one or more pregnancy tissue components with an exponential equation at different days of gestation, and then to apply an assumed k_{preg}, typically 0.13 to 0.14. Equations to predict fetal weight such as those of Koong et al. (1975) require input of predicted birth weight. In this regard, Freetly and Leymaster (2004) recently noted differences among sheep breeds in the relationship between litter size and birth weight. The manner in which pregnancy tissue mass increases with advancing gestation is thought to be similar for sheep and goats, as also seems to be the case for k_{preg} (INRA, 1989; SCA, 1990; AFRC, 1998). The value k_{preg} is commonly assumed to be constant regardless of dietary ME concentration, although potential for an effect of diet was discussed by SCA (1990). However, SCA (1990) also suggested that the efficiency of use of mobilized tissue energy for pregnancy is greater than of dietary ME, thus preventing k_{preg} from deviating markedly from 0.13 to 0.14 with low-quality diets. Also, k_{preg} is normally not thought to vary with litter size. In support, Robinson et al. (1980) did not observe a significant effect of litter size in sheep on efficiency of ME use for fetal growth; however, small differences between litter size of 1 and 2 in sheep of opposite direction were noted by Lodge and Heaney (1970) and Rattray et al. (1974a).

NRC (1981b) recommended an additional 76 kcal/kg $BW^{0.75}$ (318 kJ/kg $BW^{0.75}$) of ME in the last 2 months of gestation for goats, and a 20 percent increase was proposed for multiple births. AFRC (1998) based pregnancy ME re-

TABLE 4-2 Energy and Protein Requirements of Small Ruminants for Pregnancy of SCA (1990), AFRC (1993, 1998), Sahlu et al. (2004), and NRC (1985)[a]

			SCA (1990)		AFRC (1993)		Sahlu et al. (2004)				NRC (1985) AFRC (1998)		
Litter size	Birth weight per kid	Day of gestation	ME_{preg}, Mcal	NE_{preg}, Mcal	MP_{preg}, g	NP_{preg}, g	ME_{preg}, Mcal	NE_{preg}, Mcal	MP_{preg}, g	NP_{preg}, g	ME_{preg}, Mcal	NE_{preg}, Mcal	MP_{preg}, g
NRC (1985) tabular listings for sheep											NRC (1985)		
1	5	100	0.45	0.06	12	8	0.24	0.03	17	6	0.54	0.07	
1	5	120	0.82	0.11	21	15	0.91	0.12	46	15	1.12	0.15	
1	5	140	1.37	0.18	35	24	1.36	0.18	66	22	2.00	0.26	
2	4.5	100	0.81	0.11	21	15	0.42	0.05	26	9	0.96	0.13	
2	4.5	120	1.48	0.19	38	27	1.28	0.17	66	22	2.04	0.27	
2	4.5	140	2.46	0.32	63	44	1.93	0.25	96	32	3.39	0.44	
3	3.83	100	1.04	0.14	27	19	0.52	0.07	32	10	1.31	0.17	
3	3.83	120	1.89	0.25	49	34	1.49	0.19	77	25	2.65	0.35	
3	3.83	140	3.14	0.41	80	56	2.24	0.29	114	38	4.39	0.57	
AFRC (1998) tabular listings for goats											AFRC (1998)		
1	4.44	105	0.47	0.06	12	9	0.38	0.05	22	7	0.47		10
1	4.44	133	1.02	0.13	26	18	1.09	0.14	53	18	0.88		19
2	3.95	105	0.83	0.11	22	15	0.57	0.07	32	11	0.77		17
2	3.95	133	1.82	0.24	47	33	1.52	0.20	76	25	1.47		32
3	3.65	105	1.16	0.15	30	21	0.75	0.10	42	14	1.06		24
3	3.65	133	2.53	0.33	65	45	1.91	0.25	97	32	1.96		43
1	2.75	105	0.29	0.04	8	5	0.24	0.03	14	5	0.27		6
1	2.75	133	0.63	0.08	16	11	0.69	0.09	33	11	0.52		12
2	2.25	105	0.48	0.06	12	9	0.33	0.04	19	6	0.41		10
2	2.25	133	1.04	0.14	27	19	0.88	0.11	44	15	0.80		18

[a] ME_{preg} = metabolizable energy used for pregnancy; NE_{preg} = net energy used for pregnancy; MP_{preg} = metabolizable protein used for pregnancy; NP_{preg} = net protein used for pregnancy.

quirements on a k_{preg} of 0.133 (ARC, 1980), sheep tissue composition data, mean birth weights from dairy and fiber-producing goat kid data sets, and use of a Gompertz equation. The NRC (1985) recommendation for the NE for pregnancy requirement was based on reports of Rattray et al. (1974a,b) for the gravid uterus (plus contents) and mammary gland. The SCA (1990) predicted ME_{preg} for maintenance and development of the gravid uterus for cattle, sheep, and goats with a Gompertz model adapted from that of ARC (1980). Sahlu et al. (2004) proposed a system to predict ME_{preg} of goats in late gestation, based on Equation II of Koong et al. (1975) developed for sheep to predict fetal weight at different days of gestation; sheep data of Rattray et al. (1974b) to predict total energy and protein in all pregnancy tissues, including the mammary gland; and a k_{preg} of 0.133 (Rattray et al., 1974a).

Table 4-2 provides comparisons of net and metabolizable energy (NE_{preg} and ME_{preg}, respectively) and net and metabolizable protein (MP) for pregnancy (NP_{preg} and MP_{preg}, respectively) from different prediction methods. Litter size, birth weight per animal, and day of gestation are those listed in tables of NRC (1985) for sheep and AFRC (1998) for goats. For NRC (1985) tabular listings, ME_{preg} ranked NRC (1985) > SCA (1990) and AFRC (1993) > Sahlu et al. (2004). The AFRC (1998) tabular listings for ME_{preg} were also greater for SCA (1990) and AFRC (1993) than for those of Sahlu et al. (2004), although the latter values were not greatly different from those of AFRC (1998). Some NP_{preg} values of Sahlu et al. (2004) were similar to those of SCA (1990) and AFRC (1993), but many were lower. However, the lower efficiency of ME use for pregnancy (NRC, 2001) employed by Sahlu et al. (2004), as addressed in Chapter 5, resulted in considerably greater MP_{preg}. Most MP_{preg} values of AFRC (1998) were slightly lower than those of SCA (1990) and AFRC (1993).

Concepta and fetal growth curves developed for many species (Huggett and Widdas, 1951) have been generalized to cervid species since they have the same essential power function and a sigmoid growth curve (Robbins and Robbins, 1979; Robbins, 1993). Although most growth occurs in the last trimester (Robbins, 1993), growth velocities vary between species (Huggett and Widdas, 1951; Robbins and Robbins, 1979; Roine et al., 1982; Oftedal, 1985; Adam et al., 1988a,b). Therefore, estimates of fetal weight at a particular gestation age must usually be obtained from the literature. Where the fetal growth curve is not known, fetal weight (W, kg) at a particular gestation age (t, d) can be predicted from the specific fetal growth velocity (a), birth weight (W_b, kg), duration of initial stage of slow growth (t_0, d), and gestation length (t_g, d). As detailed by Oftedal

(1985), $a = W_b^{0.33}/(t_g - t_0)$ and $W_b^{0.33} = a \times (t - t_0)$ (Huggett and Widdas, 1951), where t is time since conception (days). For the four species of cervids in this study, "a" ranged between 0.0109 and 0.125, and t_0 between 45 and 70 days. Birth weight was sensitive to both variables, and neither "a" nor t_0 was correlated with maternal body size, confirming observations reported by Oftedal (1985). Among ruminants, gestation length (t_g, d) scales to maternal BW at 109 $BW^{0.19}$ (Robbins, 1993), and among artiodactyls at 120 $BW^{0.16}$ (Hudson, 1985). Both equations tend to overestimate gestation length for focal species, the former by 11–17 percent and the latter by 7–15 percent. Birth weight of north temperate cervids that regularly produce twins, but may also produce singlets, decreases from 4.5–7.0 percent with maternal BW (Robbins and Robbins, 1979; Oftedal, 1985). Allometrically, birth weight (W_b, kg) of small herbivores, including small ruminants, scales with maternal BW (kg) as 0.214 $BW^{0.793}$ (Robbins and Robbins, 1979; Robbins, 1993) or as 0.166 $BW^{0.90}$ (Oftedal, 1985).

Energy deposited during gestation is then given by the energy content of the fetus and concepta (1.03–1.20 Mcal/kg, 4.31–5.0 MJ/kg) divided by 0.82, assuming that the fetus represents 82 percent of the gravid uterus at term (Oftedal, 1985). However, Robbins and Robbins (1979) report that fetus weight as a percent of concepta weight is not constant throughout gestation, but it increases linearly from 5 percent at 20 percent of gestation to 60 percent at term (100 percent gestation). Robbins and Moen (1975) show that energy retention of the gravid uterus (NE_{preg}), expressed as a percent of fetus weight at term (Y, kcal/d per kg) during pregnancy in deer and other small to large ruminants, is given by $L_nY = -0.8393 + 0.0501 \times X$, where X = stage of gestation (0–100 percent). At term this equation gives a daily NE_{preg} of 63 kcal/kg fetus, which is in agreement for deer producing twin fetuses, but is twice the value generated by species-specific equations for caribou and elk/wapiti. A reasonable recommendation for daily NE_{preg} of cervids producing single offspring is half the estimate from Robbins and Moen (1975). At term the mean daily NE_{preg} is 32 kcal/kg fetus. In cervids, k_{preg} for sheep (0.133) is assumed in order to calculate ME_{preg} (Oftedal, 1985). In white-tailed deer, over a 200-day pregnancy period, the energy deposited in concepta is 18.6 Mcal/kg $BW^{0.75}$ (78 MJ/kg $BW^{0.75}$), which is approximately 16 percent greater than the cost for maintenance of a nonpregnant deer (Robbins, 1993; Pekins et al., 1998), and 10–20 percent is retained as new uterine tissue (Robbins, 1993). For white-tailed deer, reindeer/caribou, red deer, and elk/wapiti, mean daily ME_{preg} at term is 55 kcal/kg$BW^{0.75}$, which is approximately 43 percent of winter ME_m. Compared with early gestation or nonpregnant animals, metabolic rate increases by ~ 15 percent in roe deer (Mauget et al., 1997a), ~ 60 percent in wapiti (Pauls et al., 1981), and 45 percent in white-tailed deer (Pekins et al., 1998), supporting recommendations for use of a low value for k_{preg}.

REQUIREMENT RECOMMENDATIONS

There are different formats in which nutrient requirement recommendations can be presented. The decision regarding which means is most appropriate is probably simplest for publications dealing with only one species. For multiple species, in some respects it might be thought best to address all species within a section concerning a particular energy use, such as in AFRC (1993) and SCA (1990). However, as supported by publications specific for goats (e.g., AFRC, 1998, based primarily on AFRC, 1993), there is also logic in addressing each species separately with subsections for the various functions for which energy is metabolized. In part this is justified by different approaches in arriving at requirement expressions taken in the most up-to-date studies for the different species, as well as various expression forms (e.g., ME vs. NE). Relatedly, because environmental conditions can vary, dealing with all species together in sections could force some users to devote time to areas not of great importance or relevance to them and their species of interest.

Although stated before by others, the area of nutrient requirements is not static. The relationships recommended today are felt most appropriate given the information available and interpretation possible at this point in time. Recommendations of this publication build upon the past important efforts of our predecessors. It is hoped that these nutrient requirement expressions will be useful, but it is recognized that future research will certainly lead to their enhancement or substitution with more appropriate ones.

SHEEP

Growing/Finishing Sheep

Evaluation

Cannas et al. (2004) described the CNCPS-S system and evaluated predictions of digestibility and BW change and milk production by mature sheep. To evaluate components of this method. as well as that of NRC (1985) for describing energy requirements of growing/finishing sheep, a database of treatment mean observations from the literature was constructed, which is described in Tables 4-3 and 4-4. There were 31 references used, with a final number of 156 observations representing 1,875 sheep. Observations were interaction rather than main effect means; there were two references in which main effect means were listed, with interaction means obtained from the authors. The intent for the database was to be broad in terms of genotypes, ADG, diet nutritive value, and other factors. One reference was not presented in Tables 4-3 or 4-4 and excluded from the database because of fairly short periods (28 d) coupled with substantial changes in level of intake from period to period that seemed to result in ADG substantially influenced by gut fill.

When not provided in references, dietary ingredient concentrations of ME, NE_m, NE_g, CP, rumen undegraded intake

TABLE 4-3 References, Number of Treatment Mean Observations, and Genotypes in the Database Used to Evaluate Prediction of Average Daily Gain by Methods of NRC (1985) and CNCPS-S (Cannas et al., 2004)

Reference	Number of Observations	Genotype
von Keyserlingk and Mathison (1993)	3	Dorset crossbred
Hufstedler et al. (1996)		Crossbred
Galloway et al. (1996)	16	Rambouillet × Dorset
Goetsch (1997)	5	St. Croix
Goetsch and Aiken (1999)	8	St. Croix and St. Croix crossbred
Goetsch et al. (1998)	3	Dorset and Suffolk crossbred
Animut (2004)	6	Khatadin
Sun et al. (1994)	6	Hampshire × (Rambouillet × Dorset)
Phillips et al. (2006)	5	Romonav × Polypay, Romonav × St. Croix, St. Croix, Texel × Polypay, and Texel × St. Croix
Ruder et al. (1997)	4	White face or fine wool
Haddad et al. (2001)	5	Awassi
Westendorf and Gordon (1998)	4	Dorset
Murphy et al. (1994)	6	Hampshire × Targhee
Gentry et al. (1999)	8	Suffolk
Kreikemeier et al. (1987)	5	Rambouillet × Suffolk
Glimp et al. (1989)	5	Rambouillet
Funk et al. (1986)	4	Fine wool
Turgeon et al. (1986)	6	Suffolk × Rambouillet
Dhakad et al. (2002)	3	Indigenous (India)
Fimbres et al. (2002)	4	Pelibuey
Pineda et al. (1998)	3	Pelibuey
Fluharty et al. (1999)	2	Targhee
Fluharty and McClure (1997)	8	Hampshire × Targhee
Aderibigbe and Church (1983)	5	Crossbred
Said and Tolera (1993)	6	Menz
Tolera and Sundstøl (2000)	7	Local, Southern Ethiopia
Amaning-Kwarteng and Kellaway (1987)	1	Merino × Border Leicester
Thomas et al. (1994)	3	Rambouillet
Ørskov et al. (1971)	2	Suffolk × Scottish halfbred
Pond (1989)	4	Synthetic 1: Finn × (Dorset × Rambouillet)
Willms et al. (1991)	5	Various crossbreds

TABLE 4-4 Description of the Database Used to Evaluate Prediction of Average Daily Gain by Methods of NRC (1985) and CNCPS-S (Cannas et al., 2004)[a]

Item[b]	Mean	SD	Minimum	Maximum
Length, d	67	26.7	28	207
Dietary TDN, % DM	72.7	10.24	44.9	91.9
Dietary ME, Mcal/kg DM	2.62	0.375	1.63	3.17
Dietary CP, % DM	14.8	3.87	6.2	30
Dietary NDF, % DM	33	18.64	8.9	72.4
Dietary UIP, % CP	39.8	11.37	12.4	67.7
Average full body weight, kg	33.2	8.24	13.4	48.9
Dry matter intake, kg/d	1.11	0.312	0.39	1.65
Average daily gain, g	189	103.7	6	430

[a]n = 156.
[b]TDN = total digestible nutrients; DM = dry matter; ME = metabolizable energy; CP = crude protein; NDF = neutral detergent fiber; UIP = undegraded intake protein.

protein (UIP), TDN, neutral detergent fiber (NDF), and effective NDF (eNDF) were derived from NRC (2000) to determine average dietary levels. When not available from that source, values were obtained from NRC (2001) and then, if necessary, Preston (2000). The CNCPS-S and NRC methods require estimates of full BW at maturity with a BCS of 3.0 (0–5 scale) and mature ram BW, respectively. These BW were derived from the "Breeds of Livestock" website (www.ansi. okstate.edu/breeds/) of the Animal Science Department of Oklahoma State University in December 2004.

Means were used when ranges were presented. In instances when these BW were not available, a value for a genotype thought comparable was used. Mature BW was assumed to be the same for females and male castrates. The effect of use of inaccurate mature BW values did not appear major relative to other factors, since evaluation with categorization as small, moderate, or large as listed by NRC (1985), with an assumed difference between male castrates and females compared with intact males, yielded similar results. When age was not specified, a value estimated from other information presented was employed.

To address the issue of energy rather than protein being most limiting to ADG, it was necessary to predict MP intake (MPI) and the MP requirement. Because methods such as the Level II approach of the CNCPS and that of AFRC (1993) necessitate many dietary characteristic inputs, which with such a database are difficult to derive with confidence of accuracy, a simpler approach requiring less inputs was employed. This method was deemed appropriate in regard to the purpose of this estimation and because accuracy lost may not have been great considering the uncertainty of use of nitrogen and carbohydrate characteristics available from the literature for a large number of dietary feedstuffs.

Ruminal microbial CP synthesis was estimated as described by NRC (2000, 2001). Microbial CP synthesis when ruminal availability of nitrogenous compounds was not limiting to microbial growth was determined as 13 percent of TDN intake, with a correction for eNDF intake (NRC, 2000). For limiting ruminal availability of nitrogenous compounds when rumen degraded intake CP (DIP) intake was less than 118 percent of microbial protein synthesis based on TDN intake, microbial CP was estimated at 85 percent of DIP intake. Microbial MP was calculated as 64 percent of microbial CP. Metabolizable protein from the diet was estimated from UIP intake and 80 percent small intestinal digestion of UIP. The method of CNCPS-S (Cannas et al., 2004) was largely used to derive the MP requirement for maintenance (MP_m). Since very few references reported fiber growth, in many cases scurf CP was estimated from an equation of NRC (1984): $0.2 \times \text{kg BW}^{0.6}$, with an efficiency of MP use of 0.6 assumed (Cannas et al., 2004). The difference between MPI and MP_m was assumed MP available for gain (MP_g). To derive the protein concentration in tissue gained, the CNCPS-S equation for energy concentration in tissue accretion was used in conjunction with equation 1.30 of SCA (1990), which was presented by Garrett (1987, as cited by SCA, 1990). The protein concentration in tissue accreted on a full BW or ADG basis was assumed to be 92 percent of that for the empty body. Net protein for gain (NP_g) was derived from MP_g assuming an efficiency of MP use for tissue protein accretion of 0.7 (Cannas et al., 2004). Net protein for gain divided by tissue protein concentration on an ADG basis provided a prediction of ADG based on MPI ($ADG_{pred\text{-}mp}$). Of the 185 treatment mean observations, there were 21 with $ADG_{pred\text{-}mp}$ less than ADG based on energy ($ADG_{pred\text{-}en}$) and with observed ADG (ADG_{obs}) less than $ADG_{pred\text{-}en}$, which were dropped from the database. In addition, for evaluation of the NRC (1985) method, it was necessary to remove 12 observations with negative ADG_{obs}, although 4 of these observations were deleted because of the aforementioned criterion. The remaining 156 treatment observations were used to evaluate NRC and CNCPS-S methods.

For both methods, there was no adjustment of ME_m for activity because animals in this database were confined. It was assumed that there were no effects on energy needs of cold stress or acclimatization. Furthermore, excretion of excess urea nitrogen as discussed by Cannas et al. (2004) was not addressed in the CNCPS-S method. However, projections of this cost were made and had little to no effect on observed bias.

Evaluation was conducted by regressing ADG_{obs} against $ADG_{pred\text{-}en}$. Regressions unweighted for the number of animals per treatment mean observation accounted for slightly more variability than ones weighted and, thus, are shown below. The SGE abbreviation denotes sheep growing equation.

Eqn. SGE1 (NRC):

ADG_{obs} (g) = 19.4 (SE = 9.30) + 0.916 (SE = 0.0443) × $ADG_{pred\text{-}en}$ ($R^2 = 0.73$; mean bias = 4; Figure 4-1)

Eqn. SGE2 (CNCPS-S):

ADG_{obs} (g) = 30.7 (SE = 9.58) + 1.041 (SE = 0.0551) × $ADG_{pred\text{-}en}$ ($R^2 = 0.70$; mean bias = 37; Figure 4-2)

In addition to simple linear regression, mixed model analysis was conducted to ascertain the need to consider the effect of report. First, the effect of the number of observations was not significant. For the NRC method, covariance parameter estimates for the intercept ($P < 0.11$), slope ($P < 0.10$), and intercept-slope interaction ($P < 0.34$) were not significant, and the corresponding equation was similar to Eqn. SGE1: ADG_{obs} (g) = 22.9 (SE = 16.12) + 0.896 (SE = 0.0823) × $ADG_{pred\text{-}en}$. For the CNCPS-S method, covariance parameter estimates for the intercept ($P < 0.01$), slope ($P < 0.01$), and intercept-slope interaction ($P < 0.04$) were significant, and the resulting equation was similar to Eqn. SGE2: ADG_{obs} (g) = 46.6 (SE = 20.11) + 0.944 (SE = 0.1148) × $ADG_{pred\text{-}en}$.

Both NRC and CNCPS-S exhibited prediction bias as evident in Figures 4-1 and 4-2, respectively. There were a number of factors tested to possibly explain this bias. One was the method of determining the energy concentration in tissue gain. An alternative equation of Rompala and Johnson (1985) was used (Factor EVG). A k_m that varied with dietary ME concentration (NRC, 1985) was tested with the CNCPS-S method rather than a constant value of 0.644 (Factor k_m). The possible effect of compensatory growth on ME_m was addressed (Factor COMP). References and treatment mean observations were closely scrutinized, and subjective decreases in ME_m up to 20 percent were employed. Another factor

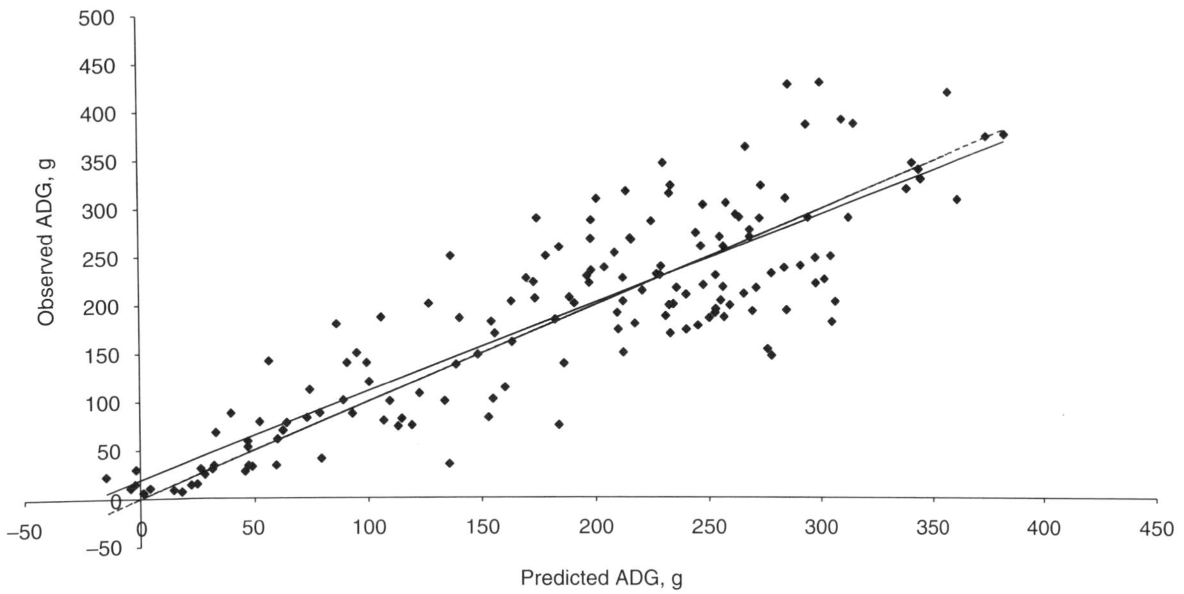

FIGURE 4-1 The relationship between observed ADG (ADG_{obs}) and ADG predicted (ADG_{pred}) by the NRC (1985) method for growing/finishing sheep. The solid line depicts Eqn. SGE1: ADG_{obs} (g) = 19.4 (SE = 9.30) + 0.916 (SE = 0.443) × $ADG_{pred\text{-}en}$ (R^2 = 0.73). The dashed line depicts $ADG_{obs} = ADG_{pred\text{-}en}$.

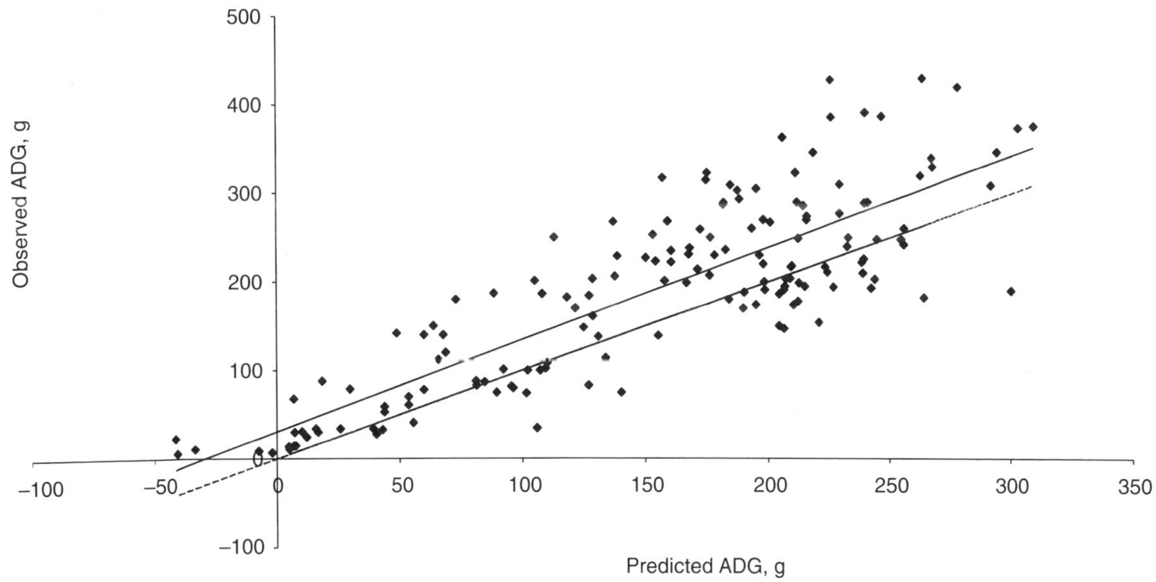

FIGURE 4-2 The relationship between observed ADG (ADG_{obs}) and ADG predicted (ADG_{pred}) by the CNCPS-S method (Cannas et al., 2004) for growing/finishing sheep. The solid line depicts Eqn. SGE2: ADG_{obs} (g) = 30.7 (SE = 9.58) + 1.041 (SE = 0.0551) × $ADG_{pred\text{-}en}$ (R^2 = 0.70). The dashed line depicts $ADG_{obs} = ADG_{pred\text{-}en}$.

viewed was level of MEI relative to ME_m (Factor INT). This adjustment was included for observations with MEI less than 200 percent of ME_m, with a linear increase in the downward adjustment of ME_m up to 20 percent at MEI of 100 percent of ME_m (i.e., 0.8 × ME_m with MEI = ME_m). Also, for CNCPS-S the visceral organ component (Factor VO) of the ME_m equation was omitted for all observations or when COMP and INT factors were included. In all other cases the VO factor is included. Another factor tested for CNCPS-S was the assumed unadjusted energy requirement for fasting metabolism, which is 0.062 Mcal per kg of shrunk $BW^{0.75}$, with shrunk BW being 96 percent of full or unshrunk BW. As discussed earlier, ME_m in sheep decreases with increasing age, but the change is in accordance with that in the proportion of mature size. Hence, the age component of the ME_m equation was removed, and the function of Freetly et al. (1995b, 2002a,b [Factor PMW]) was used to determine the energy requirement for fasting metabolism (kcal/kg FBW = $59.5e^{-0.797(FBW/FmatBW)}$), with FBW and FmatBW being estimates of average actual BW and mature size within a fasting period of 48 to 71 hours. To estimate FBW and FmatBW, 90 percent of full or unshrunk BW was assumed (Freetly et al., 2002a). It should be mentioned, however, that Freetly et al. (2002a) determined that this function cannot be extended to sheep subjected to a nutritional restriction. These regression equations are shown below.

Eqn. SGE3 (NRC; EVG):
ADG_{obs} (g) = 24.8 (SE = 9.01) + 0.903 (SE = 0.0434) × $ADG_{pred\text{-}en}$ (R^2 = 0.74; mean bias = 7)

Eqn. SGE4 (NRC; COMP):
ADG_{obs} (g) = 17.1 (SE = 9.26) + 0.917 (SE = 0.0437) × $ADG_{pred\text{-}en}$ (R^2 = 0.74; mean bias = 2)

Eqn. SGE5 (NRC; INT):
ADG_{obs} (g) = 11.9 (SE = 9.67) + 0.945 (SE = 0.0460) × $ADG_{pred\text{-}en}$ (R^2 = 0.73; mean bias = 2)

Eqn. SGE6 (NRC; COMP, INT):
ADG_{obs} (g) = 9.5 (SE = 9.62) + 0.947 (SE = 0.0453) × $ADG_{pred\text{-}en}$ (R^2 = 0.74; mean bias = –1; Figure 4-3)

Eqn. SGE7 (CNCPS-S; EVG):
ADG_{obs} (g) = 41.8 (SE = 9.63) + 1.034 (SE = 0.0585) × $ADG_{pred\text{-}en}$ (R^2 = 0.67; mean bias = 47)

Eqn. SGE8 (CNCPS-S; k_m):
ADG_{obs} (g) = 47.0 (SE = 8.70) + 0.937 (SE = 0.0490) × $ADG_{pred\text{-}en}$ (R^2 = 0.70; mean bias = 37)

Eqn. SGE9 (CNCPS-S; VO omitted for all observations):
ADG_{obs} (g) = 17.0 (SE = 10.09) + 0.960 (SE = 0.0502) × $ADG_{pred\text{-}en}$ (R^2 = 0.70; mean bias = 10; Figure 4-4)

Eqn. SGE10 (CNCPS-S; VO omitted for COMP and INT observations):
ADG_{obs} (g) = 6.2 (SE = 10.15) + 1.094 (SE = 0.0547) × $ADG_{pred\text{-}en}$ (R^2 = 0.72; mean bias = 22)

Eqn. SGE11 (CNCPS-S; VO for COMP and INT observations, COMP, INT):
ADG_{obs} (g) = –17.7 (SE = 11.10) + 1.184 (SE = 0.0584) × $ADG_{pred\text{-}en}$ (R^2 = 0.73; mean bias = 14)

Eqn. SGE12 (CNCPS-S; PMW):
ADG_{obs} (g) = 140.2 (SE = 6.05) + 0.811 (SE = 0.0516) × $ADG_{pred\text{-}en}$ (R^2 = 0.61; mean bias = 129)

Inclusion of COMP and/or INT factors removed prediction bias with the NRC method. Significance levels for differences of the intercept from 0 and slope from 1, respec-

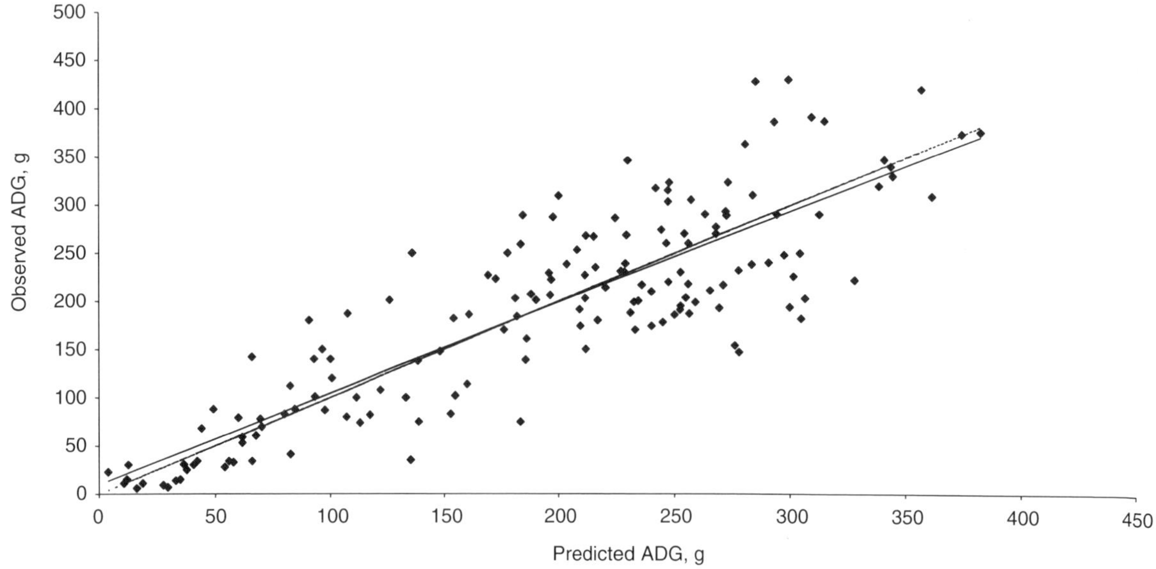

FIGURE 4-3 The relationship between observed ADG (ADG_{obs}) and ADG predicted (ADG_{pred}) by the NRC (1985) method for growing/finishing sheep. The solid line depicts Eqn. SGE6: ADG_{obs} (g) = 9.5 (SE = 9.62) + 0.947 (SE = 0.0453) × $ADG_{pred\text{-}en}$ (R^2 = 0.74). The dashed line depicts $ADG_{obs} = ADG_{pred\text{-}en}$.

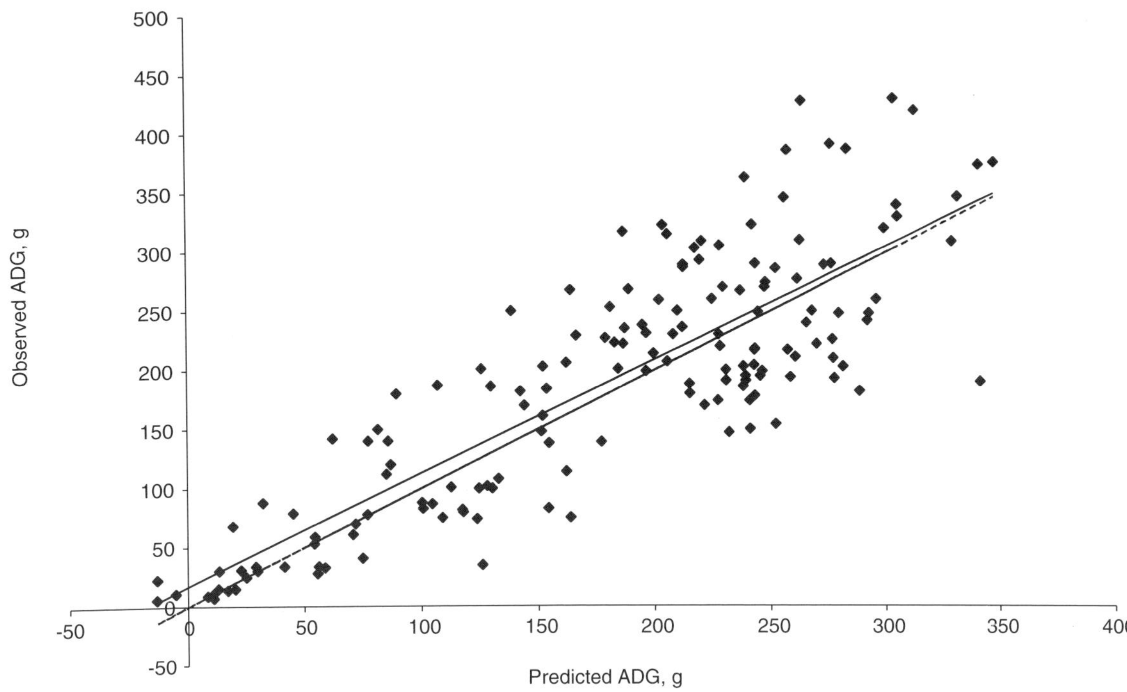

FIGURE 4-4 The relationship between observed ADG (ADG_{obs}) and ADG predicted (ADG_{pred}) by the CNCPS-S method (Cannas et al., 2004) for growing/finishing sheep. The solid line depicts Eqn. SGE9: ADG_{obs} (g) = 17.0 (SE = 10.09) + 0.960 (SE = 0.0502) × $ADG_{pred\text{-}en}$ (R^2 = 0.70; mean bias = 10). The dashed line depicts $ADG_{obs} = ADG_{pred\text{-}en}$.

tively, were 0.07 and 0.06 for Eqn. SGE4; 0.22 and 0.24 for Eqn. SGE5; and 0.33 and 0.25 for Eqn. SGE6. For the CNCPS-S method, significance levels of differences of the intercept from 0 and slope from 1 were 0.10 and 0.43 for Eqn. SGE9, and 0.55 and 0.09 for Eqn. SGE10, respectively.

Based on these evaluation equations, it is difficult to present clear justification for suggesting use of one method rather than the other. Considering the variable experimental conditions under which these observations were derived, both methods seemed to predict reasonably well. This evaluation suggests that the NRC (1985) method could continue to be used. The need to input dietary NE_m and NE_g requirements compared with CNCPS-S may not be a true disadvantage, because the CNCPS-S also relies on an equation to predict k_g (i.e., dietary NE_g/ME). It seems that prediction with the NRC method can be enhanced by adjusting ME_m for a current or previous low nutritional plane. Presently, there does not seem available a tested accurate method of decreasing ME_m for current or previous low planes of nutrition. However, as noted before, potential methods have been suggested for other ruminant species. For example, NRC (2000) proposed decreasing ME_m by 5 percent for each 1 unit BCS less than 5 on a 9-point scale, with increases of the same magnitude for BCS above 5. Sahlu et al. (2004) proposed the same adjustment for goats, though on a 5-point scale, and only for BCS below 3. However, such adjustments of ME_m for plane of nutrition seem best suited when on a constant nutritional plane at a particular BCS and may not necessarily accurately address effects of nutritional plane during the period when BCS is changing.

The CNCPS-S method without adjustment (Eqn. SGE2) slightly underpredicted ADG and, therefore, overestimated the energy requirement. In this regard, the component in the ME_m equation of the CNCPS-S method to account for in creasing energy use by visceral organs with increasing energy intake is in accordance with findings of Dawson and Steen (1998) with sheep on moderate to high planes of nutrition. However, this adjustment is based on MEI regardless of its size relative to ME_m, thus increasing ME_m above 96 kcal/kg shrunk $BW^{0.75}$ even with MEI less than ME_m. Eqn. SGE9 compared with Eqn. SGE2 suggests less biased prediction of ADG and, thus, more accurate description of energy requirements, if this adjustment is not made.

Description of Methods

Because one method was not discernibly appreciably superior to the other, with bias removed upon adjustments of ME_m (e.g., Eqn. SGE6 and SGE9), use of both methods will be overviewed below. However, since the CNCPS-S method also considers protein requirements and supplies and includes assumptions allowing prediction of negative BW change with low MEI, and also because of recommendations for use of CNCPS-S methods for other classes of sheep (e.g., energy for lactation), this method will be employed to predict energy requirements in subsequent "look-up" tables.

NRC

The NRC (1985) method of describing or predicting the energy requirement of growing/finishing sheep is overviewed below, although in the evaluation exercise ADG was predicted based on NE available after subtracting DM necessary to meet the maintenance requirement. Moreover, though not addressed below, it would seem beneficial to decrease ME_m in accordance with a present or recent past low nutritional plane.

1. Average unshrunk or full BW (FBW) within the feeding period, kg
2. ADG, kg
3. Energy requirement for fasting metabolism (NE_m), Mcal/kg $FBW^{0.75} = 0.056$
4. NE_m requirement, Mcal/d = kg $FBW^{0.75} \times NE_m$
5. Mature ram BW (MATRBW), kg
6. NE_g requirement on an ADG basis ($NE_{g\text{-}ADG}$), Mcal/(ADG × $FBW^{0.75}$) = (276 – ((MATRBW – 115) × 2.1))/1,000
7. DMI required for maintenance (DMI_m), kg/d = NE_m requirement/dietary NE_m concentration
8. DMI for gain (DMI_g), kg/d = $NE_{g\text{-}ADG}/NE_g$ concentration in the diet
9. Total DMI requirement, kg/d = $DMI_m + DMI_g$

CNCPS-S

The method of the CNCPS system (Cannas et al., 2004) to describe the energy requirement of growing/finishing sheep is given below. However, the description for the gain component is to predict the requirement for a particular ADG rather than as used in the evaluation exercise to predict ADG when energy intake is known. In addition, effects on energy requirements of cold stress, acclimatization, and excretion of excess urea nitrogen are not addressed. Moreover, the upward adjustment of ME_m in accordance with MEI (i.e., 0.09 × MEI) is included below. Inclusion may not in all instances be most appropriate, although perhaps its use would provide a safety factor in predicted requirements.

1. Shrunk BW (SBW), kg = 96 percent of full or unshrunk BW (FBW)
2. Unadjusted energy requirement for fasting metabolism (a1 or $NE_{m\text{-}SBW}$), Mcal/kg $SBW^{0.75} = 0.062$
3. Multiplicative adjustment of $NE_{m\text{-}SBW}$ for gender (S) = 1 for females and male castrates, 1.15 for intact males
4. Multiplicative adjustment of $NE_{m\text{-}SBW}$ for years of age (AGE) = e(–0.03 × years of age), with years of age greater than 6 set equal to 6
5. Additive adjustment of $NE_{m\text{-}SBW}$ for grazing activity (ACT; Mcal/d) = (0.00062 × FBW × km of flat distance traveled) + (0.00669 × FBW × km of vertical distance traveled)
6. Unadjusted net energy requirement for maintenance (UNE_m), Mcal/d = ($SBW^{0.75} \times NE_{m\text{-}SBW} \times S \times AGE$) + ACT
7. Unadjusted metabolizable energy requirement for maintenance (UME_m), Mcal/d = $UNE_m/0.644$
8. Full BW at BCS of 3.0 ($FBW_{BCS3.0}$; 0–5 scale) = FBW when skeletal development is complete, empty body fat concentration is 25 percent, and BCS is 2.8 to 3.0
9. Maturity index (P), fraction = current $FBW/FBW_{BCS3.0}$
10. Energy concentration in empty body (EB) gain (EVG), Mcal/kg EB = (27/(1 + e(–6 × P – 0.4))) × 0.239

(This equation is the same as equation [22] of Cannas et al. (2004) except for omission of the "R" term. Cannas et al. (2004) stated that "R is the adjustment for rate of gain or loss when ME intake is known and gain or loss must be predicted." Because ME requirements are being predicted here and, thus, ME intake is not known, "R" is dropped from the equation.)

11. Recovered energy (RE or NE_g), Mcal/d = ADG (kg) × EVG × 0.92
12. ME concentration in the diet (MEC), Mcal/kg DM
13. Efficiency of ME use for gain (k_g), fraction = ((1.42 × MEC) – (0.174 × MEC^2) + (0.0122 × MEC^3) – 1.65)/MEC
14. ME required for gain (ME_g), Mcal/d = RE/k_g
15. Unadjusted total ME requirement (UME_{req}), Mcal/d = $UME_m + ME_g$
16. Additive adjustment of UME_m for the effect of level of MEI on visceral organ tissue energy use (VO), Mcal/d = 0.09 × UME_{req}
17. ME requirement for maintenance (ME_m), Mcal/d = UME_m + VO
18. Net energy requirement for maintenance (NE_m), Mcal/d = $ME_m \times 0.644$
19. Total ME requirement (ME_{req}), Mcal/d = $ME_m + ME_g$

Lactating Sheep

Evaluation

Though Cannas et al. (2004) included some observations with lactating sheep in a database used to evaluate the CNCPS-S for predicting BW change of mature sheep, an independent database was constructed for further evaluation with lactating sheep. The database is described in Tables 4-5 and 4-6. Interaction rather than main effect means were used. Treatments involving factors that might influence the relationship between milk energy yield or ADG and energy intake were excluded, such as bovine somatotrophin (bST) treatment in the D'Urso et al. (1998) reference. There was a limited number of references available that reported all necessary information. Furthermore, some assumptions were made to include references providing all but one or a small

TABLE 4-5 References, Number of Treatment Mean Observations, and Genotypes in the Database Used to Evaluate Prediction of Net Energy for Lactation and Average Daily Gain by the CNCPS-S Method (Cannas et al., 2004)

Reference	Number of Observations	Genotype
Susin et al. (1995)	2	Polypay
Appeddu et al. (2004)	6	Polypay
Fegeros et al. (1995)	2	Karagouniko
D'Urso et al. (1998)	2	Comisana
Penning et al. (1988)	5	Border Leicester × Cheviot
Appeddu et al. (1995)	2	Polypay

number of inputs. Also, to address tissue mobilization in support of milk production, a k_{lt} of 0.82 was assumed.

Diet composition and FBW at maturity were determined as described for growing/finishing sheep. For the study of Fegeros et al. (1995), it was stated that there was no change in BW or BCS; therefore, zero ADG and the same final and initial BCS were assumed. Sheep were confined except in the study of D'Urso et al. (1998). Because adequate information was not available to use an existent prediction system to estimate the activity energy cost, a value of 20 percent of the ME_m requirement was used for observations of this reference. Penning et al. (1988) reported changes in BW or BCS but not initial values. Hence, it was assumed that initial BCS was 2.5 and that BW was FBW at maturity from the Oklahoma State University website. Body condition scores for the report of Appeddu et al. (1995) were estimated based on the relationship between BW and assumed mature BW and relatively minor change in BW during the experiment.

To address the issue of energy rather than protein being most limiting to milk production and BW stasis or gain, MPI was predicted as discussed previously for growing/finishing sheep. The MP requirement for maintenance was also estimated as noted earlier. In addition, an efficiency of use of MP for milk protein synthesis of 0.58 was assumed (Cannas et al., 2004). Protein in tissue mobilized or accreted was determined as described by Cannas et al. (2004) based on change in BCS. The assumed efficiency of use of mobilized tissue protein for milk protein synthesis was 0.8 and that of MPI for tissue protein accretion was 0.7 (Cannas et al., 2004). In all cases, MPI was greater than that required and, thus, milk yield was assumed dictated by energy supply.

Evaluation was conducted by two methods, regressing (1) ADG_{obs} against $ADG_{pred\text{-}en}$, with milk energy yield (NE_l) as an input, and (2) observed NE_l ($NE_{l\text{-}obs}$) against predicted NE_l ($NE_{l\text{-}pred}$), with ADG an input. Regressions were conducted unweighted and weighted by the number of observations per treatment mean. The SLE abbreviation denotes sheep lactation equation.

Eqn. SLE1 (unweighted):

ADG_{obs}, g = –32.2 (SE = 18.77) + 0.929 (SE = 0.1882) × $ADG_{pred\text{-}en}$ (R^2 = 0.59; mean bias = –28.7)

Eqn. SLE2 (weighted):

ADG_{obs}, g = –26.2 (SE = 14.31) + 1.021 (SE = 0.1710) × $ADG_{pred\text{-}en}$ (R^2 = 0.68; mean bias that of Eqn. SLE1)

Eqn. SLE3 (unweighted):

$NE_{l\text{-}obs}$, Mcal = 0.420 (SE = 0.3930) + 0.824 (SE = 0.1332) × $NE_{l\text{-}pred}$ (R^2 = 0.69; mean bias = –0.040)

TABLE 4-6 Description of the Database Used to Evaluate Prediction of Average Daily Gain and Net Energy for Lactation by the CNCPS-S Method (Cannas et al., 2004)[a]

Item[b]	Mean	SD	Minimum	Maximum
Length, d	40	11.81	17	52
Dietary TDN, % DM	72.1	5.14	61.8	79.9
Dietary ME, Mcal/kg DM	2.81	0.427	0.23	3.64
Dietary CP, % DM	16.4	2.22	12.4	19.6
Dietary NDF, % DM	40.2	7.76	18	48.5
Dietary UIP, % CP	27.6	5.54	13	36.3
Initial full body weight, kg	72.1	13.77	45.7	84.8
Final full body weight, kg	68	10.98	46.2	81
Initial body condition score[c]	2.9	0.56	2.1	3.8
Final body condition score	2.5	0.61	1.5	3.5
Milk yield, kg	2.2	0.83	0.67	3.17
Milk fat concentration, %	8.5	1.61	6.1	12.1
Milk protein concentration, %	4.7	0.44	4.3	5.9
Dry matter intake, kg	2.46	0.545	1.41	3.34
Average daily gain, g	–86	100.7	–293	58

[a]n = 19.
[b]TDN = total digestible nutrients; DM = dry matter; ME = metabolizable energy; CP = crude protein; NDF = neutral detergent fiber; UIP = undegraded intake protein;
[c]body condition score = 0–5, with 0 extremely thin and 5 extremely obese.

Eqn. SLE4 (weighted):
$NE_{l\text{-}obs}$, Mcal = 0.157 (SE = 0.2805) + 0.846 (SE = 0.1058) × $NE_{l\text{-}pred}$ (R^2 = 0.80; mean bias that of Eqn. SLE3)

Bias existed in prediction of NE_l but not ADG. However, there were some instances of unrealistic estimates of the energy concentration in tissue accreted or mobilized, which was based on inputs of initial and final BW and BCS. On a FBW basis, the energy concentration in tissue lost or gained (TECFBW) averaged 8.1 Mcal/kg but ranged from –18.4 to 23.3 Mcal/kg. Such extreme values resulted from instances where changes in inputs of FBW and BCS were not in close agreement, such as no change in BW and substantial increase or decrease in BCS or vice versa. Hence, data were reanalyzed, first with TECFBW set at 5.7 Mcal/kg for all observations (Eqn. SLE5, SLE6, SLE7, and SLE8), and second when the calculated TECFBW based on BCS was less than 2 or greater than 8 Mcal/kg (Eqn. SLE9, SLE10, SLE11, and SLE12). Alternative equations based on data of Sanson et al. (1993) were used to predict TECFBW, although regression equations with and without setting extreme TECFBW at 5.7 Mcal/kg had lower R^2 and did not lessen bias compared with those shown below with TECFBW based on equations of CNCPS-S (Cannas et al., 2004).

Eqn. SLE5 (TECFBW = 5.7 Mcal/kg; unweighted):
ADG_{obs}, g = –44.9 (SE = 22.27) + 0.499 (SE = 0.1497) × $ADG_{pred\text{-}en}$ (R^2 = 0.39; mean bias = –3.2)

Eqn. SLE6 (TECFBW = 5.7 Mcal/kg; weighted):
ADG_{obs}, g = –30.1 (SE = 18.19) + 0.588 (SE = 0.1469) × $ADG_{pred\text{-}en}$ (R^2 = 0.49; mean bias that of Eqn. SLE5)

Eqn. SLE7 (TECFBW = 5.7 Mcal/kg; unweighted):
$NE_{l\text{-}obs}$, Mcal = 0.247 (SE = 0.4209) + 0.949 (SE = 0.1539) × $NE_{l\text{-}pred}$ (R^2 = 0.69; mean bias = 0.129)

Eqn. SLE8 (TECFBW = 5.7 Mcal/kg; weighted):
$NE_{l\text{-}obs}$, Mcal = –0.064 (SE = 0.2826) + 1.047 (SE = 0.1161) × $NE_{l\text{-}pred}$ (R^2 = 0.83; mean bias that of Eqn. SLE7)

Eqn. SLE9 (TECFBW = 5.7 Mcal/kg when the value based on change in FBW and BCS was less than 2 or greater than 8 Mcal/kg; unweighted):
ADG_{obs}, g = –48.4 (SE = 22.21) + 0.517 (SE = 0.1618) × $ADG_{pred\text{-}en}$ (R^2 = 0.38; mean bias = –13.2; Figure 4-5)

Eqn. SLE10 (TECFBW = 5.7 Mcal/kg when the value based on change in FBW and BCS was less than 2 or greater than 8 Mcal/kg; weighted):
ADG_{obs}, g = –34.4 (SE = 18.19) + 0.601 (SE = 0.1566) × $ADG_{pred\text{-}en}$ (R^2 = 0.46; mean bias that of Eqn. SLE9; Figure 4-6)

Eqn. SLE11 (TECFBW = 5.7 Mcal/kg when the value based on change in FBW and BCS was less than 2 or greater than 8 Mcal/kg; unweighted):
$NE_{l\text{-}obs}$, Mcal = 0.278 (SE = 0.4128) + 0.919 (SE = 0.1479) × $NE_{l\text{-}pred}$ (R^2 = 0.69; mean bias = 0.174; Figure 4-7)

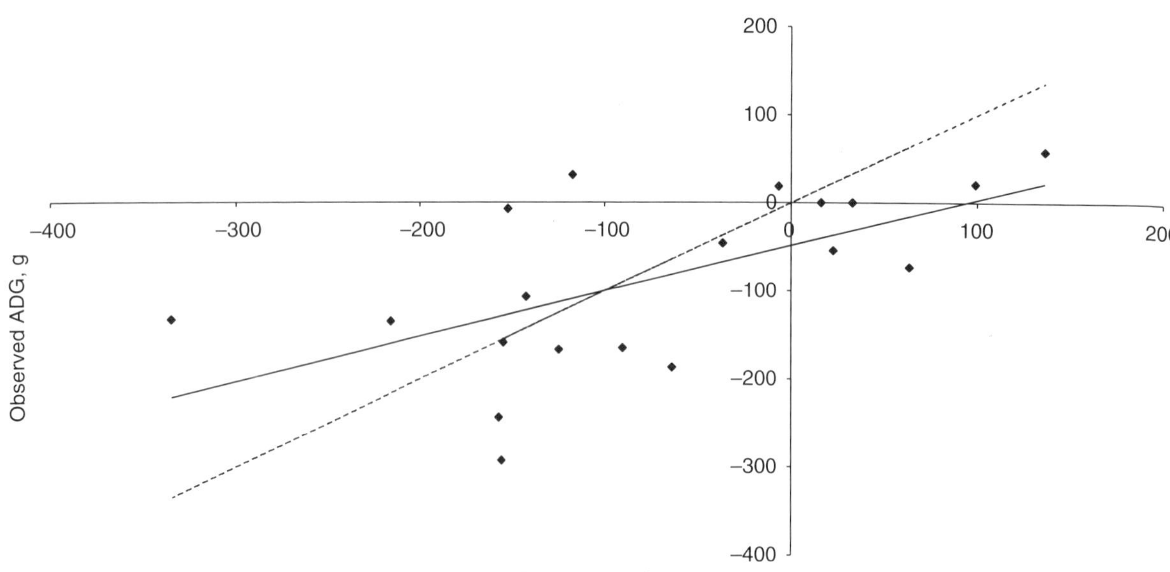

FIGURE 4-5 The relationship between observed ADG (ADG_{obs}) and ADG predicted (ADG_{pred}) by the CNCPS-S method (Cannas et al., 2004) for lactating sheep. The solid line depicts Eqn. SLE9 (unweighted for the number of observations per treatment mean): ADG_{obs}, g = –48.4 (SE = 22.21) + 0.517 (SE = 0.1618) × $ADG_{pred\text{-}en}$ (R^2 = 0.38). The dashed line depicts $ADG_{obs} = ADG_{pred\text{-}en}$.

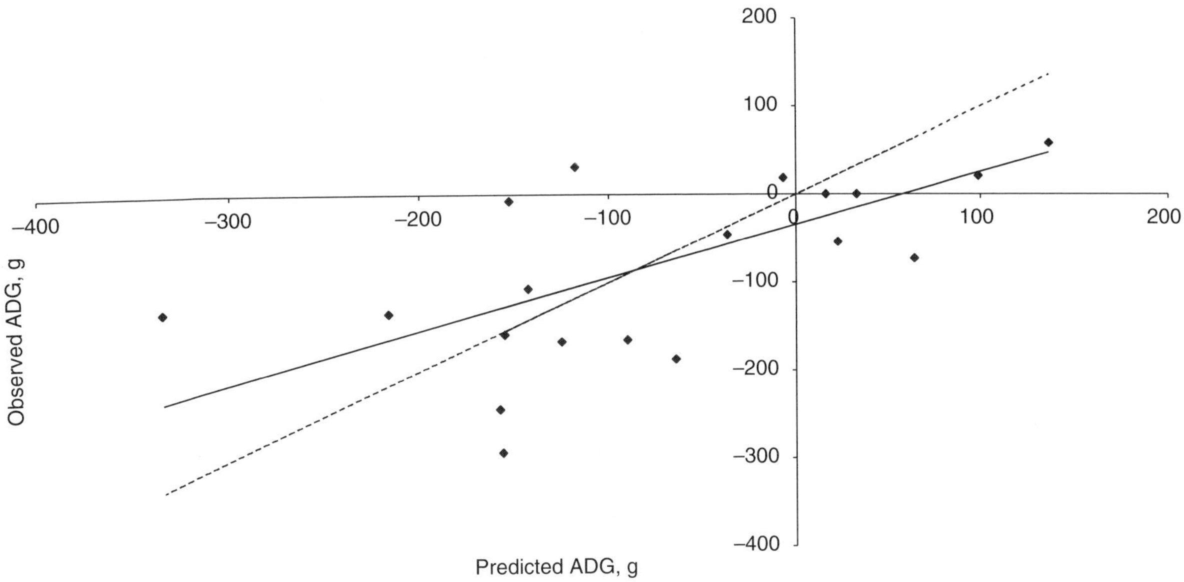

FIGURE 4-6 The relationship between observed ADG (ADG_{obs}) and ADG predicted (ADG_{pred}) by the CNCPS-S method (Cannas et al., 2004) for lactating sheep. The solid line depicts Eqn. SLE10 (weighted for the number of observations per treatment mean): ADG_{obs}, g = –34.4 (SE = 18.19) + 0.601 (SE = 0.1566) × $ADG_{pred\text{-}en}$ (R^2 = 0.46). The dashed line depicts $ADG_{obs} = ADG_{pred\text{-}en}$.

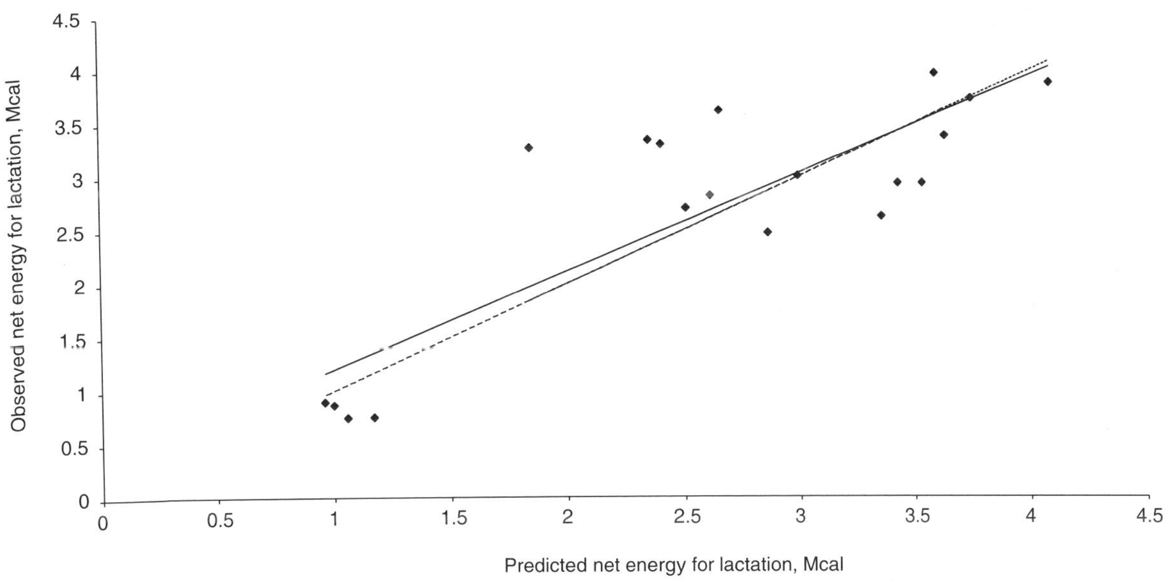

FIGURE 4-7 The relationship between observed NE_l ($NE_{l\text{-}obs}$) and NE_l predicted ($NE_{l\text{-}pred}$) by the CNCPS-S method (Cannas et al., 2004) for lactating sheep. The solid line depicts Eqn. SLE11 (unweighted for the number of observations per treatment mean): $NE_{l\text{-}obs}$, Mcal = 0.278 (SE = 0.4128) + 0.919 (SE = 0.1479) × $NE_{l\text{-}pred}$ (R^2 = 0.69). The dashed line depicts $ADG_{obs} = ADG_{pred\text{-}en}$

Eqn. SLE12 (TECFBW = 5.7 Mcal/kg when the value based on change in FBW and BCS was less than 2 or greater than 8 Mcal/kg; weighted):

$NE_{l\text{-}obs}$, Mcal = –0.022 (SE = 0.2810) + 1.013 (SE = 0.1134) × $NE_{l\text{-}pred}$ (R^2 = 0.82; mean bias that of Eqn. SLE11; Figure 4-8)

These equations suggest the appropriateness of the CNCPS-S assumptions for predicting NE_l when ADG is known and the estimate of TECFBW is reasonable. However, this does not appear to be the case for predicting ADG when NE_l is an input. This finding may involve the relatively small number of observations in the database, inaccuracy of

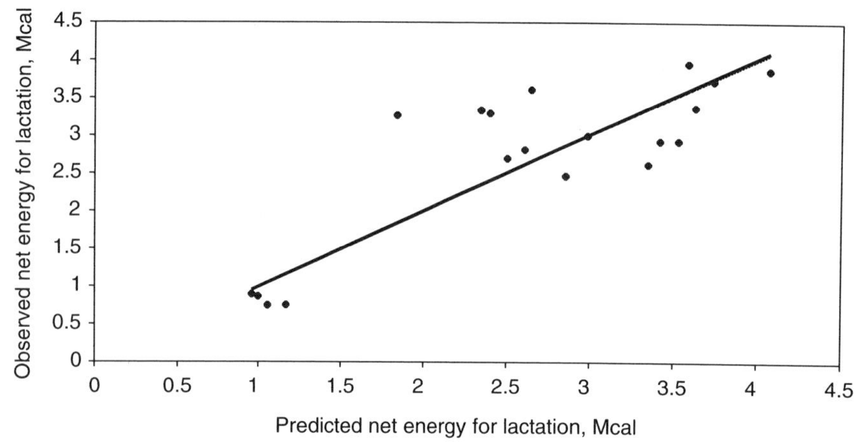

FIGURE 4-8. The relationship between observed NE_l ($NE_{l\text{-obs}}$) and NE_l predicted ($NE_{l\text{-pred}}$) by the CNCPS-S method (Cannas et al., 2004) for lactating sheep. The solid line depicts Eqn. SLE12 (weighted for the number of observations per treatment mean): $NE_{l\text{-obs}}$, Mcal = –0.022 (SE = 0.2810) + 1.013 (SE = 0.1134) × $NE_{l\text{-pred}}$ (R^2 = 0.82). The dashed line depicts $NE_{l\text{-obs}} = NE_{l\text{-pred}}$.

inputs, short experimental periods in some instances, and other factors. But, the method of estimating ME used for lactation, in equation [4] of Cannas et al. (2004), could have had an influence as well. This equation determines total NE_l based on milk yield and concentrations of fat and protein in milk, followed by estimating ME_l by assuming a k_l of 0.644 regardless of the origin of energy fueling milk synthesis. Energy balance is calculated (equation [15] of Cannas et al., 2004) by subtracting the sum of ME_m and ME_l from energy balance. In equation [37] of Cannas et al. (2004), ADG is then predicted by dividing energy balance adjusted for factor k_r by the predicted energy concentration in tissue mobilized or accreted. Cannas et al. (2004) define k_r as the ratio between reserves in NE and ME, and is set at 0.6. Inclusion of k_r with tissue accretion might be appropriate if one assumes a k_g of 0.6. But this may not be desirable with tissue mobilization for support of lactation, with an assumed efficiency of energy use for lactation of 0.644 previously employed in equation [4] to estimate ME_l needed to determine energy balance (Cannas et al., 2004). Relatedly, in other components of the CNCPS-S, k_g varies with dietary ME concentration and the efficiency of use of mobilized tissue energy for lactation is 0.82.

Description of Methods

The CNCPS-S method (Cannas et al., 2004) to describe the energy requirement of lactating sheep is given below. However, the description given is to predict the requirement for particular ADG and milk energy yield rather than as used in the evaluation exercise to predict milk energy yield when ADG is known and vice versa. In addition, a k_{lt} of 0.82 is assumed.

1. FBW_{init}, kg = initial full or unshrunk BW (FBW)
2. FBW_{fin}, kg = final FBW
3. Average shrunk BW (SBW), kg = 96 percent of the average of FBW_{init} and FBW_{fin}
4. Unadjusted energy requirement for fasting metabolism (a1 or $NE_{m\text{-SBW}}$), Mcal/kg $SBW^{0.75}$ = 0.062
5. Multiplicative adjustment of $NE_{m\text{-SBW}}$ for gender (S) = 1 for females
6. Multiplicative adjustment of $NE_{m\text{-SBW}}$ for years of age (AGE) = e(–0.03 × years of age), with years of age greater than 6 set equal to 6
7. Additive adjustment of $NE_{m\text{-SBW}}$ for grazing activity (ACT; Mcal/d) = (0.00062 × FBW × km of flat distance traveled) + (0.00669 × FBW × km of vertical distance traveled)
8. Unadjusted net energy requirement for maintenance (UNE_m), Mcal/d = ($SBW^{0.75}$ × $NE_{m\text{-SBW}}$ × S × AGE) + ACT
9. Unadjusted metabolizable energy requirement for maintenance (UME_m), Mcal/d = UNE_m/0.644
10. FBW at BCS of 3.0 ($FBW_{BCS3.0}$; 0–5 scale) = FBW when skeletal development is complete, empty body fat concentration is 25 percent, and BCS is 2.8 to 3.0
11. Maturity index (P), fraction = average FBW within the feeding period/$FBW_{BCS3.0}$
12. Initial BCS (BCS_{init}) = 0 to 5, with 0 and 5 extremely thin and obese, respectively
13. Initial fraction of fat in the empty body ($FatFr_{init}$) = 0.0269 + (0.0869 × BCS_{init})
14. Initial fraction of protein in the empty body ($ProFr_{init}$) = 0.1449 + (0.0279 × BCS_{init}) – (0.0039 × BCS_{init}^2)
15. Initial empty BW (EBW_{init}), kg = 0.851 × 0.96 × FBW_{init}
16. Initial fat mass ($FatM_{init}$), kg = $FatFr_{init}$ × EBW_{init}

17. Initial protein mass ($ProM_{init}$), kg = $ProFr_{init}$ × EBW_{init}
18. Initial tissue energy (TE_{init}), Mcal = (9.4 × $FatM_{init}$) + (5.7 × $ProM_{init}$)
19. Final BCS (BCS_{fin}) = 0 to 5, with 0 and 5 extremely thin and obese, respectively
20. Final fraction of fat in the empty body ($FatFr_{fin}$) = 0.0269 + (0.0869 × BCS_{fin})
21. Final fraction of protein in the empty body ($ProFr_{fin}$) = 0.1449 + (0.0279 × BCS_{fin}) – (0.0039 × BCS_{fin}^2)
22. Final empty BW (EBW_{fin}), kg = 0.851 × 0.96 × FBW_{fin}
23. Final fat mass ($FatM_{fin}$), kg = $FatFr_{fin}$ × EBW_{fin}
24. Final protein mass ($ProM_{fin}$), kg = $ProFr_{fin}$ × EBW_{fin}
25. Final tissue energy (TE_{fin}), Mcal = (9.4 × $FatM_{fin}$) + (5.7 × $ProM_{fin}$)
26. Average energy concentration on a FBW basis during the feeding period (TEC_{avg}), Mcal/kg = (TE_{fin} – TE_{init})/(FBW_{fin} – FBW_{init})
27. NE requirement for gain when ADG is positive (NE_g), Mcal/d = ADG (kg) × TEC_{avg}
28. ME requirement for gain when ADG is positive (ME_g), Mcal/d = NE_g/0.6
29. Mobilized tissue energy used for lactation when ADG is negative ($ME_{l\text{-}t}$), Mcal/d = (ADG (negative, kg) × TEC_{avg}) × –1
30. NE_l from $ME_{l\text{-}t}$ ($NE_{l\text{-}t}$), Mcal/d = $ME_{l\text{-}t}$ × 0.82
31. MFC, % = milk fat concentration
32. MPC, % = milk true protein concentration
33. MY, kg/d = milk yield
34. NE_l (total), Mcal/d = (251.73 + (89.64 × MFC) + (37.85 × (MPC/0.95))) × 0.001 × MY
35. Dietary NE for lactation ($NE_{l\text{-}d}$), Mcal/d = NE_l – $NE_{l\text{-}t}$
36. Dietary ME for lactation ($ME_{l\text{-}d}$), Mcal/d = $NE_{l\text{-}d}$ / 0.644
37. Total ME for lactation (ME_l), Mcal/d = $ME_{l\text{-}d}$ + $ME_{l\text{-}t}$
38. Unadjusted total ME requirement (UME_{req}), Mcal/d = UME_m + ME_g+ $ME_{l\text{-}d}$
39. Additive adjustment of UME_m for the effect of level of MEI on visceral organ tissue energy use (VO), Mcal/d = 0.09 × UME_{req}
40. ME requirement for maintenance (ME_m), Mcal/d = UME_m + VO
41. Net energy requirement for maintenance (NE_m), Mcal/d = ME_m × 0.644
42. Total ME requirement (ME_{req}), Mcal/d = ME_m + ME_g + $ME_{l\text{-}d}$

Mature Sheep (Nonpregnant) or in Early and Mid-Gestation

Cannas et al. (2004) conducted an evaluation of the CNCPS-S method for mature sheep, with a database also including some lactating animal observations. Shrunk BW gain was accurately predicted with positive ruminal nitrogen balance. Based on this and the aforementioned evaluation for lactating sheep, the CNCPS-S method of describing energy requirements of mature sheep is recommended, as overviewed above for lactating sheep but with omission of the requirement for milk production. As noted above, the upward adjustment of ME_m in accordance with MEI (i.e., 0.09 × MEI) is included, but this may not be most appropriate in all instances. Perhaps, however, inclusion would provide a safety factor in predicted requirements.

Sheep in Late Gestation

Energy requirements for late gestation (ME_{preg}) are predicted as in the CNCPS-S method (Cannas et al., 2004), which is overviewed below:

$$ME_{preg}\ (\text{Mcal/d}) = (36.9644 \times e(-11.465 \times e(-0.00643 \times T) - 0.00643 \times T) \times (LBW/4))/0.13$$

where T = day of gestation and LBW = total litter birth weight (kg) or the product of litter size and birth weight per lamb.

Acclimatization

The recommended optional adjustment of ME_m for acclimatization is the same as that used in other systems, such as SCA (1990) and NRC (2000), as shown below but for ME_m with an assumed k_m of 0.644:

$$ME\ (\text{Mcal/d}) = ((0.00293 \times (20 - Tp)) \times 0.322\ \text{MJ/kg}\ BW^{0.75})/(0.644 \times 0.239)$$

where Tp is the average ambient temperature in the preceding month (°C) and 20 is the mid-point thermoneutral zone temperature (°C). For adjustment in MJ/d, multiplication by 0.239 can be omitted. There may be more appropriate midpoint thermoneutral zone temperatures for various sheep and climatic conditions.

Heat and Cold Extremes

Recommendations for adjusting ME_m for heat and cold extremes are those of NRC (1981a). As noted before, with heat stress, ME_m could be increased by 7 and by 11–25 percent for rapid, shallow breathing and for deep, open-mouth panting, respectively. For cold stress, total insulation (IN) = tissue insulation (TI) + external insulation (EI). NRC (2000) indicated TI values of 2.5, 6.5, 5.5–8.0, and 6.0–12.0 for newborn calves, 1-month-old calves, yearling cattle, and adult cattle, respectively, based on subcutaneous fat and skin thickness. Appropriate values for sheep can be extrapolated from these, based on BCS, fiber growth as influencing skin thickness, and time of shearing. External insulations is estimated as: ((1.759 – 0.0707 × WIND + 0.6095 × HAIR) ×

MUD × HIDE) × 0.239. EI is °C/Mcal/m^2, WIND is km/h, HAIR (effective) is cm, and MUD and HIDE are fractional adjustments for thicknesses. For EI in °C/MJ/m^2, multiplication by 0.239 can be omitted. It is doubtful most sheep production scenarios would require a MUD input.

Lower critical temperature (LCT; °C) is estimated as:

$$39 - IN \times ((HE/SA) - H_e)$$

where HE is heat energy (Mcal or MJ), SA is surface area (m^2 = 0.09 × kg BW$^{0.67}$), and H_e is the minimal evaporative heat loss (HE/SA × 0.15). Effective ambient temperature (EAT) is then determined from skin exposure to the environment (i.e., increase with exposure to sunlight and decrease on cold clear nights). The increase in ME_m (Mcal) is estimated as: (SA × ((LCT – EAT) / IN)) × 0.239. For the adjustment in MJ, multiplication by 0.239 can be omitted.

Season

As noted before, season may impact ME_m. Since such effects in sheep have not been extensively studied, no standard adjustment can be recommended.

Parasitism

Subclinical parasitism can influence nutrient requirements, although such impacts have not been well characterized, such as regarding site of infestation (e.g., abomasum vs. small intestine for internal parasites) and level (e.g., linear, quadratic change). Likewise, type of infection could have an impact, with parasites eliciting primarily blood loss (e.g., ticks) or ingesting nutrients from the gut lumen (e.g., tapeworms) presumably impacting energy loss relatively more than ones principally causing gastrointestinal tract tissue damage.

Internal parasitism has a relatively greater effect on the requirement for MP vs. ME and typical management practices are such to avoid high levels of internal parasitism that noticeably impact performance. Thus, at present no recommendation is made to adjust the ME_m requirement other than that associated with an increase in MP_m with internal parasites increasing gastrointestinal tract tissue protein turnover.

GOATS

Introduction

Recommendations for energy requirements of goats are based primarily on reports summarized by Sahlu and coworkers (Luo et al., 2004a,b,d,e; Moore et al., 2004; Nsahlai et al., 2004a; Sahlu et al., 2004). These studies entailed regression analyses with a database of treatment mean observations compiled from the literature. Whenever possible, the expressions were evaluated with independent databases; none of those presented showed significant prediction bias. It was felt preferable to propose these expressions, rather than unevaluated simple means determined in small numbers of individual studies, since they were developed from a database with a broad array of goats and diets. Similarly, other systems entailing recommendations for goats based largely on, or extrapolated from, data for other ruminant species are not proposed since they have not been evaluated to the extent of those of Sahlu et al. (2004) and/or require inputs that some users might not be able to accurately provide.

Maintenance

Metabolizable energy for maintenance requirements listed below is on a full or unshrunk BW basis (FBW). Values determined in reports summarized by Sahlu et al. (2004) were:

Suckling or preweaning
 116 kcal/kg FBW$^{0.75}$ (485 kJ/kg FBW$^{0.75}$)

Growing (weaning to 1.5 years of age)
 Meat (50 percent Boer)
 117 kcal/kg FBW$^{0.75}$ (489 kJ/kg FBW$^{0.75}$)
 Dairy (selected for milk production)
 139 kcal/kg FBW$^{0.75}$ (580 kJ/kg FBW$^{0.75}$)
 Indigenous or local
 117 kcal/kg FBW$^{0.75}$ (489 kJ/kg FBW$^{0.75}$)

Mature (dairy and indigenous)
 110 kcal/kg FBW$^{0.75}$ (462 kJ/kg FBW$^{0.75}$)

Angora (> 1 year of age)
 113 kcal/kg FBW$^{0.75}$ (473 kJ/kg FBW$^{0.75}$)

For values listed below, a 15 percent difference in ME_m between intact males compared with females and male castrates or wethers was assumed (NRC, 2000) and was applied to values listed above in accordance with the gender makeup of the data sets used. In addition, an ME_m 5 percent greater for growing vs. mature Angora goats was assumed as suggested by Sahlu et al. (2004). The same relative difference in ME_m between biotypes of growing goats was extended to the mature goat ME_m, since the latter data set was relatively small.

Suckling or preweaning
 Intact males
 125 kcal/kg FBW$^{0.75}$ (521 kJ/kg FBW$^{0.75}$)
 Females and wethers
 107 kcal/kg FBW$^{0.75}$ (449 kJ/kg FBW$^{0.75}$)

- Growing
  - Meat
    - Intact males
      - 126 kcal/kg $FBW^{0.75}$ (526 kJ/kg $FBW^{0.75}$)
    - Females and wethers
      - 108 kcal/kg $FBW^{0.75}$ (452 kJ/kg $FBW^{0.75}$)
  - Dairy
    - Intact males
      - 149 kcal/kg $FBW^{0.75}$ (624 kJ/kg $FBW^{0.75}$)
    - Females and wethers
      - 128 kcal/kg $FBW^{0.75}$ (537 kJ/kg $FBW^{0.75}$)
  - Indigenous
    - Intact males
      - 126 kcal/kg $FBW^{0.75}$ (526 kJ/kg $FBW^{0.75}$)
    - Females and wethers
      - 108 kcal/kg $FBW^{0.75}$ (452 kJ/kg $FBW^{0.75}$)
  - Angora
    - Intact males
      - 128 kcal/kg $FBW^{0.75}$ (534 kJ/kg $FBW^{0.75}$)
    - Females and wethers
      - 110 kcal/kg $FBW^{0.75}$ (459 kJ/kg $FBW^{0.75}$)

- Mature
  - Meat
    - Intact males
      - 116 kcal/kg $FBW^{0.75}$ (486 kJ/kg $FBW^{0.75}$)
    - Females and wethers
      - 101 kcal/kg $FBW^{0.75}$ (423 kJ/kg $FBW^{0.75}$)
  - Dairy
    - Intact males
      - 138 kcal/kg $FBW^{0.75}$ (576 kJ/kg $FBW^{0.75}$)
    - Females and wethers
      - 120 kcal/kg $FBW^{0.75}$ (501 kJ/kg $FBW^{0.75}$)
  - Indigenous
    - Intact males
      - 116 kcal/kg $FBW^{0.75}$ (486 kJ/kg $FBW^{0.75}$)
    - Females and wethers
      - 101 kcal/kg $FBW^{0.75}$ (423 kJ/kg $FBW^{0.75}$)
  - Angora
    - Intact males
      - 130 kcal/kg $FBW^{0.75}$ (544 kJ/kg $FBW^{0.75}$)
    - Females and wethers
      - 113 kcal/kg $FBW^{0.75}$ (473 kJ/kg $FBW^{0.75}$)

Sahlu et al. (2004) suggested, in accordance with NRC (2000) recommendations for beef cattle, that ME_m be decreased by as much as 20 percent because of low nutritional planes for a period 2 to 3 months in length. In a goat nutrient requirement calculation system (www2.luresext.edu/goats/research/nutreqgoats.html) complementary to the report of and studies summarized by Sahlu et al. (2004), the following formula based on the time (week, WK) after change in nutritional plane from a limiting to nonlimiting level and BCS (1 to 5, with 1 being emaciated and 5 quite obese) was used to derive an adjustment factor (AF) to be multiplied by the ME_m based on $BW^{0.75}$:

$$AF = 0.68305 + (0.093975 \times BCS) + (0.022850 \times WK) + (0.0031006 \times BCS^2) + (0.000065720 \times WK^2) - (0.0053890 \times BCS \times WK) - (0.000054958 \times BCS \times WK^2) + (0.0037706 \times WK \times BCS^2) - (0.0012983 \times BCS \times WK \times BCS^2) - (0.0000013703 \times BCS \times WK \times WK^2) + (0.0000008396 \times BCS \times WK \times BCS^2 \times WK^2).$$

This equation was derived from adjustment factors in Table 4-7.

Production

ME_g requirements are:

- Suckling
  - 3.20 kcal/g ADG (13.4 kJ/g ADG)
- Growing
  - Meat 5.52 kcal/g ADG (23.1 kJ/g ADG)
  - Dairy 5.52 kcal/g ADG (23.1 kJ/g ADG)
  - Indigenous
    - 4.73 kcal/g ADG (19.8 kJ/g ADG)
- Mature
  - 6.81 kcal/g ADG (28.5 kJ/g ADG)

TABLE 4-7 Adjustment Factors

	Week after low nutritional plane stops and adequate nutritional plane starts										
BCS	1	2	3	4	5	6	7	8	9	10	11
1.0	0.800	0.820	0.840	0.860	0.880	0.900	0.920	0.940	0.960	0.980	1.000
1.5	0.850	0.869	0.887	0.906	0.925	0.944	0.963	0.981	1.000	1.000	1.000
2.0	0.900	0.917	0.933	0.950	0.966	0.983	1.000	1.000	1.000	1.000	1.000
2.5	0.950	0.962	0.975	0.987	1.000	1.000	1.000	1.000	1.000	1.000	1.000
3.0	1.000	1.000	1.000	1.000	1.000	1.000	1.000	1.000	1.000	1.000	1.000
3.5	1.000	1.000	1.000	1.000	1.000	1.000	1.000	1.000	1.000	1.000	1.000
4.0	1.000	1.000	1.000	1.000	1.000	1.000	1.000	1.000	1.000	1.000	1.000
4.5	1.000	1.000	1.000	1.000	1.000	1.000	1.000	1.000	1.000	1.000	1.000
5.0	1.000	1.000	1.000	1.000	1.000	1.000	1.000	1.000	1.000	1.000	1.000

For Angora goats, ME requirements were determined for nonfiber tissue gain (ME_{tg}) and for clean mohair fiber gain (ME_f). ME_l was determined for 1 kg of 4 percent fat-corrected milk (FCM; 3.079 MJ/kg).

ME_{tg} 8.89 kcal/g ADG (37.2 kJ/g)
ME_f 37.5 kcal/g ADG (157 kJ/g)
ME_l 1.25 Mcal/kg 4 percent fat-corrected milk (5.22 MJ/kg)

Parity

As noted by Sahlu et al. (2004), additional energy is required for yearling lactating goats for continual growth and development, which can be addressed by use of the mature goat ME_g of 6.81 kcal/g ADG (28.5 kJ/g).

Mobilized Tissue

In determining ME_l, a factorial approach was taken, with use of the appropriate mature goat ME_m and assuming a k_{lt} of 0.84 and k_g of 0.75. Luo et al. (2004c) assumed that mobilized tissue energy was used with the same efficiency as dietary energy (i.e., k_m), which was determined with an AFRC (1993, 1998) equation (0.503 + (0.0795 × dietary ME, Mcal/kg DM)). Tissue accreted or mobilized by mature and lactating goats was assumed to have an energy concentration of 5.71 Mcal/kg (AFRC, 1998). For growing and Angora goats, tissue energy concentration (Mcal/kg) was estimated with the AFRC (1998) equation of 1.188 + (1.370 × BW, kg). For lactating and Angora goats, it was assumed that all mobilized tissue energy was used for milk production and fiber accretion, respectively.

Activity

Metabolizable energy for maintenance requirements noted earlier includes an activity energy cost of goats in confinement in pens, stalls, or yards. The manner in which HjE is predicted by various other energy systems was addressed earlier. However, neither these methods nor the one proposed has been thoroughly evaluated. Because of the relationship between time spent grazing and HjE, the following equation developed from the method suggested by Sahlu et al. (2004) is proposed to determine an adjustment factor (AF_{act}) to be multiplied by the ME_m of confined goats to account for HjE:

$$AF_{act} = -0.138896 + (0.058056 \times GWT) - (0.002906 \times DIG) + (0.30129925926 \times DT) + (0.000597 \times TER) + (0.0034375 \times TER^2)$$

where GWT = grazing plus walking time (h), DIG = digestibility of organic matter or TDN (%), DT = distance traveled (km), and TER = terrain score (1 to 5, with 1 having little or no vertical ascent and little or no movement other than associated with grazing and 5 being very rugged and mountainous). Values for GWT of 4, 5, 6, 7, 8, 9, 10, 11, 12, and 13 h result in AF_{act} of 0.05, 0.10, 0.15, 0.20, 0.25, 0.30, 0.35, 0.40, 0.45, and 0.50, respectively. Values for DIG below 60 percent, DT above 5 km, and TS above 3 result in increased AF_{act}, and opposite values elicit lower estimates based on GWT. Predictions with typical inputs are in line with the few available estimates of HjE for goats in the literature. This simple equation was derived from AF_{act} presented by Sahlu et al. (2004), although a more complex regression equation would be required for an exact match of all values.

Pregnancy

The method of predicting ME_{preg} of Sahlu et al. (2004), used later for "look-up" tables, can be described as:

$$ME_{preg}\ (Mcal/d) = (-15.467 - (1.1439 \times BIRWT) + (0.26316 \times DAY) - (0.0021667 \times LS) - (0.0010963 \times DAY^2) + (0.011772 \times BIRWT \times DAY) - (0.98352 \times BIRWT \times LS) + (0.011735 \times BIRWT \times DAY \times LS)) \times 0.239$$

where BIRWT = average birth weight (kg) per kid, DAY = day of gestation, and LS = litter size. For ME_{preg} in MJ/d, multiplication by 0.239 can be omitted. This estimate includes energy metabolized by all components of the gravid uterus and the mammary gland and, therefore, should be added to ME_m of a nonpregnant goat of the same BW or that of the pregnant goat before the last 2 months of gestation. Alternatively, the method of SCA (1990), used by Cannas et al. (2004) in the CNCPS-S, could be employed to predict ME required for maintenance and development of the gravid uterus, which is highlighted below.

$$ME_{preg}\ (Mcal/d) = (36.9644 \times e(-11.465 \times e(-0.00643 \times T) - 0.00643 \times t) \times (LBW/4))/0.13$$

where T = day of gestation and LBW = total litter birth weight (kg) or the product of litter size and birth weight per kid. This method does not seem to partition mammary gland energy use with that of other pregnancy tissues. Thus, efficiency of ME use by existing mammary gland tissue for maintenance may be assumed that for nonpregnancy tissues and RE by the developing mammary gland not addressed.

Acclimatization

The recommended optional adjustment of ME_m for acclimatization is the same as that used in other systems, such as SCA (1990) and NRC (2000), as shown below but for ME_m with an assumed k_m of 0.70:

$$\text{ME (Mcal/day)} = ((0.00293 \times (20 - \text{Tp})) \times 0.322 \text{ MJ/kg BW}^{0.75})/(0.70 \times 0.239)$$

where Tp is the average ambient temperature in the preceding month (°C) and 20 is the mid-point thermoneutral zone temperature (°C). For adjustment in MJ/day, division by 4.184 can be omitted. Sahlu et al. (2004) suggested that there may be more appropriate mid-point thermoneutral zone temperatures for various goats and climatic conditions.

Heat and Cold Extremes

Recommendations for adjusting ME_m for heat and cold extremes are those of Sahlu et al. (2004), which were based on NRC (1981a, 2000). As noted before, with heat stress, ME_m could be increased by 7 and by 11–25 percent for rapid, shallow breathing and for deep, open-mouth panting, respectively. For cold stress, total insulation (IN) = tissue insulation (TI) + external insulation (EI). The NRC (2000) indicated TI values of 2.5, 6.5, 5.5–8.0, and 6.0–12.0 for newborn calves, 1-month-old calves, yearling cattle, and adult cattle, respectively, based on subcutaneous fat and skin thickness. Appropriate values for goats can be extrapolated from these, based on BCS, fiber growth as influencing skin thickness, and time of shearing. The value for EI is estimated as: ((1.759 – 0.0707 × WIND + 0.6095 × HAIR) × MUD × HIDE) × 0.239 where EI is °C/Mcal/m^2, WIND is km/h, HAIR (effective) is cm, and MUD and HIDE are fractional adjustments for thicknesses. For EI in °C/MJ/m^2, multiplication by 0.239 can be omitted. It is doubtful that in most goat production scenarios would require a MUD input.

Lower critical temperature (LCT; °C) is estimated as:

$$39 - \text{IN} \times ((\text{HE/SA}) - H_e)$$

where HE is heat energy (Mcal or MJ), SA is surface area (m^2 = 0.09 × kg BW$^{0.67}$), and H_e is the minimal evaporative heat loss (HE/SA × 0.15). Effective ambient temperature (EAT) is then determined from skin exposure to the environment (i.e., increase with exposure to sunlight and decrease on cold clear nights). The increase in ME_m (Mcal) is estimated as: (SA × ((LCT – EAT) / IN)) × 0.239. For the adjustment in MJ, multiplication by 0.239 can be omitted.

Season

As noted before, season may affect ME_m. However, since such effects in goats have not been extensively studied, no standard adjustment can be recommended.

Parasitism

Subclinical parasitism can influence nutrient requirements, although such effects have not been well characterized, such as regarding site of infestation (e.g., abomasum vs. small intestine for internal parasites) and level (e.g., linear, quadratic change). Likewise, type of infection could have an influence, with parasites eliciting primarily blood loss (e.g., ticks) or ingesting nutrients from the gut lumen (e.g., tapeworms) presumably increasing energy loss relatively more than ones principally causing gastrointestinal tract tissue damage. The ME requirement recommendations listed earlier were for confined animals, which would suggest low levels of parasitism compared with grazing goats. However, some reports did not specify internal parasite control methods, and with anthelmintic resistance, it is likely that even with confinement there were subclinical levels of internal parasites in some cases. Hence, it is presumed that the recommendations do encompass an influence of low levels of parasitism. In addition, internal parasitism has a relatively greater effect on the requirement for MP vs. ME, and typical management practices are such to avoid high levels of internal parasitism that noticeably impact performance. Hence, at present, no recommendation is made to adjust the ME_m requirement other than associated with an increase in the MP requirement for maintenance with internal parasites increasing gastrointestinal tract tissue protein turnover.

Adjustment of Feed Intake

Sahlu et al. (2004) suggested adjusting estimates of feed intake required to meet ME needs for effects of dietary ME concentration (MEC) on efficiencies of metabolism. The method is based on MEC relative to the mean of 2.39 Mcal/kg DM (10 MJ/kg DM) in the database used and the level of MEI relative to estimated requirements for ME_m and production by growing and mohair fiber growth (Angora goats). Given below are equations derived from values of Sahlu et al. (2004) to estimate an AF for correction of estimated DM intake to meet ME requirements.

Growing goat

$$\text{AF} = 1.474800751 - (0.093205211 \times \text{MEC} \times 4.184) + (0.266851028 \times \text{MEI}/ME_m) + (0.004336355 \times (\text{MEC} \times 4.184)^2) - (0.025700525 \times \text{MEC} \times 4.184 \times \text{MEI}/ME_m)$$

Angora goat

$$\text{AF} = 1.13042 - (0.024343 \times \text{MEC} \times 4.184) + (0.37085 \times \text{MEI}/ME_m) + (0.30621 \times ME_f/ME_g) + (0.0010615 \times (\text{MEC} \times 4.184)^2) - (0.036237 \times \text{MEC} \times 4.184 \times \text{MEI}/ME_m) - (0.029841 \times \text{MEC} \times 4.184 \times ME_f/ME_g) - (0.43464 \times \text{MEI}/ME_m \times ME_f/ME_g) + (0.042421 \times \text{MEC} \times 4.184 \times \text{MEI}/ME_m \times ME_f/ME_g)$$

ME_f/ME_g is the proportion (e.g., 0.5) of ME for gain (i.e., nonfiber plus fiber) used for fiber growth, and MEC is in Mcal/kg.

CERVIDS

Introduction

Recommendations for energy requirements of cervids whenever possible are based on published values for the four focal species: white-tailed deer, reindeer/caribou, red deer, and elk/wapiti. Attempts to use the sheep and goat models, the CNCPS-S system (Cannas et al., 2004), to calculate maintenance and production requirements of cervids were not successful. Therefore, pragmatic use of published values combined with estimates using allometry to interpolate and extrapolate to required BW have been used. Thus, within and between species, estimates for ME_m requirements of cervids were assumed to scale to $BW^{0.75}$. Published estimates of ME_m for adult females in winter may include a portion of the pregnancy requirement (ME_{preg}), but are not affected by fiber/hair growth. Estimates of ME_m in summer and ME_g, ME_f, and ME_l were not always available, and extrapolation was made from other closely related species, depending on body size similarities. For all cervid males and for female reindeer/caribou, an estimate of energy requirement for antler growth (ME_a) was based on organic matter deposition assuming k_g (Moen and Pastor, 1998). Estimates of daily ME_m in animals in the summer are assumed to include scurf, ME_f, which is ~12 kcal/kg $BW^{0.75}$. Unless otherwise stated, efficiency in use of ME (k_m, k_g, k_f, k_{preg}, k_{gest}, k_l) were taken from ARC (1980) and NRC (1981b, 1985, 2001).

Maintenance

Due to a lack of studies designed to estimate daily ME_m of neonate fawns and calves, use of the estimate for goats is recommended. Also included is the estimate from White and Luick (1984) for free-ranging maternally nursed reindeer.

Suckling or preweaned	
Penned	116 kcal/kg $BW^{0.75}$
Field-maternally raised	230 kcal/kg $BW^{0.75}$

Growing (weaning to 1.5 years of age)	
Winter	a kcal/kg $BW^{0.75}$

where a = 125–131 for white-tailed deer yearlings (Ullrey et al., 1970; Thompson et al., 1973); 103 and 87 for Norwegian and Svalbard reindeer yearlings, respectively (Nilssen et al., 1984); and 108 for red deer calves (Simpson et al., 1978a,b).

Mature	
Winter	a kcal/kg $BW^{0.75}$

where a = 135 for white-tailed deer does (Ullrey et al., 1969; Thompson et al., 1973), 118 for female reindeer (Larsen and Blix, 1985), 134–140 for female caribou (McEwan, 1970; Fancy and White, 1985b), 124–136 for red deer hinds and stags (Brockway and Maloiy, 1968; Fennessy et al., 1981; Kay and Staines, 1981; Suttie et al., 1987), and 137 and 122 for elk/wapiti hinds and stags, respectively (Jiang and Hudson, 1992; Haigh and Hudson, 1993).

Growing (weaning to 1.5 years of age)	
Summer	a kcal/kg $BW^{0.75}$

where a = 192 for white-tailed deer yearlings (Thompson et al., 1973), 120 for red deer calves (Simpson et al., 1978b), and 224 and 210 for yearling wapiti hinds and stags housed outdoors (Jiang and Hudson 1992; Wairimu et al., 1992).

Mature	
Summer	b kcal/kg $BW^{0.75}$

where b = 173 for white-tailed deer does (Thompson et al., 1973), 145 for female reindeer (Mesteig et al., 2000), 183 for female caribou (Fancy and White, 1985b), and 203 for red deer stags (Fennessy et al., 1981). Summer ME_m could include components of gain (ME_g) and fiber (ME_f).

Production

ME_g requirements are:

Suckling (free-range reindeer, White and Luick, 1984)
5.33 kcal/g ADG

Growing	
Weaned (Jiang and Hudson, 1992)	4.7 kcal/g ADG
Yearling hinds (Jiang and Hudson, 1992)	9.2 kcal/g ADG
Yearling males (Wairimu et al., 1992)	8.0 kcal/g ADG

Mature	
Reindeer/caribou, nonlactating (Chan-McLeod et al., 1994)	10.3 kcal/g ADG
Red deer hinds (Fennessy et al., 1981)	13.1 kcal/g ADG
Lactating (rein/caribou, Chan-McLeod et al., 1994)	11.1 kcal/g ADG

Antler growth (add to ME_m in summer)	
Males	21 kcal/kg $BW^{0.75}$
Female reindeer/caribou	4.2 kcal/kg $BW^{0.75}$

Pregnancy

The NE_{preg} at day t during the second half of gestation (100–130 d depending on species) was estimated as daily energy retention of the gravid uterus per kg parturition fetus weight, times parturition fetus weight:

$$NE_{preg}\, t = LBW \times Yt$$

where LBW = parturition fetus weight (kg) and Yt = energy retention (kcal/d) per kg fetus produced at t (day of gestation). Separate equations for white-tailed deer (Robbins and Moen, 1975), reindeer/caribou (Robbins and Moen, 1975), red deer (Adam et al., 1988a,b) and elk/wapiti (Robbins and Moen, 1975) relate Yt to days pregnant:

$L_n\,Yt = -0.8393 + 0.0257 \times X$	white-tailed deer
$L_n\,Yt = -1.6198 + 0.0226 \times X$	reindeer/caribou
$L_n\,Yt = -1.6198 + 0.0226 \times X$	red deer
$L_n\,Yt = -1.7938 + 0.0193 \times X$	wapiti/elk

where Y = energy retention (kcal/d) per kg fetus produced, t = day of gestation, and X = day of gestation. From data in Robbins and Moen (1975), at term NE_{preg} was related to maternal weight, which allowed estimation of NE_{preg} for species other than those listed above:

$$Yterm = 120 + 1.319 \times X$$

where Yterm = energy retention (NE_{preg}, kcal/d) at term, and X = maternal body weight (kg).

ME_{preg} was estimated assuming a k_{preg} of 0.13. For the four cervid species examined, the mean daily ME_{preg} (Y, kcal/kg $BW^{0.75}$) was less than NRC recommendations (NRC, 1981b).

$ME_{preg} = 55$ kcal/kg $BW^{0.75}$	Single offspring
$ME_{preg} = 115$ kcal/kg $BW^{0.75}$	Twins

ME_{preg} in the last trimester represented 43 percent of ME_m for singlets and 85 percent for twins.

For pen-fed cervids with a single fetus, ME_{preg} + winter ME_m gives a mean ME requirement of 183 kcal/kg $BW^{0.75}$ (190 white-tailed deer, 192 reindeer/caribou, 167 red deer, 173 elk/wapiti), and 250 kcal/kg $BW^{0.75}$ for a white tailed deer bearing twin fetuses.

Thus, a female with a single fetus of weight W_b has the following ME requirement (Mcal/d) for the gravid uterus and winter maintenance:

	$ME_{preg} + ME_m$
white-tailed deer (W_b = 3.2 kg)	3.57
reindeer/caribou (W_b = 5.9/7 kg)	4.42/5.80
red deer (W_b = 7.5 kg)	4.47
elk/wapiti (W_b = 17.5 kg)	10.42

Lactation

Energy requirements for lactation depend on the amount and composition of milk (Oftedal, 1984; Robbins, 1993). Peak lactation occurs at 1.5–3 weeks postpartum in cervids that are pen-raised and declines exponentially thereafter (Arman et al., 1974; Robbins et al., 1981; Loudon et al., 1983; White and Luick, 1984; Hudson and Adamczewski, 1990). However for a lower plane of nutrition, especially in free-range conditions, an exponential decline occurs from the first week (Loudon et al., 1983; White and Luick 1984). Thus changes in daily NE_l and ME_l as a function of postpartum age are not simply combinable into a single equation according to Wood (1967). Under some conditions in the wild, dams nurse offspring for an entire year (Russell et al., 1998). Currently there are no estimates of overwinter NE_l and ME_l for nursing females.

Efficiency of use of ME for lactation is usually expressed as Mcal/kg milk corrected to 4 percent fat, but this simplification is difficult to justify, given that milk of cervids is more concentrated in both fat (6–12 percent) and protein (5–10 percent) and is low in lactose (< 4.5 percent) compared with milk of cattle and sheep. However, within and among species, protein (P, percent) and fat (F, percent) contents are highly interrelated (Luick et al., 1974):

$$P = 1.05 + 0.57 \times F$$

In the absence of direct measure for cervids, $k_l = 0.65$ is assumed when body stores are not used. Otherwise use of maternal tissue (k_{lt}) of 0.84 is assumed.

For a female with one offspring peak daily milk net energy output (NE_l) scales to maternal BW (Oftedal, 1984):

$$\text{Peak } NE_l = 104 \text{ kcal/kg } BW^{0.70}$$

This equation gives a mean estimate of NE_l at 94 percent of observed theoretical estimates values for peak NE_l (white-tailed deer 120, reindeer 73, caribou 84, red deer 76, elk/wapiti 112). For conditions where peak milk production occurs at 3–6 weeks (Type I curve), initial milk production is 85 percent of the peak, and the exponential decline after the peak is approximately 0.52 percent per day (range of 0.45–1.60: Robbins et al., 1981; Loudon et al., 1983; White and Luick, 1984; Parker et al., 1990; García et al., 1999; Reese and Robbins, 1994) with little difference between Type I and Type II curves (García et al., 1999; Landete-Castillejos et al., 2000). Using this procedure, net energy requirement on any particular day of lactation, and hence ME_l, can be estimated. Where only milk yield (Y_m, L/d) is known, energy content of the milk (Q, kcal/mL) at all stages of lactation for reindeer/caribou (White and Luick, 1984) approximates:

$$Q = (12 - 3.33 \times Y_m)/4.184$$

Or for cervids, where daily Y_m is in mL/kg $BW^{0.75}$:

$$Q = 4.24 - 0.6202 \times \text{Ln } Y_m$$

Thus daily ME_l from diet was calculated as:

$ME_l = NE_l / k_{l\text{-}d}$ $\quad$ $k_{l\text{-}d} = 0.644$

$= 161$ kcal/kg $BW^{0.75}$

Daily ME_l from tissue mobilization was calculated as:

$ME_l = NE_l / k_{l\text{-}t}$ $\quad k_{l\text{-}t} = 0.82$
$= 127$ kcal/kg $BW^{0.75}$

Milk production of females with a single offspring is assumed to be 65 percent of that with twins (Oftedal, 1984). Thus, ME_l is divided by 0.65 to account for the requirement of twins and 0.55 for triplets.

For female cervids with single offspring, the following metabolizable energy requirements (Mcal/d) were estimated for milk production (ME_l) and milk production plus summer maintenance ($ME_l + ME_m$):

	ME_l	$ME_l + ME_m$
white-tailed deer	2.47	5.73
reindeer/caribou	2.97/3.88	6.29/9.44
red deer	3.44	8.25
elk/wapiti	7.31	18.1

Free-ranging and Wild Cervids

Considerably more research is needed to make confident estimations of the energy requirements of cervids in the field, whether they are free ranging or in the wild. With a limited data set, several approaches are possible: regression analysis of animals taken from the field (Jiang and Hudson, 1992; Wairimu et al., 1992); computer simulation modeling using activity budgets (Swift, 1983; Boertje, 1985; Hudson and White, 1985; Parker et al., 1996; Moen and Pastor, 1998; Russell et al., 2005); and extrapolation from results of DEE estimated with the doubly labeled isotope technique. Comparison of red deer stags in pens and outdoors in winter gives a 49 percent increase in ME_m (Fennessey et al., 1981; Suttie et al., 1987), for wapiti hinds in pens compared with outdoors in winter gives a 63 percent increase (Jiang and Hudson, 1992; Wairimu et al., 1992), and for wapiti stags in summer gives an 88 percent increase (Wairimu et al., 1992; Haigh and Hudson, 1993). The DEE of free-ranging animals is ~ 64 percent higher than those in pens (Gotaas et al., 2000; Haggarty, 2000). For young and adult cervids at maintenance in winter, the mean increase in outdoors requirements is 67–87 kcal/kg $BW^{0.75}$ and is 88 kcal/kg $BW^{0.75}$ in summer. When a mean 64 percent increase in outdoors cost is applied to ME_m in pens, the range in costs is 50–170 kcal/kg $BW^{0.75}$, depending on level of productivity:

Winter (maintenance)	= 130/0.64	= 200 kcal/kg $BW^{0.75}$
Summer (maintenance)	= 175/0.64	= 275 kcal/kg $BW^{0.75}$
Summer (growth)	= 250/0.64	= 390 kcal/kg $BW^{0.75}$
Peak lactation	= 300/0.64	= 470 kcal/kg $BW^{0.75}$

CAMELIDS

Recently, Van Saun (2006) reviewed research of the nutrient requirements of llamas and alpacas. When direct estimates of energy requirements were not available, which was the case in most instances, Van Saun (2006) presented rationale for assuming requirements similar to ones of other ruminant species, in order to use a factorial approach to estimate total energy needs as well as requirements for protein, minerals, and vitamins. Van Saun (2006) also identified the many areas in which additional research is needed to derive more accurate nutrient requirements. These energy requirements are overviewed below. The review of Van Saun (2006) should be consulted for a more detailed accounting.

Van Saun (2006) suggested an ME_m of 72.85 kcal/kg of $FBW^{0.75}$, which was derived from the mean of two estimates with llamas (Schneider et al., 1974; Carmean et al., 1992). However, for comparison purposes, requirements based on the higher ME_m were also given in tabular form. A slightly lower ME_m for alpacas (66 kcal/kg $BW^{0.75}$) was reported by Newman and Paterson (1994), but findings of Russel and Redden (1997) suggested a greater value.

Because llamas and alpacas typically graze and move freely, Van Saun (2006) pointed out the importance of accounting for energy used in activity. There would be no activity adjustment of ME_m for llamas and alpacas confined in pens, stalls, or small lots. The system of projecting the activity energy cost of NRC (1981b) for goats was proposed as appropriate for use with grazing animals until more information becomes available. As stated by Van Saun (2006), ME_m can be increased by 25, 50, or 75 percent based on pasture characteristics (i.e., intensive management or typical range, semiarid rangeland, and arid rangeland, respectively) and nature of the terrain (flat, slightly hilly, and mountainous, respectively). It was also proposed that similar projections could be made for the intensity and duration of work performed by pack llamas.

To an even greater extent than for goats, there is little knowledge available on the composition of tissue being accreted or mobilized by llamas and alpacas. Because of this and because ADG by llamas and alpacas seems generally within the range for goats, Van Saun (2006) suggested use of the ME requirement for growth by goats of NRC (1981b), which is 7.25 kcal/g ADG and similar to the value suggested by Fowler (1998).

Van Saun (2006) used the method of predicting the pregnancy ME cost for sheep of NRC (1985) at 100, 120, and 140 days of gestation to develop a comparable system for llamas and alpacas in 8, 9, and 10 months of gestation. The prediction equations are shown below.

8 months: pregnancy ME (kcal/d) = $-33.50 + (65.34 \times$ total birth weight, kg)
9 months: pregnancy ME (kcal/d) = $-39.74 + (131.68 \times$ total birth weight, kg)
10 months: pregnancy ME (kcal/d) = $86.12 + (203.51 \times$ total birth weight, kg)

For the ME requirement of lactation by llamas and alpacas, Van Saun (2006) first cited llama milk composition values of Morin et al. (1995; 13.1 percent total solids, 6.5 percent lactose, 3.4 percent protein, and 2.7 percent fat) to estimate an average milk energy concentration of 700.2 kcal/kg. Then an efficiency of ME use for milk synthesis of 74 percent was assumed to obtain a ME requirement for lactation of 946.2 kcal/kg of milk. Van Saun (2006) noted that milk production by llamas and alpacas has not been extensively studied, listing a range of 0.75 to 2.5 kg/d.

To address the ME cost for fiber growth, Van Saun (2006) used the requirement for sheep of NRC (1985), which is 30 kcal/g of greasy fleece. This value is not greatly different from the requirement suggested for goats of 37.5 kcal/g of clean fiber.

The recommended energy requirements for llamas and alpacas are summarized below.

ME for maintenance (ME_m):	72.85 kcal/kg $FBW^{0.75}$
ME for activity:	0 to 75 percent of ME_m, depending on pasture and terrain conditions
ME for gain:	7.25 kcal/g ADG

ME for pregnancy (kcal/d)

8 months:	–33.50 + (65.34 × total birth weight, kg)
9 months:	–39.74 + (131.68 × total birth weight, kg)
10 months:	86.12 + (203.51 × total birth weight, kg)

ME for lactation:	946.2 kcal/kg milk, assuming a milk energy concentration of 700.2 kcal/kg
ME for fiber production:	30 kcal/g greasy fleece

REFERENCES

Adam, C. L., I. McDonald, C. E. Moir, and K. Pennie. 1988a. Foetal development in red deer (Cervus elaphus) 1. Growth of the foetus and associated tissues. Anim. Prod. 46:131–138.

Adam, C. L., I. McDonald, C. E. Moir, and R. I. Smart. 1988b. Foetal development in red deer (Cervus elaphus) 2. Chemical composition of the foetus and associated tissues. Anim. Prod. 46:139–146.

Adamczewski, J. Z., C. C. Gates, R. J. Hudson, and M. A. Price. 1987. Seasonal changes in body composition of mature female caribou and calves (*Rangifer tarandus groenlandicus*) on an arctic island with limited-winter resources. Can. J. Zool. 65:1149–1157.

Adams, N. R., and S. M. Liu. 2003. Principles of nutrient partitioning for wool, growth and reproduction: Implications for nematode parasitism. Aust. J. Exp. Agric. 43:1399–1407.

Adams, N. R., S. Liu, and D. G. Masters. 2000. Regulation of protein synthesis for wool growth. Pp. 255–272 in Ruminant Physiology: Digestion, Metabolism, Growth, and Reproduction, P. B. Cronjé, ed. New York: CABI Publishing.

Aderibigbe, A. O., and D. C. Church. 1983. Feather and hair meals for ruminants. II. Comparative evaluation of feather and hair meals as protein supplements. J. Anim. Sci. 57:473–482.

AFRC (Agriculture and Food Research Council). 1993. Energy and Protein Requirements of Ruminants. Pp. 5–55 in An Advisory Manual Prepared by the AFRC Technical Committee on Responses to Nutrients. Wallingford, UK: CAB International.

AFRC. 1998. The Nutrition of Goats. New York: CAB International.

Alam, M. R., D. P. Poppi, and A. R. Sykes. 1991. Comparative energy and protein utilization in kids and lambs. J. Agric. Sci. 117:121–127.

Albon, S. D., A. Stein, R. J. Irvine, R. Langvatn, E. Ropstad, and O. Halvorsen. 2002. The role of parasites in the dynamics of a reindeer population. Proc. R. Soc. Lond. B. 269:1625–1632.

Alexander, G. 1962. Temperature regulation in the newborn lamb. IV. The effect of wind and evaporation of water from the coat on metabolic rate and body temperature. Aust. J. Agric. Res. 13:82–89.

Amaning-Kwarteng, K., and R. C. Kellaway. 1987. Influence of cottonseed meal and barley grain supplements on intake, digestion, liveweight gain and wool growth in sheep fed NaOH-treated oat and wheat straw diets. J. Agric. Sci. 108:211–219.

Anderson, A. E., D. E. Medin, and D. C. Bowden. 1974. Growth and morphometry of the carcass, selected bones, organs, and glands of mule deer. Wildl. Monog. 39:1–122.

Anderson, R. M., and R. M. May. 1978. Regulation and stability of host-parasite population interactions. J. Anim. Ecol. 47:219–247.

Animut, G. 2004. Evaluation of stocking rate effects with pastures that contain various forbs and grasses being co-grazed by goats and sheep and subsequent performance with an energy-rich diet. Ph.D. dissertation. Oklahoma State University, Stillwater, OK.

Appeddu, L. A., D. G. Ely, D. K. Aaron, W. P. Deweese, and E. Fink. 1995. Supplementing ewe diets with the calcium salts of palm oil fatty acids during lactation. Sheep Goat Res. J. 11:132–139.

Appeddu, L. A., D. G. Ely, D. K. Aaron, W. P. Deweese, and E. Fink. 2004. Effects of supplementing with calcium salts of palm oil fatty acids or hydrogenated tallow on ewe milk production and twin lamb growth. J. Anim. Sci. 82:2780–2789.

ARC (Agricultural Research Council). 1980. The Nutrient Requirements of Ruminant Livestock. Slough, UK: Commonwealth Agricultural Bureaux.

Arman, P., R. N. B. Kay, E. D. Goodall, and G. A. M. Sharman. 1974. The composition and yield of milk from captive red deer (Cervus elaphus L.). J. Reprod. Fertil. 37:67–84.

Armstrong, E., D. Euler, and G. Racey. 1983. Winter bed-site selection by white-tailed deer in central Ontario. J. Wildl. Manage. 47:880–884.

Arnold, W., T. Ruff, S. Reimoser, F. Tataruch, K. Onderscheka, and F. Schober. 2003. Nocturnal hypometabolism as an overwintering strategy of red deer (*Cervus elphus*). Am. J. Physiol. Regul. Integr. Comp. Physiol. 286:R174–R181.

Ash, A. J., and B. W. Norton. 1987. Studies with the Australian cashmere goat. II. Effects of dietary protein concentration and feeding level on body composition of male and female goats. Aust. J. Agric. Res. 38:957–969.

Aziz, N. N., D. M. Murray, and R. O. Ball. 1994. The effect of live weight gain and live weight loss on body composition of Merino wethers: Chemical composition of the noncarcass organs and the empty body. J. Anim. Sci. 72:3098–3109.

Baker, D. L., D. E. Johnson, L. H. Carpenter, O. C. Wallmo, and R. B. Gill. 1979. Energy requirements of mule deer fawns in winter. J. Wildl. Manage. 43:162–169.

Bandy, P. J., I. McT. Cowan, and A. J. Wood. 1970. Comparative growth in four races of black-tailed deer (*Odocoileus hemionus*). Part I. Growth in body weight. Can. J. Zool. 48:1401–1410.

Barboza, P. S., and K. L. Parker. 2006. Body protein stores and isotopic indicators of N balance in female reindeer (*Ranfifer tarandus*) during winter. Physiol. Biochem. Zool. 79:628–644.

Beaver J. M., B. E. Olson, and J. M. Wraith. 1996. A simple index of standard operative temperature for mule deer and cattle in winter. J. Thermal Biol. 21:345–352.

Bell, A. W. 1986. Efficiency of prenatal growth and the heat increment of pregnancy. Pp. 64–67 in Proceedings of the Cornell Nutrition Conference for Feed Manufacturers. Ithaca, NY: Cornell Univ. Agric. Exp. Sta.

Blanchard, J. M., and Hauer, W. E. 1986. Reproductive performance of reindeer fed all-grain and hay-grain rations. Rangifer Spec. Iss. No.1: 39–41.

Blanchard, J. M., W. E. Hauer, and J. R. Luick. 1984. The effects of feeding whole-grain barley to free-ranging and penned reindeer. Agroborealis 15:57–60.

Blaxter, K. L., J. L. Clapperton, and F. W. Wainman. 1966. The extent of differences between six British breeds of sheep in their metabolism, feed intake and utilization, and resistance to climatic stress. Br. J. Nutr. 20:282–294.

Blaxter. K. L., R. N. B. Kay, G. A. M. Sharman, J. M. M. Cunningham, and W. J. Hamilton. 1974. Farming red deer. Dept. Agric. Fish. Scotland. Edinburgh: Her Majesty's Stationary Office. 93 pp.

Blix, A. S., and J. B. Steen. 1979. Temperature regulation in newborn polar homeotherms. Physiol. Rev. 59:285–304.

Boertje, R. D. 1985. An energy model for adult female caribou of the Denali herd, Alaska. J. Range. Manage. 38:468–473.

Brockway, J. M., and G. M. O. Maloiy. 1968. Energy metabolism of the red deer. J. Physiol. 194:22P–24P.

Brown, R. D. 1990. Nutrition and antler development. Pp. 426–441 in Horns, Pronghorns and Antlers, G. A. Bubenik and A. B. Bubenik, eds. New York: Springer-Verlag.

Bubenik, G. A., D. Schams, R. G. White, J. Rowell, J. Blake, and L. Bartos. 1997. Seasonal levels of reproductive hormones and their relationship to the antler cycle of male and female reindeer (*Rangifer tarandus*). Comp. Biochem. Physiol. 116B:269–277.

Bubenik, G. A., D. Schams, R. G. White, J. Rowell, J. Blake and L. Bartos. 1998. Seasonal levels of metabolic hormones and substrates in male and female reindeer (*Rangifer tarandus*). Comp. Biochem. Physiol. 120 C:307–315.

Bubenik, G. A., R. G. White and L. Bartos. 2000. Antler growth in male and female reindeer and its relationship to seasonal blood levels of alkaline phosphatase. Folia Zool. 49:161–166.

Cameron, R. D., and R. G. White. 1996. Importance of summer weight gain to the reproductive success of caribou in arctic Alaska. Rangifer Spec. Iss. No. 9:397.

Cameron, R. D., W. T. Smith, R. G. White, and B. Griffith. 2005. Central Arctic caribou and petroleum development: Distributional, nutritional, and reproductive implications. Arctic 58:1–9.

Cannas, A., L. O. Tedeschi, D. G. Fox, A. N. Pell, and P. J. Van Soest. 2004. A mechanistic model for predicting the nutrient requirements and feed biological values for sheep. J. Anim. Sci. 82:149–169.

Carmean, B. R., K. A. Johnson, D. E. Johnson, and L. W. Johnson. 1992. Maintenance energy requirement of llamas. Am. J. Vet Res. 53: 1696–1698.

Chan-McLeod, A. C. A., R. G. White, and D. F. Holleman. 1994. Effects of protein and energy intake, body condition, and season on nutrient partitioning and milk production in caribou and reindeer. Can. J. Zool. 72:938–947.

Chan-McLeod, A. C. A., R. G. White, and D. E. Russell. 1999. Comparative body composition strategies of breeding and non-breeding female caribou. Can. J. Zool. 77:1901–1907.

Clutton-Brock, T. H., and S. D. Albon. 1989. Red deer in the highlands. Oxford: BSP Professional Books.

Cook, J. G., L. L. Irwin, L. D. Bryant, R. A. Biggs, and J. W. Thomas. 1998. Relations of forest cover and condition of elk: A test of the thermal cover hypothesis in summer and winter. Wildl. Monog. 141:1–61.

Cook, R. C., J. G. Cook, D. L. Murray, P. Zager, B. K. Johnson, and M. W. Gratson. 2001a. Development of apredictive models of nutritional condition for Rocky Mountain elk. J. Wildl. Manage. 65:973–987.

Cook, R. C., J. G. Cook, D. L. Murray, P. Zager, B. K. Johnson, and M. W. Gratson. 2001b. Nutritional condition models for elk: Which are the most sensitive, accurate, and precise? J. Wildl. Manage. 65:988–997.

Cool, N., and R. J. Hudson. 1996. Requirements for maintenance and live weight gain of moose and wapiti calves during winter. Rangifer 16:41–45.

Corbett, J. L., and M. Freer. 2003. Past and present definitions of the energy and protein requirements of ruminants. Asian-Aust. J. Anim. Sci. 16:609–624.

Cuyler, C., and N. A. Øritsland. 2004. Rain more important than windchill for insulation loss in Svalbard reindeer fur. Rangifer 24:7–13.

Dauphiné, T. C. 1976. Biology of the Kaminuriak population of barren-ground caribou. Part 4. Growth, reproduction and energy reserves. Can. Wildl. Serv. Rep. Ser. No. 38.

Dawson, L. E. R., and R. W. J. Steen. 1998. Estimation of maintenance energy requirements of beef cattle and sheep. J. Agric. Sci. 131:477–485.

Demarchi, M. W., and F. L. Bunnell. 1993. Estimating forest canopy effects on summer thermal cover for Cervidae (deer family). Can. J. For. Res. 23:2419–2426.

Dhakad, A., A. K. Garg, P. Singh, and D. K. Agrawal. 2002. Effect of replacement of maize grain with wheat bran on the performance of growing lambs. Small Ruminant Res. 43:227–234.

Dove, H. 1988. Estimation of the intake of milk by lambs, from the turnover of deuterium- or tritium-labelled water. Br. J. Nutr. 60: 375–387.

Dove, H., and M. Freer. 1979. The accuracy of tritiated water turnover rate as an estimate of milk intake in lambs. Aust. J. Agric. Res. 30:725–739.

Drochner, W., G. Flachowsky, J. Pallauf, E. Pfeffer, M. Rodehutscond, and W. Staudacher. 2003. Recommendations for the Supply of Energy and Nutrients to Goats. Frankfurt, Germany: DLG-Verlag.

Drouillard, J. S., T. J. Klopfenstein, R. A. Britton, M. L. Bauer, S. M. Gramlich, T. J. Wester, and C. L. Ferrell. 1991. Growth, body composition, and visceral organ mass and metabolism in lambs during and after metabolizable protein or net energy restrictions. J. Anim. Sci. 69: 3357–3375.

D'Urso, G., M. Avondo, S. Bordonaro, D. Marletta, and A. M. Guastella. 1998. Effect of sustained-release somatotropin on performance and grazing behavior of ewes housed at different stocking rates. J. Dairy Sci. 81:958–965.

Eilertsen, S. M., I. Schjelderup, G. McL. Dryden, and S. D. Mathiesen. 2001. High protein pastures in spring–effects on body composition in reindeer. Rangifer 21:13–19.

Emmans, G. C. 1994. Effective energy: A concept of energy utilisation applied across species. Br. J. Nutr. 71:801–821.

Fancy, S. G., and R. G. White. 1985a. The incremental cost of activity. Pp.143–159 in Bioenergetics of Wild Herbivores, R. J. Hudson and R. G. White, eds. Boca Raton, FL: CRC Press.

Fancy, S. G., and R. G. White. 1985b. Energy expenditures by caribou while cratering in snow. J. Wildl. Manage. 49:987–993.

Fancy, S. G., J. M. Blanchard, D. R. Holleman, K. J. Kokjer, and R. G. White. 1986. Validation of doubly labeled water method using a ruminant. Am. J. Physiol. 251:R143–R149.

Fauchald, P., T. Tveraa, C. Henaug, and N. Yoccoz. 2004. Adaptive regulation of body reserves in reindeer, *Rangifer tarandus*: A feeding experiment. Oikos 107:583–591.

Fegeros, K., G. Zervas, S. Stamouli, and E. Apostolaki. 1995. Nutritive value of dried citrus pulp and its effect on milk yield and milk composition of lactating ewes. J. Dairy Sci. 78:1116–1121.

Fennessy, P. F., G. J. Greer, and D. A. Forbes. 1980. Voluntary intake and digestion in red deer and sheep. Proc. NZ Soc. Anim. Prod. 40: 158–162.

Fennessy, P. F., G. H. Moore, and I. D. Corson. 1981. Energy requirements of red deer. Proc. NZ Soc. Anim. Prod. 41:167–173.

Ferrell, C. L., and L. P. Reynolds. 1987. Oxidative metabolism of gravid uterine tissues of the cow. Energy Metab. Proc. Symp. 32:298–301.

Fimbres, H., G. Hernández-Vidal, J. F. Picón-Rubio, J. R. Kawas, and C. D. Lu. 2002. Productive performance and carcass characteristics of lambs fed finishing ration containing various forage levels. Small Ruminant Res. 43:283–288.

Finstad, G. L., and A. K. Pritchard. 2000. Growth and body weight of free-ranging reindeer in western Alaska. Rangifer 20:221–227.

Fluharty, F. L., and K. E. McClure. 1997. Effects of dietary energy intake and protein concentration on performance and visceral organ mass in lambs. J. Anim. Sci. 75:604–606.

Fluharty, F. L., K. E. McClure, M. B. Solomon, D. D. Clevenger, and G. D. Lowe. 1999. Energy source and ionophore supplementation effects on lamb growth, carcass characteristics, visceral organ mass, diet digestibility, and nitrogen metabolism. J. Anim. Sci. 77:816–823.

Fowler, M. E. 1998. Feeding and nutrition. Pp. 12–48 in Medicine and Surgery of South American Camelids: Llama, Alpaca, Vicuna, Guanaco, 2nd ed. Ames: Iowa State University Press.

Freetly, H. C., and C. L. Ferrell. 1997. Oxygen consumption by and blood flow across the portal-drained viscera and liver of pregnancy ewes. J. Anim. Sci. 75:1950–1955.

Freetly, H. C., and K. A. Leymaster. 2004. Relationship between litter birth weight and litter size in six breeds of sheep. J. Anim. Sci. 82:612–618.

Freetly, H. C., C. L. Ferrell, T. G. Jenkins, and A. L. Goetsch. 1995a. Visceral oxygen consumption during chronic restriction and realimentation in sheep. J. Anim. Sci. 73:843–852.

Freetly, H. C., J. A. Nienaber, K. A. Leymaster, and T. G. Jenkins. 1995b. Relationships among heat production, body weight, and age in Suffolk and Texel ewes. J. Anim. Sci. 73:1030–1037.

Freetly, H. C., J. A. Nienaber, and T. M. Brown-Brandl. 2002a. Relationship between aging and nutritionally controlled growth rate on heat production of ewe lambs. J. Anim. Sci. 80:2759–2763.

Freetly, H. C., J. A. Nienaber, and T. M. Brown-Brandl. 2002b. Relationships among heat production, body weight, and age in Finnsheep and Rambouillet ewes. J. Anim. Sci. 80:825–832.

Funk, M. A., M. L. Galyean, and T. T. Ross. 1986. Potassium and lasalocid effects on performance and digestion in lambs. J. Anim. Sci. 63: 685–691.

Galloway, D. L., Sr., A. L. Goetsch, and D. M. Hallford. 1996. Effects of supplementing moderate- to low-quality grass hay with maize and (or) rumen-undegradable protein on growth of wethers. Small Ruminant Res. 21:181–193.

García, A., T. Landete-Castillejos, A. Molina, B. Albiñana, C. Fernández, J. Garde, and L. Gallego. 1999. Lactation curves in captive Iberian red deer (*Cervus elaphus hispanicus*). J. Anim. Sci. 77:3150–3155.

Gates, C. C., and R. J. Hudson. 1979. Effect of posture and activity on metabolic responses of wapiti to cold. J. Wildl. Manage. 43:564–567.

Gentry, L. R., J. M. Fernandez, T. L. Ward, T. W. White, L. L. Southern, T. D. Bidner, D. L. Thompson, Jr., D. W. Horohov, A. M. Chapa, and T. Sahlu. 1999. Dietary protein and chromium tripicolinate in Suffolk wether lambs: Effects on production characteristics, metabolic and hormonal responses, and immune status. J. Anim. Sci. 77:1284–1294.

Gerhart, K. L., R. G. White, R. D. Cameron, and D. E. Russell. 1996a. Body composition and nutrient reserves of arctic caribou. Can. J. Zool. 74:136–146.

Gerhart, K. L., R. G. White, R. D. Cameron, and D. E. Russell. 1996b. Estimating fat content of caribou from body condition scores. J. Wildl. Manage. 60:713–718.

Gillingham, M. P., K. L. Parker, and T. A. Hanley. 1997. Forage intake by black-tailed deer in a natural environment: Bout dynamics. Can. J. Zool. 75:1118–1128.

Glimp, H. A., S. P. Hart, and D. VonTungeln. 1989. Effect of altering nutrient density (concentrate to roughage ratio) and restricting energy intake on rate, efficiency and composition of growing lambs. J. Anim. Sci. 67:865–871.

Goetsch, A. L. 1997. Growing and finishing performance and body composition for St. Croix wethers consuming growing diets differing in grain and protein levels. J. Anim. Feed Sci. 6:319–332.

Goetsch, A. L. 1998. Splanchnic tissue energy use in ruminants that consume forage-based diets ad libitum. J. Anim. Sci. 76:2737–2746.

Goetsch, A. L., and G. E. Aiken. 1999. Effects of limited concentrate intake following forage on subsequent performance of lambs consuming concentrate. Sheep Goat Res. J. 15:147–153.

Goetsch, A. L., S. W. Coleman, and W. A. Phillips. 1998. Growth and body composition of two crossbred wether types fed different quality grasses. Sheep Goat Res. J. 4:138–143.

Goss, R. J. 1963. Inhibition of growth and shedding of antlers by sex hormones. Nature 220:83–85.

Goss, R. J. 1995. Future directions in antler research. Anatom. Rec. 241:291–302.

Gotaas, G., E. Milne, P. Haggarty, and N. J. C. Tyler. 2000. Energy expenditure of free-living reindeer estimated by the doubly labelled water method. Rangifer 20:211–219.

Graham, N. McC. 1968. The metabolic rate of Merino rams bred for high or low wool production. Aust. J. Agric. Res. 19:821–824.

Graham, N. McC., and T. W. Searle. 1982. Energy and nitrogen utilization for body growth in young sheep from two breeds with differing capacities for wool growth. Aust. J. Agric. Res. 33:607–615.

Graham, N. McC., T. W. Searle, and D. A. Griffiths. 1974. Basal metabolic rate in lambs and young sheep. Aust. J. Agric. Res. 25:957–971.

Gulland, F. M. D. 1995. The impact of infectious diseases on wild populations: A review. Pp. 20–51 in Ecology of Infectious Diseases in Natural Populations, B. T. Grenfell and A. P. Dobson, eds. Cambridge, UK: Cambridge University Press.

Haddad, S. G., R. E. Nasr, and M. M. Muwalla. 2001. Optimum dietary crude protein level for finishing Awassi lambs. Small Ruminant Res. 39(1):41–46.

Haggarty, P. 2000. Quantifying the free living energy exchange of Arctic ungulates with stable isotopes. Rangifer 20:59–69.

Haggarty, P., J. J. Robinson, J. Ashton, E. Milne, C. L. Adam, C. E. Kyle, S. L. Christie, and A. J. Midwood. 1998. Estimation of energy expenditure in free–living red deer (*Cervus elaphus*) with the doubly labelled water method. Br. J. Nutr. 80:263–272.

Haigh, J. C., and R. J. Hudson. 1993. Farming Wapiti and Red Deer. St. Louis, MO: Mosby.

Halvorsen, O., A. Stein, J. Irvine, R. Langvatn, and S. Albon. 1999. Evidence for continued transmission of parasitic nematodes in reindeer during the Arctic winter. Inter. J. Parasit. 29:567–579.

Hammel, H. T. 1955. Thermal properties of fur. Am. J. Physiol. 182: 369–376.

Hart, J. S., O. Heroux, W. H. Cottle, and C. A. Mills. 1961. The influence of climate on metabolic and thermal responses of infant caribou. Can. J. Zool. 39:845–856.

Helle, T., and L. Tarvainen. 1984. Effects of insect harassment on weight gain and survival in reindeer. Rangifer 4:24–27.

Herselman, M. J., and W. A. Smith. 1991. The energy requirements of Angora goats. Karoo Agric. 4:18–20.

Hissa, R., S. Saarela, and M. Nieminen. 1981. Development of temperature regulation in newborn reindeer. Rangifer 1:29–38.

Hobbs, N. T. 1989. Linking energy balance to survival in mule deer: Development and test of a simulation model. Wildlife Monog. 101:1–39.

Holter, J. B., W. E. Urban, and H. H. Hayes. 1977. Nutrition of northern white-tailed deer throughout the year. J. Anim. Sci. 45:365–376.

Hudson, R. J. 1985. Body size, energetics , and adaptive radiation. Pp. 1–24 in Bioenergetics of Wild Herbivores, R. J. Hudson and R. G. White, eds. Boca Raton, FL: CRC Press.

Hudson, R. J., and J. Adamczewski. 1990. Effect of supplementing summer ranges on lactation and growth of wapiti (*Cervus elaphus*). Can. J. Anim. Sci. 70:551–560.

Hudson, R. J., and R. J. Christopherson. 1985. Maintenance metabolism. Pp. 143–159 in Bioenergetics of Wild Herbivores, R. J. Hudson and R. G. White, eds. Boca Raton, FL: CRC Press.

Hudson, R. J., and R. G. White. 1985. Computer simulation of energy budgets. Pp. 261–290 (Chapter 12) in Bioenergetics of Wild Herbivores, R. J. Hudson and R. G. White, eds. Boca Raton, FL: CRC Press.

Hudson, R. J., W. G. Watkins, and R. W. Pauls. 1985. Seasonal bioenergetics of wapiti in western Canada. Pp. 447–452 in Biology of Deer Production, P. F. Fennessy and K. R. Drew, eds. Royal Society of New Zealand, Bulletin 22.

Hufstedler, G. D., P. L. Gillman, G. E. Carstens, L. W. Greene, and N. D. Turner. 1996. Physiological and hormonal responses of lambs repeatedly implanted with zeranol and provided two levels of feed intake. J. Anim. Sci. 74:2376–2384.

Huggett, A. St. G., and W. F. Widdas. 1951. The relationship between mammalian foetal weight and conception age. J. Physiol. (Lond.) 114:306–317.

Hundertmark, K. J., and C. C. Schwartz. 1998. Predicting body mass of Alaskan moose (Alces alces gigas) using body measurements and condition assessment. Alces 34:83–89.

Huot, J. 1989. Body composition of the George River caribou (*Rangifer tarandus caribou*) in fall and late winter. Can. J. Zool. 67:103–107.

Hutchings, N. J. 1997. Estimating the metabolizable energy requirement for pregnancy in sheep. Anim. Sci. 64:463–467.

INRA (Institut National de la Recherche Agronomique). 1989. Ruminant Nutrition. Recommended Allowances and Feed Tables, R. Jarrige, ed. Paris: INRA.

Jacobsen, N. K. 1980. Differences of thermal properties of white-tailed deer pelage between seasons and body regions. J. Therm. Biol. 5:151–158.

Jenness, R., and R. E. Sloan. 1970. The composition of milks of various species: A review. Dairy Sci. Abstr. 32:599–612.

Jensen, P. G., P. J. Pekins, and J. B. Holter. 1999. Compensatory effect of the heat increment of feeding on thermoregulation costs of white-tailed deer fawns in winter. Can. J. Zool. 77:1474–1485.

Jiang, Z., and R. J. Hudson. 1992. Estimating forage intake and energy requirements of free-ranging wapiti (*Cervus elaphus*). Can. J. Zool. 70:675–679.

Jiang, Z., and R. J. Hudson. 1994. Seasonal energy requirements of wapiti (*Cervus elaphus*) for maintenance and growth. Can. J. Anim. Sci. 74:97–102.

Johnson, K. A., and D. E. Johnson. 1995. Methane emissions from cattle. J. Anim. Sci. 3:2483–2492.

Kay, R. N. B. 1979. Seasonal changes of appetite in deer and sheep. Agric. Res. Council Res. Rev. 5:13–15.

Kay, R. N. B., and E. D. Goodall. 1976. The intake digestibility and retention time of roughage diets by red deer (*Cervus elaphus*) and sheep. Proc. Nutr. Soc. 35:98A.

Kay, R. N. B., and B. W. Staines. 1981. The nutrition of the red deer (*Cervus elaphus*). Nutr. Abst. Rev. 5:601–622.

Kearl, L. C. 1982. Nutrient Requirements of Ruminants in Developing Countries. International Feedstuffs Institute. Logan: Utah State University.

Keech, M. A., T. S. Stephenson, R. T. Bowyer, V. van Ballenberghe, and J. M. Ver Hoef. 1998. Relationships between blood-serum variables and rump fat in Alaskan moose. Alces 34:173–179.

Kelsall, J. P. 1968. The Caribou. Ottawa, Canada: Queen's Printer.

Koong, L. J., W. N. Garrett, and P. V. Rattray. 1975. A description of the dynamics of fetal growth in sheep. J. Anim. Sci. 41:1065–1068.

Knott, K. K., P. S. Barboza, R. T. Bowyer, and J. E. Blake. 2004. Nutritional development of feeding strategies in arctic ruminants: Digestive morphometry of reindeer, *Rangifer tarandus*, and muskoxen, *Ovibos moschatus*. Zoology 107:315–333.

Knott, K. K., P. S. Barboza, and R. T. Bowyer. 2005. Growth in arctic ungulates: Postnatal development and organ maturation in *Rangifer tarandus* and *Ovibos moschatus*. J. Mamm. 86:121–130.

Kreikemeier, K. K., R. A. Stock, D. R. Brink, and R. A. Britton. 1987. Feeding combinations of dry corn and wheat to finishing lambs and cattle. J. Anim. Sci. 65:1647–1654.

Lachica, M., C. Prieto, and J. F. Aguilera. 1997. The energy cost of walking on the level and on negative and positive slopes in the Granadina goat (*Capra hircus*). Br. J. Nutr. 77:73–81.

Landete-Castillejos, T., A. Garcia, J. Garde, and L. Gallegos. 2000. Milk intake and production curves and allosuckling in captive Iberian red deer, *Cervus elaphus hispanicus*. Anim. Behav. 60:679–687.

Landete-Castillejos, T., A. Garcia, and L. Gallego. 2001. Calf growth in captive Iberian red deer (*Cervus elaphus hispanicus*): Effects of birth date and hind milk production and composition. J. Anim. Sci. 79:1085–1092.

Langlands, J. P., and J. E. Bowles. 1974. Herbage intake and production of Merino sheep grazing native and improved pastures at different stocking rates. Aust. J. Exp. Agric. Anim. Husb. 14:307–315.

Larsen, T. S., and A. S. Blix. 1985. Seasonal changes in body water; body composition and water turnover in reindeer. Rangifer 5:2–9.

Larsen, T. S., N. Ø. Nilsson, and A. S. Blix. 1985. Seasonal changes in lipogenesis and lipolysis in isolated adipocytes from Svalbard and Norwegian reindeer. Acta Physiol. Scand. 123:97–104.

Lentz, C. P., and J. S. Hart. 1960. The effect of wind and moisture on heat loss through the fur of newborn caribou. Can. J. Zool. 38:679–688.

Lenvik, D., E. Bø, and A. Fjellheim. 1988. Relationship between the weight of reindeer calves in autumn and their mother's age and weight in the previous spring. Rangifer 8:20–24.

Lincoln, G. A., F. Guinness, and R. V. Short. 1972. The way in which testosterone controls the social and sexual behaviour of the red deer stag (*Cervus elaphus*). Horm. Behav. 3:375–396.

Litherland, A. J., C. Toerien, T. Sahlu, and A. L. Goetsch. 2000. Effects of season on fleece traits of Angora does in the US. Small Ruminant Res. 38:63–70.

Liu, S. M., D. G. Masters, and N. R. Adams. 2003. Potential impact of nematode parasitism on nutrient partitioning for wool production, growth and reproduction in sheep. Aust. J. Exp. Agric. 43:1409–1417.

Lodge, G. A., and D. P. Heaney. 1970. Energy cost of pregnancy in the ewe. Pp. 109–112 in Energy Metabolism of Farm Animals, A. Schürch and C. Wenk, eds. Zurich, Switzerland: Juris Druck + Verlag.

Loudon, A. S. I., and R. N. B. Kay. 1984. Lactational constraints on a seasonal breeding mammal: The red deer. Symp. Zool. Soc. Lond. No. 51:233–225.

Loudon, A. S. I., A. S. McNeilly, and J. A. Milne. 1983. Nutritional and lactational control of fertility in red deer. Nature 302:145–147.

Loudon A. S. I., A. D. Darrock, and J. A. Milne. 1984. The lactation performance of red deer on hill and improved species pastures. J. Agric. Sci. 102:149–158.

Luick, J. R., R. G. White, A. M. Gau, and R. Jenness. 1974. Compositional changes in the milk secreted by reindeer. I. Gross composition and ash. J. Dairy Sci. 57:1325–1333.

Luo, J., A. L. Goetsch, J. E. Moore, Z. B. Johnson, T. Sahlu, C. L. Ferrell, M. L. Galyean, and F. N. Owens. 2004a. Prediction of endogenous urinary nitrogen of goats. Small Ruminant Res. 53:293–308.

Luo, J., A. L. Goetsch, I. V. Nsahlai, Z. B. Johnson, T. Sahlu, J. E. Moore, C. L. Ferrell, M. L. Galyean, and F. N. Owens. 2004b. Maintenance energy needs of goats: Predictions based on observations of heat and recovered energy. Small Ruminant Res. 53:221–230.

Luo, J., A. L. Goetsch, I. V. Nsahlai, J. E. Moore, M. L. Galyean, Z. B. Johnson, T. Sahlu, C. L. Ferrell, and F. N. Owens. 2004c. Prediction of voluntary feed intake by lactating, Angora, growing and mature goats. Small Ruminant Res. 53:357–378.

Luo, J., A. L. Goetsch, I. V. Nsahlai, T. Sahlu, C. L. Ferrell, F. N. Owens, M. L. Galyean, J. E. Moore, and Z. B. Johnson. 2004d. Prediction of metabolizable energy and protein requirements for maintenance, gain and fiber growth of Angora goats. Small Ruminant Res. 53:339–356.

Luo, J., A. L. Goetsch, T. Sahlu, I. V. Nsahlai, Z. B. Johnson, J. E. Moore, M. L. Galyean, F. N. Owens, and C. L. Ferrell. 2004e. Prediction of metabolizable energy requirements for maintenance and gain of preweaning, growing, and mature goats. Small Ruminant Res. 53:231–252.

MAFF (Ministry of Agriculture, Fisheries and Food). 1984. Energy Allowances and Feeding Systems for Ruminants. Pp. 57–61 in UK Ministry of Agriculture, Fisheries and Food, Reference Book 433. London: HMSO.

Markussen, K. A., A. Rognmo, and A. S. Blix. 1985. Some aspects of thermoregulation in newborn reindeer calves (*Rangifer tarandus tarandus*). Acta Physiol. Scand. 123:215–220.

Mauget, C., R. Mauget, and P. Duncan. 1997a. Metabolic rate and body mass in female European roe deer (*Capreolus capreolus*): Incidence of reproduction. Can. J. Zool. 75:731–739.

Mauget, C., R. Mauget, and A. Sempéré. 1997b. Energy expenditure in European roe deer fawns during the suckling period and its relationship with maternal reproductive cost. Can. J. Zool. 77:389–396.

Mautz, W. W., J. Kanter, and P. J. Pekins. 1992. Seasonal metabolic rhythms of captive female white-tailed deer: A reexamination. J. Wildl. Manage. 56:656–661.

McEwan, E. H. 1968. Growth and development of the barren-ground caribou. II. Postnatal growth rates. Can. J. Zool. 46:1023–1029.

McEwan, E. H. 1970. Energy metabolism of barren ground caribou (*Rangifer tarandus*). Can. J. Zool. 48:391–392.

McEwan, E. H., and P. E. Whitehead. 1971. Measurement of the milk intake of reindeer and caribou calves using tritiated water. Can. J. Zool. 49:443–447.

McMahon C. D., I. D. Corson, R. P. Littlejohn, S. K. Stuart, B. A. Veenvliet, J. R. Webster, and J. M. Suttie. 1997. Prolactin does not enhance glucose-stimulated insulin release in red deer stags. Domestic Anim. Endocrin. 14:47–61.

Meissner, H. H. 1976. A note on the energy requirements of young, growing blesbock. S. Afr. J. Wildlife Res. 6:51–52.

Mesteig, K., N. J. C. Tyler, and A.S. Blix. 2000. Seasonal changes in heart rate and food intake in reindeer (*Rangifer tarandus tarandus*). Acta Physiol. Scand. 170:145–151.

Miller, F. L., and A. Gunn. 1986. Effect of adverse weather on neonatal caribou survival—a review. Rangifer, Spec. Iss. No. 1:211–217.

Milne, J. A., J. C. MacRae, A. M. Spence, and S. Wilson. 1978. A comparison of the voluntary intake and digestion of a range of forages at different times of the year by the sheep and the red deer (*Cervus elaphus*). Br. J. Nutr. 40:347–357.

Mitchell. B., D. McCowan, and I. A. Nicholson. 1976. Annual cycles of body weight and condition in Scottish red deer. J. Zool. 180:107–127.

Moen, A. N. 1968a. Energy exchange of white-tailed deer, Western Minnesota. Ecology 49:676–682.

Moen, A. N. 1968b. Surface temperatures and radiant heat loss from white-tailed deer. J. Wildl. Manage. 32:338–344.

Moen, A. N. 1973. Wildlife Ecology. San Francisco: W. H. Freeman.

Moen, A. N. 1976. Energy conservation by white-tailed deer in the winter. Ecology 57:192–198.

Moen, R., and J. Pastor. 1998. Simulating antler growth and energy, nitrogen, calcium and phosphorus metabolism in caribou. Rangifer Spec. Iss. No. 10:85–97.

Moen, R., J. Pastor, and Y. Cohen. 1997. A spatially explicit model of moose foraging and energetics. Ecology 78:505–521.

Moen, R., Y. Cohen, and J. Pastor. 1998. Linking moose population and plant growth models with a moose energetics model. Ecosystems 1:52–63.

Moore, J. E., A. L. Goetsch, J. Luo, F. N. Owens, M. L. Galyean, Z. B. Johnson, T. Sahlu, and C. L. Ferrell. 2004. Prediction of fecal crude protein excretion of goats. Small Ruminant Res. 53:275–292.

Morin, D. E., L. L. Rowan, W. L. Hurley, and W. E. Braselton. 1995. Composition of milk from llamas in the United States. J. Dairy Sci. 78:1713–1720.

Murphy, T. A., S. C. Loerch, K. E. McClure, and M. B. Solomon. 1994. Effects of restricted feeding on growth performance and carcass composition of lambs. J. Anim. Sci. 72:3131–3137.

Newman, S. A. N., and D. J. Paterson. 1994. Effect of level of nutrition and season on fibre growth in alpacas. Proc. NZ Soc. Anim. Prod. 54: 147–150.

Nieminen, M., S. Kellokumpu, P. Väyrynen, and H. Hyvärinen. 1980. Rumen function of the reindeer. Pp. 213–223 in Proc. 2nd Int'l. Reindeer and Caribou Symp., E. Reimers, E. Gaare, and S. Skjenneberg, eds. Trondheim, Norway: Directoratet for vilt og ferskvannsfisk.

Nieminen, M., V. Ojutkangas, J. Timisjärvi, and R. Hissa. 1984. Serum lipids, thyroxine and catecholamine levels in the reindeer with reference to the annual climate cycle. Comp. Biochem. Physiol. 60 A:123–126.

Nieminen, M., A-S. Pokka, and U. Heiskari. 1987. Artificial feeding and nutritional status of semi-domesticated reindeer during winter. Rangifer 7:51–58.

Nilssen, K. J., J. A. Sundsfjord, and A. S. Blix. 1984. Regulation of metabolic rate in Svalbard and Norwegian reindeer. Am. J. Physiol. 247:R837–841.

Nilssen, K. L., S. D. Mathiesen, and A. S. Blix. 1994. Metabolic rate and plasma T_3 in *ad lib.* fed and starved muskoxen. Rangifer 14:79–81.

Nilssen, A., Ö. Danell, M. Murphy, K. Olsson, and B. Åhman. 2000. Health, body condition and metabolites in reindeer after submaintenance feed intake and subsequent feeding. Rangifer 20:187–200.

Nordan, H. C., I. McT. Cowan, and A. J. Wood. 1970. Feed intake and heat production of the young black-tailed deer (*Odocoileus hemionus columbianus*). Can. J. Zool. 48:275–282.

NRC (National Research Council). 1981a. Effect of Environment on Nutrient Requirements of Domestic Animals. Washington, DC: National Academy Press.

NRC. 1981b. Nutrient Requirements of Goats: Angora, Dairy, and Meat Goats in Temperate and Tropical Countries. Washington, DC: National Academy Press.

NRC. 1984. Nutrient Requirements of Beef Cattle, 6th ed. Washington, DC: National Academy Press.

NRC. 1985. Nutrient Requirements of Sheep, 6th rev. ed. Washington, DC: National Academy Press.

NRC. 2000. Nutrient Requirements of Beef Cattle (Update 2000). Washington, DC: National Academy Press.

NRC. 2001. Nutrient Requirements of Dairy Cattle, 7th rev. ed. Washington, DC: National Academy Press.

Nsahlai, I. V., P. O. Osuji, and N. N. Umunna. 1997. Digestible organic matter requirements of Ethiopian Menz sheep: Model and application. J. Appl. Anim. Res. 11:83–100.

Nsahlai, I. V., A. L. Goetsch, J. Luo, Z. B. Johnson, J. E. Moore, T. Sahlu, C. L. Ferrell, M. L. Galyean, and F. N. Owens. 2004a. Energy requirements of lactating goats. Small Ruminant Res. 53:253–274.

Ockenfels, R. A., and D. E. Brooks. 1994. Summer diurnal bed sites of Coues white-tailed deer. J. Wildl. Manage. 58:70–75.

Oftedal, O. T. 1984. Milk composition, milk yield and energy output at peak lactation: A comparative review. Symp. Zool. Soc. Lond. 51:33–85.

Oftedal, O. T. 1985. Pregnancy and lactation. Pp. 215–218 (Chapter 10) in Bioenergetics of Wild Herbivores, R. J. Hudson and R. G. White, eds. Boca Raton, FL: CRC Press.

Olthoff, J. C., G. E. Dickerson, and J. A. Nienaber. 1989. Energy utilization in mature ewes from seven breeds with diverse production potentials. J. Anim. Sci. 67:2550–2564.

Ørskov, E. R., C. Fraser, J. C. Gill, and E. L. Corse. 1971. The effect in an intensive production system of type of cereal and time of weaning on the performance of lambs. Anim. Prod. 13:485–492.

Parker, K. L. 1987. Body-surface measurements of mule deer and elk. J. Wildl. Manage. 51:630–633.

Parker, K. L. 1988. Effects of heat, cold, and rain on coastal black-tailed deer. Can. J. Zool. 66:2475–2483.

Parker, K. L. 1989. Growth rates and morphological measurements of Porcupine caribou calves. Rangifer 9:9–13.

Parker, K. L. 2003. Advances in the nutritional ecology of cervids at different scales. Ecoscience 10:395–411.

Parker, K.L., and M. P. Gillingham. 1990. Estimates of critical thermal environments for mule deer. J. Range Manage. 43:73–81.

Parker, K. L., and C. T. Robbins. 1984. Thermoregulation in mule deer and elk. Can. J. Zool. 62:1409–1422.

Parker, K. L., and C. T. Robbins. 1985. Thermoregulation in ungulates. Pp. 161–182 in Bioenergetics of Wild Herbivores, R. J. Hudson and R. G. White, eds. Boca Raton, FL: CRC Press.

Parker, K. L., R. G. White, M. P. Gillingham, and D. F. Holleman. 1990. Comparison of energy metabolism in relation to daily activity and milk consumption by caribou and muskox neonates. Can. J. Zool. 68:106–114.

Parker, K. L., M. P. Gillingham, T. A. Hanley, and C. T. Robbins. 1993. Seasonal patterns in body mass, body composition, and water transfer rates of free-ranging and captive black-tailed deer (*Odocoileus hemionus sitkensis*) in Alaska. Can. J. Zool. 71:1397–1404.

Parker, K. L., M. P. Gillingham, T. A. Hanley, and C. T. Robbins. 1996. Foraging efficiency: Energy expenditure versus energy gain in free-ranging black-tailed deer. Can. J. Zool. 74:442–450.

Parker, K. L., M. P. Gillingham, T. A. Hanley, and C. T. Robbins. 1999. Energy and protein balance of free-ranging black-tailed deer in a natural forest environment. Wildl. Monog. 143:1–47.

Parker, K.L., P. S. Barboza, and T. R. Stephenson. 2005. Protein conservation in female caribou (*Rangifer tarandus*): Effects of decreasing diet quality during winter. J. Mamm. 86:610–622.

Pauls, R. W., R. J. Hudson, and S. Sylvén. 1981. Energy expenditure of free-ranging wapiti. Pp. 87–90 in 60th Annual Feeders Day Report. University of Alberta, Edmonton.

Peltier, T. C., P. S. Barboza, and J. E. Blake. 2003. Seasonal hyperphagia does not reduce digestive efficiency in an arctic grazer. Physiol. Biochem. Zool. 76:471–483.

Pekins, P. J., K. S. Smith, and W. W. Mautz. 1998. The energy cost of gestation in white-tailed deer. Can. J. Zool. 76:1091–1097.

Penning, P. D., R. J. Orr, and T. T. Treacher. 1988. Responses of lactating ewes, offered fresh herbage indoors and when grazing, to supplements containing differing protein concentrations. Anim. Prod. 46:403–415.

Phillips, W. A., M. A. Brown, G. H. Dolezal, and G. Q. Fitch. 2006. Feedlot performance and carcass characteristics of crossbred lambs sired by Texel, Romonav, St. Croix or Dorset rams from Polypay and St. Croix ewes. Sheep Goat Res. J. (In press.)

Pineda, J., J. M. Palma, G. F. W. Haenlein, and M. A. Galina. 1998. Fattening of Pelibuey hair sheep and crossbreds (Rambouillet-Dorsect × Pelibuey) in the Mexican tropics. Small Ruminant Res. 27:263–266.

Pond, W. G. 1989. Effects of dietary protein level and clinoptilolite on the weight gain and liver mineral response of growing lambs to copper supplementation. J. Anim. Sci. 67:2772–2781.

Preston, R. L. 2000. Typical composition of feeds for cattle and sheep. Beef (Intertec Publ. Co.) 36(10):10–20.

Puchala, R., S. G. Pierzynowski, T. Wuliji, A. L. Goetsch, T. Sahlu, M. Lachica, and S. A. Soto-Navarro. 2002. Effects of small peptides or amino acids infused to a perfused area of the skin of Angora goats on mohair growth. J. Anim. Sci. 80:1097–1104.

Puchala, R., S. G. Pierzynowski, T. Wuliji, A. L. Goetsch, S. A. Soto-Navarro, and T. Sahlu. 2003. Effects of prolactin administered to a perfused area of the skin of Angora goats. J. Anim. Sci. 81:279–284.

Pulina, G., A. Cappio-Borlino, N. Macciotta, C. Di Maurio, and A. Nudda. 2001. Empirical and mechanistic models of temporal evolution of milk production in ruminants. Biology Forum 94:331–344.

Rattray, P. V., W. N. Garrett, N. E. East, and N. Hinman. 1974a. Efficiency of utilization of metabolizable energy during pregnancy and the energy requirements for pregnancy in sheep. J. Anim. Sci. 38:383–393.

Rattray, P. V., W. N. Garrett, N. E. East, and N. Hinman. 1974b. Growth, development and composition of the ovine conceptus and mammary gland during pregnancy. J. Anim. Sci. 38:613–626.

Reese, E. O., and C. T. Robbins. 1994. Characteristics of moose lactation and neonatal growth. Can. J. Zool. 72:953–957.

Regelin, W. L., C. C. Schwartz, and A. W. Franzmann. 1985. Seasonal energy metabolism of adult moose. J. Wildl. Manage. 49:388–393.

Reimers, E. 1972. Growth in domestic and wild reindeer. J. Wildl. Manage. 36:612–619.

Reimers, E. 1980. Activity pattern; The major determinant for growth and fattening in *Rangifer*. Pp. 466–475 in Proc. 2nd Int'l. Reindeer and Caribou Symp., E. Reimers, E. Gaare and S. Skjenneberg, eds. Trondheim, Norway: Directoratet for vilt og ferskvannsfisk.

Reimers, E. 1983. Growth rate and body size differences in *Rangifer*, a study of causes and effects. Rangifer 3:3–15.

Reimers, E., T. Ringberg, and R. Sørumgård. 1982. Body composition of Svalbard reindeer. Can. J. Zool. 60:1812–1821.

Renecker, L. A., and R. J. Hudson. 1986. Seasonal energy expenditures and thermoregulatory responses of moose. Can. J. Zool. 64:322–327.

Renecker, L. A., and W. M. Samuel. 1991. Growth and seasonal weight changes as they relate to spring and autumn set points in mule deer. Can. J. Zool. 69:744–747.

Rhind, S. M., Z. A. Archer, and C. L. Adam. 2002. Seasonality of food intake in ruminants: Recent developments in understanding. Nutr. Res. Rev. 15:43–65.

Robbins, C. T. 1993. Wildlife Feeding and Nutrition. New York: Academic Press.

Robbins, C. T., and A. N. Moen. 1975. Uterine composition and growth in pregnant white-tailed deer. J. Wildl. Manage. 39:684–691.

Robbins, C. T., and B. L. Robbins. 1979. Fetal and neonatal growth patterns and maternal reproductive effort in ungulates and subungulates. Am. Nat. 114:101–116.

Robbins, C. T., A. N. Moen, and J. T. Reid. 1974. Body composition of white-tailed deer. J. Anim. Sci. 38:871–876.

Robbins, C. T., R. S. Podbielancik-Norman, D. L. Wilson, and E. Mould. 1981. Growth and nutrient consumption of elk calves compared to other ungulate species. J. Wildl. Manage. 45:172–186.

Robbins, C. T., O. Oftedal, and K. I. O'Rourke. 1987. Lactation, early nutrition, and hand-rearing of wild ungulates, with special reference to deer. Pp. 429–442 in Biology and Management of the Cervidae, C. M. Wemmer, ed. Washington, DC: Smithsonian Institute Press.

Robelin, J., and Y. Geay. 1984. Body composition of cattle as affected by physiological status, breed, sex and diet. Pp. 525–548 in Herbivore Nutrition in the Subtropics and Tropics, F. M. C. Gilchrist and R. I. Mackie, eds. Craighall, South Africa: The Science Press.

Robinson, J. J., I. McDonald, C. Fraser, and J. G. Gordon. 1980. Studies on reproduction in prolific ewes. 6. The efficiency of energy utilization for conceptus growth. J. Agric. Sci. 94:331–338.

Roine, K. M., M. Nieminen, and J. Timisjarvi. 1982. Foetal growth in the reindeer. Acta Vet. Scand. 23:107–117.

Rompala, R. E., and D. E. Johnson. 1985. The influence of empty body weight and mature weight of the genotype on energy density of empty body gain in growing lambs. J. Anim. Sci. 61(4): 802–806.

Ruder, R. P., L. A. Burgwald-Balstad, D. W. Sanson, M. L. Riley, and W. C. Russell. 1997. Performance, intake and digestibility of lambs fed alfalfa hay and various levels of barley. Sheep Goat Res. J. 13:60–66.

Russel, A. J. F., and H. L. Redden. 1997. The effect of nutrition on fibre growth in the alpaca. Anim. Sci. 64:509–512.

Russel, A. J. F., J. M. Doney, and R. G. Gunn. 1969. Subjective assessment of body fat in live sheep. J. Agric. Sci. 72:451–454.

Russell, D. E., A. M. Martell, and W. A. C. Nixon. 1993. Range ecology of the porcupine caribou herd in Canada. Rangifer Spec. Iss. No. 8:3–167.

Russell, D. E., D. van de Wetering, R. G. White, and K. L. Gerhart. 1996. Oil and the porcupine caribou herd—can we quantify the impacts? Rangifer Spec. Iss. No. 9:255–257.

Russell, D. E., K. L. Gerhart, R. G. White, and D. Van De Wetering. 1998. Detection of early pregnancy in caribou: Evidence for embryonic mortality. J. Wildl. Manage. 62:1066–1075.

Russell, D. E., R. G. White, and C. J. Daniel. 2005. Energetics of the porcupine caribou herd: A computer simulation model. Canadian Wildlife Service, Ottawa, Ontario, Technical Report Series 431:1–64.

Ryder, M. L. 1977. Seasonal coat changes in grazing red deer (*Cervus elaphus*). J. Zool. 181:137–143.

Ryg, M. 1983a. Effect of testosterone on antler growth in yearling male reindeer. Rangifer 3:6–9.

Ryg, M. 1983b. Relationships between hormone-induced and compensatory weight changes in reindeer (*Rangifer tarandus tarandus*). Comp. Biochem. Physiol. 74A:33–35.

Sadleir, R. M. F. S. 1980. Milk yield of black-tailed deer. J. Wildl. Manage. 44:472–477.

Sadleir, R. M. F. S. 1982. Energy consumption and subsequent partitioning in lactating black-tailed deer. Can. J. Zool. 60:382–386.

Sahlu, T., A. L. Goetsch, J. Luo, I. V. Nsahlai, J. E. Moore, M. L. Galyean, F. N. Owens, C. L. Ferrell, and Z. B. Johnson. 2004. Energy and protein requirements of goats: Developed equations, other considerations and future research to improve them. Small Ruminant Res. 53:191–220.

Said, A. N., and A. Tolera. 1993. The supplementary value of forage legume hays in sheep feeding: Feed intake, nitrogen retention and body weight change. Livest. Prod. Sci. 33:229–237.

Sainz, R. D., and B. E. Bentley. 1997. Visceral organ mass and cellularity in growth-restricted and refed beef steers. J. Anim. Sci. 75:1229–1236.

Sanson, D. W., T. R. West, W. R. Tatman, M. L. Riley, M. B. Judkins, and G. E. Moss. 1993. Relationship of body condition of mature ewes with condition score and body weight. J. Anim. Sci. 71:1112–1116.

Sauer, P. R. 1984. Physical characteristics. Pp. 73–90 in White-Tailed Deer: Ecology and Management, L. K. Halls, ed. Harrisburg, PA: Stackpole Books.

SCA (Standing Committee on Agriculture, Ruminants Subcommittee). 1990. Feeding Standards for Australian Livestock. Ruminants. East Melbourne, Australia: CSIRO Publications.

Schneider, W., R. Hauffe, and W. von Engelhardt. 1974. Energy and nitrogen exchange in the llama. Pp. 127–130 in Proc. Sixth Symp. Energy Metabolism of Farm Animals. European Assoc. Anim. Prod. Pub. No. 14.

Scholander, P. F., V. Walters, R. Hock, and L. Irving. 1950. Body insulation of some Arctic and tropical mammals and birds. Biol. Bull. 99: 225–236.

Schwartz, C. C., W. L. Regelin, A. W. Franzmann, and M. Hubbert. 1987. Nutritional energetics of moose. Swedish Wildlife Res. Suppl. 1:265–279.

Silanikove, N. 2000. The physiological basis of adaptation in goats to harsh environments. Small Ruminant Res. 35:181–193.

Silver, H., N. F. Colovos, J. B. Holter, and H. H. Hayes. 1969. Fasting metabolism of white-tailed deer. J. Wildl. Manage. 33:490–498.

Simpson, A. M., A. J. F. Webster, J. S. Smith, and C. A. Simpson. 1978a. The efficiency of utilization of dietary energy for growth in sheep (*Ovis ovis*) and red deer (*Cervus elaphus*). Comp. Biochem. Physiol. 59A: 95–99.

Simpson, A. M., A. J. F. Webster, J. S. Smith, and C. A. Simpson. 1978b. Energy and nitrogen metabolism of red deer (*Cervus elaphus*) in cold environments: A comparison with cattle and sheep. Comp. Biochem. Physiol. 60A:251–256.

Soppela, P., M. Nieminen, and J. Timisjärvi. 1986a. Thermoregulation in reindeer. Rangifer Spec. Iss. No. 1:273–278.

Soppela, P., M. Nieminen, S. Saarela, and R. Hissa. 1986b. The influence of ambient temperature on metabolism and body temperature of newborn and growing reindeer calves (*Rangifer tarandus tarandus* L.). Comp. Biochem. Physiol. 83A:317–386.

Soppela, P., M. Nieminen, S. Saarela, J. S. Keith, J. N. Morrison, F. MacFarlane, and P. Trayhurn. 1991. Brown fat-specific mitochondrial uncoupling protein in adipose tissue of newborn reindeer. Am. J. Physiol. 260:R1229–R1234.

Stein, A., R. J. Irvine, R. Langvatn, S. D. Albon, and O. Halvorsen. 2002. The population dynamics of *Ostertagia gruehneri* in reindeer: A model for the seasonal and intensity dependent variation in nematode fecundity. Inter. J. Parasit. 32:991–996.

Stein, A., R. J. Irvine, R. Langvatn, and E. Ropstad. 2003. Evaluation of ultrasound scanning as a method for measuring subcutaneous fat in Svalbard reindeer. Rangifer 23:71–73.

Stephenson, T. R., K. J. Hundertmark, C. C. Schwartz, and V. Van Ballenberghe. 1998. Predicting body fat and body mass with ultrasonography. Can. J. Zool. 76:712–722.

Stephenson, T. R., V. C. Bleich, B. M. Pierce, and G. P. Mulcahy. 2002. Validation of mule deer body composition using in vivo and post-mortem indices of nutritional condition. Wildl. Soc. Bull. 30:557–564.

Sun, W., A. L. Goetsch, L. A. Forster, Jr., D. L. Galloway, Sr., and P. K. Lewis, Jr. 1994. Forage and splanchnic tissue mass in growing lambs: Effects of dietary forage levels and source on splanchnic tissue mass in growing lambs. Br. J. Nutr. 71:141–151.

Susin, I., S. C. Loerch, and K. E. McClure. 1995. Effects of feeding a high-grain diet at a restricted intake on lactation performance and rebreeding of ewes. J. Anim. Sci. 73:3199–3205.

Suttie, J. M. 1980. Influence of nutrition on growth and sexual maturation of captive red deer stags. Pp. 341–349 in Proc. 2nd Int'l. Reindeer and Caribou Symp., E. Reimers, E. Gaare, and S. Skjenneberg, eds. Trondheim, Norway: Directoratet for vilt og ferskvannsfisk.

Suttie, J. M., and R. N. B. Kay. 1982 The influence of nutrition and photoperiod on the growth of antlers of young red deer. Pp. 61–71 in Antler Development in Cervidae, R. D. Brown, ed. Kingsville, TX: Caesar Kleberg Wildl. Res. Inst.

Suttie, J. M., and A. M. Simpson. 1985. Photoperiodic control of appetite, growth, antlers, and endocrine status of red deer. Royal Soc. New Zealand Bull. 22:429–432.

Suttie, J. M., and J. R. Webster. 1995. Extreme seasonal growth in Arctic deer: Comparisons and control mechanisms. Amer. Zool. 35:215–221.

Suttie, J. M., and J. R. Webster. 1998. Are arctic ungulates physiologically unique? Rangifer 18:99–118.

Suttie, J. M., E. D. Goodall, K. Pennie, and R. N. B. Kay. 1983. Winter food restriction and summer compensation in red deer stags (*Cervus elaphus*). Br. J. Nutr. 50:737–747.

Suttie, J. M., P. F. Fennessy, B. A.VeenVliet, R. P. Littlejohn, M. W. Fisher, I. D. Corson, and R. E. Labes, 1987. Energy nutrition of young red deer *(Cervus elaphus)* hinds and a comparison with young stags. Proc. NZ Soc. Anim. Prod. 47:111–114.

Swift, D. M. 1983. A simulation model of energy and nitrogen balance for free-ranging ruminants. J. Wildl. Manage. 47:620–645.

Swift, D. M., J. E. Ellis, and N. T. Hobbs. 1980. Nitrogen and energy requirements of North American cervids in winter: A simulation study. Pp. 244–251 in Proc. 2nd Int'l. Reindeer and Caribou Symp., E. Reimers, E. Gaare and S. Skjenneberg, eds. Trondheim, Norway: Directoratet for vilt og ferskvannsfisk.

Sykes, A. R. 1994. Parasitism and production in farm animals. Anim. Prod. 59:155–172.

Sykes, A. R., and A. W. Greer. 2003. Effects of parasitism on the nutrient economy of sheep: An overview. Aust. J. Exp. Agric. 43:1393–1398.

Thomas, V. M., C. K. Clark, and C. M. Schuldt. 1994. Effects of substituting feather meal for soybean meal on ruminal fiber fermentation and lamb and wool growth. J. Anim. Sci. 72:509–514.

Thompson, C. B., J. B. Holter, H. H. Hayes, H. Silver, and W. E. Urban. 1973. Nutrition of white-tailed deer. 1. Energy requirements of fawns. J. Wildl. Manage. 37:301–311.

Timisjärvi, J., M. Nieminen, and A. L. Sippola. 1984. The structure and insulation properties of the reindeer fur. Comp. Bioch. Physiol 79A:601–609.

Tolera, A., and F. Sundstøl. 2000. Supplementation of graded levels of *Desmodium intortum* hay to sheep feeding on maize stover harvested at three stages of maturity. 1. Feed intake, digestibility and body weight change. Anim. Feed Sci. Technol. 85:239–257.

Tolkamp, B. J., and J. J. M. H. Ketelaars. 1992. Toward a new theory of feed intake regulation in ruminants. 2. Costs and benefits of feed consumption: An optimization approach. Livest. Prod. Sci. 30:297–317.

Torbit, S. C., L. H. Carpenter, D. M. Swift, and A. W. Alldredge. 1985. Differential loss of fat and protein by mule deer during winter. J. Wildl. Manage. 49:80–85.

Turgeon, O. A., Jr., D. R. Brink, S. J. Bartle, T. J. Klopfenstein, and C. L. Ferrell. 1986. Effects of growth rate and compensatory growth on body composition in lambs. J. Anim. Sci. 63:770–780.

Tyler, N. J. C. 1987. Body composition and energy balance of pregnant and non-pregnant Svalbard reindeer during winter. Zool. Soc. London Symp. 57:203–229.

Tyler, N. J. C., and A. S. Blix. 1990. Survival strategies in arctic ungulates. Rangifer Spec. Iss. No. 3:211–230.

Tyler, N. J. C., P. Fauchald, O. Johansen, and H. R. Christiansen. 1999. Seasonal inappetance and weight loss in female reindeer in winter. Ecol. Bull. 47:105–116.

Ullrey, D. E. 1982. Nutrition and antler development in white-tailed deer. Pp. 49–59 in Antler Development in Cervidae, R. D. Brown, ed. Kingsville, TX: Caesar Kleberg Wildl. Res. Inst.

Ullrey, D. E., W. G. Youatt, H. E. Johnson, L. D. Fay, B. L. Schoepke, and W. T. Magee. 1969. Digestible energy requirements for winter maintenance of Michigan white-tailed does. J. Wildl. Manage. 33:482–490.

Ullrey, D. E., W. G. Youatt, H. E. Johnson, L. D. Fay, B. L. Schoepke, and W. T. Magee. 1970. Digestible and metabolizable energy requirements for winter maintenance of Michigan whitetailed does. J. Wildl. Mgt. 34:863–869.

Van Saun, R. J. 2006. Nutrient requirements of South American camelids: A factorial approach. Small Ruminant Res. 61:165–186.

von Keyserlingk, G. E. M., and G. W. Mathison. 1993. The effect of ruminal escape protein and ambient temperature on the efficiency of utilization of metabolizable energy by lambs. J. Anim. Sci. 71:2206–2217.

Wairimu, S., R. J. Hudson, and M. A. Price. 1992. Catch-up growth of yearling wapiti stags (*Cervus elaphus*). Can. J. Anim. Sci. 72: 619–631.

Watkins, W. G., R. J. Hudson, and P. Fargey. 1991. Compensatory growth of wapiti (Cervus elaphus) on spring ranges. Can. J. Zool. 69:1682–1688.

Weber, M. L., and J. M. Thompson 1998. Seasonal patterns in food intake, live mass, and body composition of mature female fallow deer (*Dama dama*). Can. J. Zool. 76:1141–1152.

Webster, A. J. F. 1980. The energetic efficiency of growth. Livest. Prod. Sci. 7:243–252.

Webster, A. J. F., A. M. Hicks, and F. L. Hays. 1969. Cold climate and cold temperature induced changes in the heat production and thermal insulation of sheep. Can. J. Physiol. Pharmacol. 47:553–562.

Webster, A. J. F., J. Chlumecky, and B. A. Young. 1970. Effects of cold environments on the energy exchanges of young beef cattle. Can. J. Anim. Sci. 50:89–100.

Weiner, J. 1977. Energy metabolism of the roe deer. Acta Theriol. 22:3–24.

Wesley, D. A., K. L. Knox, and J. G. Nagy. 1973. Energy metabolism of pronghorn antelopes. J. Wildl. Manage. 37:563–573.

Westendorf, M. L., and R. Gordon. 1998. Effect of undegradable intake protein when sheep are fed diets low in protein. Prof. Anim. Sci. 14:16–21.

Wester, T. J., R. A. Britton, T. J. Klopfenstein, G. A. Ham, D. T. Hickok, and C. R. Krehbiel. 1995. Differential effects of plane of protein or energy nutrition on visceral organs and hormones in lambs. J. Anim. Sci. 73:1674–1688.

White, R. G. 1983. Foraging patterns and their multiplier effects on productivity of northern ungulates. Oikos 40:377–384.

White, R. G. 1992. Nutrition in relation to season, lactation and growth of north temperate deer. Pp. 407–417 in The Biology of Deer, R. D. Brown, ed. New York: Springer-Verlag.

White, R. G., and J. R. Luick. 1984. Plasticity and constraints in the lactational strategy of reindeer and caribou. Symp. Zool. Soc. Lond. 51: 215–232.

White, R. G., D. F. Holleman, and B. A. Tiplady. 1989. Seasonal body weight, body condition, and lactational trends in muskoxen. Can. J. Zool. 67:1125–1133.

Wika, M., and J. Krog. 1980. Thermoregulation and brown adipose tissue in the newborn reindeer calf. Pp. 425–431 in Proc. 2nd Int'l. Reindeer and Caribou Symp., E. Reimers, E. Gaare, and S. Skjenneberg, eds. Trondheim, Norway: Directoratet for vilt og ferskvannsfisk.

Williams, C. B., and T. G. Jenkins. 2003. A dynamic model of metabolizable energy utilization in growing and mature cattle. I. Metabolizable energy utilization for maintenance and support metabolism. J. Anim. Sci. 81:1371–1381.

Willms, C. L., L. L. Berger, N. R. Merchen, and G. C. Fahey, Jr. 1991. Effects of supplemental protein source and level of urea on intestinal amino acid supply and feedlot performance of lambs fed diets based on alkaline hydrogen peroxide-treated wheat straw. J. Anim. Sci. 69:4925–4938.

Wislocki, G. B., J. C. Aub, and C. M. Waldo. 1947. The effects of gonadectomy and the administration of testosterone propionate on the growth of antlers in male and female deer. Endocrinol. 40:202–224.

Wood, A. J., I. McT. Cowan, and H. C. Nordan. 1962. Periodicity of growth in ungulates as shown by deer of the genus *Odocoileus*. Can. J. Zool. 40:593–603.

Wood, P. D. P. 1967. Algebraic model of the lactation curve in cattle. Nature 216:164–165.

Worden, K. A., and P. J. Pekins. 1995. Seasonal changes in feed intake, body composition, and metabolic rate of white-tailed deer. Can. J. Zool. 73:452–457.

Wuliji, T., A. L. Goetsch, T. Sahlu, R. Puchala, S. Soto-Navarro, R. C. Merkel, G. Detweiler, and T. Gipson. 2003a. Effects of different quality diets consumed continuously or after a lower quality diet on characteristics of growth of young Spanish goats. Small Ruminant Res. 50:83–96.

Wuliji, T., A. L. Goetsch, R. Puchala, T. Sahlu, R. C. Merkel, G. Detweiler, S. Soto-Navarro, J. Luo, and T. Shenkoru. 2003b. Relationships between body composition and shrunk body weight and urea space in growing goats. J. Appl. Anim. Res. 23:1–24.

Yates, N. G., W. V. Macfarlane, and R. Ellis. 1971. The estimation of milk intake and growth of beef calves in the field by using tritiated water. Aust. J. Agric. Res. 22:91–306.

Young, B. A. 1975. Effect of winter acclimatization on resting metabolism of beef cows. Can. J. Anim. Sci. 55:619–625.

Young, B. A. 1976. Effect of cold environments on nutrient requirements of ruminants. Feedstuffs 48:24–33.

Young, B. A., and J. L. Corbett. 1972. Maintenance energy requirement of grazing sheep in relation to herbage availability. I. Calorimetric estimates. Aust. J. Agric. Res. 23:57–76.

Zhigunov, P. 1968. Reindeer Husbandry. 2nd ed., 343 pp. Jerusalem, Israel: Program for Scientific Translations.

5

Protein

PROTEIN REQUIREMENTS FOR MAINTENANCE

Protein requirements are often determined by factorial approaches, with maintenance requirements considered first. Maintenance protein needs in most metabolizable protein (MP) systems include losses of nitrogen (N) in feces and urine and from skin as scurf and fiber.

Metabolic Fecal Crude Protein

The fecal maintenance crude protein (CP) loss is termed metabolic fecal nitrogen or CP (MFCP). It is classically determined by regressing digestible CP concentration in the diet against total CP concentration, with the slope representing truly digestible CP and the intercept describing MFCP as a percent of dry matter intake (DMI). However, in some cases expressions relative to indigestible DMI have proven more accurate. Additional considerations of whether to express MFCP on a DMI or indigestible DMI basis are the need to predict both DMI and digestibility and potential for double accounting (i.e., accounting for microbial residues in feces twice) with the latter method (Cannas et al., 2004).

Metabolic fecal CP as determined by regression includes CP sources such as enzymes and epithelial cells; however, microbial cells formed in the hindgut and microbial cell fragments of ruminal origin also contribute CP, which are not true endogenous losses. This has led to corrections of MFCP estimates derived by regression for microbial CP (e.g., NRC, 2001). Though this is an appropriate consideration in theory, marked benefits have not been conclusively shown. In this regard, regressions of digestible against total CP typically explain considerable variation (e.g., Moore et al., 2004), perhaps reflecting relatively little variability in the microbial contribution at least with typical diets. Regression of digested protein against dietary CP content in cervids (white-tailed deer: Holter et al., 1977; elk: Mould and Robbins, 1981) gives close estimates of uncorrected MFCP, and the study with elk shows the major effect of plants high in phenolics on increasing fecal CP loss and lowering the amount of digestible CP relative to CP content. The dairy NRC (2001) adjustment does not seem to be influenced by hindgut microbial cell production, but rather is based on the estimate of ruminally synthesized microbial true protein not digested in the small intestine (i.e., 20 percent of the quantity entering) and digested in the hindgut to an extent of 50 percent of the quantity entering. Another related factor in evaluating need for such adjustments is the efficiency of metabolizable protein use for maintenance (k_{pm}), for which there are marked differences. The NRC (2001) assumes a k_{pm} of 0.67 compared with 1.0 of Luo et al. (2004b,c) and Nsahlai et al. (2004) based on AFRC (1993, 1998). Different k_{pm} assumptions may partially compensate for correcting MFCP for microbial CP.

Estimates of MFCP (uncorrected) as a percentage of DMI by regression analyses are fairly similar among domesticated ruminant species and cervids (Holter et al., 1977; Mould and Robbins, 1981; Schwartz et al., 1987; Robbins, 1993; Asleson et al., 1996). However, because of the need to predict DMI to estimate MFCP, and because other endogenous losses (i.e., urinary and scurf plus fiber) are usually based on body weight (BW), in some cases MFCP has been predicted from BW. This seems acceptable within species and biotypes of species not differing markedly in BW, but may not be appropriate with substantial BW variation. In addition, some estimates of the total maintenance requirement relative to BW or $BW^{0.75}$ have been determined by regression of intake against performance (e.g., NRC, 2000; Luo et al., 2004b,c). This has the advantage of not requiring a prediction of DMI.

Plant secondary metabolites, notably condensed tannins (CT), are dietary constituents that can affect fecal CP excretion. Fecal nitrogen (CP) excretion can increase, and apparent digestion of nitrogen decrease, due to the presence of CT in a diet (Mould and Robbins, 1981; Robbins et al., 1987). One effect of CT is to increase rumen outflow, which could be responsible for an increase in apparent net absorption of essential amino acids (AA) (Waghorn et al., 1987). Silanikove et al. (2001) indicated that adverse effects of high dietary levels of CT are due to decreased activity of intestinal enzymes (i.e., trypsin and amylase) and interaction of CT with the epithelium lining of the digestive tract, leading to decreased true protein digestion. Similarly, other reports indicate that effects of CT on fecal CP are primarily via influence on true CP digestibility (Robbins et al., 1987; Reed, 1995; Hove et al., 2001; Moore et al., 2004), although effect on MFCP is conceivable with extensive CT tissue binding. Several types of CT are capable of binding to epithelial tissues, and not all studies report the levels and types of CT. In large part, this is due to high variability and inadequacy of current assay procedures. Thus, it is not presently possible to predict accurately the influences of CT and their types on digestibility.

Endogenous Urinary Crude Protein

The endogenous urinary CP loss (EUCP) is appreciable but usually less than MFCP. The EUCP arises from obligatory oxidation of AA and maintenance costs associated with the protein turnover process, resulting in urinary excretion of urea, creatinine, bilirubin, allantoin, hippuric acid, uric acid, and the amino acid 3-methyl-histidine (SCA, 1990). Because EUCP is related to energy metabolism, it is scaled by a function of BW, with the function recommended possibly differing among species (Brody, 1945). For example, NRC (2001) recommended that the EUCP loss for dairy cattle be scaled by $BW^{0.50}$, compared with $BW^{0.75}$ determined for goats by Luo et al. (2004a). The EUCP of cervids scales to $BW^{0.75}$ (Robbins, 1993) and is in the same range as sheep and cattle; however, that for elk/wapiti (Mould and Robbins 1981) is 45–75 percent higher than white-tailed deer and red deer (Robbins et al., 1975; Mould and Robbins, 1981). Male white-tailed deer appear to have an 18 percent greater daily EUCP production than females (Robbins et al., 1975; Asleson et al., 1996).

Endogenous urinary CP has been estimated by feeding very low CP diets and regressing urinary nitrogen excretion against total or digestible nitrogen intake. Luo et al. (2004a) discussed different considerations regarding choice of method. Regression against digestible CP intake results in a greater estimate of EUCP than use of total CP intake. However, choice of an assumed k_{pm} also has a marked impact.

Scurf and Fiber Crude Protein

Dermal losses of CP as scurf and fiber are described as functions of BW. For example, AFRC (1993) recommended a scurf and hair protein loss for cattle and goats of 0.1125 g/kg $BW^{0.75}$, whereas NRC (1984, 2001) for beef and dairy cattle proposed the estimate of 0.2 g/kg $BW^{0.60}$. Scaling by $BW^{0.60}$ is in accordance with the assumption of a relationship with surface area. For lactating goats, Nsahlai et al. (2004) used the assumption of 0.2 g/kg $BW^{0.60}$ of NRC (1984, 2001). However, because fiber production can be affected by season, breed type, species, and frequency of shedding, scurf and fiber CP can vary and could be a significant consideration for wool- and hair-producing ruminants. Certainly, there is need for research and evaluation of the metabolizable protein needs for hair/wool production. As detailed in Chapter 4, in cervids, fiber growth occurs in summer, following shedding of the thick winter coat. In most species the initial thin coat is then shed (Jacobsen, 1980). A longer coat grown in late summer/autumn is associated with growth of wool-like fibers, termed underwool, and is grown from secondary follicles (Sauer, 1984). In winter no growth occurs and scurf loss is assumed to be that for skin shedding and replacement (~ 2 mg/kg $BW^{0.6}$). Hair weight in mammals approximates 2 percent of BW and weight of hair scales at 0.035 g/g $BW^{0.92}$ (Robbins, 1993). Daily net protein for fiber (NP_f) for growing white-tailed deer fawns is estimated at 5.4–13 g protein (Robbins et al., 1974b). Assuming a 135-day growing period, a daily metabolizable protein for fiber (MP_f; hair fiber) for sub-adult and adult cervids is 0.25 gCP/kg $BW^{0.75}$, using a fiber CP content of 0.89–0.91g/gDM (Robbins et al., 1974b; Gerhart et al., 1996) and an efficiency of metabolizable protein use for fiber growth (k_{pf}) of 0.6.

Efficiency of Metabolizable Protein Use

As noted before, there are considerable differences among metabolizable protein systems in assumed k_{pm} (e.g., 0.67 vs. 1.0). Typically, k_{pm} for MFCP, EUCP, and scurf CP is assumed to be similar, although Cannas et al. (2004) used a k_{pm} for dermal and wool losses of sheep of 0.6, slightly lower than that employed for MFCP and EUCP (i.e., 0.67). For cervids, efficiency in use of metabolizable protein was assumed to be as for sheep.

The k_{pm} value seems deserving of future research attention. There should be consideration given to the source of metabolizable protein being metabolized. For example, one might suppose relatively efficient metabolizable protein use in a well-fed state, given the availability of amino acids from the diet and normal turnover of proteinaceous tissue, making the amino acid profile of each origin less important than otherwise. Conversely, with low nutrient intake and mobilization of proteinaceous tissue to support maintenance of other tissues, k_{pm} might be lower than with greater intake, since efficiency would be dependent upon how well the amino acid profile of mobilized protein (mostly muscle) matches amino acid needs of the "maintenance" tissues (e.g., liver, skin, gastrointestinal tract, heart, brain). This does not consider potential for effects of level of alimentation on the efficiency with which specific amino acids are conserved.

In Chapter 4 it was noted that the maintenance requirement decreases with increasing age, which seems primarily attributable to change in fasting heat production. It is not known if k_{pm} varies with age.

Parasitism

The abomasal nematodes *Haemonchus contortus*, *Ostertagia* (*Teladorsagia*) *circumcincta* and *Trichostrongylus axei* and the small intestinal species of *Trichostrongylus*, *Nematodirus*, and *Cooperia* are generally associated with production losses and clinical diseases. These nematodes are more prevalent in grazing ruminants (Sykes, 1994). Effects of such parasitism on metabolizable energy (ME) requirements were briefly addressed in Chapter 4. The effect on the metabolizable protein requirement seems to be related to the greater use of amino acids to mount the immune response (e.g., synthesis of immunoglobulins and cytokines), repair and replacement of gastrointestinal tract tissues (i.e., leakage of plasma protein, sloughing of epithelial cells, secreted mucoproteins), and, relatedly, support of higher rates of liver export protein synthesis (Sykes and Coop, 2001; Liu et al., 2003). In sheep, gastrointestinal parasite infection increases nitrogen flow into the gastrointestinal tract and reduces the efficiency of dietary nutrient use for production (Sykes, 2000). Thus, in general, subclinical internal parasitism has relatively greater impact on MP than on ME requirements with, in consequence, influences on the optimum or required dietary MP:ME ratio (Brown et al., 1991; Liu et al., 2003). Liu et al. (2003) estimated that the immunity-associated response to an infection of sheep with the small intestinal parasite *Trichostrongylus colubriformis* increases the metabolizable protein requirement for maintenance (MP_m) by 0.69-fold for ewes in late pregnancy and by 2.5-fold for ewes in early lactation. In addition to the increased competition for metabolizable protein with internal parasitism, there are effects on the profile of amino acids (e.g., lower sulfur-amino acids) available to nonvisceral tissues, with likely impact on the efficiencies of metabolizable protein utilization.

Numerous studies now support the view that providing supplemental metabolizable protein to sheep with subclinical infections of gastrointestinal parasites improves their resilience and resistance to parasites (van Houtert et al., 1995; Kyriazakis et al., 1996; Coop and Kyriazakis, 1999). In addition, for the most part, the response to supplementation is greater when the protein source is not extensively degraded in the rumen, such as in fish meal. For example, worm burdens (*T. colubriformis* and *T. circumcincta)* were dramatically reduced (3- to 4-fold) in sheep in late pregnancy given supplemental (8 percent) fish meal, accompanied by positive effects on BW change and condition (Donaldson et al., 1998). Feed selection is also influenced during parasitism, presumably as part of a coordinated effort to counter the effects of infestation and to mount an effective immune response. Thus, parasitized sheep and goats, if given the choice, will select for a relatively high dietary protein concentration (e.g., 21 vs. 9 percent CP: (Aumont et al., 1984; Kyriazakis et al., 1994, 1996). The primary immune response to infection involves increased hepatic synthesis (e.g., acute phase proteins, albumin) and gastrointestinal losses of proteins high in sulfur-amino acids, and so it is expected that the requirement for sulfur-amino acids will be greater during infestation. In consequence, synthesis of proteins high in sulfur-amino acid such as wool and milk proteins will be reduced. Coop et al. (1997) showed that in lambs exposed to a trickle infection of *T. colubriformis*, supplemental rumen-protected methionine improved live weight gain and wool growth, and overall the adverse effects of the continuous infection were reduced.

The ability of animals to express immunity to gastrointestinal nematodes includes decreased establishment and arrested development of incoming larvae, decreased fecundity, and enhanced expulsion of the worm burden (Barnes and Dobson, 1993). Adams and Liu (2003) predicted that the animal's ability to resist parasite infestation is most likely to be compromised during physiological states where the demand for protein by tissues is barely met by either protein reserves or the animal's feed intake. For example, during pregnancy and early lactation, when priorities for nutrient partition favor fetal growth and milk production, respectively, relaxation in immunity is most likely to occur that compromises the ability to resist parasite infestation. Periparturient relaxation, or breakdown in immunity, is more prevalent in ewes carrying multiple fetuses and suckling multiple lambs (i.e., with greater milk production demands: Houdijk et al., 2001) and in high- versus low-producing dairy goats (Hoste and Chartier, 1993; Chartier et al., 2000). These are situations where consumption of feed often places a limit on intake of metabolizable protein to support production. In these situations, expression of immunity was enhanced in sheep and goats fed greater amounts of MP.

There is need for more information on the consequences of internal parasitism on metabolizable protein requirements and development of practical indicators of the types and levels of infestation, including associated effects on level of feed intake. For example, decreased feed intake in response to internal parasitism would entail an increased metabolizable protein requirement both on absolute and dietary concentration bases. Furthermore, relaxation in immunity seems to be parasite species-dependent (Coop and Holmes, 1996) and season-dependent. Therefore, the nutrient requirements to support necessary components of the protective immune system may also vary with the stage of parasite development. At present, and in the future, these areas of research will be of greater importance in light of the increasing development of anthelmintic resistance in farm animals. That is, producers should not only weigh the cost of increasing metabolizable protein intake to maintain desired levels of performance with internal parasite infections and cost of treatment with any remaining effective anthelmintics, but also must consider effects of treatment today on future efficacy.

For cervids, few experimental studies confirm such effects of parasites on reproduction (Chapter 4; Albon et al.,

2002), even though levels of infection at the end of winter and spring (Halvorsen et al., 1999) suggest the possibility of an effect on protein metabolism. Accounting for effects of parasites on protein metabolism is confounded because high infestation may influence energy metabolism and appetite as well as protein. Thus, climate and forage biomass and quality are important factors in field experimentation, and simulation modeling is required to account for effects of pasture contamination, parasite fecundity, and host density on infection (Stein et al., 2002). Cervids also are affected seasonally by external parasites that influence nutrient requirements directly through blood loss (Zhigunov, 1968), protein costs of immune responses, and energy-protein costs of responding behaviorally to minimize parasite infection rates (Reimers, 1980; White, 1983; Russell et al., 1993). Therefore, energy and protein costs of external parasites may adversely influence postnatal growth rates (Helle and Tarvainen, 1984) and compensatory growth of free-ranging adults (Cameron et al., 2005).

Other Influencing Factors

Effects of gender on metabolizable protein requirements appear related primarily to protein concentration in tissue being accreted and maintained as reflected by stage of maturity and growth rate. The effects on the ME requirement for maintenance (ME_m) of the tissues being maintained were addressed in Chapter 4. Comparable influences on MP_m have not been extensively studied. Nonetheless, one intuitively would expect greater EUCP for lean vs. fat animals per unit of BW at the same stage of maturity.

There have been relatively fewer studies that have examined the effects of previous nutritional plane on MP requirements compared with ME requirements. Current metabolizable protein systems do not address potential effects, which in part may be because of counteracting changes in maintenance and production needs. For example, with decreased ME and MP needs for maintenance after a low nutritional plane, there is increased metabolizable protein available for greater levels of production, with generally greater protein accretion early in the period of compensation.

Effects of extreme heat and cold conditions on metabolizable protein requirements have not been well defined. However, with cold stress and the associated increased ME_m requirement, less ME available for gain seems to be accompanied by a decreased requirement of MP for gain or growth (MP_g). An increased ME_m with acclimatization to nonextreme cold temperatures would represent a decreased MP requirement relative to that for ME. The decrease in feed intake with extreme heat stress and decreased production indicates a decrease in the MP requirement, assuming that ME is more limiting than or co-limiting with MP. With metabolizable protein relatively more limiting, however, the metabolizable protein requirement on a dietary concentration basis would be elevated depending on the magnitude of decline in feed intake. A decrease in ME_m in response to acclimatization to a nonextreme high temperature would depend on how ratios of MP:ME for maintenance and productive functions compare, with relatively small differences in most practical settings.

PROTEIN REQUIREMENTS FOR PRODUCTION

Growth

The two general factors necessary to predict MP_g with many metabolizable protein systems are protein concentration in tissue gain and efficiency of metabolizable protein use (k_{pg}). Protein concentration decreases with increasing energy content as rate of growth increases, and metabolizable protein systems have equations in addition to ones for energy to predict protein concentration based on rate of change in BW, retained energy, and/or BW adjusted to standard body condition score (BCS) relative to mature weight (SCA, 1990; NRC, 2000). Such approaches are preferred given the existence of accurate means of predicting protein concentration in tissue gain or protein accretion and application of an appropriate k_{pg}. For the latter factor, assumed k_{pg} vary among metabolizable protein systems (e.g., 0.7 for SCA, 1990; and 0.5 for NRC, 1985b). Research is needed to gain a better understanding of k_{pg}. In this regard, to address potential change in k_{pg} with increasing age, based on data from two experiments, NRC (2000) adjusted k_{pg} for equivalent BW (adjusted for BCS) of beef steers up to 300 kg, assuming constant k_{pg} (near 0.50) with BW above 300 kg.

Luo et al. (2004b,c) determined metabolizable protein requirements for tissue growth by growing goats based on change in BW with a method similar to that of Wilkerson et al. (1993). Though protein concentration in tissue gain could not be addressed, given the few serial slaughter experiments reported, uncertainty regarding k_{pg}, typical marketing at relatively young age, and general reliance on herbage rather than concentrate-based diets, this approach seems the most realistic and appropriate possible for goats at present.

In cervid species the protein content of tissue gain remains constant from birth to weaning at 20.2 and 20.5 percent protein for females and males, respectively (Robbins et al., 1974a) and is higher in adults ranging from 23 percent in white-tailed deer (Robbins, 1993) to between 24 and 46 percent in adult female Arctic caribou depending on reproductive condition (calculated from Adamczewski et al., 1987; Chan-McLeod et al., 1999). For males, regain of both protein and fat occurs during spring through autumn, and protein in the regain approximates 23 percent (Clutton-Brock et al., 1982; Barboza et al., 2004). Efficiency in deposition net protein, k_{pg}, was assumed to be 0.7 (CSIRO, 1990). Thus MP requirements for BW gain varied with animal group, with a range of 0.3–0.5 g/g BW gain depending on protein deposition in the gain. Adult male and female cervids make an average daily gain (ADG) in summer that attempts to compensate for weight losses associated with breeding. For males most weight loss occurs during the autumn-winter rut, and involves protein loss of approximately 23 percent over a 70–80 day rut (~ 77 g/d: Barboza et al., 2004). Fat losses exceed protein, and regain of both protein and fat occurs during spring through autumn (Clutton-Brock et al., 1982; Barboza et al., 2004). Since the period over which ADG occurs exceeds the loss period, a maximum net protein gain of 46 g/day was assumed. For reproductive females, maternal weight loss involves both fat and protein during pregnancy (Gerhart et al., 1996; Parker et al., 2005). Protein loss approximates 3 percent of BW (calculated from data of Parker et al., 2005), and compensatory gain over 150 days following a decline in milk production in midsummer was approximately 150 g/day and was dominated by protein gain (Parker et al., 1990; Gerhart et al., 1996). For nonlactating females, a 208-day period was assumed for a growth rate of approximately 208 g/d. Amplitude of the proportional change in body weight of males was about twice that of females (Leader-Williams and Ricketts, 1981). Because the k_{pg} estimate is not known for cervids, calculating MP_g and the MP requirements of the growing cervid, and those making seasonal body compensatory gain, are first approximates of real values. Validation studies are needed.

Lactation

Efficiencies of metabolizable protein use for lactation (k_{pl}) assumed by many metabolizable protein systems are similar: for example, 0.67, 0.70, and 0.68 of NRC (2001), SCA (1990), and AFRC (1993), respectively. INRA (1989) and Cannas et al. (2004) employed a lower value of 0.58 for sheep, which Cannas et al. (2004) explained was because of fiber growth and its high demand for sulfur-containing AA. For goats, INRA (1989) recommended use of a k_{pl} of 0.64 and Nsahlai et al. (2004) found a value of 0.69. However, in some cases, it is not so clear which k_{pl} is assumed for use of mobilized tissue protein for milk production ($k_{pl\text{-}t}$) or which k_{pg} is appropriate for dietary metabolizable protein used in tissue replenishment in mid- and late lactation. In this regard, Nsahlai et al. (2004) assumed that k_{pl} was similar regardless of origin of metabolizable protein (i.e., diet vs. tissue) and a k_{pg} of 0.59. Furthermore, a constant tissue protein concentration of 14.3 percent was assumed for mobilization and accretion. As high milk-producing ruminants are either losing or gaining protein throughout a large proportion of the lactation period, future research is needed to characterize more thoroughly efficiency of mobilized tissue protein for milk production ($k_{pl\text{-}t}$) and k_{pg}, as well as the concentration of protein in tissue mobilized and accreted. In regard to the latter factor, it is suggested that tissue protein concentration be based on BCS, with consideration for potential differences in tissue protein concentration for mobilization vs. accretion.

For cervids, protein requirements vary with maternal BW, number of offspring, and stage of lactation, provided other nutrients are in adequate supply. For females with one offspring, milk production scales to maternal $BW^{0.75}$ (Oftedal, 1984), and milk protein content is highly related to both the lipid content (Luick et al., 1974) and milk yield in cervids. Based on postnatal BW changes, most cervids are highly dependent on body protein stores until after peak milk production, after which body protein is deposited concomitant with a decrease in milk production (Chapter 4). Thus, a k_{pl} representing tissue mobilization of 0.65 likely represents early to peak lactation and a k_{pl} of 0.84 when most milk protein is derived from feed resources. Other researchers (Nsahlai et al., 2004) assumed that k_{pl} is similar regardless of origin of MP (i.e., diet vs. tissue) and a k_{pg} of 0.59 is assumed.

Fiber Growth

There is considerable variability among metabolizable protein systems in assumed metabolizable protein requirements or efficiencies of metabolizable protein use for fiber growth (k_{pf}). For example, k_{pf} are 0.26, 0.50, and 0.60 for AFRC (1993), NRC (1985a), and SCA (1990), respectively. Luo et al. (2004b) reported a metabolizable protein requirement for clean mohair fiber growth of 1.65 g/g, with suggested equivalence to a k_{pf} of about 0.48 assuming a clean fiber protein concentration of 80 percent.

There is need for future study of k_{pf}, including the testing of appropriateness of assuming similar values for wool-producing sheep and Angora goats. Moreover, because of the high sulfur-amino acid concentration in fiber, there should be consideration for potential differences between major origins of metabolizable protein (i.e., diet vs. mobilized tissue). Likewise, how rate of nonfiber tissue gain by growing animals, with impacts on amino acid partitioning, may affect k_{pf} should be studied. It is possible that such factors contribute to the different k_{pf} used in various metabolizable protein systems.

Factors associated with timing of pelage growth and contribution to protein requirements of cervids are reviewed in Chapter 4, and under the section on scurf and fiber crude protein above.

Pregnancy

As summarized in Chapter 4 for energy, metabolizable protein systems vary somewhat in how metabolizable protein requirements for pregnancy or gestation are addressed. A primary difference is in the assumed efficiency of metabolizable protein use (k_{ppreg}), with values of 0.85 (AFRC, 1993, 1998), 0.65 (NRC, 2000), 0.7 (SCA, 1990), 0.4 (sheep; INRA, 1989), and 0.33 (NRC, 2001; Sahlu et al., 2004). Research is needed to define more clearly k_{ppreg}, including closer scrutiny of potential species differences.

Metabolizable protein systems include equations to predict the increase in gestation tissue total and protein mass with advancing pregnancy. In some cases it is unclear if or how total BW should be adjusted for pregnancy tissue mass to estimate the amount of metabolizable protein used for maintenance. Not adjusting for pregnancy tissue mass might overestimate MP_m. For systems not including development of the mammary gland as a part of gestation, it would seem that its mass would contribute to the estimate of BW used to calculate the maintenance metabolizable protein requirement and that an efficiency of metabolizable protein use the same as that for accretion of nonpregnancy tissues is being assumed.

For cervids, daily rate of deposition of nitrogen during pregnancy was based on data for white-tailed deer (equation [2], Robbins and Moen, 1975). For reindeer/caribou and wapiti, nitrogen deposition per kg fetus at term was used as estimated in Table 5 of Robbins and Moen (1975). For red deer, daily rate nitrogen deposition per kg fetus was estimated using a modification of the generalized cervid equation (equation [4], Robbins and Moen, 1975). Thus:

$$L_n\, Y(t) = -3.3856 + 0.0275 \times X \qquad \text{white-tailed deer}$$

where Y = N retention (g/d), t = day of gestation, and X = day of gestation.

$$L_n\, Y(t) = -5.4794 + 0.0231 \times X \qquad \text{reindeer/caribou}$$
$$L_n\, Y(t) = -5.3602 + 0.0218 \times X \qquad \text{red deer}$$
$$L_n\, Y(t) = -5.6555 + 0.0197 \times X \qquad \text{wapiti/elk}$$

where Y = N retention (g/d) per kg fetus produced, t = day of gestation and X = day of gestation.

Retention of nitrogen was converted to protein and divided by $k_{ppreg} = 0.33$ (NRC, 2001; Sahlu et al., 2004) to determine MP_{ppreg}. Protein requirement for conceptus at term relates to both maternal BW and BW (Robbins and Moen, 1975). Estimation of the development of fetus weight during pregnancy is reviewed in Chapter 4. Given that most fetal tissue may be derived from maternal protein (Gerhart et al., 1996; Parker et al., 2005; Barboza and Parker, 2006), it is possible that k_{ppreg} may be high, at 0.7–0.85 as proposed by AFRC (1993, 1998), CSIRO (1990), and NRC (2000).

Antler Growth

Adult male cervids grow antlers, shed velvet, and cast antlers in response to day length under an endogenous rhythm (Goss 1969a,b) that ensures growth in summer. This timing appears similar for most cervid species (Suttie and Kay, 1982). However, timing of casting of antlers by males is influenced by nutrition (Long et al., 1959; Watson, 1971). Initiation of the first antler growth is determined by BW rather than photoperiod for red deer fawns, which suggests a strong nutritional influence (Suttie and Kay, 1982). Access to adequate nutrition also affects antler size (French et al., 1956; Ullrey, 1983; Wolfe, 1983; Brown, 1990) and in extreme undernutrition males may not grow antlers (Lincoln, 1971). However, Asleson et al. (1997) showed that a 12-week restriction in protein intake in early or late antlerogenesis did not result in a reduction in BW or antler size in white-tailed deer. Compensatory growth following restriction in early antlerogenesis could have accounted for the lack of an effect in this treatment. Supplemental feeding in winter has been especially successful in increasing antler size of red deer (Peek et al., 2002). This suggests that body reserves of protein and minerals may be the preferred sources for antlerogenesis. The antler growth period lasts 10–15 weeks in young deer and approximates 22 weeks in adult reindeer/caribou (Bergerud, 1976), at which time antlers are fully ossified (Banks et al., 1968). Changes in antler weight during antlerogenesis have rarely been measured; however, Muir et al. (1987) report that mass and ash content increases as a power function, and these equations have been used in an experimental estimate of protein requirements and antler growth of white-tailed deer (Asleson et al., 1996) and for modeling of nutrient requirements for antler growth in caribou (Moen and Pastor, 1998). The Muir et al. (1987) relationships can be scaled to other cervids based on the antler-growing period and maximum antler weight (Moen and Pastor, 1998). Maximum antler size increases with age in cervids (Hyvarinen et al., 1977; Wolfe, 1983). In early antlerogenesis, protein content of the velvet antler is high at 80 percent DM (Ullrey, 1983), and in the harvested velvet antler, CP is 67–69 percent DM (Sim and Hudson, 1991). The hardened antler contains 32 percent protein, and this protein is in the organic matter component, which is 80 percent CP (Asleson et al., 1997). A distinguishing feature of the genus *Rangifer* (reindeer/caribou) is that both males and females grow antlers (Kelsall, 1968). Antlers of female reindeer/caribou are proportionally much smaller than males. Antlers of male caribou are proportionally greater than other cervids (Geist, 1987). Measurements of CP requirements for antler growth are difficult to achieve (Brown, 1990; Asleson et al., 1996), and estimates have been made using factorial studies (Verme and Ullrey, 1984; Brown, 1990) and modeling (Moen and Pastor, 1998). In some studies involving estimation of nitrogen requirements for growth, a positive nitrogen balance has been recorded when animals are at 0 BW change or losing weight (Holter et al., 1977; Asleson et al., 1996), which complicates making a precise estimate of nitrogen requirement. In addition, unaccounted-for nitrogen losses as pelage, hoof growth, and skin-sloughing limit the ability to accurately apportion nitrogen retention to antlers (Asleson et al., 1996). Protein requirement for antler growth is considered small compared with that for maintenance (Verme and Ullrey, 1984; Brown, 1990; Robbins, 1993). Asleson et al. (1996) determined the mean daily nitrogen deposition in antlers of white-tailed deer at 29 mg/kg $BW^{0.75}$ (maximum 60 mg/kg $BW^{0.75}$), considerably less than that deduced for male caribou (mean 105 mg/kg $BW^{0.75}$, calculated from Moen and Pastor, 1998) with total antler weight of 10 kg. Asleson et al. (1996) estimated that maintenance nitrogen requirement was raised by 0.04 g/kg $BW^{0.75}$ (a 7 percent increase) during antlerogenesis, giving a MP requirement of 0.25 g/kg $BW^{0.75}$. If the factorial approach is used to estimate MP requirement of this study, the mean daily nitrogen retention of 29 mg/kg $BW^{0.75}$ gives a daily MP requirement of 0.26 g/kg $BW^{0.75}$, and the maximum rate of nitrogen deposition, 60 mg/kg $BW^{0.75}$ gives a daily MP requirement of 0.54 g/kg $BW^{0.75}$. A k_{pg} for antlers of 0.7 was used assuming antler protein was derived from body protein. For male caribou, mean daily MP was determined to be 0.90 g/kg $BW^{0.75}$, assuming $k_{pg} = 0.7$. For the female caribou, using a nitrogen retention of 1 g/d (Moen and Pastor, 1998), the daily MP requirement for antlerogenesis was estimated at 0.31 g/kg $BW^{0.75}$. Both antler size and rate of growth affect MP requirements. Therefore, there are possible species and nutritional effects that have not been determined.

AMINO ACID REQUIREMENTS

Essential vs. Nonessential

There are 20 amino acids commonly found in animal and plant proteins. The terms "essential" and "nonessential" are the classical divisions of amino acids that define the metabolic capability of an animal to synthesize the amino acids in these groups. Thus, essential amino acids are those that the animal cannot synthesize at a sufficient rate to meet needs and must be supplied in the diet, and include histidine, lysine, methionine, phenylalanine, threonine, tryptophan, arginine, and the branched-chain amino acids isoleucine, leucine, and valine. By contrast, the nonessentials are ones that the animal can synthesize at an adequate rate and include proline, aspartate, asparagine, glutamate, glutamine, tyrosine, alanine, serine, glycine, and cysteine. Rumen microbes are capable of synthesizing all amino acids for microbial protein synthesis as long as sufficient carbon skeletons (from dietary protein and carbohydrates), nonprotein nitrogen, and inorganic sulfur are available (Atasoglu et al., 1998). In this respect, ruminants do not have a dietary requirement for amino acids because the rumen microbes degrade and subsequently synthesize all amino acids. However, studies conducted in vitro indicate that for many rumen microbes to grow and function at maximum rates, intact (undegraded) amino acids (Maeng and Baldwin, 1976; Atasoglu et al., 1999, 2001) and peptides (Maeng et al., 1976; Cotta and Russell, 1982) supplied by the diet seem to be obligate requirements, in addition to ammonia. Similarly, rumen microbial growth and fiber digestion are enhanced in steers (McAllan, 1991) and sheep (Chikunya et al., 1996) fed diets containing higher levels of either rumen degradable (casein) or undegradable (fish meal) protein sources.

For ruminants fed highly rumen degradable protein, a large portion of the amino acid supply for absorption will be in the form of microbial protein. In this case, the rumen microbial protein supply to the small intestines delivers a good quality pattern of essential and nonessential amino acids sufficient to support maintenance and normal, but not maximal, growth and milk production (Virtanen, 1966; Storm and Ørskov, 1984). However, to optimize production of meat, milk, conceptus, and wool protein, certain amino acids may limit (e.g., lysine and methionine for milk production, cysteine and methionine for wool growth) attainment of optimal production levels. Under these conditions supplemental feed sources high in rumen undegraded intake protein (UIP) or rumen-protected amino acids can be fed to complement the supply of amino acids from microbial protein and balance the supply of essential amino acids to meet protein synthetic needs.

Limiting Amino Acids

Unlike nonruminant species or species lacking pregastric fermentation, ruminants harbor a highly active microbial population in the rumen that leads to extensive and often variable degrees of dietary protein breakdown. In consequence, the relative supplies of microbial vs. dietary protein to the small intestines vary, and so, too, will the pattern of essential amino acids available for absorption. This latter presents a challenge to ruminant nutritionists when it comes to predicting the composition of essential, potentially limiting, amino acids that will be available to meet productive tissue (e.g., muscle, mammary gland, skin) requirements. In this regard, it has proven difficult to establish sound predictions and recommendations of the limiting amino acids for ruminant production when anything other than highly degradable nitrogen sources are fed, and where microbial protein is the predominant amino acid source (Storm and Ørskov, 1984). However, because the microbial protein biomass supplies 50–90 percent of the essential amino acids absorbed from the small intestine (Smith, 1975), and given the relatively constant proportions of essential amino acids in protein of mixed microbial populations (Table 5-1), the starting point for assessing limiting amino acids for maintenance, growth, and milk and wool production begins with the pattern of essential amino acids in microbial protein. Data in Table 5-1 provide a comparison of the amino acid composition of mixed microbial biomass protein with carcass, milk, skin, and wool proteins. Based on this simple comparison, microbial protein will supply a fairly balanced supply of essential amino acids for net synthesis of proteins accreted or secreted by sheep and goats. Two exceptions are methionine and histidine, which will be limiting, especially at high rates of milk casein or carcass protein synthesis.

Tissue and Muscle Growth

In general, the amino acid needs of sheep and goats for growth of muscle, conceptus development, and milk pro-

TABLE 5-1 Essential Amino Acid Composition (grams of amino acid per 100 grams protein) of Mixed Microbial Protein Compared with Carcass Tissue, Milk Casein, Skin, and Wool

Amino Acid	Rumen Microbes[a,b]	Carcass[c] (sheep)	Casein[d] (goat)	Skin[c] (sheep)	Whole Wool[c] (sheep)
Methionine	1.6–2.5	1.8	2.54	1	0.6
Lysine	8.1–11.5	7	6.7	4.8	3.5
Histidine	1.6–2.1	2.6	2.5	1.4	1.2
Phenylalanine	4.9–5.7	3.9	4.44	3.2	3.6
Tryptophan	na	na	(1.36)	na	na
Threonine	5.2–6.6	5	4.35	3.9	6
Leucine	7.4–8.3	7.5	8.15	5.7	7.4
Isoleucine	5.4–6.2	3.8	4.39	2.4	3
Valine	5.3–6.5	4.9	6.39	0.3	5.5
Arginine	4.6–5.3	7.3	2.57	7.9	9.1
Cyst(e)ine	2.0–2.6	0.9	0.7	3.5	9.8

na = tryptophan is destroyed during acid hydrolysis. The value for casein tryptophan is based on gene sequences of bovine caseins.
[a]Storm and Ørskov (1983).
[b]Martin et al. (1996.
[c]MacRae et al. (1993).
[d]Bequette (unpublished data).

duction do not differ greatly from that reported for beef (NRC, 2000) and dairy cattle (NRC, 2001). One exception is the greater requirement for sulfur-amino acids to support wool and mohair growth (see below), both of which contain a high content of cyst(e)ine. In terms of tissue growth and nitrogen retention, a number of studies in sheep have examined growth responses to single amino acids, groups of amino acids, and intact proteins. The qualitative importance of these results, however, depends largely upon the types and amounts of the basal diets fed in the studies. In studies where the ingredients in the basal diet were highly degradable in the rumen, and where microbial protein was probably the predominant source of protein for digestion, significant responses in growth and nitrogen retention were observed in lambs when additional methionine and/or lysine was supplied (Schelling and Hatfield, 1968; Nimrick et al., 1970a,b). The most complete evaluation of the order of limiting amino acids in microbial protein for lamb growth was conducted by Storm and Ørskov (1984), and here the most limiting amino acids were, in descending order, methionine, lysine, arginine, and histidine. Even in studies where barley, corn, or corn gluten meal constituted part of the diet, and where some degree of rumen bypass occurred, lysine and methionine were found to be first- or co-limiting AA (Schelling et al., 1973; Matras et al., 2000). Similar results have been derived from studies in growing calves fed soybean hull-based diets and where most of the MP supply was represented by ruminal microbes. Here, the limiting amino acids were, in descending order, methionine, lysine, histidine, and at least one of the branched-chain amino acids (Greenwood and Titgemeyer, 2000).

Milk Protein Production

The qualitative and quantitative requirements for milk protein synthesis are mostly determined by the amino acid composition and milk output of casein. Because the pattern of amino acids in milk protein of lactating sheep and goats is comparable to that of lactating dairy cows and beef cattle (Davis et al., 1994), it is likely that when similar diets are fed to these species either methionine, lysine, or both will be the first limiting AA.

In recent years, the practice of providing protected amino acids in lactating ewe and dairy goat diets has become more common. In ewes (Lacaune, Dorset), addition of protected amino acids was found to increase milk production during the suckling (0.11 percent methionine + 0.28 percent lysine: Lynch et al., 1991; 0.2 percent methionine: Baldwin et al., 1993) and milking periods (3–6 g/d methionine: Bocquier et al., 1994). The response to methionine was higher when the basal diet was based on silage than on hay, indicating that methionine content could be the limiting AA in this last diet. Milk yield and milk fat content were unaffected by the supplementation.

Wool Protein Production

In mature animals, the daily production of clean wool by sheep can be 8–21 g/d; for goats clean mohair production can be 10–22 g/d (see Reis and Sahlu, 1994). For both fiber types, the most important quality factor in pricing is fiber diameter, followed by fiber length and fiber strength. Wool fiber is primarily comprised of protein with 0.5 percent each of lipid and minerals (Williams, 1995). Wool protein is

TABLE 5-2 Wool Protein Composition (grams of amino acid per 100 grams protein)

		Type of Wool Protein[b]		
	Whole Wool[a]	Low-Sulfur Proteins	High-Sulfur Proteins	High-Tyrosine Proteins
Histidine	0.8–1.3	0.6	0.7–1.3	0
Isoleucine	2.7–3.2	3.8	1.7–2.6	0
Leucine	6.7–7.9	10.2	1.4–3.4	3.5–6.4
Lysine	2.7–3.5	4.1	0.6–0.9	0
Methionine	0.44–0.63	0.6	0	0
Phenylalanine	2.5–3.6	2	0.5–1.6	2.7–9.6
Threonine	5.4–6.6	4.8	10.2–11.1	0–3.4
Valine	4.6–5.7	6.4	4.3–5.3	0–4.7
Alanine	3.2–5.2	7.7	2.0–2.9	0–3.1
Arginine	6.2–9.1	7.8	6.2–6.9	3.5–4.7
Aspartate	5.5–6.6	9.6	0.6–2.3	1.9–2.2
Cyst(e)ine	8.6–13.1	6	22.1–22.9	6.4–10.2
Glutamate	11.1–14.2	16.9	7.9	0
Glycine	4.6–8.6	5.2	4.2–6.2	26.5–38.8
Proline	5.3–7.5	3.3	12.6–12.8	1.7–6.7
Serine	8.3–10.8	8.1	12.7–13.2	12.4–12.6
Tyrosine	3.8–6.3	2.7	1.8–2.1	18.0–20.8

[a]MacRae et al. (1993).
[b]Reis (1979).

grouped into three main types (Table 5-2): (1) low-sulfur proteins constituting 60–70 percent of total proteins, (2) high-sulfur proteins constituting 20–40 percent of total proteins that contain very high levels of cyst(e)ine but no methionine, and (3) high-tyrosine proteins constituting approximately 1–12 percent of total proteins characterized by high levels of tyrosine but no methionine, lysine, isoleucine, histidine, or glutamic acid (Reis, 1979). Cysteine accounts for approximately 10 percent (8.6–13.1 percent) of amino acids in wool protein (Reis, 1979), compared with 1.3 percent in whole body tissues (MacRae et al., 1993), whereas methionine content in wool is low at about half that in whole body tissues. Mohair protein has an amino acid content similar to that of wool proteins, in particular with a high content of sulfur-amino acids (Parris and Swart, 1975). Thus, wool and mohair have a sulfur-amino acids concentration that is much higher than muscle and significantly greater than microbial protein and other typical protein supplements, such as fish meal and soybean meal proteins.

Given their high sulfur-amino acid contents, it is not surprising that the quantity and quality of wool and mohair fibers are strongly affected by level of nutrition and feed intake (Allden, 1979; Reis, 1979; Russel, 1992), with the amount and quality of dietary protein the most influential. Linear increases in the growth and diameter of mohair have been observed in Angora wether goats given increasing levels of dietary protein (Sahlu et al., 1992; Shahjalal et al., 1992). Increased growth rate of mohair fibers has also been observed when formaldehyde-treated casein (Throckmorton et al., 1982) and heat-treated soybean meal (Sahlu et al., 1992) were supplemented. Specifically, the responses to additional UIP are due to the increased supplies of methionine and cysteine. Bassett et al. (1981) observed increased mohair growth when polymer-encapsulated methionine was added to diets at 0.1 percent and 0.2 percent. Sahlu and Fernandez (1992) administered L-methionine and L-lysine intraperitoneally to Angora goats, and observed small, but significant, increases in clean fiber growth and fiber diameter in response to methionine, but not lysine. Current evidence suggests that methionine can be converted to cysteine in the skin, but that the rates of this conversion are insufficient to optimize wool growth under normal feeding conditions (Liu and Masters, 2003). In fact, intravenous or abomasal infusion of cysteine not only increases the abundance of cysteine-rich keratin-associated proteins in sheep wool, but also acts as a regulator at the cellular level to increase the gene expression in the follicle paracortical cells of these cysteine-rich wool proteins (Fratini et al., 1994).

Partition of amino acids between wool growth and weight gain of growing animals can be determined by comparison of their relative growth rates. Black et al. (1973) observed that nitrogen retained in wool accounted for 0.34–0.49 of total body nitrogen accreted (including wool) in Merino wethers (32 kg BW) in response to increasing levels of casein (20–100 g/d) infused into the abomasum. The linear increases in wool nitrogen and total body nitrogen retention suggested that dietary protein level does not alter the partition of amino acids between wool and other body tissues (Black et al., 1973). MacRae et al. (1993) found a similar relationship in Suffolk-Finn Dorset lambs. From 25–40 kg BW, wool nitrogen and total body nitrogen retentions increased in the relationship 0.34:1 and from 40–55 kg the relationship was similar at 0.36:1. In cashmere-yielding and Angora goats (Souri et al., 1998), nitrogen accretion in fiber accounted for 37 percent of total body nitrogen accretion (including fiber), and this relationship did not change (38 percent) when fiber growth was increased by 69 percent in response to supplemental (2.5 g/d) rumen-protected methionine (Galbraith, 1998). Thus, it appears that in weight-gaining, wool-producing breeds, the partition of nitrogen to wool or fiber growth is reasonably stable with respect to BW gain.

PROTEIN AND AMINO ACID REQUIREMENT RECOMMENDATIONS

SHEEP

Growing/Finishing Sheep

Evaluation

As noted by NRC (2000) and in many other publications, there have been fewer studies conducted in which protein is more limiting than energy, and no one study with growing/finishing sheep on which metabolizable protein requirements could be based was identified. Therefore, to evaluate protein requirements of growing/finishing sheep using the Cornell Net Carbohydrate and Protein System for Sheep method (CNCPS-S; Cannas et al., 2004), a database of treatment mean observations was constructed. The initial database entailed 31 references and 174 treatment mean observations. The final database selected consisted of 48 treatment mean observations from 14 references, representing 335 sheep (Tables 5-3 and 5-4).

To determine observations to be used, MP intake (MPI) was estimated as described in Chapter 4 with an approach similar to that of NRC (2000, 2001). The MP_m of CNCPS-S was based on estimates of MFCP, EUCP (Cannas et al., 2004), and scurf (without fiber). The scurf CP loss was estimated as $0.2 \times \text{kg BW}^{0.6}$ (NRC, 1984). The efficiency of metabolizable protein use for scurf CP was 0.6. The MFCP was estimated as 15.2 g/kg DMI, with an efficiency of metabolizable protein use of 0.67, and EUCP (g/d) was derived from the equation 3.375 + (0.147 × full or unshrunk BW, kg), also with an efficiency of metabolizable protein use of 0.67. The difference between MPI and MP_m was assumed to be metabolizable protein available for gain ($MP_{g\text{-avail}}$), which would include both fiber and nonfiber tissue.

To derive the protein concentration in BW gained or lost, the CNCPS-S equation for tissue energy concentration was used in conjunction with equation [1.30] of SCA (1990), which was derived from Garrett (1987, as cited by SCA, 1990). The protein concentration in tissue accreted or mobilized on a full BW (FBW) or average daily gain (ADG) basis was assumed to have 92 percent of that on an empty BW basis, which along with ADG was used to determine net protein gained or replacing maintenance protein with tissue mobilization ($NP_{g\text{-used}}$). The $NP_{g\text{-used}}$ was divided by an efficiency of metabolizable protein use for accretion or maintenance of 0.7 to derive metabolizable protein used for gain or mobilized ($MP_{g\text{-used}}$). Cannas et al. (2004) did not identify an assumed efficiency of use of mobilized tissue protein for maintenance in the CNCPS-S method, and one is not clearly indicated by SCA (1990). The value of 0.7 is employed here because it is similar to ones of the CNCPS-S for maintenance protein and that used by SCA (1990) for maintenance and growth, along with the assumption of NRC (1985b) of similar efficiencies of protein use regardless of derivation from the diet or mobilized tissue. Lastly, $NP_{g\text{-used}}$ divided by body protein concentration on an ADG basis provided a prediction of ADG based on MPI (ADG_{pred}).

The database used for evaluation consisted of 23 observations for which ADG_{pred} based on metabolizable protein was less than that based on energy as predicted by CNCPS-S and of 14 and 11 observations with ADG_{pred} based on metabolizable protein within 15 and 30 g/d, respectively, of observed ADG (ADG_{obs}). There were two observations of the Dixon and Egan (2000) reference (FM/L-1 and FM/L-3 treatments) that fit the criteria to be included in the database but were omitted because of very poor agreement with other observations in the relationship between $MP_{g\text{-avail}}$ and $MP_{g\text{-used}}$. Factors responsible for this finding are unknown, although supplementation in this study was twice weekly.

Evaluation of the description of metabolizable protein requirements of growing/finishing sheep by CNCPS-S (Cannas et al., 2004) was through regressing $MP_{g\text{-avail}}$ against $MP_{g\text{-used}}$. Regressions unweighted and weighted for the number of observations per treatment mean resulted in very similar equations, although the weighted equation had a slightly higher R^2 (0.01) and, thus, was chosen. As shown by the regression equation below, there was close agreement between $MP_{g\text{-avail}}$ and $MP_{g\text{-used}}$, without significant bias.

Eqn. SGP1

$MP_{g\text{-avail}}$ (g) = 1.41 (SE = 1.629) + 0.962 (SE = 0.0526) × $MP_{g\text{-used}}$ (R_2 = 0.88; mean bias = 0.9; Figure 5-1)

In addition to simple linear regression, mixed model analysis was conducted to ascertain the need to consider the effect of report. The effect of the number of observations was not significant. Covariance parameter estimates for the intercept ($P < 0.07$), slope ($P < 0.19$), and intercept-slope interaction ($P < 0.50$) were not significant, and the resulting equation was similar to Eqn. SGP1: $MP_{g\text{-avail}}$ (g) = 3.10 (SE = 3.880) + 0.997 (SE = 0.1432) × $MP_{g\text{-used}}$.

Eqn. SGP1 suggests appropriateness of CNCPS-S assumptions of metabolizable protein requirements of growing/finishing sheep. Nonetheless, there were a number of alternatives tested, such as use of a lower efficiency of metabolizable protein use for gain or replacing maintenance protein, a higher efficiency of metabolizable protein use for maintenance, and a different equation, not requiring the

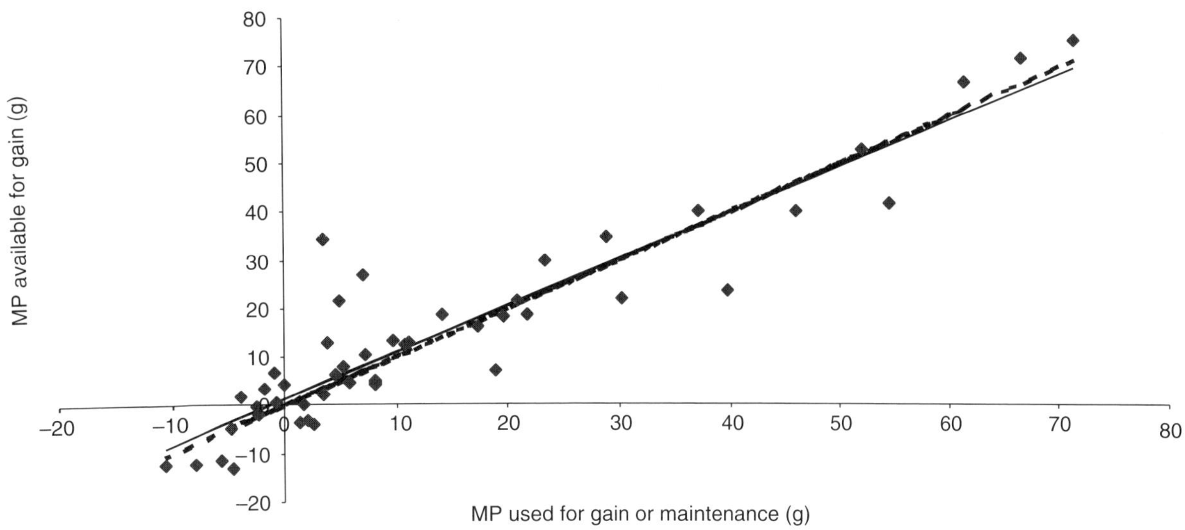

FIGURE 5-1 The relationship between metabolizable protein (MP) available (based on the difference between predicted metabolizable protein intake and metabolizable protein used for maintenance; $MP_{g\text{-avail}}$) and used for gain or maintenance (based on predicted metabolizable protein accreted in tissue or mobilized and used for maintenance; $MP_{g\text{-used}}$) for evaluation of the CNCPS-S method (Cannas et al., 2004) of describing protein requirements of growing/finishing sheep. The solid line depicts Eqn. SGP1: $MP_{g\text{-avail}}$, g = 1.41 (SE = 1.629) + 0.962 (SE = 0.0526) × $MP_{g\text{-used}}$ (R^2 = 0.88; mean bias = 0.9). The dashed line depicts $MP_{g\text{-avail}} = MP_{g\text{-used}}$.

input of tissue energy concentration, to predict the protein concentration in tissue accreted or mobilized. As expected given the high R^2 of Eqn. SGP1 and no significant bias, none of these alternatives improved prediction.

Although the CNCPS-S system considers mature weight of genotypes and the proportion of maturity to facilitate casual comparisons with values for other ruminant species, MPI (total) was regressed against ADG, with both scaled by $BW^{0.75}$ (MPI_{mbw} and ADG_{mbw}, respectively).

Eqn. SGP2

MPI_{mbw} (g/kg $BW^{0.75}$) = 2.51 (SE = 0.146) + 0.225 (SE = 0.0124) × ADG_{mbw} (R^2 = 0.88)

Based on this approach, the metabolizable protein requirement for maintenance was 2.51 g/kg $BW^{0.75}$ and that for gain was 0.225 g/g ADG. This MP_m estimate is that recommended for sheep by INRA (1989). The estimates are slightly less than those noted by Wilkerson et al. (1993) for growing beef cattle and Luo et al. (2004b) for growing goats. However, for goats, Luo et al. (2004b) used a database without exclusion of observations for which energy might have been more limiting than protein. It was stated that these estimates should be considered as maximums, without increases included as a safety factor. Moreover, with protein being more limiting to ADG than energy or co-limiting, as for observations of this database, nitrogen recycling relative to nitrogen intake and perhaps efficiency of metabolizable protein use would be greater than with energy most limiting. Hence, it may be reasonable to consider the requirements of CNCPS-S evaluated here as minimum to average ranges, and that additional metabolizable protein as a safety factor could be appropriate.

Description of Methods

The method of CNCPS-S (Cannas et al., 2004) to describe protein requirements of growing/finishing sheep is given below, with use of a SCA (1990) equation from Garrett (1987, as cited by SCA, 1990) to predict body protein concentration from the level of energy. The description given is to predict the requirement for a particular set of conditions, including known ADG and DMI, rather than to predict ADG based on estimated $MP_{g\text{-avail}}$, as was performed as a part of the evaluation exercise. Relatedly, it is necessary to consider needs for accretion of both fiber and nonfiber tissues. To do so, clean wool growth or production can be a direct input as in the CNCPS-S (Cannas et al., 2004). Alternatively, the method of SCA (1990) is given to predict clean wool growth, if an estimate is not available, based on a standard fleece weight relative to mature size adjusted for age for sheep less than 2 years of age. For hair sheep, the scurf or dermal loss of NRC (1984) is available. In addition, there are some inputs necessary to determine the energy concentration in tissue accreted or mobilized, listed earlier in Chapter 4, that must be repeated here.

1. Average unshrunk or full BW within the feeding period (FBW), kg
2. FBW at a BCS of 3.0 ($FBW_{BCS3.0}$; 0–5 scale) = FBW when skeletal development is complete, empty body fat concentration is 25 percent, and BCS is 2.8 to 3.0

3. DMI, kg/d
4. ME intake, Mcal/d
5. Maturity index (P), fraction = current $FBW/FBW_{BCS3.0}$
6. Energy concentration in empty body gain (EVG), Mcal/kg = (27/(1 + e(–6 × (P – 0.4)))) × 0.239
7. Age (AGEM), months (less than 24)
8. Wool age adjustment factor (WAAF) = 1 if > 24 months and otherwise (1 + e(–0.33 × AGEM)) × $P^{0.67}$
9. SFW (kg/year) = standard fleece weight (greasy) for an adult sheep (> 2 years of age) with good climatic conditions for pasture growth
10. Scurf and fiber CP (dermal plus clean fiber; $SF\text{-}CP_E$), g/d = wool sheep: direct entry of clean fiber growth or ME intake × 33.472 × ($SFW/FBW_{BCS3.0}$) × WAAF; hair sheep: 0.2 × kg $BW^{0.6}$
11. Endogenous urinary CP ($U\text{-}CP_E$), g/d = 3.375 + (0.147 × kg FBW)
12. Metabolic fecal CP ($F\text{-}CP_E$), g/d = 15.2 × kg DMI
13. MP requirement for maintenance plus fiber (MP_m), g/d = ($SF\text{-}CP_E$/0.6) + ($U\text{-}CP_E$/0.67) + ($F\text{-}CP_E$/0.67)
14. Protein concentration in tissue accreted or mobilized on an empty BW basis (TPFr), fraction = 0.256 – (0.0067 × (EVG, Mcal/kg × 4.184))
15. ADG on an FBW basis, g
16. Protein accretion or replacing maintenance protein (NP_g), g/d = ADG × TPFr × 0.92
17. MP requirement for gain, or mobilized protein used for maintenance (MP_g), g/d = NP_g/0.7
18. Total metabolizable protein requirement (MP_{req}), g/d = MP_m + MP_g

Mature Sheep (Nonpregnant) or Sheep in Early and Mid-Gestation

The CNCPS-S method (Cannas et al., 2004) plus additional considerations for fiber growth described for growing/finishing sheep are recommended for mature sheep in early and mid-gestation. Justification is based on the aforementioned evaluation conducted with growing/finishing sheep. An efficiency of use of mobilized tissue protein for maintenance with BW loss in the CNCPS-S method was not identified by Cannas et al. (2004); hence, an efficiency of 0.7 is assumed. For growing/finishing sheep, it was suggested that these requirements may be minimums and that additional protein could be supplied as a safety factor. Because protein turnover decreases with advancing stage of maturity and extensive AA recycling, it is proposed that supplying additional protein for mature sheep would not be necessary. This method is described below.

1. Average unshrunk or full BW within the feeding period (FBW), kg
2. FBW at a BCS of 3.0 ($FBW_{BCS3.0}$; 0–5 scale) = FBW when skeletal development is complete, empty body fat concentration is 25 percent, and BCS is 2.8 to 3.0
3. DMI, kg/g
4. ME intake, Mcal/d
5. Maturity index (P), fraction = current $FBW/FBW_{BCS3.0}$
6. SFW (kg/year) = standard fleece weight (greasy) for an adult sheep (> 2 years of age) with good climatic conditions for pasture growth
7. Scurf and fiber CP (dermal plus clean fiber; $SF\text{-}CP_E$), g/d = wool sheep: direct entry of clean fiber growth or ME intake × 33.472 × ($SFW/FBW_{BCS3.0}$); hair sheep: 0.2 × kg $BW^{0.6}$
8. Endogenous urinary CP ($U\text{-}CP_E$), g/d = 3.375 + (0.147 × kg FBW)
9. Metabolic fecal CP ($F\text{-}CP_E$), g/d = 15.2 × kg DMI
10. MP requirement for maintenance plus fiber (MP_m), g/d = ($SF\text{-}CP_E$/0.6) + ($U\text{-}CP_E$/0.67) + ($F\text{-}CP_E$/0.67)
11. FBW_{init}, kg = initial FBW
12. FBW_{fin}, kg = final FBW
13. Initial BCS (BCS_{init}) = 0 to 5, with 0 and 5 extremely thin and obese, respectively
14. Initial fraction of protein in the empty body ($ProFr_{init}$) = 0.1449 + (0.0279 × BCS_{init}) – (0.0039 × BCS_{init}^2)
15. Initial empty BW (EBW_{init}), kg = 0.851 × 0.96 × FBW_{init}
16. Initial protein mass ($ProM_{init}$), kg = $ProFr_{init}$ × EBW_{init}
17. Final BCS (BCS_{fin}) = 0 to 5, with 0 and 5 extremely thin and obese, respectively
18. Final fraction of protein in the empty body ($ProFr_{fin}$) = 0.1449 + (0.0279 × BCS_{fin}) – (0.0039 × BCS_{fin}^2)
19. Final empty BW (EBW_{fin}), kg = 0.851 × 0.96 × FBW_{fin}
20. Final protein mass ($ProM_{fin}$), kg = $ProFr_{fin}$ × EBW_{fin}
21. Average protein concentration as a fraction on a FBW basis during the feeding period ($TPFr_{avg}$) = (($ProM_{fin}$ – $ProM_{init}$)/(FBW_{fin} – FBW_{init})
22. ADG on a FBW basis, g
23. Protein accretion or replacing maintenance protein (NP_g), g/d = ADG × $TPFr_{avg}$
24. MP requirement for gain, or mobilized protein used for maintenance (MP_g), g/d = NP_g/0.7
25. Total metabolizable protein requirement (MP_{req}), g/d = MP_m + MP_g

Lactating Sheep

The CNCPS-S method (Cannas et al., 2004) plus additional considerations described for other sheep are recommended for describing protein requirements of lactating sheep. Justification for the proposed method is that the evaluation of the CNCPS-S indicated an acceptable description of protein requirements of growing/finishing sheep. This suggests that the CNCPS-S should likewise be appropriate for maintenance requirements of lactating sheep. The efficiency of MP use for milk protein synthesis of CNCPS-S is somewhat lower than that assumed for most other ruminant livestock species (i.e., 0.58 vs. 0.64–0.70), which Cannas et al. (2004) based on sulfur-amino acid use for fiber growth by sheep regardless of wool or hair growth rate. Because of this relatively low efficiency, it would not seem appropriate to add additional protein as a safety factor.

In the description of methods below, there may be a small deviation from that of Cannas et al. (2004) depending on interpretation. In equation [12] of Cannas et al. (2004), the efficiency of 0.58 is applied to total milk protein yield regardless of contributions of metabolizable protein from dietary origin and mobilized tissue. However, the report later states that the CNCPS-S assumes an efficiency of use of mobilized tissue protein for milk protein synthesis of 0.8 (SCA, 1990). Different efficiencies of use for lactation of metabolizable protein from the diet and mobilized tissue are employed in the following description.

1. Average unshrunk or full BW within the feeding period (FBW), kg
2. FBW at a BCS of 3.0 ($FBW_{BCS3.0}$; 0–5 scale) = FBW when skeletal development is complete, empty body fat concentration is 25 percent, and BCS is 2.8 to 3.0
3. DMI, kg/d
4. ME intake, Mcal/d
5. Dietary ME used for lactation ($ME_{l\text{-}d}$), Mcal/d
6. Maturity index (P), fraction = current $FBW/FBW_{BCS3.0}$
7. SFW (kg/year) = standard fleece weight (greasy) for an adult sheep (> 2 years of age) with good climatic conditions for pasture growth
8. Scurf and fiber CP (dermal plus clean fiber; $SF\text{-}CP_E$), g/d = wool sheep: direct entry of clean fiber growth or (ME intake – $ME_{l\text{-}d}$) × 33.472 × ($SFW/FBW_{BCS3.0}$); hair sheep: 0.2 × kg $BW^{0.6}$
9. Endogenous urinary CP ($U\text{-}CP_E$), g/d = 3.375 + (0.147 × kg FBW)
10. Metabolic fecal CP ($F\text{-}CP_E$), g/d = 15.2 × kg DMI
11. MP requirement for maintenance plus fiber (MP_m), g/d = ($SF\text{-}CP_E$/0.6) + ($U\text{-}CP_E$/0.67) + ($F\text{-}CP_E$/0.67)
12. FBW_{init}, kg = initial FBW
13. FBW_{fin}, kg = final FBW
14. Initial BCS (BCS_{init}) = 0 to 5, with 0 and 5 extremely thin and obese, respectively
15. Initial fraction of protein in the empty body ($ProFr_{init}$) = 0.1449 + (0.0279 × BCS_{init}) – (0.0039 × BCS_{init}^2)
16. Initial empty BW (EBW_{init}), kg = 0.851 × 0.96 × FBW_{init}
17. Initial protein mass ($ProM_{init}$), kg = $ProFr_{init}$ × EBW_{init}
18. Final BCS (BCS_{fin}) = 0 to 5, with 0 and 5 extremely thin and obese, respectively
19. Final fraction of protein in the empty body ($ProFr_{fin}$) = 0.1449 + (0.0279 × BCS_{fin}) – (0.0039 × BCS_{fin}^2)
20. Final empty BW (EBW_{fin}), kg = 0.851 × 0.96 × FBW_{fin}
21. Final protein mass ($ProM_{fin}$), kg = $ProFr_{fin}$ × EBW_{fin}
22. Average protein concentration as a fraction on a FBW basis during the feeding period ($TPFr_{avg}$) = ($ProM_{fin}$ – $ProM_{init}$)/(FBW_{fin} – FBW_{init})
23. ADG on a FBW basis, g
24. Protein accretion when ADG is positive (NP_g), g/d = ADG × $TPFr_{avg}$
25. Mobilized tissue protein used for lactation when ADG is negative ($MP_{l\text{-}t}$), g/d = (ADG × TPFr) × –1
26. Milk protein from $MP_{l\text{-}t}$ ($NP_{l\text{-}t}$), g = $MP_{l\text{-}t}$ × 0.8
27. MTPC, % = milk true protein concentration
28. MY, kg/d = milk yield
29. Total milk protein yield (NP_l), g/d = (10 × MTPC × MY)
30. Milk protein from the diet ($NP_{l\text{-}d}$), /g/d = NP_l – $NP_{l\text{-}t}$
31. Dietary (including microbial) metabolizable protein used or required for lactation ($MP_{l\text{-}d}$), g/d = $NP_{l\text{-}d}$/0.58
32. Total metabolizable protein used for lactation (MP_l), g/d = $MP_{l\text{-}d}$ + $MP_{l\text{-}t}$
32. Total dietary metabolizable protein requirement (MP_{req}), g/d = MP_m + MP_g + $MP_{l\text{-}d}$

Sheep During Late Gestation

The metabolizable protein requirement for late gestation of sheep is that of the CNCPS-S method (Cannas et al., 2004):

$$MP_{preg} = ((LBW/4) \times 0.0674 \times e(11.347 - 11.22 \times e(-0.00601 \times T) - 0.00601 \times T))/0.7$$

where T = day of gestation, LBW = total litter birth weight, and a k_{ppreg} of 0.7. To determine clean fiber growth of sheep in late gestation with the method of SCA (1990) based on SFW, ME intake should be corrected or adjusted for ME used for pregnancy, in the same manner as the adjustment for $ME_{l\text{-}d}$ with lactating sheep.

Metabolizable and Crude Protein

Even though MP requirements are strongly preferred compared with CP, for some users application of MP requirements may be difficult. Hence, Sahlu et al. (2004) used a simple conversion of MP to CP stated by NRC (2000). The NRC (2000) indicated that MP intake or concentration in the diet ranges from 64–80 percent of CP with diets of 0–100 percent UIP. Thus, a possible conversion of requirements of MP to CP is: CP = MP/((64 + (0.16 × % UIP))/100). For example, with an MP requirement of 100 g and a dietary UIP concentration of 70 percent of CP, the CP requirement is 145 g. This method seems a useful means of deriving CP from MP needs unless there is a factor restricting microbial growth such as ruminal nitrogenous compound availability.

Rumen Degraded Intake Protein

In the evaluation of protein requirements of the CNCPS-S system, of the 48 observations used, 37 entailed dietary levels of DIP that limited microbial protein synthesis. Since the evaluation indicated that the assumptions used were reasonably accurate, the method employed to estimate microbial protein synthesis when DIP was limiting, or the DIP requirement, is recommended. This DIP requirement was that used for beef cattle (NRC, 2000), which is based on the dietary total digestible nutrients (TDN) concentration plus a correction for low dietary concentrations of effective neutral detergent fiber (eNDF), as shown below:

DIP requirement (% TDN) = (0.13 × TDN, % DM) – 0.022 × (20 – eNDF, % DM), when eNDF < 20

GOATS

Metabolizable Protein for Maintenance, Growth, Lactation, and Mohair Fiber

Recommendations for protein requirements of goats are based primarily on reports summarized by Sahlu and coworkers (Luo et al., 2004a,b,c; Moore et al., 2004; Nsahlai et al., 2004; Sahlu et al., 2004). These studies entailed regression analyses with a database of treatment mean observations compiled from the literature. Metabolizable protein intake was determined by an approach very similar to those of AFRC (1993). Whenever possible the expressions were evaluated with independent databases, with none of the ones to be presented showing significant prediction bias. It was felt preferable to propose these expressions rather than unevaluated simple means determined in small numbers of individual studies since they were developed from a database with a broad array of goats and diets. Similarly, other systems entailing recommendations for goats based largely on, or extrapolated from, data for other ruminant species are not presented since they have not been evaluated to the extent of those of Sahlu et al. (2004) and/or require inputs that some users might not be able to provide accurately.

Metabolizable Protein for Maintenance

Mature and lactating	
MFCP	2.67 percent DMI
True CP digestibility	88 percent
EUCP	1.031 g/kg $BW^{0.75}$
MP_m	MFCP + EUCP + (0.2 g/kg $BW^{0.60}$)
Growing	3.07 g/kg $BW^{0.75}$
Angora	3.35 g/kg $BW^{0.75}$

Metabolizable Protein for Body or Tissue Gain

Growing	
Dairy	0.290 g/g ADG
Indigenous	0.290 g/g ADG
Meat	0.404 g/g ADG
Angora	0.281 g/g tissue gain

Metabolizable Protein for Milk Protein

1.45 g/g

Metabolizable Protein for Clean Mohair Fiber

1.65 g/g

Growing goats were categorized as < 1.5 years of age. The estimate for Angora is for both growing and mature goats. The dairy biotype includes genotypes selected for milk production, such as Saanen, Alpine, and Nubian. Meat goats are those with ≥ 50 percent Boer genetics. Indigenous or local goats are ones other than dairy, meat, and Angora. In addition, there were some assumptions employed in arriving at the requirements listed above:

1. efficiency of use of dietary for maintenance functions: 1.0,
2. efficiency of use of dietary metabolizable protein for tissue gain by lactating goats: 0.59,
3. efficiency of use of mobilized metabolizable protein for milk protein synthesis: 0.69 or 1.45 g/g, and
4. efficiency of use of mobilized metabolizable protein for clean mohair fiber synthesis: 1.65 g/g.

Metabolizable Protein for Pregnancy

The method of predicting MP_{preg} of Sahlu et al. (2004) can be described by this equation:

$$MP_{preg}\,(g) = (-155.62 - (8.6668 \times BIRWT) + (2.6495 \times DAY) + (0.0041667 \times LS) - (0.011049 \times DAY2) + (0.097691 \times BIRWT \times DAY) - (12.136 \times BIRWT \times LS) + (0.14631 \times BIRWT \times DAY \times LS))/0.33$$

where BIRWT = average birth weight (kg) per kid, DAY = day of gestation, LS = litter size, and 0.33 k_{ppreg}. This estimate includes metabolizable protein metabolized by all components of the gravid uterus and the mammary gland and, therefore, should be added to ME_{preg} of a nonpregnant goat of the same BW or that of the pregnant goat before the last 2 months of gestation. Alternatively, Cannas et al. (2004) used the method of CSIRO (1990) to predict MP_{preg} for sheep in the CNCPS-S, with a k_{ppreg} of 0.70:

$$MP_{preg} = ((LBW/4) \times 0.0674 \times e(11.347 - 11.22 \times e(-0.00601 \times T) - 0.00601 \times T))/0.7$$

where T = day of gestation, LBW = total litter birth weight, and a k_{ppreg} of 0.7. Though this estimate of ME_{preg} is for the total pregnancy requirement, it would seem most appropriate for calculating MP_m to adjust BW for predicted weight of the gravid uterus.

Parasitism

Metabolizable protein requirement recommendations listed earlier were for confined animals, which would suggest low levels of parasitism compared with grazing goats. However, some reports did not specify internal parasite control methods, and with anthelmintic resistance it is likely that even with confinement, there were subclinical levels of internal parasites in some cases. Hence, it is presumed that the recommendations do encompass an influence of low levels of parasitism. Nonetheless, there are no clear recommendations in the various metabolizable protein systems available for effects of subclinical levels of parasitism on metabolizable protein requirements.

Requirements for goats presented by Luo et al. (2004b,c) and Nsahlai et al. (2004) were via regression analyses with animals in fairly typical production settings. It was suggested that in some cases ME intake may have been slightly more limiting than metabolizable protein and, thus, inclusion of safety factors above determined requirements would be unnecessary. Hence, these values either would not require additional metabolizable protein required for subclinical levels of parasitism or would necessitate less of an adjustment than with other systems.

Metabolizable and Crude Protein

Even though MP requirements are strongly preferred compared with CP, application of metabolizable protein requirements may be difficult for some users. Hence, Sahlu et al. (2004) used a simple conversion of metabolizable protein to CP stated by NRC (2000). The NRC (2000) indicated that metabolizable protein intake or concentration in the diet ranges from 64–80 percent of CP with diets of 0–100 percent UIP. Thus, a possible conversion of requirements of MP to CP is: $CP = MP/((64 + (0.16 \times \%\ UIP))/100)$. For example, with a metabolizable protein requirement of 100 g and a dietary UIP concentration of 70 percent of CP, the CP requirement is 145 g. This method seems a useful means of deriving CP from metabolizable protein needs unless there is a factor restricting microbial growth such as ruminal nitrogenous compound availability.

Rumen Degraded Intake Protein

The DIP requirement of goats has not been extensively studied, though goats seem able to recycle more nitrogen than other ruminant species (Silanikove, 2000). To evaluate the DIP requirement for goats, a database of treatment mean observations from the literature was constructed from some of the studies used in reports summarized by Sahlu et al. (2004). Goats were classified as growing or mature, with a division age of 1.5 years. There were 41 reports for growing goats with 197 observations representing 1,810 goats, and 11 reports for mature goats with 39 observations representing 315 goats. All reports included ADG and DMI, with DMI being ad libitum in all instances. The dietary DIP concentration was determined from UIP values listed by Preston (2005). The intent was to regress the DIP concentration as a percentage of TDN intake against ADG and DMI scaled by kg $BW^{0.75}$. Theoretically, ADG and DMI should increase with increasing DIP when values are low up to the point at which DIP is no longer limiting. However, as noted in Figures 5-2, 5-3, 5-4, and 5-5, this approach was not effective, probably because of factors such as variability in methods among studies and in measures within reports and limited numbers of observations with low DIP concentrations. An inability to determine accurately the dietary DIP concentration could have also been involved, as well as a DIP requirement not necessarily constant across different types of diets. In addition, the degree to which TDN concentration is related to energy derived from ruminal fermentation varies among diets.

NRC (2000) considered the DIP requirement for beef cattle equal to microbial CP synthesis, estimated as 13 percent of TDN intake plus a correction for decreased microbial protein synthesis with diets low in effective fiber concentra-

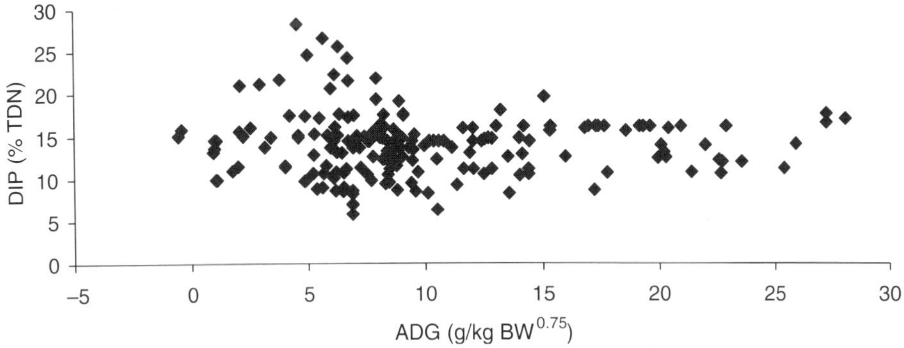

FIGURE 5-2 The relationship between rumen degraded intake protein (DIP) as a percent of total digestible nutrients (TDN) and average daily gain (ADG) relative to body weight $(BW)^{0.75}$ with a database of treatment mean observations from the literature for growing goats.

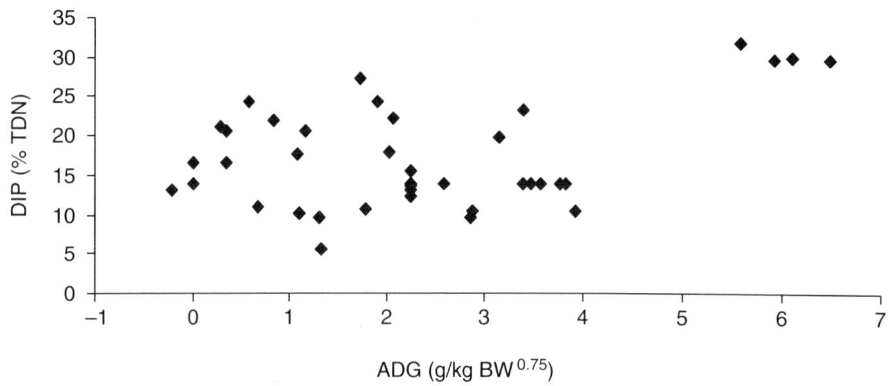

FIGURE 5-3 The relationship between rumen degraded intake protein (DIP) as a percent of total digestible nutrients (TDN) and average daily gain (ADG) relative to body weight $(BW)^{0.75}$ with a database of treatment mean observations from the literature for mature goats.

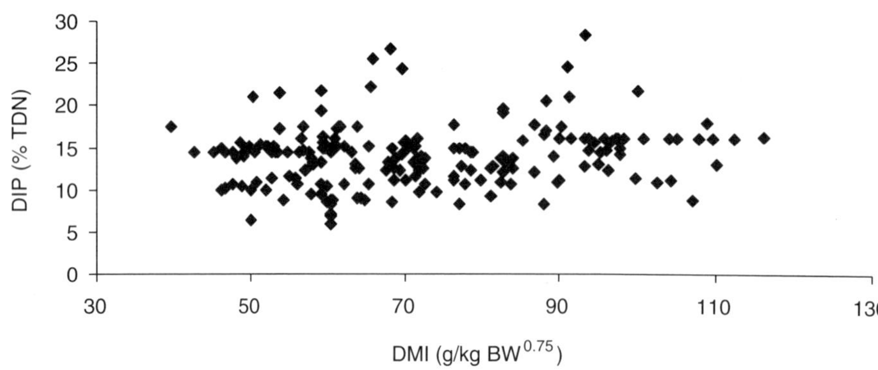

FIGURE 5-4 The relationship between rumen degraded intake protein (DIP) as a percent of total digestible nutrients (TDN) and dry matter intake (DMI) relative to body weight $(BW)^{0.75}$ with a database of treatment mean observations from the literature for growing goats.

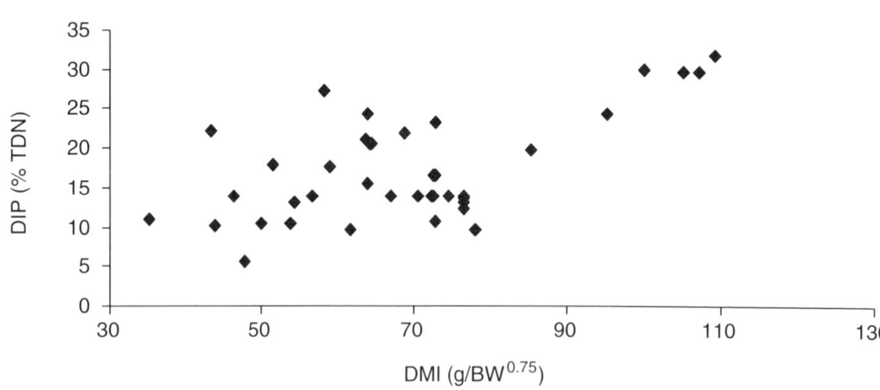

FIGURE 5-5 The relationship between rumen degraded intake protein (DIP) as a percent of total digestible nutrients (TDN) and dry matter intake (DMI) relative to body weight $(BW)^{0.75}$ with a database of treatment mean observations from the literature for mature goats.

tion. Recently, Soto-Navarro et al. (2003, 2004) did not observe limitations in ruminal digestion or performance of goats consuming concentrate-based diets with DIP levels of 7 percent and 9 percent of TDN. Prieto et al. (2000), however, reported a tendency for lower BW gain and a considerably lower ruminal ammonia concentration in growing meat goats consuming a diet with a DIP level of 8 percent of TDN compared with dietary levels of 11.5 percent to 13.8 percent. Hence, the current recommended DIP requirement for goats is 9 percent of TDN intake. However, it should be noted that many factors influence the DIP requirement and the ability to recycle nitrogen to the rumen.

This DIP requirement can be considered as a general guideline only. That is, in the method of predicting microbial protein synthesis with the database used to determine the metabolizable protein requirement expressions (Luo et al., 2004b,c; Nsahlai et al., 2004), a DIP requirement per se was not employed. Rather, as noted earlier, microbial protein synthesis was predicted based on an estimate of ruminally fermented energy intake and effective ruminally degraded CP. When the latter estimate was greater than the former, DIP was considered inadequate and microbial protein synthesis was set equal to effective ruminally degraded CP.

CERVIDS

Metabolizable Protein for Maintenance

Recommendations for fecal daily CP loss were based on DMI because of the dependency of MFCP on DMI (mean 39.1 g/kg DMI: Holter et al., 1977; Mould and Robbins, 1981; Robbins, 1993). Using a winter voluntary DMI of 35 g/kg$^{0.75}$ and assuming a k_{pm} of 0.67, the mean daily MFCP for cervids was 2.04 g/kg$^{0.75}$.

	MFCP (g/kg DMI)	MFCP (g/d)	MFCP (g/kg$^{0.75}$ × d^{-1})
white-tailed deer	38.8	40.3	2.02
red deer	43.6	61.0	2.28
reindeer/caribou	39.1	46.8/62.2	2.04
elk/wapiti	34.9	96.9	1.82

Assuming a mean true CP digestibility of 94 percent (Robbins et al., 1974b; Robbins, 1993), the expected daily CP intake to meet MFCP loss was 2.17 g/kg$^{0.75}$.

True CP digestibility	(g/100 g DM)
white-tailed deer	93
red deer	96
reindeer/caribou	92
elk/wapiti	98

Since daily endogenous urinary CP (EUCP) loss scales to metabolic body weight (0.76 g/kg BW$^{0.75}$: Robbins, 1993), mean winter daily metabolic urinary crude protein (MUCP) for cervids was 1.12 g/kg BW$^{0.75}$. The daily EUCP of male white-tailed deer (0.85 g/kg BW$^{0.75}$: Asleson et al., 1996) is higher than females (0.72 g/kg BW$^{0.75}$: Robbins et al., 1975).

	BW (kg)	EUCP (g/kg BW$^{0.75}$)	MUCP (g/d)	MUCP (g/kg BW$^{0.75}$ × d^{-1})
white-tailed deer	54	0.72	21.4	1.07
red deer	80	0.56	22.5	0.84
reindeer/caribou	65/95	0.75	25.6/34.1	1.12
elk/wapiti	200	1.00	79.4	1.49

Nitrogen loss due to fiber and skin losses scales to BW$^{0.60}$, but CP loss in winter was assumed to be very small, attributable to skin loss (2 mg/kg BW$^{0.60}$). For calculation of MP_m, SCURF losses were rescaled to BW$^{0.75}$, and a mean winter SCURF metabolizable protein loss (SLMP) of 1.7 mg/kg BW$^{0.75}$ was assumed. The assumed $k_{p\text{-}scurf}$ was 0.6. During spring, summer, and autumn, CP losses were calculated assuming linear growth of the coat. Mean summer metabolizable protein for SCURF for cervids was 250 mg/kg BW$^{0.75}$.

SUMMER	SCURF (g CP/kg BW$^{0.6}$)	Scurf loss metabolizable protein (g/d)	(g/kg BW$^{0.75}$ × d^{-1})
white-tailed deer	0.25	4.56	0.23
red deer	0.25	5.78	0.22
reindeer/caribou	0.36	7.34/9.22	0.31
elk/wapiti	0.25	10.0	0.30

Maintenance requirement (MP_m) was estimated as:

$$MP_m = MFCP + MUCP + SLMP$$

For winter the mean daily MP_m estimate was 3.17 g/kg BW$^{0.75}$, requiring a CP intake of 3.37 g/kg BW$^{0.75}$ to meet this MP_m requirement. At a daily DMI of 35 g/kg BW$^{0.75}$, the mean dietary CP concentration required to meet MP_m is 9.6 percent. This estimate of CPI (3.37 g/kg BW$^{0.75}$) is 37 percent lower than published estimates of daily CPI to meet nitrogen balance (4.64 g/kg BW$^{0.75}$: Robbins, 1993), and the winter MP_m of female white-tailed deer (below) is 15 percent less than for males (Asleson et al., 1996).

In summary:

	Expected CPI at N balance (g/kg BW$^{0.75}$ × d^{-1})	MP_m (g/kg BW$^{0.75}$ × d^{-1}) WINTER	MP_m (g/kg BW$^{0.75}$ × d^{-1}) SUMMER
white-tailed deer	4.44	3.10	4.19
red deer	4.25	3.12	4.49
reindeer/caribou	5.12	3.16	4.74
elk/wapiti	4.25	3.32	4.72

Thus, although winter MP_m appears underestimated when a winter DMI of 35 g/kg BW$^{0.75}$ is assumed, a daily DMI of 55 g/kg BW$^{0.75}$ increases MFCP excretion to 3.21 g/kg BW$^{0.75}$, and MP_m to 4.34 g/kg BW$^{0.75}$, and gives a crude protein intake (CPI) required to meet nitrogen balance (4.61 g/kg BW$^{0.75}$) equivalent to the findings of Robbins (1993) at 4.64 g/kg BW$^{0.75}$. The dietary CP content required to meet MP_m is 8.4 percent for a daily DMI of 55 g/kg BW$^{0.75}$. This is the same level of intake that satisfies ME_m for a diet of approximately 70 percent energy digestibility and ME content of 2.4 kcal/g (Chapter 4).

In summer, a daily DMI of 50 g/kg $BW^{0.75}$ meets theoretical ME_m. At this level of intake, mean daily metabolic fecal CP for maintenance ($MFCP_m$) was 2.92 g/kg $BW^{0.75}$, metabolic urinary CP for maintenance ($MUCP_m$) was 1.13 g/kg $BW^{0.75}$, and metabolic protein used for scurf (MP-SCURF) was 0.27 g/kg $BW^{0.75}$ (1.52 g/g hair growth), giving an MP_m of 4.30 g/kg $BW^{0.75}$ for cervids. Assuming a true protein digestibility of 94 percent, the daily dietary CP intake to meet this MP_m is 4.57 g/kg $BW^{0.75}$, which is only slightly less than the reported CP intake required to meet nitrogen balance in cervids (4.64 g/kg $BW^{0.75}$: Robbins, 1993). At a daily DMI of 50 g/kg $BW^{0.75}$, the minimal dietary CP content required to satisfied MP_m is 9.1 percent. However, because young cervids are growing, and older animals are lactating or making compensatory growth in early summer, voluntary DMI usually exceeds 50 g/kg $BW^{0.75}$ and can be as high as 140 g/kg $BW^{0.75}$ (Verme and Ozoga, 1980).

Metabolizable Protein for Tissue Gain

Among cervids and other ruminants, neonatal growth rate (Y, g/d) is related to maternal body weight (X, kg) (Robbins and Robbins, 1979):

$$Y = -1162.4 + 333.47 \times L_n X$$

For white-tailed deer, reindeer/caribou, and wapiti, predicted ADG is approximately 67 percent of reported maxima (Verme and Ozoga, 1980; Robbins et al., 1981; Parker et al., 1990; Knott et al., 2005), but is representative of most studies (Cook et al., 1996) given the wide range of ADG related to both maternal and range-nutrition effects (Loudon et al., 1984). Alternately, relative ADG of neonates, birth to 4 weeks, scales to daily milk protein intake (Robbins et al., 1981) as:

$$Y = -0.0227 + 0.0257 \times L_n X$$

where Y = relative ADG (kg/kg BW), and X = daily milk protein intake (g CP/kg BW).

For other calculations, ADG was based on ingesta-free BW (IFBW). The percent of ADG being CP was estimated from available data or values were taken from Adamczewski et al. (1987), Robbins (1993), and Chan-McLeod et al. (1999), and a k_{pg} of 0.7 was assumed in converting net protein gain to MP. Expressed as g/g BW gain, MP_g ranged from less than 0.3 in adult males and neonates, to as high as 0.53 in lactating females making compensatory gain in late summer. The very high value appeared related to the low level of fat regain (Chan-McLeod et al., 1999). When expressed on a metabolic body size basis, average daily MP_g exceeded 10 g/kg $BW^{0.75}$ for neonates and declined with BW to as low as 1–3 g/kg $BW^{0.75}$ for animals older than yearlings.

MP requirement for compensatory growth in males and females was estimated as summer MP_m + MP_g.

	ADG (g/d)	CP in ADG (%)	MP_g (g/g)	MP_g (g/kg $BW^{0.75}$)
Neonate (0–21 d)	382	20	0.29	19
Weaned (> 20 wk)	310	25	0.35	9
Yearling	130	25	0.31	2
Two years	46	23	0.36	1
Lactating	150	37	0.53	3
Nonlactating	208	27	0.38	3
Adult males	358	23	0.29	2

Metabolizable Protein for Pregnancy

Rate of daily deposition of nitrogen during pregnancy for white-tailed deer (eq. 2 of Robbins and Moen, 1975), and reindeer/caribou and wapiti was determined from equations Table 5 in Robbins and Moen (1975). For red deer using a

TABLE 5-3 References, Number of Treatment Mean Observations, and Genotypes in the Database Used to Evaluate Metabolizable Protein Requirements of the CNCPS-S Method (Cannas et al., 2004)

Reference	Number of observations	Genotype
von Keyserlingk and Mathison (1993)	1	Dorset crossbred
Goetsch (1997)	1	St. Croix
Goetsch et al. (1998)	3	Dorset and Suffolk crossbreds
Haddad et al. (2001)	1	Awassi
Gentry et al. (1999)	3	Suffolk
Kreikemeier et al. (1987)	2	Rambouillet × Suffolk
Dhakad et al. (2002)	3	Indigenous (India)
Pineda et al. (1998)	3	Pelibuey
Fluharty and McClure (1997)	1	Hampshire × Targhee
Aderibigbe and Church (1983)	1	Crossbred
Said and Tolera (1993)	7	Menz
Tolera and Sundstøl (2000)	12	Local, southern Ethiopia
Dixon and Egan (2000)	9	Merino × Border Leicester
Amaning-Dwarteng and Kellaway (1987)	1	Merino × Border Leicester

TABLE 5-4 Description of the Database Used to Evaluate Metabolizable Protein (MP) Requirements of the CNCPS-S Method (Cannas et al., 2004)[a]

Item[b]	Mean	SD	Minimum	Maximum
Length, d	72	18.7	42	120
Dietary TDN, % DM	61	17.44	31.1	83.8
Dietary ME, Mcal/kg DM	2.18	0.471	1.12	3.03
Dietary CP, % DM	10.2	4.02	3.1	20.6
Dietary NDF, % DM	55.2	19.54	10.1	80.1
Dietary UIP, % CP	30.4	13.3	12.4	70
Average full BW, kg	24.2	7.97	13.4	48.8
TEC, Mcal/kg (empty BW basis)	3.08	0.61	2.26	4.68
TPC, % (empty BW basis)	17	1.73	12.5	19.3
DM intake, g	696	341.6	326	1,600
Average daily gain, g	71	104.6	–42	376
CP intake, g	77	56.1	10	263
MP intake, g	44	29.8	6	128
MP from the diet, g	19	17.3	2	72
MP from microbial cells, g	25	14.5	2	58

[a]n = 48.
[b]TDN = total digestible nutrients; DM = dry matter; ME = metabolizable energy; CP = crude protein; NDF = neutral detergent fiber; UIP = rumen undegraded intake protein; BW = body weight; TEC = energy concentration in tissue accreted or mobilized; TPC = protein concentration in tissue accreted or mobilized.

modification of the generalized cervid equation (eq. 4, Robbins and Moen, 1975):

$$L_n Y(t) = -3.3856 + 0.0275 \times X \qquad \text{white-tailed deer}$$

where Y = nitrogen retention (g/d), t = day of gestation, and X = day of gestation.

$$L_n Y(t) = -5.4794 + 0.0231 \times X \qquad \text{reindeer/caribou}$$
$$L_n Y(t) = -5.3602 + 0.0218 \times X \qquad \text{red deer}$$
$$L_n Y(t) = -5.6555 + 0.0197 \times X \qquad \text{wapiti/elk}$$

where Y = nitrogen retention (g/d) per kg fetus produced, t = day of gestation, and X = day of gestation. Estimation of MP_{preg} at time t during pregnancy was estimated from nitrogen content of protein (6.25) and k_{ppreg} (0.33):

$$MP_{preg}(t) = Yt \times 6.25/0.33$$

At term MP_{preg} (g/d) for females with single offspring was related to maternal weight (kg) (calculated from data in Robbins and Moen, 1975), which allowed estimation at term of MP_{preg} for species other than those listed above.

$$MP_{preg}\ \text{term} = 56.9 + 0.614 \times X$$

Although a less precise estimate, MP_{preg} at term also was related to birth weight (X, kg):

$$MP_{preg}\ \text{term} = 65.1 + 6.93 \times X$$

Daily requirements of metabolizable protein (Y, g) were calculated during pregnancy (Y(t)) and at term (Yterm) as:

$$Y(t) = MP_m + MP_{preg}(t), \text{ and}$$
$$\text{Yterm} = MP_m + MP_{preg}\ \text{term}.$$

where MP_m is winter maintenance metabolic protein requirement.

In summary, the requirements for pregnancy at term for different cervid species are as follows:

	BW (kg)	Term Fetus (kg)	MP_{gest} (g/d)	MP_{gest} (g/kg $BW^{0.75}$)	Yterm (g/kg $BW^{0.75}$)
white-tailed deer	50	5.8	88	4.66	7.8
red deer	80	7.5	106	3.96	7.1
reindeer/ caribou	65/95	7.0/9.0	97/115	4.23/3.79	7.4/7.0
elk/wapiti	235	16.0	201	3.35	6.7

Metabolizable Protein for Lactation

Metabolic protein requirement for lactation (MP_l) was calculated from an estimate of milk yield, nitrogen (or protein) content, and k_l or k_{lt}. For a female with one offspring, peak milk yield (Y, L/d) scales to maternal BW (Oftedal, 1984):

$$Y = 48 - 72 \text{ g/kg } BW^{0.75}$$

Values for red deer, reindeer, caribou, and wapiti are respectively 72, 48, 55, and 65 (mean 60) g/kg $BW^{0.75}$ (Oftedal, 1985; Parker et al., 1990). It was assumed, as shown for red deer and reindeer (Loudon and Kay, 1984; White and

Luick, 1984), that milk protein content is inversely related to milk yield:

$$P = 14 - 0.340 \times Y$$

where P = milk protein (g/100 g milk), and Y = daily milk yield (mL/kg). Thus daily net milk protein yield (NPy, g) was calculated as:

$$NPy = (P/100) \times Y \times BW, \text{ or}$$
$$NPy = (0.14 \times Y - 0.00340 \times Y^2) \times BW$$

Daily MP_l (g) for dietary protein was calculated as:

$MP_l = NPy/k_{p\text{-}l}$, and for body protein as the main source $MP_l = NPy/k_{p\text{-}lt}$

In the absence of direct measure for cervids, $k_{p\text{-}l} = 0.65$ is assumed when body stores are not used. Otherwise use of maternal tissue ($k_{p\text{-}lt}$) of 0.84 is assumed.

Using this procedure, net CP requirement on any particular day of lactation, and hence MP_l, was estimated. Milk production of females with a single offspring is assumed to be 65 percent of that with twins (Oftedal, 1984); thus, MP_l is divided by 0.65 to account for the requirement of twins and 0.55 for triplets. Average MP_l increased from 1.14 g/g milk protein at 20 percent derived from dietary CP, 80 percent from maternal protein, to 1.45 g/g at 100 percent from the diet. For female cervids with single offspring, the following daily MP requirement (MPR) estimated for milk production (MP_l) and milk production plus summer maintenance including scurf (MPR = $MP_l + MP_m$) was 9.7 g/kg $BW^{0.75}$. Milk production accounted for ~ 53 percent of MPR. Assumed BW for these calculations are: white-tailed deer, 50 kg; reindeer, 65 kg; caribou, 95 kg; red deer, 80 kg; and elk/wapiti, 235 kg.

Estimates of MP_l and MPR for the focal cervid species at peak lactation BW gain = 0:

	MP_l (g/d)	MPR (g/d)	MPR ($g/kg^{0.75} \times d^{-1}$)
white-tailed deer	38	162	8.6
reindeer/caribou	108/160	211/296	9.2/9.7
red deer	133	260	9.7
elk/wapiti	388	671	11.2

Metabolizable Protein for Antler Growth

Experimentally determined mean daily MP for antler growth (MP_{antler})by Asleson et al. (1996) for male white-tailed deer was 0.25 g CP/kg $BW^{0.75}$. In a modeling study to determine energy, nitrogen, calcium, and phosphorus requirements for antler growth of caribou, a daily MP requirement of 1.8 g/kg $BW^{0.75}$ can be estimated during peak antler growth that occurs at 70 days from initiation (Moen and Pastor, 1998). Thus, for this study values used for all male white-tailed deer was 0.25 g/kg $BW^{0.75}$ and 0.54 for other cervids, assuming the maximum antler growth rate reported by Asleson et al. (1996) is achieved. Because the value for caribou was extremely high, a value of 0.9 g/kg $BW^{0.75}$ was assumed. These estimates of MP requirements for antler growth are 6–18 percent of MP for maintenance plus pelage growth and 3–9 percent of MP requirements of males making average ADG. Moen and Pastor (1998) also modeled antler growth in female caribou, and from this simulation a daily MP requirement of 0.31 g/kg $BW^{0.75}$ was estimated.

MPR of sub-adult/adult males assuming low spring BW and high ADG is as follows:

Spring	BW (kg)	ADG (g/d)	MP_m (g/d)	MP_{antler} (g/d)	MPR (g/d)	MPR ($g/kg^{0.75} \times d^{-1}$)
white-tailed deer	50	575	79	4.7	167	8.9
reindeer/ caribou	60/70	525/470	97/115	19.4/21.8	225/259	10.4/10.7
red deer	60	520	102	11.6	217	10.1
elk/wapiti	100	930	149	17.1	325	10.3

CAMELIDS

As noted in Chapter 4, Van Saun (2006) recently reviewed the literature available regarding nutrient requirements of llamas and alpacas. There were two approaches given to address the protein requirement for maintenance. The first was to use a digestible protein estimate of Huasaquiche (1974) relative to $FBW^{0.75}$ (i.e., 2.38 g digestible protein/kg $FBW^{0.75}$) and then convert to a CP basis with an assumed apparent total tract protein digestibility (i.e., yielding 3.5 g CP/kg $FBW^{0.75}$). Estimates of metabolizable protein needs of llamas and alpacas are not available. This maintenance CP requirement is slightly less than recommended for growing goats when the metabolizable protein requirements are converted to a CP basis (e.g., 4.7 and 4.3 g/kg $FBW^{0.75}$ for Angora and other goats, respectively, assuming an efficiency of conversion of CP to metabolizable protein of 72 percent). The second method used was based on a CP requirement of 31 g/Mcal digestible energy (DE) suggested by Fowler (1998), to be applied to maintenance and pregnancy requirements. By assuming that ME is 82 percent of DE, this requirement is 37.8 g CP/Mcal ME. The maintenance requirement estimated by both methods for example llama and alpaca conditions of Van Saun (2006) were similar. Because of this and because few direct estimates of ME_m for llamas and alpacas are available, the first suggested requirement of CP for maintenance of Van Saun (2006), 3.5 g/kg $FBW^{0.75}$, is recommended.

With the paucity of information available, Van Saun (2006) suggested that the NRC (1981) CP requirement for gain of goats (i.e., 0.284 g/g ADG) be used until further research is conducted. For pregnancy, Van Saun (2006) first cited the suggestion of Hospinal (1997) that the CP requirement for maintenance and gestation is 68 percent greater than for maintenance alone, which equates to 5.88 g CP/kg FBW$^{0.75}$, given the maintenance requirement noted above. However, it was pointed out that one requirement for the last 3 months of gestation would result in overfeeding early in the period and underfeeding later. Thus, Van Saun (2006) calculated CP requirements of pregnancy based on energy requirements described in Chapter 4 and an assumed CP to ME ratio of 48 g/Mcal. This value appears to be the result of a comparison with a lower one (i.e., 42.4) derived from the protein requirement of Hospinal (1997), the energy requirement of pregnancy of Fowler (1998), and the ME$_m$ recommended earlier. Van Saun (2006) suggested that 42.4 g CP/Mcal ME was too low for camelids given the importance of protein and amino acids in fetal development; therefore, the higher value of 48 g CP/Mcal ME was employed. The resulting pregnancy CP requirement prediction equations are given below.

8 months:	pregnancy CP (g/d) = 0.95 g/kg FBW$^{0.75}$
9 months:	pregnancy CP (g/d) = 1.94 g/kg FBW$^{0.75}$
10 months:	pregnancy CP (g/d) = 3.23 g/kg FBW$^{0.75}$

The Van Saun (2006) CP requirement for lactation was based on an average milk protein concentration of 3.4 percent for llamas reported by Morin et al. (1995), although it was pointed out that this value included nonprotein nitrogen that seems to be high relative to levels for other ruminant species. A total tract protein digestibility of 85 percent and biological value of 66 percent were assumed, which yielded a CP requirement of 60.6 g/kg milk. Van Saun (2006) listed a CP requirement for fiber of 4.283 g/kg of greasy fleece, which was derived from the NRC (1981) value for goats.

The recommended protein requirements for llamas and alpacas are summarized below.

CP for maintenance:	3.5 g CP/kg FBW$^{0.75}$
CP for gain:	0.284 g/g ADG
CP for pregnancy (g/d)	
8 months:	0.95 g/kg FBW$^{0.75}$
9 months:	1.94 g/kg FBW$^{0.75}$
10 months:	3.23 g/kg FBW$^{0.75}$
CP for lactation:	60.6 g/kg milk, assuming a milk CP concentration of 3.4 percent
CP for fiber production:	4.283 g/g greasy fleece

REFERENCES

Adamczewski, J. Z., C. C. Gates, R. J. Hudson, and M. A. Price. 1987. Seasonal changes in body composition of mature female caribou and calves (*Rangifer tarandus groenlandicus*) on an Arctic island with limited-winter resources. Can. J. Zool. 65:1149–1157.

Adams, N. R., and S. M. Liu. 2003. Principles of nutrient partitioning for wool, growth and reproduction: Implications for nematode parasitism. Austral. J. Exp. Ag. 43:1399–1407.

Aderibigbe, A. O., and D. C. Church. 1983. Feather and hair meals for ruminants. II. Comparative evaluation of feather and hair meals as protein supplements. J. Anim. Sci. 57:473–482.

AFRC (Agriculture and Food Research Council). 1993. Energy and Protein Requirements of Ruminants. An Advisory Manual Prepared by the AFRC Technical Committee on Responses to Nutrients. Wallingford, UK: CABI Publishing.

AFRC. 1998. The Nutrition of Goats. Technical Committee on Responses to Nutrients. Report 10. Wallingford, UK: CABI Publishing.

Albon, S. D., A. Stein, R. J. Irvine, R. Langvatn, E. Ropstad, and O. Halvorsen. 2002. The role of parasites in the dynamics of a reindeer population. Proc. R. Soc. Lond. B. 269:1625–1632.

Allden, W. G. 1979. Feed intake, diet composition and wool growth. P. 61 in Physiological and Environmental Limitations to Wool Growth, J. L. Black and P. J. Reis, eds. Armidale, Australia: University of New England.

Amaning-Kwarteng, K., and R. C. Kellaway. 1987. Influence of cottonseed meal and barley grain supplements on intake, digestion, liveweight gain and wool growth in sheep fed NaOH-treated oat and wheat straw diets. J. Agric. Sci. 108:211–219.

Asleson, M. A., E. C. Hellgren, and L. W. Varner. 1996. Nitrogen requirements for antler growth and maintenance in white-tailed deer. J. Wildl. Manage. 60:744–752.

Asleson, M. A., E. C. Hellgren, and L. W. Varner. 1997. Effects of seasonal protein restriction on antlerogenesis and body mass in adult male white-tailed deer. J. Wildl. Manage. 61:1098–1107.

Atasoglu, C., C. Valdés, N. D. Walker, C. J. Newbold, and R. J. Wallace. 1998. *De novo* synthesis of amino acids by the ruminal bacteria *Prevotella bryantii* B14, *Selenomonas ruminantium* HD4, and *Streptococcus bovis* ES1. Appl. Environ. Microbiol. 64:2836–2843.

Atasoglu, C., C. Valdés, C. J. Newbold, and R. J. Wallace. 1999. Influence of peptides and amino acids on fermentation rate and *de novo* synthesis of amino acids by mixed rumen micro-organisms from the sheep rumen. Br. J. Nutr. 81:307–314.

Atasoglu, C., C. J. Newbold, and R. J. Wallace. 2001. Incorporation of [^{15}N]ammonia by the cellulolytic ruminal bacteria *Fibrobacter succinogenes* BL2, *Ruminococcus albus* SY3, and *Ruminococcus flavefaciens* 17. Appl. Environ. Microbiol. 67:2819–2822.

Aumont, G., P. Yvox, and A. Esnault. 1984. Experimental coccidiosis in goats. 1. Experimental model: Effects of parasitism on the feeding behaviour and the growth of animals; intestinal lesions. Ann. Recherche Vet. 15:467–473.

Baldwin, J. A., G. M. J. Horton, J. E. Wholt, D. D. Palatini, and S. M. Emanuele. 1993. Rumen protected methionine for lactation, wool and growth in sheep. Small Ruminant Res. 12:125–132.

Banks, W. J., G. P. Epling, R. A. Kainer, and R. W. Davis. 1968. Antler growth and osteoporosis. I. Morphological and morphometric changes in the costal compacta during the antler growth cycle. Anat. Rec.162:387–398.

Barboza, P. S., D. W. Hartbauer, W. E. Hauer, and J. E. Blake. 2004. Polygynous mating impairs body condition and homeostasis in male reindeer (*Rangifer tarandus*). J. Comp. Physiol. 174B:309–317.

Barboza, P. S., and K. L. Parker. 2006. Body protein stores and isotopic indicators of N balance in female reindeer (*Rangifer tarandus*) during winter. Physiol. Biochem. Zool. 79:628–644.

Barnes, E. H., and R. J. Dobson. 1993. Persistence of acquired immunity to *Trichostrongylus colubriformis* in sheep after termination of infection. Inter. J. Parasit. 23:1019–1026.

Bassett, J. W., B. C. Baldwin, M. C. Calhoun, and R. H. Stobart. 1981. Plasma methionine and mohair response to dietary rumen-protected methonine in Angora goats, p. 68. Texas Agric. Exp. Sta., PR 3904, Texas A&M Univ.

Bergerud, A. T. 1976. The annual antler cycle in Newfoundland caribou. Can. Field-Nat. 90:449–463.

Black, J. L., G. E. Robards, and R. Thomas. 1973. Effects of protein and energy intakes on the wool growth of Merino wethers. Aust. J. Agric. Res. 24:399–412.

Bocquier F., G. Delmas, B. Sloan, C. Vacaresse, and E. Van Quackebeke. 1994. Effet de la supplémentation en méthionine protégée sur la production et la composition du lait de brebis Lacaune. (Effect of protected methionine supplementation on production and the composition of ewe's milk from Lacaune). Renc. Rech. Rum. 1:101–104.

Brody, S. 1945. Bioenergetics and Growth (pp. 352–404). New York: Reinhold Publ. Corp.

Brown, M. D., D. P. Poppi, and A. R. Sykes. 1991. The effect of post-ruminal infusion of protein or energy on the pathophysiology of *Trichostrongylus colubriformis* infection and body composition in lambs. Aust. J. Agric. Res. 42:253–267.

Brown, R. D. 1990. Nutrition and antler development. Pp. 426–441 in Horns, Pronghorns and Antlers, G. A. Bubenik and A. B. Bubenik, eds. New York: Springer-Verlag.

Cameron, R. D., W. T. Smith, R. G. White, and B. Griffith. 2005. Central Arctic caribou and petroleum development: Distributional, nutritional, and reproductive implications. Arctic 58:1–9.

Cannas, A., L. O. Tedeschi, D. G. Fox, A. N. Pell, and P. J. Van Soest. 2004. A mechanistic model for predicting the nutrient requirements and feed biological values for sheep. J. Anim. Sci. 82:149–169.

Chan-McLeod, A. C. A., R. G. White, and D. E. Russell. 1999. Comparative body composition strategies of breeding and non-breeding female caribou. Can. J. Zool. 77:1901–1907.

Chartier, C., E. Etter, H. Hoste, I. Pors, M-P. Mallereau, C. Broqua, S. Mallet, C. Koch, and A. Massé. 2000. Effects of the initial level of milk production and of the dietary protein intake on the course of natural nematode infection in dairy goats. Vet. Parasitol. 92:1–13.

Chikunya, S., C. J. Newbold, L. Rode, X. B. Chen, and R. J. Wallace. 1996. Influence of dietary rumen-degradable protein on bacterial growth in the rumen of sheep receiving different energy sources. Anim. Feed Sci. Technol. 63:333–340.

Clutton-Brock, T. H., F. E. Guinness, and S. D. Albon. 1982. The rutting behavior of stags. Pp. 104–142 in Red Deer: Behavior and Ecology of Two Sexes, T. H. Clutton–Brock, F. E. Guinness, and S. D. Albon, eds. Chicago: The University of Chicago Press.

Cook, J. G., L. J. Quinlan, L. L. Irwin, L. D. Bryant, R. A. Riggs, and J. W. Thomas. 1996. Nutrition-growth relations of elk calves during late summer and fall. J. Wildl. Manage. 60:528–541.

Coop, R. L., and P. H. Holmes. 1996. Nutrition and parasite interaction. Inter. J. Parasit. 26: 951–962.

Coop, R. L., and I. Kyriazakis. 1999. Nutrition—Parasite interaction. Vet. Parasitol. 84:187–204.

Coop, R. L., I. Kyriazakis, J. F. Huntley, E. Jackson, and F. Jackson. 1997. The influence of protein and amino acid on the resilience of sheep to intestinal parasitism. Pp. 196–198 in Proc. 4th Int. Congress for Sheep Veterinarians, Armidale, NSW, Australia.

Cotta, M. A., and J. B. Russell. 1982. Effect of peptides and amino acids on efficiency of rumen bacterial protein synthesis in continuous culture. J. Dairy Sci. 65:226–234.

CSIRO (Commonwealth Scientific and Industrial Research Organization). Standing Committee on Agriculture, Ruminants Subcommittee. 1990. Feeding Standards for Australian Livestock. Ruminants. East Melbourne, Australia: CSIRO Publications.

Davis, T. A., H. V. Nguyen, R. Garcia-Bravo, M. L. Fiorotto, E. M. Jackson, D. S. Lewis, D. R. Lee, and P. J. Reeds. 1994. Amino acid composition of human milk is not unique. J. Nutr. 124:1126–1132.

Dhakad, A., A. K. Garg, P. Singh, and D. K. Agrawal. 2002. Effect of replacement of maize grain with wheat bran on the performance of growing lambs. Small Ruminant Res. 43:227–234.

Dixon, R. M., and A. R. Egan. 2000. Response of lambs fed low quality roughage to supplements based on urea, cereal grain, or protein meals. Aust. J. Agric. Res. 51:811–821.

Donaldson, J. D., M. F. J. van Houtert, and A. R. Sykes. 1998. The effect of nutrition on the periparturient parasite status of mature sheep. Anim. Sci. 67:523–533.

Fluharty, F. L., and K. E. McClure. 1997. Effects of dietary energy intake and protein concentration on performance and visceral organ mass in lambs. J. Anim. Sci. 75:604–606.

Fowler, M. E. 1998. Feeding and nutrition. Pp. 12–48 in Medicine and Surgery of South American Camelids: Llama, Alpaca, Vicuna, Guanaco, 2nd ed. Ames: Iowa State University Press.

Fratini, A, B. C. Powell, P. I. Hynd, R. A. Keough, and G. E. Rogers. 1994. Dietary cysteine regulates the levels of mRNAs encoding a family of cysteine-rich proteins of wool. J. Invest. Dermatol. 102:178–185.

French, C. E., L. E. McEwan, N. D. Magruder, R. H. Ingram, and R. W. Swift. 1956. Nutrient requirements for growth and antler development in the white-tailed deer. J. Wildl. Manage. 20:221–232.

Galbraith, H. 1998. Nutritional and hormonal regulation of hair follicle growth and development. Proc. Nutr. Soc. 57:195–205.

Geist, V. 1987. On the evolution of optical signals in deer: A preliminary analysis. Pp. 235–255 in Biology and Management of Cervidae, C. M. Wemmer, ed. Washington, DC; London: Smithsonian Institution Press.

Gentry, L. R., J. M. Fernandez, T. L. Ward, T. W. White, L. L. Southern, T. D. Bidner, D. L. Thompson, Jr., D. W. Horohov, A. M. Chapa, and T. Sahlu. 1999. Dietary protein and chromium tripicolinate in Suffolk wether lambs: Effects on production characteristics, metabolic and hormonal responses, and immune status. J. Anim. Sci. 77:1284–1294.

Gerhart, K. L., R. G. White, R. D. Cameron, and D. E. Russell. 1996. Body composition and nutrient reserves of Arctic caribou. Can. J. Zool. 74:136–146.

Goetsch, A. L. 1997. Growing and finishing performance and body composition for St. Croix wethers consuming growing diets differing in grain and protein levels. J. Anim. Feed Sci. 6:319–332.

Goetsch, A. L., S. W. Coleman, and W. A. Phillips. 1998. Growth and body composition of two crossbred wether types fed different quality grasses. Sheep Goat Res. J. 4:138–143.

Goss, R. J. 1969a. Photoperiodic control of antler cycles in deer. 1. Phase shift and frequency changes. J. Exp. Zool. 171:233–234.

Goss, R. J. 1969b. Photoperiodic control of antler cycles in deer. 2. Alterations in amplitude. J. Exp. Zool. 170:311–324.

Greenwood, R. H., and E. C. Titgemeyer. 2000. Limiting amino acids for growing Holstein steers limit-fed soybean hull-based diets. J. Anim. Sci. 78:1997–2004.

Haddad, S. G., R. E. Nasr, and M. M. Muwalla. 2001. Optimum dietary crude protein level for finishing Awassi lambs. Small Ruminant Res. 39(1):41–46.

Halvorsen, O., A. Stein, J. Irvine, R. Langvatn, and S. Albon. 1999. Evidence for continued transmission of parasitic nematodes in reindeer during the Arctic winter. Inter. J. Parasit. 29:567–579.

Helle, T., and L. Tarvainen. 1984. Effects of insect harassment on weight gain and survival in reindeer. Rangifer 4:24–27.

Holter, J. B., W. E. Urban, and H. H. Hayes. 1977. Nutrition of northern white-tailed deer throughout the year. J. Anim. Sci. 45:365–376.

Hospinal, R. S. 1997. Capítulo IV. Nutrición y Alimentación de Alpacas. Pp. 163–203 in Produción de Camélidos Sudamericanos. Huancayo, Peru: Imprenta Rios.

Hoste, H., and C. Chartier. 1993. Comparison of the effects on milk production of concurrent infection with *Haemonchus contortus* and *Trichostrongylus colubriformis* in high- and low-producing dairy goats. Am. J. Vet. Res. 54:1886–1893.

Houdijk, J. G. M., I. Kyriazakis, F. Jackson, and R. L. Coop. 2001. The relationship between protein nutrition, reproductive effort and breakdown in immunity to *Teladorsagia circumcincta* in periparturient ewes. Anim. Sci. 72:595–606.

Hove, L., J. H. Topps, S. Sibanda, and L. R. Ndlovu. 2001. Nutrient intake and utilisation by goats fed dried leaves of the shrub legumes (*Acacia angustissima, Calliandra calothyrsus* and *Leucaena leucocephala*) as supplements to native pasture hay. Anim. Feed Sci. Technol. 91:95–106.

Huasaquiche, A. 1974. Nitrogen balance and digestibility in alpacas and sheep. B.S. Thesis. Prog. Acad. Med. Vet., Univ. Nac. Mayor de San Marcos, Lima, Peru.

Hyvarinen, H., R. N. B. Kay, and W. J. Hamilton. 1977. Variation in the weight, specific gravity, and composition of the antlers of red deer (*Cervus elaphus* L.). Br. J. Nutr. 28:301–311.

Jacobsen, N. K. 1980. Differences of thermal properties of white-tailed deer pelage between seasons and body regions. J. Therm. Biol. 5: 151–158.

Kelsall, J. P. 1968. The Caribou. Ottawa, Canada: Queen's Printer.

INRA (Institut National de la Recherche Agronomique). 1989. Ruminant Nutrition. Recommended Allowances and Feed Tables, R. Jarrige, ed. Paris: INRA.

Knott, K. K., P. S. Barboza, and R. T. Bowyer. 2005. Growth in arctic ungulates: Postnatal development and organ maturation in *Rangifer tarandus* and *Ovibos moschatus*. J. Mamm. 86:121–130.

Kreikemeier, K. K., R. A. Stock, D. R. Brink, and R. A. Britton. 1987. Feeding combinations of dry corn and wheat to finishing lambs and cattle. J. Anim. Sci. 65:1647–1654.

Kyriazakis, I., J. D. Oldham, R. L. Coop, and F. Jackson. 1994. The effect of subclinical intestinal nematode infection on the diet selection of growing sheep. Br. J. Nutr. 72:665–677.

Kyriazakis, I., D. H. Anderson, J. D. Oldham, R. L. Coop, and F. Jackson. 1996. Long-term subclinical infection with *Trichostrongylus colubriformis*: Effects on food intake, diet selection and performance of growing lambs. Vet. Parasitol. 61:297–313.

Leader-Williams, N., and C. Ricketts. 1981. Seasonal and sexual patterns of growth and condition of reindeer introduced into South Georgia. Oikos 38:27–39.

Lincoln, G. A. 1971. Puberty in a seasonally breeding male; the red deer stag (*Cervus elaphus* L.). J. Reprod. Fert. 25:41–54.

Liu, S. M., and D. G. Masters. 2003. Amino acid utilization for wool growth. Pp. 309–328 in Amino Acids in Animal Nutrition, J. P. F. D'Mello, ed. Wallingford, UK: CABI Publishing.

Liu, S. M., D. G. Masters, and N. R. Adams. 2003. Potential impact of nematode parasitism on nutrient partitioning for wool production, growth and reproduction in sheep. Aust. J. Exp. Agric. 43:1409–1417.

Long, T. A., R. L. Cowan, C. W. Wolfe, T. Rader, and R. W. Swift. 1959. Effect of seasonal feed restriction on antler development of white-tailed deer. Penn. Agr. Exp. Sta. Progress Report 209.

Loudon, A. S. I., and R. N. B. Kay. 1984. Lactational constraints on a seasonal breeding mammal: The red deer. Symp. Zool. Soc. Lond. No. 51:233–252.

Loudon A. S. I., A. D. Darroch, and J. A. Milne. 1984. The lactation performance of red deer on hill and improved species pastures. J. Agric. Sci. 102:149–158.

Luick, J. R., R. G. White, A. M. Gau, and R. Jenness. 1974. Compositional changes in the milk secreted by grazing reindeer. I. Gross composition and ash. J. Dairy Sci. 57:1325–1333.

Luo, J., A. L. Goetsch, J. E. Moore, Z. B. Johnson, T. Sahlu, C. L. Ferrell, M. L. Galyean, and F. N. Owens. 2004a. Prediction of endogenous urinary nitrogen of goats. Small Ruminant Res. 53:293–308.

Luo, J., A. L. Goetsch, I. V. Nsahlai, T. Sahlu, C. L. Ferrell, F. N. Owens, M. L. Galyean, J. E. Moore, and Z. B. Johnson. 2004b. Metabolizable protein requirements for maintenance and gain of growing goats. Small Ruminant Res. 53:309–326.

Luo, J., A. L. Goetsch, I. V. Nsahlai, T. Sahlu, C. L. Ferrell, F. N. Owens, M. L. Galyean, J. E. Moore, and Z. B. Johnson. 2004c. Prediction of metabolizable energy and protein requirements for maintenance, gain and fiber growth of Angora goats. Small Ruminant Res. 53:339–356.

Lynch, G. P., T. H. Elsasser, C. Jackson, Jr., T. S. Rumsey, and M. J. Camp. 1991. Nitrogen metabolism of lactating ewes fed rumen-protected methionine and lysine. J. Dairy Sci. 74:2268–2276.

MacRae, J. C., A. Walker, D. Brown, and G. E. Lobley. 1993. Accretion of total protein and individual amino acids by organs and tissues of growth lambs and the ability of nitrogen balance techniques to quantitate protein retention. Anim. Prod. 57:237–245.

Maeng, W. J., and R. L. Baldwin. 1976. Factors influencing rumen microbial growth rates and yields: Effects of amino acid additions to a purified diet with nitrogen from urea. J. Dairy Sci. 59:648–655.

Maeng, W. J., C. J. van Nevel, R. L. Baldwin, and J. G. Morris. 1976. Rumen microbial growth rates and yields: Effect of amino acids and protein. J. Dairy Sci. 59:68–79.

Martin, C., L. Bernard, and B. Michalet-Doreau. 1996. Influence of sampling time and diet on amino acid composition of protozoal and bacterial fractions from bovine ruminal contents. J. Anim. Sci. 74: 1157–1163.

Matras, J., R. L. Preston, and S. J. Bartle. 2000. Influence of continuous intravenous lysine and methionine infusion on nitrogen balance in growing sheep fed diets that differ in ruminal degradable protein. J. Anim. Feed. Sci. 9:81–89.

McAllan, A. B. 1991. Carbohydrate and nitrogen metabolism in the forestomachs of steers given untreated or ammonia treated barley straw diets supplemented with urea or urea plus fishmeal. Anim. Feed Sci. Technol. 33:195–208.

Moen, R., and J. Pastor. 1998. Simulating antler growth and energy, nitrogen, calcium and phosphorus metabolism in caribou. Rangifer Spec. Iss. No. 10:85–97.

Moore, J. E., A. L. Goetsch, J. Luo, F. N. Owens, M. L. Galyean, Z. B. Johnson, T. Sahlu, and C. L. Ferrell. 2004. Prediction of fecal crude protein excretion of goats. Small Ruminant Res. 53:275–292.

Morin, D. E., L. L. Rowan, W. L. Hurley, and W. E. Braselton. 1995. Composition of milk from llamas in the United States. J. Dairy Sci. 78:1713–1720.

Mould, E. D., and C. T. Robbins. 1981. Nitrogen metabolism in elk. J. Wildl. Manage. 45:323–334.

Muir, P. D., A. R. Sykes, and G. K. Barrell. 1987. Growth and mineralization of antlers in red deer (Cervus elaphus). NZ J. Agric. Res. 30: 305–315.

Nimrick, K., E. E. Hatfield, J. Kaminski, and F. N. Owens. 1970a. Qualitative assessment of supplemental amino acid needs for growing lambs fed urea as the sole nitrogen source. J. Nutr. 100:1293–1300.

Nimrick, K., E. E. Hatfield, J. Kaminski, and F. N. Owens. 1970b. Quantitative assessment of supplemental amino acid needs for growing lambs fed urea as the sole nitrogen source. J. Nutr. 100:1301–1306.

NRC (National Research Council). 1981. Nutrient Requirements of Goats: Angora, Dairy, and Meat Goats in Temperate and Tropical Countries. Washington, DC: National Academy Press.

NRC. 1984. Nutrient Requirements of Beef Cattle, 6th ed. Washington, DC: National Academy Press.

NRC. 1985a. Nutrient Requirements of Sheep, 6th rev. ed. Washington, DC: National Academy Press.

NRC. 1985b. Ruminant Nitrogen Usage. Washington, DC: National Academy Press.

NRC. 2000. Nutrient Requirements of Beef Cattle (Update 2000). Washington, DC: National Academy Press.

NRC. 2001. Nutrient Requirements of Dairy Cattle, 7th rev. ed. Washington, DC: National Academy Press.

Nsahlai, I. V., A. L. Goetsch, J. Luo, Z. B. Johnson, J. E. Moore, T. Sahlu, C. L. Ferrell, M. L. Galyean, and F. N. Owens. 2004. Metabolizable protein requirements of lactating goats. Small Ruminant Res. 53:327–338.

Oftedal, O.T. 1984. Milk composition, milk yield and energy output at peak lactation: A comparative review. Symp. Zool. Soc. Lond. 51:33–85.

Oftedal, O. T. 1985. Pregnancy and Lactation. Pp. 215–238 (Chapter 10) in Bioenergetics of Wild Herbivores, R. J. Hudson and R. G. White, eds. Boca Raton, FL: CRC Press.

Parker, K. L., R. G. White, M. P. Gillingham, and D. F. Holleman. 1990. Comparison of energy metabolism in relation to daily activity and milk consumption by caribou and muskox neonates. Can. J. Zool. 68: 106–114.

Parker, K. L., P. S. Barboza, and T. R. Stephenson. 2005. Protein conservation in female caribou (*Rangifer tarandus*): Effects of decreasing diet quality during winter. J. Mamm. 86:610–622.

Parris, D., and L. S. Swart. 1975. Studies on the high-sulphur proteins of reduced mohair. The isolation and amino acid sequence of protein scmkb-m1.2. Biochem. J. 145:459–467.

Peek, J. M., K. T. Schmidt, M. J. Dorrance, and B. L. Smith. 2002. Supplemental feeding and farming of elk. Pp. 614–647 in North American Elk: Ecology and Management, D. E. Toweill and J. W. Thomas, eds. Washington, DC; London: Smithsonian Institution Press.

Pineda, J., J. M. Palma, G. F. W. Haenlein, and M. A. Galina. 1998. Fattening of Pelibuey hair sheep and crossbreds (Rambouillet-Dorset × Pelibuey) in the Mexican tropics. Small Ruminant Res. 27:263–266.

Preston, R. L. 2005. 2005 feed composition tables. Beef (Intertec Publ. Co.) 47(7):48–60.

Prieto, I., A. L. Goetsch, V. Banskalieva, M. Cameron, R. Puchala, T. Sahlu, L. J. Dawson, and S. W. Coleman. 2000. Effects of dietary protein concentration on postweaning growth of Boer crossbred and Spanish goat wethers. Small Ruminant Res. 78:2275–2281.

Reed, J. 1995. Nutritional toxicology of tannins and related polyphenols in forage legumes. J. Anim. Sci. 73:1516–1528.

Reimers, E. 1980. Activity pattern; the major determinant for growth and fattening in *Rangifer*. Pp. 466–475 in Proc. 2nd Int'l. Reindeer and Caribou Symp., E. Reimers, E. Gaare and S. Skjenneberg, eds. Trondheim, Norway: Directoratet for vilt og ferskvannsfisk.

Reis, P. J. 1979. Effects of amino acids on the growth and properties of wool. Pp. 223–242 in Physiological and Environmental Limitations to Wool Growth, J. L. Black and P. J. Reis, eds. Armidale, Australia: University of New England Publishing Unit.

Reis, P. J., and T. Sahlu. 1994. The nutritional control of the growth and properties of mohair and wool fibers: A comparative review. J. Anim. Sci. 72:1899–1907.

Robbins, C. T. 1993. Wildlife Feeding and Nutrition. New York: Academic Press.

Robbins, C. T., and A. N. Moen. 1975. Uterine composition and growth in pregnant white-tailed deer. J. Wildlife Manage. 39:684–691.

Robbins, C. T., and B. L. Robbins. 1979. Fetal and neonatal growth patterns and maternal reproductive effort in ungulates and subungulates. Am. Nat. 114:101–116.

Robbins, C. T., A. N. Moen, and J. T. Reid. 1974a. Body composition of white-tailed deer. J. Anim. Sci. 38:871–876.

Robbins, C. T., R. L. Prior, A. N. Moen, and W. J. Visek. 1974b. Nitrogen metabolism of white-tailed deer. J. Anim. Sci. 38:186–191.

Robbins, C. T., P. J. Van Soest, W. W. Mautz, and A. N. Moen. 1975. Feed analysis and digestion with reference to white-tailed deer. J. Wildl. Manage. 39:67–79.

Robbins, C. T., R. S. Podbielancik-Norman, D. L. Wilson, and E. D. Mould. 1981. Growth and nutrient consumption of elk calves compared to other ungulate species. J. Wildl. Manage. 45:172–186.

Robbins, C. T., T. A. Hanley, A. E. Hagerman, O. Hjeljord, D. L. Baker, C. C. Schwartz, and W. W. Mautz. 1987. Role of tannins in defending plants against ruminants: Reduction in protein availability. Ecology 68: 98–107.

Russel. A. J. F. 1992. Fiber production from sheep and goats. P. 235 in Progress in Sheep and Goat Research, A. W. Speedy, ed. Wallingford, UK: CABI Publishing.

Russell, D. E., A. M. Martell, and W. A. C. Nixon. 1993. Range ecology of the porcupine caribou herd in Canada. Rangifer Spec. Iss. No. 8: 3–167.

Sahlu, T., and J. M. Fernandez. 1992. Effect of intraperitoneal administration of lysine and methionine on mohair yield and quality in Angora goats. J. Anim. Sci. 70:3188–3193.

Sahlu, T., J. M. Fernandez, C. D. Lu, and R. Manning. 1992. Dietary protein level and ruminal degradability for mohair production in Angora goats. J. Anim. Sci. 70:1526–1533.

Sahlu, T., A. L. Goetsch, J. Luo, I. V. Nsahlai, J. E. Moore, M. L. Galyean, F. N. Owens, C. L. Ferrell, and Z. B. Johnson. 2004. Energy and protein requirements of goats: Developed equations, other considerations and future research to improve them. Small Ruminant Res. 53:191–220.

Said, A. N., and A. Tolera. 1993. The supplementary value of forage legume hays in sheep feeding: Feed intake, nitrogen retention and body weight change. Livest. Prod. Sci. 33:229–237.

Sauer, P. R. 1984. Physical characteristics. Pp. 73–90 in White-Tailed Deer: Ecology and Management, L. K. Halls, ed. Harrisburg, PA: Stackpole Books.

SCA (Standing Committee on Agriculture, Ruminants Subcommittee). 1990. Feeding Standards for Australian Livestock. Ruminants. East Melbourne, Australia: CSIRO Publications.

Schelling, G. T., J. E. Chandler, and G. C. Scott. 1973. Postruminal supplemental methionine infusion to sheep fed high quality diets. J. Anim. Sci. 37:1034–1039.

Schelling, G. T., and E. E. Hatfield. 1968. Effect of abomasally infused nitrogen sources on nitrogen retention in growing lambs. J. Nutr. 96: 319–326.

Schwartz, C. C., W. L. Regelin, and A. W. Franzmann. 1987. Protein digestion in moose. J. Wildl. Manage. 51:352–357.

Shahjalal, M. D., H. Galbraith, and J. H. Topps. 1992. The effect of changes in dietary protein and energy on growth, body composition and mohair fibre characteristics of British Angora goats. Anim. Prod. 54:405–412.

Silanikove, N. 2000. The physiological basis of adaptation in goats to harsh environments. Small Ruminant Res. 35:181–193.

Silanikove, N., A. Perevolotsky, and F. D. Provensa. 2001. Use of tannin-binding chemicals to assay for tannins and their negative postingestive effects in ruminants. Anim. Feed Sci. Technol. 91:69–81.

Sim, J. S., and R. J. Hudson. 1991. Chemical characteristics and processing technology of Alberta wapiti antlers. Proc. Intern. Wildl. Ranch. Symp. 2:533–535.

Smith, R. H. 1975. Digestion and metabolism in the ruminant. Pp. 399–415 in Proceedings of the IV International Symposium on Ruminant Physiology. Armidale, Australia: New England University Press.

Soto-Navarro, S. A., A. L. Goetsch, T. Sahlu, R. Puchala, and L. J. Dawson. 2003. Effects of ruminally degraded nitrogen source and level in a high concentrate diet on site of digestion in yearling Boer × Spanish wether goats. Small Ruminant Res. 50:117–128.

Soto-Navarro, S. A., A. L. Goetsch, T. Sahlu, and R. Puchala. 2004. Effects of level and source of supplemental protein in a concentrate-based diet on growth performance of Boer × Spanish wether goats. Small Ruminant Res. 51:101–106.

Souri M., H. Galbraith, and J. R. Scaife. 1998. Comparisons of the effect of genotype and protected methionine supplementation on growth, digestive characteristics and fiber yield in cashmere-yielding and Angora goats. Anim. Sci. 66:217–223.

Stein, A., R. J. Irvine, R. Langvatn, S. D. Albon, and O. Halvorsen. 2002. The population dynamics of *Ostertagia gruehneri* in reindeer: A model for the seasonal and intensity dependent variation in nematode fecundity. Inter. J. Parasit. 32:991–996.

Storm, E., and E. R. Ørskov. 1983. The nutritive value of rumen micro-organisms in ruminants. 1. Large-scale isolation and chemical composition of rumen micro-organisms. Br. J. Nut. 50:463–470.

Storm, E., and E. R. Ørskov. 1984. The nutritive value of rumen micro-organisms in ruminants. 4. The limiting amino acids of microbial protein in growing sheep determined by a new approach. Br. J. Nutr. 52:613–620.

Suttie, J. M., and R. N. B. Kay. 1982 The influence of nutrition and photoperiod on the growth of antlers of young red deer. Pp. 61–71 in Antler Development in Cervidae, R. D. Brown, ed. Kingsville, TX: Caesar Kleberg Wildl. Res. Inst.

Sykes, A. R. 1994. Parasitism and production in farm animals. Anim. Prod. 59:155–172.

Sykes, A. R. 2000. Environmental effects on animal production: The nutritional demands of nematode parasite exposure in sheep. Asian-Australas. J. Anim. Sci. 13 (Suppl.):343–350.

Sykes, A. R., and R. L. Coop. 2001. Interactions between nutrition and gastrointestinal parasitism in sheep. New Zealand Vet. J. 49:222–226.

Throckmorton, J. C., D. F. Foulkes, R. A. Leng, and J. V. Evans. 1982. Response to bypass protein and starch in Merino sheep and Angora goats. Proc. Aust. Soc. Anim. Prod. 14:661–665.

Tolera, A., and F. Sundstøl. 2000. Supplementation of graded levels of Desmodium intortum hay to sheep feeding on maize stover harvested at three stages of maturity. 1. Feed intake, digestibility and body weight change. Anim. Feed Sci. Technol. 85:239–257.

Ullrey, D. E. 1983. Nutrition and antler development in white-tailed deer. Pp. 49–59 in Antler Development in Cervidae, R. D. Brown, ed. Kingsville, TX: Caesar Kleberg Wildl. Res. Inst.

van Houtert, M. F. J., I. A. Barger, J. W. Steel, R. G. Windon, and D. L. Emery. 1995. Effects of dietary protein intake on responses of young sheep to infection with *Trichostrongylus colubriformis*. Vet. Parasitol. 56:163–180.

Van Saun, R. J. 2006. Nutrient requirements of South American camelids: A factorial approach. Small Ruminant Res. 61(2/3):165–186.

Verme, J. L., and J. J. Ozoga. 1980. Effects of diet on growth and lipogenesis in deer fawns. J. Wildl. Manage. 44:315–324.

Verme, L. J., and D. E. Ullrey. 1984. Physiology and Nutrition. Pp. 91–128 in White-Tailed Deer: Ecology and Management, L. K. Halls, ed. Harrisburg, PA: Stackpole Books.

Virtanen, A. I. 1966. Milk production of cows on protein-free feed. Science 153(3744):1603–1614.

von Keyserlingk, G. E. M., and G. W. Mathison. 1993. The effect of ruminal escape protein and ambient temperature on the efficiency of utilization of metabolizable energy by lambs. J. Anim. Sci. 71:2206– 2217.

Waghorn, G. C., M. J. Ulyatt, A. John, and M. T. Fisher. 1987. The effect of condensed tannins on the site of digestion of amino acids and other nutrients in sheep fed on *Lotus corniculatus* L. Br. J. Nutr. 57:115–126.

Watson, A. 1971. Climate and antler shedding and performance of red deer in North East Scotland. J. Appl. Ecol. 8:53–67.

White, R. G. 1983. Foraging patterns and their multiplier effects on productivity of northern ungulates. Oikos 40:377–384.

White, R. G., and J. R. Luick. 1984. Plasticity and constraints in the lactational strategy of reindeer and caribou. Symp. Zool. Soc. Lond. 51:215–232.

Wilkerson, V. A., T. J. Klopfenstein, R. A. Britton, R. A. Stock, and P. S. Miller. 1993. Metabolizable protein and amino acid requirements of growing cattle. J. Anim. Sci. 71:2777–2784.

Williams, A. J. 1995. Wool growth. Pp. 224–242 in Australian Sheep and Wool Handbook, D. J. Cottle, ed. Melbourne, Australia: Inkata Press.

Wolfe, G. J. 1983. The relationship between age and antler development in wapiti. Pp. 29–36 in Antler Development in Cervidae, R. D. Robert, ed. Kingsville, TX: Caesar Kleberg Wildl. Res. Inst.

Zhigunov, P. 1968. Reindeer Husbandry. 2nd. ed., 343 pp. Jerusalem, Israel: Program for Scientific Translations.

6

Essential Fatty Acids

INTRODUCTION

The classical description of essential fatty acids includes fatty acids that are required for specific physiological processes but are not synthesized by the body. Small ruminants, like other mammals, lack the Δ12 and Δ15-desaturase enzymes needed to generate the *n*-6 and *n*-3 double bonds required for the biosynthesis of the polyunsaturated fatty acids linoleic and α-linoleic acid. Linoleic acid may be classified as an *n*- or ω-6 fatty acid, whereas α-linoleic acid belongs to the *n*- or ω-3 family. These two 18-carbon fatty acids are vital components of cell membranes and serve as precursors for multiple biologically active metabolites collectively known as the eicosanoids. Eicosanoid is a term used to describe a 20-carbon fatty acid derivative. Although there is a correlation between essential fatty acid activity and the potential to be converted to eicosanoids, an essential fatty acid deficiency cannot be cured by infusion of eicosanoids because they have a very short half-life and because different cells produce their own pattern of eicosanoids (Gurr et al., 2002). Thus, this committee, the Committee on Nutrient Requirements of Small Ruminants, concurs with the NRC (2003) committee who considered the most common dietary *n*-6 and *n*-3 fatty acids, linoleate and α-linolenate, as truly essential. The only significant sources of the longer chain *n*-3 fatty acids are marine algae and fish products, neither of which are common constituents in the diets of small ruminants.

DEFINING REQUIREMENTS

The extensive review by Holman (1971) established the basis for linoleate requirements in animals. This author used the technique of plasma fatty acid profiling where the minimal triene to tetraene ratio was inferred to be the point of linoleate sufficiency. The premise behind this technique is that the Δ6-desaturase enzyme produces proportionally more 20:3*n*-9 relative to 20:4*n*-6 as availability of linoleate decreases. Clinical signs of essential fatty acid deficiency were noticeable when the triene:tetraene ratio exceeded a value of 0.4. Consequently, a minimum linoleate requirement of about 1 percent of dietary energy intake was recommended for nonruminant animals.

The triene:tetraene ratio is a valid indicator of essential fatty acid status only when *n*-6 fatty acids are the principal unsaturated fatty acids (NRC, 1995) because the Δ6-desaturase enzyme has a higher affinity for *n*-3 vs. *n*-6 fatty acid substrates (Johnston, 1985). Thus, Cunnane (2003) argued that the requirement for linoleate cannot be determined in the absence of ω-3 polyunsaturated fatty acids. In a study in which dietary α-linolenic acid was adequate, Bourre et al. (1990) noted that the rat's linoleate requirement was 0.15 percent of the diet or about 0.3 percent of energy intake. This recommendation is consistent with the value of 0.1 percent of the diet adopted by the NRC (1998) for swine.

The amount of *n*-3 polyunsaturated fatty acids required is less than the requirement for linoleic acid. Previous NRC (1995, 1998) committees recognized that animals require *n*-3 fatty acids, but specific requirements were not defined. Subsequent recommendations for α-linoleic acid ranged from 25 percent of linoleate for nonhuman primates (NRC, 2003) to roughly 10 percent of linoleate for humans (Institute of Medicine of the National Academies, 2002). Although small ruminants undoubtedly have a physiological requirement for *n*-3 polyunsaturated fatty acids, the essential fatty acid status of ruminants has been less extensively researched (Noble and Shand, 1982). Thus, recommendations for *n*-3 polyunsaturated fatty acid requirements for small ruminants are not possible due to the paucity of published data on the subject.

Although small ruminants have a physiological requirement for *n*-3 and *n*-6 fatty acids, the process of ruminal biohydrogenation (Chapter 2) complicates matters by markedly altering the composition of dietary fatty acids before they are absorbed and available for metabolism. Even without considering extensive metabolism of dietary essential fatty acids in the rumen, the induction of essential fatty acid deficiencies in adult ruminants cannot be demonstrated readily using 20:3*n*-9 as a marker (Palmquist et al., 1977). Extensive secretion of bile acids, cholesterol esters, phospholipids, triglycerides, free fatty acids, and lipase accompanied by rapid resorption resulted in a doubling of fatty acid fluxes through the duodenum of sheep (Sklan et al., 1985). A distinctive preference for available linoleate to be incorporated into phospholipids and cholesterol esters, in addition to reacylation of the hydrolytic endogenous secretory products and recycling via capillary filtrate, contribute to the ruminant's ability to make very efficient use of essential fatty acids (Noble, 1984). The efficient utilization of essential fatty acids apparently evolved from the need to counterbalance ruminal biohydrogenation (Van Soest, 1994).

RECOMMENDATIONS

Ruminants seem to have an essential fatty acid requirement approximately one-half that of nonruminants (Mattos and Palmquist, 1977). Linoleate requirements for swine range from 0.11 g/kg of body weight $(BW)^{0.75}$ for newly weaned pigs to 0.085 g/kg $BW^{0.75}$ for 120 kg finishing hogs (NRC, 1998). The presumed linoleate requirement for growing small ruminants would thus range from 0.055 g/kg $BW^{0.75}$ to 0.043 g/kg $BW^{0.75}$. Neonatal ruminants have an immediate and high requirement for essential fatty acids during the period just after birth (Noble et al., 1972). For example, newborn lambs and kids had triene: tetraene ratios of 1.7 and 2.8, respectively (Leat, 1966). Bruckner et al. (1984) observed that artificially reared lambs consuming linoleate at 0.054 g/kg $BW^{0.75}$ had triene: tetraene ratios in plasma and liver of 0.8 and 0.7, respectively. However, the unsatisfactory essential fatty acid status of the nursing ruminant is rectified within 3 to 4 days after birth (Noble, 1980; Noble and Shand, 1982) when the concentration of linoleate in colostrum and milk is at least 25 percent greater (Noble et al., 1970) than the dietary level used in the study of Bruckner et al. (1984). The minimum linoleate requirement for neonatal small ruminants is thus estimated to be 0.068 g/kg of $BW^{0.75}$. The young ruminant animal seems to be extremely efficient in utilizing and conserving the linoleate obtained from the diet (Noble, 1984), and consumption of the dam's milk is expected to meet the essential fatty acid requirements of nursing small ruminants. Essential fatty acid requirements of 7-day-old kid goats were satisfied by feeding milk replacer reconstituted with amounts of linoleate and α-linolenic acid comparable to goat's milk (Yeom et al., 2002).

Due to extensive metabolism of dietary essential fatty acids in the rumen and minimal long-chain fatty acid absorption from the rumen, linoleate requirements for fully functional small ruminants must represent the fatty acid reaching the duodenum. The maximum linoleate requirement of the growing small ruminant postweaning is expected to be 0.055 g/kg $BW^{0.75}$. It is highly probable that small ruminants fed diets allowing for moderately high gain will be able to satisfy their estimated requirement. In a study conducted by Jenkins and Adams (2002), lambs were fed a conventional, low-fat grower diet formulated to permit 300 g of daily gain. The diet fed in the first experiment averaged 2.2 percent fatty acids, whereas the diet fed in the second experiment averaged 1.92 percent fatty acids. Lambs began the study weighing 36 kg, in which case, their theoretical requirement for linoleate would be 0.81 g/d. Dry matter (DM) intake was 1,097 g/d during the first experiment. Assuming an apparent ruminal DM digestibility of 70 percent and the 2.5 mg/g linoleate in duodenal digesta reported by the authors, the lambs would have received 0.82 g/d linoleate. If these lambs consumed the diet at the same rate during the second experiment, their average body weight would be 61 kg with a theoretical maximum linoleate requirement of 1.2 g/d. With an apparent ruminal DM digestibility of 70 percent and the reported 2.8 mg/g linoleate in duodenal digesta, the lambs would have received 1.54 g/d linoleate. The abovementioned linoleate supply is likely underestimated because apparent ruminal digestibility was 50 percent for lambs consuming a comparable diet (Ikwuegbu and Sutton, 1982). Additionally, 40 kg lambs limit-fed a 75 percent corn diet (3.9 percent total fatty acids) at approximately 46 percent of ad libitum intake had 1.9 g/d of linoleate flowing to the duodenum (Kucuk et al., 2004). Hence, the amount of linoleic acid reaching the small intestine should be more than adequate for small ruminants fed conventional grower diets.

Essential fatty acid requirements of mature small ruminants are expected to decrease substantially as the physiological demand would shift from cellular growth to maintenance of cell membrane lipids. Adjusting the NRC (1998) linoleate requirement of a gestating sow to a metabolic body weight basis equates to 0.04 $g/kg^{0.75}$, which would presumably equate to 0.02 $g/kg^{0.75}$ for small ruminants. A 70 kg small ruminant consuming 1.8 kg of vegetation with 1.2 mg/g of linoleate (Whitney et al., 1999) could be in jeopardy of experiencing a linoleate deficiency because the extent of ruminal biohydrogenation averages 87 percent (Jenkins, 1994). Whereas noticeable depletion of arachidonic acid stores requires long-term depletion diets (Gurr et al., 2002), prostaglandin $F_{2\alpha}$ production in early- and late-pregnant ewes increased by feeding a rumen-protected lipid source with 53 percent linoleate (Cheng et al., 2005). In a related study, Elmes et al. (2003) noted that a similar linoleate-supplemented diet was associated with earlier delivery in ewes induced with dexamethasone. Cheng et al. (2005) estimated that intestinal supply of linoleate increased from 1.3 g/d to 8.5 g/d for ewes in early gestation. Linoleate reaching the small intestine was estimated to be increased from 2.5 to 13.7 g/d for ewes in late gestation.

Recommendations for the linoleate requirement cannot be estimated currently, but evidence suggests that the small ruminant's linoleate requirement may increase during gestation. Moreover, lamb survivability improved by increasing dietary linoleate approximately 2.3 percentage units (total fat increased 3 percentage units) during the last 45 days of gestation (Encinias et al., 2004). This response may be due to increased linoleate status of the neonatal lambs. Linoleic acid status of the neonate improved significantly by providing the late-gestational sheep (Noble et al., 1978; Shand et al., 1978) and goats (Soares, 1986) lipid supplements that greatly increased maternal plasma levels of linoleic acid.

Increasing linoleate available to the lactating small ruminant animal itself during early lactation does not seem plausible because of the inherent homeorhetic regulation involved with mammary uptake of circulating fatty acids. Rations supplemented with linoleic acid-rich seeds increase mammary output of linoleate (Chilliard and Ferlay, 2004). Supplementing with lipids will increase dietary energy (Chapter 4) and may be more feasible when energy is limiting during lactation (Appeddu et al., 2004). Milk yield and fat content increased with almost all fat supplements studied in goats (Chilliard et al., 2003).

Limitations to Evaluating Supply of Essential Fatty Acids

The problem of essential fatty acid insufficiency is easily resolved in nonruminant animals because inclusion of linoleate or ω-3 fatty acids into the diet will readily increase the amount of these fatty acids available for tissue metabolism. In contrast, the process of ruminal biohydrogenation (Chapter 2) significantly alters the composition of dietary fatty acids before they are absorbed and available for metabolism. Nutritionists would be in a better position to evaluate supply of essential fatty acids and to formulate diets to satisfy essential fatty acid requirements if mechanistic models were developed to predict ruminal metabolism and intestinal supply/availability of fatty acids. Numerous primary research papers have illustrated the impact of ruminal biohydrogenation on availability of essential fatty acids, but quantitative models to describe these processes in small ruminants are lacking. However, such models have been developed for dairy cattle.

The complex dynamic rumen model of Dijkstra et al. (1992) represented long-chain fatty acid dynamics by a lipid pool that received input from the feed and from lipid released upon the death of microbes in the rumen, in addition to a single output of lipids from the rumen. This model was later refined by Dijkstra et al. (2000) to include three pools of lipid: unhydrolyzed lipid, saturated free long-chain fatty acids, and free unsaturated long-chain fatty acids. The models of Dijkstra et al. (1992, 2000) were primarily developed to predict nutrient degradation in the rumen, and have not been evaluated for the purpose of predicting essential fatty acid flow to the small intestine of small ruminants.

A more recent model published by Moate et al. (2004) was designed as a submodel for the Cornell-Penn-Miner Dairy System. This lipid submodel considers six processes which influence the amounts of essential fatty acids and other lipid fractions that are absorbed from the intestines: (1) intake of dietary lipid, (2) ruminal lipolysis of dietary lipid, (3) biohydrogenation of individual fatty acids, (4) de novo production of specific fatty acids in the rumen, (5) ruminal passage of individual long-chain fatty acids, and (6) intestinal absorption of individual long-chain fatty acids. The model showed good concordance between measured and predicted duodenal flows in the evaluation of 36 diets from eight published papers. Development of a comparable model for small ruminants is warranted to examine productivity in terms of individual fatty acids and to allow nutritionists to more accurately formulate diets that will alter fatty acid composition of food products derived from small ruminant animals.

Quality of Small Ruminant Food Products

Small ruminants are an important source of food for humans throughout the world (Haenlein, 2001). Although food products derived from small ruminants contain a multitude of nutrients, the ensuing discussion will concentrate on these products as a source of fatty acids. The marked differences in fatty acid composition of ruminant tissues compared with tissues of other food-producing animals consuming comparable diets has been well established (Body, 1988). Differences in fatty acid profile of milk and tissue of sheep, goats, cervids, and ruminant-like animals have been reported (Christie, 1978); however, location of the tissue samples and diet consumed by the animals likely accounted for much of the differences. In reviewing data of Miller et al. (1986), Rule et al. (1995) noted that muscle fatty acid compositions were quite similar among three game species (pronghorn, deer, and elk) and range steers. Species variation for samples collected from the *longissimus dorsi* was similar to that reported for the *biceps femoris*, and slight differences within muscles probably reflected differences in diets selected by the animals (Rule et al., 1995). Greater concentrations of *n*-3 polyunsaturated fatty acids in muscle tissues of wild ruminants compared with muscle tissue of domestic ruminants may be attributable to less total fat in muscle tissue of wild ruminants (Cordain et al., 2002).

Regardless of which ruminant animal species is considered, the process of biohydrogenation alters the animal's dietary *n*-6 and *n*-3 fatty acids such that the amounts of essential fatty acids available for incorporation into tissues and milk are relatively low. Given the distinct involvement of these two families of fatty acids in cardiovascular health in humans (Wijendran and Hayes, 2004), dietary manipulation to alter lipid composition of small ruminants has been the subject of immense investigations and literature reviews (Nürnberg et al., 1998; Bas and Morand-Fehr, 2000; Banskalieva et al., 2000; Chilliard et al., 2003; Dewhurst et al., 2003; Wood et al., 2003; Chilliard and Ferlay, 2004; Dhiman et al., 2005; MacRae et al., 2005). A variety of nutritional regimens have been used to effectively change the milk and tissue fatty acid composition. In general, proportions of *n*-6 fatty acids increase when animals receive diets containing linoleate. Proportions of *n*-3 fatty acids are increased by feeding forage, marine algae, and feedstuffs derived from fish products. Although the effect of dietary manipulation on fatty acid profile can be quite dramatic, it is critically important to recognize that many regimens also influence total fat content or milk fat yield in a manner that may greatly reduce the effect when evaluated on a mass basis. Expressing polyunsaturated fatty acids in terms of mass is a more optimal approach to dietary *n*-6 and *n*-3 fatty acid balance than a simple ratio (Wijendran and Hayes, 2004).

Fatty Acids Unique to Ruminant Animal Food Products

The process of biohydrogenation clearly influences the fatty acids available to ruminant animals. A high proportion of naturally occurring 18-carbon unsaturated fatty acids in the diet are converted predominantly in the rumen to stearic acid but are accompanied also by a spectrum of geometrical and positional di- and monoenoic isomers. As a result, food products derived from these animals contain isomeric *trans* fatty acids not commonly found in food derived from nonruminant animals (Aro et al., 1998). Discovery of potential health benefits attributed to some of these unique fatty acids has prompted the suggestion that foods derived from ruminants be considered functional foods (Bauman et al., 2000; McGuire and McGuire, 2000).

Geometrical and positional isomers of linoleic acid are referred collectively to as conjugated linoleic acid (CLA). Over the past two decades, numerous health benefits have been attributed to CLA in experimental animal models (Belury, 2002). In fact, "conjugated linoleic acid (CLA) is the only fatty acid shown unequivocally to inhibit carcinogenesis in experimental animals" (NRC, 1996). Food products derived from ruminant animals are the major source of CLA in human diets (McGuire and McGuire, 2000). Current evidence suggests that the predominate CLA isoform *cis*-9, *trans*-11 CLA (rumenic acid) possesses anticarcinogenic properties.

Although the potential health benefits have largely been attributed to the 18-carbon dienoic *trans* fatty acids, the 18-carbon monoenic *trans* fatty acids formed by the action of bacteria in the rumen are of particular importance. The quantity of *trans* 18:1 reaching the small intestine far exceeds that of CLA (Bauman et al., 2003), with *trans*-11 18:1 (*trans* vaccenic acid) representing the most abundant 18-carbon monoenic *trans* fatty acid. Activity of the Δ9-desaturase enzyme in the intestinal mucosa (Archibeque et al., 2005), adipose tissues (Palmquist et al., 2004) or mammary gland (Griinari et al., 2000) gives rise to the majority of CLA in small-ruminant animal food products. The 18-carbon monoenic *trans* fatty acids constitute 52 to 75 percent of the total *trans* fatty acids, compared with 15 percent for CLA (Aro et al., 1998). Whereas only a trace of rumenic acid was detected, *trans* vaccenic acid was 1.23 to 6.06 percent of the fatty acids detected in the *biceps fermoris* muscle of wild cervids (Cordain et al., 2002). Turpeinen et al. (2002) estimated that 19 percent of dietary *trans* vaccenic acid was desaturated to rumenic acid in human subjects. Thus, the contribution of *trans* vaccenic acid desaturation to total rumenic acid supplies of the human body can be substantial.

There is no direct evidence of an anticarcinogenic effect of CLA in human subjects, but epidemiological studies suggest that CLA may be relevant as a natural anticarcinogen (Azain, 2003; Weiss et al., 2004). Although the content of CLA in food products derived from ruminants may be inadequate to make a meaningful contribution (Wahle et al., 2004; MacRae et al., 2005), the potential health benefits associated with CLA have caused research to focus on methods to enhance the CLA content in food products. Diet-related factors appear to have the most profound effect on CLA content in milk and meat from ruminants (Khanal and Dhiman, 2004). Dietary manipulation to alter CLA composition of small-ruminant animal food products has been reviewed (Chilliard et al., 2003; Chilliard and Ferlay, 2004; Khanal and Olson, 2004; Weiss et al., 2004; Dhiman et al., 2005). Manipulation of the animal's diet primarily involves supplying linoleate or α-linoleic acid as substrates for rumen biohydrogenation, but including dietary fatty acids of marine origin can also increase the proportion of CLA in milk fat. As with dietary manipulations to alter *n*-6 and *n*-3 fatty acids, however, many dietary strategies may reduce the effect when evaluated on a mass basis. A low-roughage ration supplemented with oils high in linoleate (Palmquist et al., 2004) or corn silage as the roughage source (Chilliard and Ferlay, 2004) favors the accumulation of *trans*-10 18:1; however, the effect of *trans*-10 18:1 has yet to be elucidated fully. Overall, CLA-rich dairy products likely will have a greater impact (Belury, 2002) than is possible by enriching the content of CLA in meat of small ruminants (Bolte et al., 2002).

Specific recommendations for feeding strategies to enhance CLA in food products derived from ruminant animals will be possible as the understanding of CLA biosynthesis continues to advance. The development of mathematical models to predict exogenous and endogenous contributions to rumenic acid in several tissues (Palmquist et al., 2004) is an initial step toward evaluating potential changes in tissue rumenic acid through dietary manipulation. The model of Palmquist et al. (2004), which was developed from a limited number of lambs fed four different diets, has only been evaluated using milk fatty acid profiles in an independent data set that consisted of 114 dairy cows with nine dietary treatments. This model should be challenged with data from studies with small ruminants. Evaluation of this model will invariably lead to refinements in the knowledge of CLA biosynthesis, and with appropriate adjustments, nutritionists may be able to utilize the model as a method to develop dietary regimens to enhance CLA production of food-producing small ruminants. However, the food industry must be cognizant of the decreased sensorial quality of dairy (Chilliard et al., 2003; Chilliard and Ferlay, 2004) and meat (Duckett and Kuber, 2001) products from small ruminants that have experienced dietary manipulation to alter fatty acid composition.

REFERENCES

Appeddu, L. A., D. G. Ely, D. K. Aaron, W. P. Deweese, and E. Fink. 2004. Effects of supplementing with calcium salts of palm oil fatty acids or hydrogenated tallow on ewe milk production and twin lamb growth. J. Anim. Sci. 82:2780–2789.

Archibeque, S. L., D. K. Lunt, C. D. Gilbert, R. K. Tume, and S. B. Smith. 2005. Fatty acid indices of stearoly-CoA desaturase do not reflect actual stearoyl-CoA desaturase enzyme activities in adipose tissues of beef steers finished with corn-, flaxseed-, or sorghum-based diets. J. Anim. Sci. 83:1153–1166.

Aro, A., J. M. Antoine, L. Pizzoferrato, O. Reykdal, and G. van Poppel. 1998. *Trans* fatty acids in dairy and meat products from 14 European countries: The TRANSFAIR study. J. Food Comp. Anal. 11:150–160.

Azain, M. J. 2003. Conjugated linoleic acid and its effects on animal products and health in single-stomached animals. Proc. Nutr. Soc. 62: 319–328.

Banskalieva, V., T. Sahlu, and A. L. Goetsch. 2000. Fatty acid composition of goat muscles and fat depots: A review. Small Ruminant Res. 37: 255–268.

Bas, P., and P. Morand-Fehr. 2000. Effect of nutritional factors on fatty acid composition of lamb fat deposits. Livest. Prod. Sci. 64:61–79.

Bauman, D. E., L. H. Baumgard, B. A. Corl, and J. M. Griinari. 2000. Biosynthesis of conjugated linoleic acid in ruminants. Proc. Am. Soc. Anim. Sci., 1999. Available at http://www.asas.org/jas/symposia/proceedings/0937.pdf. Accessed April 4, 2006.

Bauman, D. E., B. A. Corl, and D. G. Peterson. 2003. The biology of conjugated linoleic acid in ruminants. Pp. 146–173 in Advances in Conjugated Linoleic Acid Research, Vol. 2, J-L. Sebedio, W. W. Christie, and R. Adlof, eds. Champaign, IL: AOCS Press.

Belury, M. A. 2002. Dietary conjugated linoleic acid in health: Physiological effects and mechanisms of action. Annu. Rev. Nutr. 22:505–531.

Body, D. R. 1988. The lipid composition of adipose tissue. Prog. Lipid Res. 27:39–60.

Bolte, M. R., B. W. Hess, W. J. Means, G. E. Moss, and D. C. Rule. 2002. Feeding lambs high-oleate or high-linoleate safflower seeds differentially influences carcass fatty acid composition. J. Anim Sci. 80:609–616.

Bourre, J. M., M. Piciotti, O. Dumont, G. Pascal, and G. Durand. 1990. Dietary linoleic acid and polyunsaturated fatty acids in rat brain and other organs: Minimal requirements of linoleic acid. Lipids 25:465–472.

Bruckner, G., K. K. Grunewald, R. E. Tucker, and G. E. Mitchell, Jr. 1984. Essential fatty acid status and characteristics associated with colostrum-deprived gnotobiotic and conventional lambs. Growth, organ development, cell membrane integrity and factors associated with lower bowel function. J. Anim. Sci. 58:971–978.

Cheng, Z., M. Elmes, S. E. Kirkup, E. C. Chin, D. R. E. Abayasekara, and D. C. Wathes. 2005. The effect of a diet supplemented with the *n*-6 polyunsaturated fatty acid linoleic acid on prostaglandin production in early- and late-pregnant ewes. J. Endocrinol. 184:165–178.

Chilliard, Y., and A. Ferlay. 2004. Dietary lipids and forage interactions on cow and goat milk fatty acid composition and sensory properties. Reprod. Nutr. Dev. 44:467–492.

Chilliard, Y., A. Ferlay, J. Rouel, and G. Lamberet. 2003. A review of nutritional and physiological factors affecting goat milk lipid synthesis and lipolysis. J. Dairy Sci. 86:1751–1770.

Christie, W. W. 1978. The composition, structure and function of lipids in the tissues of ruminant animals. Prog. Lipid Res. 17:111–205.

Cordain, L., B. A. Watkins, G. L. Florant, M. Kelher, L. Rogers, and Y. Li. 2002. Fatty acid analysis of wild ruminant tissues: Evolutionary implications for reducing diet-related chronic disease. Eur. J. Clin. Nutr. 56:181–191.

Cunnane, S. C. 2003. Problems with essential fatty acids: Time for a new paradigm? Prog. Lipid Res. 42:544–568.

Dewhurst, R. J., N. D. Scollan, M. R. F. Lee, H. J. Ougham, and M. O. Humphreys. 2003. Forage breeding and management to increase the beneficial fatty acid content of ruminant products. Proc. Nutr. Soc. 62:329–336.

Dhiman, T. R., S-H. Nam, and A. L. Ure. 2005. Factors affecting conjugated linoleic acid content in milk and meat. Crit. Rev. Food Sci. Nutr. 45:463–482.

Dijkstra, J., H. D. StC. Neal, D. E. Beever, and J. France. 1992. Simulation of nutrient digestion, absorption and outflow in the rumen: Model description. J. Nutr. 122:2239–2256.

Dijkstra, J., W. J. J. Gerrits, A. Bannink, and J. France. 2000. Modelling lipid metabolism in the rumen. Pp. 25–36 in Modelling Nutrient Utilization in Farm Animals, J. P. McNamara, J. France, and D. E. Beever, eds. New York: CABI Publishing.

Duckett, S. K., and P. S. Kuber. 2001. Genetic and nutritional effects on lamb flavor. J. Anim. Sci. 79(E. Suppl.):E249–E259.

Elmes, M., K. Poore, J. Newman, L. R. Green, D. Cheng, D. R. E. Abayasekara, M. A. Hanson, and D. C. Wathes. 2003. Prostaglandin production and timing of parturition in sheep fed a diet high in *n*-6 polyunsaturated fatty acids. Endocrine Abstr. 6:61.

Encinias, H. B., G. P. Lardy, A. M. Encinias, and M. L. Bauer. 2004. High linoleic acid safflower seed supplementation for gestating ewes: Effects on ewe performance, lamb survival, and brown fat stores. J. Anim. Sci. 82:3654–3661.

Griinari, J. M., B. A. Corl, S. H. Lacy, P. Y. Chouinard, K. V. V. Nurmela, and D. E. Bauman. 2000. Conjugated linoleic acid is synthesized endogenously in lactating dairy cows by Δ^9-desaturase. J. Nutr. 130:2285–2291.

Gurr, M. I., J. L. Harwood, and K. N. Frayn. 2002. Lipid Biochemistry: An Introduction, 5th ed. Oxford, UK: Blackwell Science.

Haenlein, G. F. 2001. Past, present, and future perspectives of small ruminant dairy research. J. Dairy Sci. 84:2097–2115.

Holman, R. T. 1971. Essential fatty acid deficiency. Prog. Chem. Fats Other Lipids 9:275–348.

Ikwuegbu, O. A., and J. D. Sutton. 1982. The effect of varying the amount of linseed oil supplementation on rumen metabolism in sheep. Br. J. Nutr. 48:365–375.

Institute of Medicine of the National Academies. 2002. Dietary Reference Intakes for Energy, Carbohydrate, Fiber, Fat, Fatty Acids, Cholesterol, Protein, and Amino Acids. Washington, DC: The National Academies Press.

Jenkins, T. C. 1994. Regulation of lipid metabolism in the rumen. J. Nutr. 124:1372S–1376S.

Jenkins, T. C., and C. S. Adams. 2002. The biohydrogenation of linoleamide in vitro and its effects on linoleic acid concentration in duodenal contents of sheep. J. Anim. Sci. 80:533–540.

Johnston, P. V. 1985. Dietary fat, eicosanoids, and immunity. Adv. Lipid Res. 21:103–141.

Khanal, R. C., and T. R. Dhiman. 2004. Biosynthesis of conjugated linoleic acid (CLA): A review. Pakistan J. Nutr. 3:72–81.

Khanal, R. C., and K. C. Olson. 2004. Factors affecting conjugated linoleic acid (CLA) content in milk, meat, and egg: A review. Pakistan J. Nutr. 3:82–98.

Kucuk, O., B. W. Hess, and D. C. Rule. 2004. Soybean oil supplementation of a high-concentrate diet does not affect site and extent of organic matter, starch, neutral detergent fiber, or nitrogen digestion, but influences both ruminal metabolism and intestinal flow of fatty acids in limit-fed lambs. J. Anim. Sci. 82:2985–2994.

Leat, W. M. F. 1966. Fatty acid composition of plasma lipids of new-born and maternal ruminants. Biochem. J. 98:598–603.

MacRae, J., L. O'Reilly, and P. Morgan. 2005. Desirable characteristics of animal products from a human health perspective. Livest. Prod. Sci. 94:95–103.

Mattos, W., and D. L. Palmquist. 1977. Biohydrogenation and availability of linoleic acid in lactating cows. J. Nutr. 107:1755–1761.

McGuire, M. A., and M. K. McGuire. 2000. Conjugated linoleic acid (CLA): A ruminant fatty acid with beneficial effects on human health. Proc. Am. Soc. Anim. Sci., 1999. Available at http://www.asas.org/JAS/symposia/proceedings/0938.pdf. Accessed April 4, 2006.

Miller, G. J., R. A. Field, M. L. Riley, and J. C. Williams. 1986. Lipids in wild ruminant animals and steers. J. Food Qual. 9:331–343.

Moate, P. J., W. Chalupa, T. C. Jenkins, and R. C. Boston. 2004. A model to describe ruminal metabolism and intestinal absorption of long chain fatty acids. Anim. Feed Sci. Technol. 112:79–105.

Noble, R. C. 1980. Lipid metabolism in the neonatal ruminant. Prog. Lipid Res. 18:179–216.

Noble, R. C. 1984. Essential fatty acids in the ruminant. Pp. 185–200 in Fats in Animal Nutrition, J. Wiseman, ed. London: Butterworths.

Noble, R. C., and J. H. Shand. 1982. Fatty acid metabolism in the neonatal ruminant. Adv. Nutr. Res. 4:287–337.

Noble, R. C., W. Steele, and J. H. Moore. 1970. The composition of ewe's milk fat during early and late lactation. J. Dairy Res. 37:297–301.

Noble, R. C., W. Steele, and J. H. Moore. 1972. The metabolism of linoleic acid by the young lamb. Br. J. Nutr. 27:503–508.

Noble, R. C., J. H. Shand, J. T. Drummond, and J. H. Moore. 1978. "Protected" polyunsaturated fatty acid in the diet of the ewe and the essential fatty acid status of the neonatal lamb. J. Nutr. 108:1868–1876.

NRC (National Research Council). 1995. Nutrient Requirements of Laboratory Animals, 4th ed. Washington, DC: National Academies Press.

NRC. 1996. Carcinogens and Anticarcinogens in the Human Diet. Washington, DC: National Academy Press.

NRC. 1998. Nutrient Requirements of Swine, 10th rev. ed. Washington, DC: National Academy Press.

NRC. 2003. Nutrient Requirements of Nonhuman Primates, 2nd ed. Washington, DC: National Academy Press.

Nürnberg, K., J. Wegner, and K. Ender. 1998. Factors influencing fat composition in muscle and adipose tissue of farm animals. Livest. Prod. Sci. 56:145–156.

Palmquist, D. L., W. Mattos, and R. L. Stone. 1977. Absence of eicosatrienoic acid in plasma of sheep parenterally infused with a high glucose fat-free solution. Lipids 12:235–238.

Palmquist, D. L., N. St-Pierre, and K. E. McClure. 2004. Tissue fatty acid profiles can be used to quantify endogenous rumenic acid synthesis in lambs. J. Nutr. 134:2407–2414.

Rule, D. C., S. B. Smith, and J. R. Romans. 1995. Fatty acid composition of muscle and adipose tissue of meat animals. Pp. 144–165 in The Biology of Fat in Meat Animals, S. B. Smith and D. R. Smith, eds. Champaign, IL: American Society of Animal Science.

Shand, J. H., R. C. Noble, and J. H. Moore. 1978. Dietary influences on fatty acid metabolism in the liver of the neonatal lamb. Biol. Neonate 34:217–224.

Sklan, D., A. Arieli, W. Chalupa, and D. S. Kronfeld. 1985. Digestion and absorption of lipids and bile acids in sheep fed stearic acid, oleic acid, or tristearin. J. Dairy Sci. 68:1667–1675.

Soares, M. C. 1986. Effect of dietary protected lipids on the essential fatty acid status of the newborn kid. J. Nutr. 116:1473–1479.

Turpeinen, A. M., M. Mutanen, A. Aro, I. Salminen, S. Basu, D. L. Palmquist, and J. M. Griinari. 2002. Bioconversion of vaccenic acid to conjugated linoleic acid in humans. Am. J. Clin. Nutr. 76:504–510.

Van Soest, P. J. 1994. Nutritional Ecology of the Ruminant, 2nd ed., p. 331. Ithaca, NY: Cornell University Press.

Wahle, K. W. J., S. D. Heys, and D. Rotondo. 2004. Conjugated linoleic acids: Are they beneficial or detrimental to health? Prog. Lipid Res. 43:553–587.

Weiss, M. F., F. A. Martz, and C. L. Lorenzen. 2004. Review: Conjugated linoleic acid: Historical context and implications. Prof. Anim. Sci. 20:118–126.

Whitney, M. B., B. W. Hess, J. E. Kaltenbach, H. J. Harlow, and D. C. Rule. 1999. Direct transesterification of lipids from feedstuffs and ruminal bacteria. Can. J. Anim. Sci. 79:247–249.

Wijendran, V., and K. C. Hayes. 2004. Dietary *n*-6 and *n*-3 fatty acid balance and cardiovascular health. Annu. Rev. Nutr. 24:597–615.

Wood, J. D., R. I. Richardson, G. R. Nute, A. V. Fisher, M. M. Campo, E. Kasapidou, P. R. Sheard, and M. Enser. 2003. Effects of fatty acids on meat quality: A review. Meat Sci. 66:21–32.

Yeom, K. H., G. Van Trierum, R. Hovenier, A. B. Schellingerhout, K. W. Lee, and A. C. Beynen. 2002. Fatty acid composition of adipose tissue in goat kids fed milk replacers with different contents of α-linolenic and linoleic acid. Small Ruminant Res. 43:15–22.

7

Minerals

INTRODUCTION

Mineral nutrition must be a priority to all who manage small ruminants and New World camelids (NWC). Animal production, reproduction, immunity, and survival may be curtailed when a mineral is outside the adequate range. There are 14 elements that are essential and may be added to the diet under practical conditions. They are separated into macrominerals and microminerals, or trace minerals, according to the amounts required by the animals. The macrominerals include calcium, phosphorus, sodium, chlorine, potassium, magnesium, and sulfur. The microminerals are cobalt, copper, iodine, iron, manganese, selenium, and zinc. Thirteen other elements are considered essential for certain types of animals under some conditions: aluminum, arsenic, boron, chromium, fluorine, lead, lithium, molybdenum, nickel, rubidium, silicon, tin, and vanadium (Underwood and Suttle, 1999). The elements fluorine, molybdenum, lead, arsenic, aluminum, cadmium, and mercury are better known for their toxic effects.

The main sources of minerals are feeds. However, under certain circumstances, water can contribute significant amounts of some minerals like iodine, manganese, iron, sulfur, sodium, chlorine, and magnesium (Tomlinson, 2002). Management practices (grazing pressure) or weather (rainsplash, flooding) can cause consumption of substantial amounts of soil that may provide important amounts of cobalt, iodine, iron, manganese, or selenium (Whitehead, 2000) to grazing animals. For cervids in the wild, soil may be ingested at locations that constitute a mineral "lick," supplying sodium among other minerals (Cowan and Brink, 1949; Calef and Lortie, 1975; Weeks and Kirkpatrick, 1976). In wild ruminants, use of licks is particularly high in spring as they begin to consume the spring flush of vegetation. Fecal pellets are almost pure clay and it has been suggested that besides replacing minerals lost during scouring, the presence of the clay particles may help to control the scouring.

Forages are the main feeds for small ruminants and camelids under grazing conditions and many confinement arrangements. Cereals are the main feeds under confinement for intensive finishing of animals. In general, forages are rich sources of potassium and iron, deficient in sodium, and have variable concentrations of the rest of the minerals. Forages near coastlines often contain high levels of sodium (Låg, 1963; Staaland and White, 2001). Cereals are rich sources of phosphorus and poor sources of calcium, sodium, and probably iron, potassium, copper, zinc, manganese, iodine, and cobalt. Protein feeds derived from legume seeds are invariably richer in all minerals than forages or cereals (Underwood and Suttle, 1999).

Mineral concentrations in forages depend on soil pH and fertility, forage species and maturity stage, season and climate, irrigation water, and atmospheric inputs. An acid soil (pH < 6.0) may limit absorption of phosphorus, potassium, sulfur, calcium, magnesium, and selenium by the plant. However, it may increase absorption of iron, manganese, boron, copper, and zinc (Whiteman et al., 1974; NRC, 1983). Therefore, excesses of molybdenum and selenium and deficiencies of iron, copper, zinc, boron, and manganese may be found in animals fed forages grown in alkaline soils. Sandy soils are poor sources of nutrients because of low organic matter and water retention. Forages like *Atriplex* spp. and *Kochia* spp. may accumulate great quantities of sodium and chlorine, as do some aquatic plants (Staaland and White, 2001). Some *Astragalus* species grown in seleniferous soils contain up to 5,000 mg Se kg^{-1} DM. Legumes are richer sources of all minerals, except manganese and silicon, than grasses (Underwood, 1977), and leaves of willow shrubs (*Salix*) constitute good sources of copper and cobalt on north temperate ranges (O'Hara et al., 2001; Staaland and White, 2001). Leaves are also richer than stems in all minerals (Minson, 1990). When forage maturity increases, protein and mineral contents decline. More than 50 percent of fibrous byproducts listed by NRC publications (1984, 1985, 1989) are deficient in calcium, phosphorus, sodium, magnesium, sulfur, cobalt, copper, manganese, and zinc for ruminants. These mineral deficiencies are severe and include several of them in the same forage. Climate and season of growth of forages may change mineral concentrations of forages. Climatic effects are associated with soil pH, lixiviation, and forage species and maturity. Tropical regions normally have an acid soil, high or low precipitation, and faster-maturing forages with lower quality than other regions. Season of growth may affect mineral content by its relation to maturity stage of forages, water availability, and growth rate of forages. The seasonal production of leaves and current year stem growth of vegetation in north temperate ecosystems provide a dependable rich "pulse" of protein and minerals that match coevolved life history events of small ruminants, including cervid species (White et al., 1981). Irrigation of forages with sewage water can increase the soil concentration of several minerals including copper, manganese, and iron. These minerals can accumulate and cause toxicity to the plants or animals that consume them (Whitehead, 2000). Atmospheric input of minerals can be important in some cases. Sodium and iodine are carried by rainfall. Therefore, regions with high rainfall and close to the sea may contain more of these elements. Sulfur, fluorine, and cadmium are sent into the air by factories, lead by vehicles, and volcanoes causing environmental contamination (Underwood and Suttle, 1999).

Interactions among minerals may modify their availability and can be an important cause of mineral deficiencies or excesses. These problems may arise from natural imbalances or be induced by management practices that promote soil ingestion, contamination of water sources, or inadequate mineral supplementation. Interactions may occur during absorption, transport, cellular uptake, intracellular function, or at storage or excretion sites.

Life history events place special temporal demands for minerals (Robbins, 1993). These events include lactation, skeletal growth of young, seasonal growth of wool and fiber (pelage), and the annual growth of antlers by male deer species (Ullrey, 1983) and by females of the genus *Rangifer* (reindeer/caribou) (Kelsall, 1968; Høymork and Reimers, 2002). Thus, the mineral status of classes of animals may change in association with life history events, in relation to availability of minerals in the diet (Staaland and Hove, 2000), and in relation to the availability in mineral supplements, either natural or provided through feed additives (Underwood, 1977; Underwood and Suttle 1999). Robbins (1993) cautioned against the use of mineral requirements determined on domestic species for direct application to wildlife.

The mineral requirements of the class *Cervidae* for antler growth have not previously been a product of NRC publications on livestock. Justification for including nutrient requirements for antler growth in cervids revolves around their economic importance in commercial harvest of farmed and ranched deer (Sim and Hudson, 1991, Haigh and Hudson, 1993), their role as a determinant of hunter management in wild populations (Peek et al., 2002), and as indicators of individual and herd health in wildlife and ecosystem management (Watson, 1971). Because mature antlers are bone, with the inclusion of fluoride and chloride ($Ca_5(F,Cl)P_3O_{12}$; Ullrey, 1983), the minerals of direct importance are calcium and phosphorus. Antlers are grown and shed annually with the maximum rate of mineralization occurring late in the growth cycle (Hyvarinen et al., 1977; Brown, 1990); however, antler mass and growth rate increase with animal age and body weight and is strongly influenced by winter nutrition (French et al., 1956; Lincoln, 1971; Bergerud, 1976; Ullrey, 1983; Wolfe, 1983; Brown, 1990; Grasman and Hellgren, 1993; Peek et al., 2002). During peak mineralization of antler, both calcium and phosphorus are withdrawn from the skeleton to produce a clear cyclical osteoporosis. The process also is supported by increased plasma alkaline phosphatase (Grasman and Hellgren, 1993: Bubenik et al., 2000) that is associated with the rate of bone formation and with 1,25 dihydroxyvitamin D_3 (Eiben et al., 1984) that has a strong influence over calcium absorption (Hove et al., 1986). These associations could explain a lower endogenous calcium loss during antlerogenesis of young males (Stephenson and Brown, 1984; Brown 1990). Brown (1990) calculated that calcium and phosphorus requirements for antler growth in males are less than those requirements for the entire lactation cycle. Growth of antlers by female reindeer and caribou adds to nutrient demands when the individual is lactating, though peak mineral deposition occurs following peak milk production (Moen and Pastor, 1998).

The assessment of mineral status of animals necessitates knowledge of the mineral content of water, soil where feeds are grown, diets selected, and fluids and tissues (blood, bone, liver), as well as any clinical signs shown by the animal. A diagnosis is confirmed when the problem is corrected and the animal returns to a normal condition. Improvement in the animal condition can be achieved by fertilizing the soil where feeds are grown or by supplementation with the mineral required. Fertilization can be the most desired practice for most minerals, because there is a response of the plant and the animal (Rees et al., 1974; Allaway, 1986; Minson, 1990). The exception may be iodine and sodium, because plants do not require them or the amounts needed are very small (Allaway, 1986).

CALCIUM

Calcium (Ca) is the main structural component of bone and teeth, which contain 98–99 percent of total calcium in the body. The main component of bone is hydroxyapatite ($Ca_{10}(PO_4)_6(OH)_2$), where magnesium can replace a small part of calcium, and fluorine can replace the hydroxyl group. Bone is a dynamic tissue, where osteoclast cells dissolve or reabsorb bone, and osteoblasts are bone-forming cells. The balance in activity of these cells leads to bone growth or osteoporosis. Bone formation requires iron, copper, and manganese for collagen synthesis as well as vitamin A and vitamin D_3. Calcium functions as an intracellular messenger for transmission of nerve impulses, muscular contraction, constriction and relaxation of blood vessels, and release of hormones such as insulin. Calcium is a cofactor for enzymes as in the coagulation cascade. Therefore, there is a relationship between calcium and vitamin K.

Calcium Homeostasis

Calcium homeostasis is achieved by variable absorption, renal excretion, and bone deposition and mobilization. Calcium is absorbed mainly by active transport in the small intestine. Passive transport also occurs throughout the gastrointestinal tract. Calcium losses from the body are through fecal (85–98 percent) and urinary (2–5 percent) excretions. Calcitonin, calcitriol [1,25-$(OH)_2$-cholecalciferol], and parathyroid hormone (PTH) are the hormones involved in calcium balance (Bronner, 1997). When blood calcium decreases, PTH is released to convert vitamin D_3 to calcitriol in the kidneys. Calcitriol increases calcium absorption from the small intestine. Calcitriol and PTH stimulate bone osteoclasts to release calcium, while increasing its reabsorption by the kidneys. Calcitonin prevents development of physiological hypercalcemia.

Normal calcium levels in plasma range from 8–12 mg/100 mL. When calcium levels fall below this range, hypocalcemia or milk fever ensues. When calcium levels increase above this range, hypercalcemia ensues (Puls, 1994; McDowell, 1997). Plasma ionized calcium may be more indicative of calcium status than total plasma calcium. Normal range of plasma ionized calcium is 4–5 mg/100 mL (NRC, 2001).

Calcium Requirements of Sheep

The calcium requirements were determined by the factorial method. ARC (1980) estimated requirements for maintenance based on total endogenous loss of 16 mg/kg BW per day mainly through fecal loss (AFRC, 1991). These fecal losses can be estimated by dry matter intake (DMI, kg/d) (NRC, 1985; AFRC, 1991). Absorption coefficients used to calculate dietary requirements are variable (ARC, 1980; Braithwaite, 1983; NRC, 1985; Chrisp et al., 1989; AFRC, 1991). Maintenance requirements of sheep were estimated using the equation developed by AFRC (1991) and the 0.40 absorption coefficient used in the previous edition (NRC, 1985).

$$\text{Requirement of calcium for maintenance, g/d} = \frac{0.623 \times \text{DMI} + 0.228}{0.40}$$

Calcium deposited in weight gain of lambs was estimated as 11 g/kg of empty body gain in previous recommendations (ARC, 1980; NRC, 1985). However, bone growth declines as the animal approaches maturity (AFRC, 1991). In this report, sheep maturity was considered to estimate energy and protein requirements. Therefore, the AFRC (1991) approach to estimate calcium requirements for growth was used. Calcium absorption coefficients used previously to estimate requirements for growing lambs were 0.60 (NRC, 1985) and 0.68 (ARC, 1980; AFRC, 1991). The committee adopted the value of 0.68 for calcium absorption by growing lambs.

$$\text{requirement of Ca for growth, g/d} = \frac{(0.623 \times \text{DMI} + 0.228) + (\text{ADG} \times 6.75 \times \text{MW}^{0.28} \times \text{BW}^{0.28})}{0.68}$$

where DMI = dry matter intake, kg/d; ADG = average daily weight gain, kg; MW = mature weight, kg; and BW = actual body weight, kg.

The requirements of calcium for lactating sheep were estimated considering milk yield (MY, kg/d) and 1.6 g Ca/kg milk (ARC, 1980). The absorption coefficient used was 0.50 for yearling and mature ewes. The previous recommendation used 1.8 g Ca/kg milk and 0.60 absorption coefficient (NRC, 1985).

$$\text{requirement of Ca for lactation, g/d} = \frac{(0.623 \times \text{DMI} + 0.228) + (1.6 \times \text{MY})}{0.50}$$

Calcium requirements for gestating ewes were calculated for the periods 105–133 days, and the last 14 days of gestation. It was calculated from ARC (1980) that calcium deposited in the conceptus was 0.214 and 0.329 g/day for each kg of lamb born, respectively. The absorption coefficient used was 0.50 (NRC, 1985).

$$\text{requirement of Ca for gestation (105 to 133d), g/d} = \frac{(0.623 \times \text{DMI} + 0.228) + (0.214 \times \text{LBW})}{0.50}$$

$$\text{requirement of Ca for gestation (133 to 147d), g/d} = \frac{(0.623 \times \text{DMI} + 0.228) + (0.329 \times \text{LBW})}{0.50}$$

where LBW = typical birth weight of the litter, kg.

In the case of gestating yearling ewes, an additional amount of calcium was added considering a growth rate of 75 g/day and 75 percent maturity based on the estimation of calcium deposited in weight gain.

Calcium Requirements of Goats

A number of factors in modern livestock husbandry have contributed to increased calcium requirements. These factors include (1) animal selection and genetic improvement for faster growth rates and higher milk production; (2) use of high-energy grain mixes, which are generally low in calcium; (3) use of rapidly growing improved pastures, which may dilute calcium concentration in plants; (4) early weaning and changing from a milk diet to solids with less efficient calcium utilization; (5) early breeding when animals are still growing; (6) raising animals indoors with lack of sunlight and vitamin D_3; (7) enforcing intensive grazing vs. browse with increased parasite load; and (8) use of antibiotics, hormones, or other growth stimulants.

Calcium required for maintenance, growth, pregnancy, and lactation was estimated by the factorial method and adjusted according to the latest data available (Haenlein, 1992; AFRC, 1997; Meschy, 2000). The AFRC (1997) approach was used applying adjustments using sheep and cattle data where necessary. Estimates of requirements for total daily calcium were from endogenous losses (maintenance) and requirements for gain, fetal growth during pregnancy, and lactation and using absorption coefficient estimates. Endogenous losses of calcium, the basis for estimating the maintenance requirement, are more related to DMI than body weight (Pfeffer, 1989). Maintenance calcium requirements were recommended as 20 mg/kg BW (Kessler, 1991; Haenlein, 1992). In the absence of recent data for endogenous losses of calcium in goats and with the commitment to the factorial approach, data for sheep are used in these calculations. Meschy (2000) suggested the following equation for calculating endogenous calcium losses. Calcium requirements for maintenance were calculated using the equation suggested by Meschy (2000) and a 0.40 absorption coefficient.

$$\text{requirement of Ca for maintenance, g/d} = \frac{0.623 \times \text{DMI} + 0.228}{0.40}$$

Required calcium for gain was estimated to be 9.4 g/kg live weight (LW) gain for goats (Meschy, 2000) after considering the range for sheep of 8.2–12.9 g/kg LW gain and decreasing with age. However, AFRC (1997) used requirements ranging from 10.9–16.2 g/kg LW for cattle. The committee agrees with and accepts the principle that proportion of skeletal mass decreases with age, and goats generally have higher bone ratio in the body than sheep (AFRC, 1997). New findings (Pfeffer and Keunecke, 1986; Pfeffer, 1989; Pfeffer et al., 1995) suggest that calcium accretion is slightly lower in goats than it is in sheep, which leads to the adoption of the value of 11 g/kg LW gain.

Calcium required for pregnancy depends on size and number of kids carried. This requirement is for the mineralization of fetuses and should only be considered during the last third of pregnancy. The calcium concentration in newborn fetuses is estimated at 11.5 g/kg fetal weight (Pfeffer and Keunecke, 1986; Pfeffer and Rodehutscord, 1998; Kessler, 1991). Therefore, 0.23 g Ca/kg fetus weight per day for the last 50 days of pregnancy is needed.

Calcium required for lactation depends on calcium concentration in milk and amount of milk produced. The calcium concentration of goat's milk decreases from early to late lactation and is reported to be 1.18–1.40 g/kg milk with a median of 1.26 g/kg of milk (Schmidely et al., 2002; Guéguen, 1997). The committee recommends using 1.4 g Ca required for 1 kg milk.

Several factors can contribute to variation in the absorption coefficient for calcium including source, levels of calcium and other minerals in the diet, and the mineral status and physiological state of animal. Values of 30 percent (Kessler, 1991) and 55 percent (AFRC, 1997) have been adopted. There are no sufficient data to differentiate the absorption coefficients for maintenance, gain, or lactation; therefore, the committee recommends adoption of a more moderate value of 0.45 with caution and that it should be used under normal conditions.

Calcium Requirements of Cervids

For wildlife species, calcium and phosphorus requirements have been expressed as dietary contents together because of the close ratio of Ca:P = 2:1 in the skeletal bone (Widdowson and Dickerson, 1964; Ullrey et al., 1973, 1975; Robbins, 1993). Thus, although 98 percent of calcium and 80 percent of phosphorus in the body is in bone, both minerals are important for many body functions other than structural. The composition and density of bones and antlers change with age and productivity, which limits the use of expressing requirements as a dietary concentration. Reported requirements for growing animals range from 0.4–1.2 percent Ca and 0.3–0.6 percent P on a DM basis (Ullrey et al., 1973, 1975; Ullrey, 1983; Stephenson and Brown, 1984; Robbins, 1993).

Estimation of requirements based on the factorial system has the limitation of few studies to verify the accuracy. Nevertheless, estimates have been made of calcium requirements for maintenance based on interspecies comparisons of published value for calcium intake with excretion (Robbins, 1993). Daily endogenous calcium loss was 22–28 (mean 25) mg/kg BW and 28–39 percent of the calcium intake was retained (Stephenson and Brown, 1984; Robbins, 1993). Calcium balance was achieved at a daily intake of 73 mg/kg BW.

For male cervids, antler growth has an added significant requirement for calcium; however, antler growth rates are not well documented in all species. During antler growth absorption increases to greater than the 30 percent noted at maintenance, and endogenous calcium loss decreases (Stephenson and Brown, 1984; Brown, 1990). Thus, calcium requirements for antler growth in white-tailed deer and red deer are considered to be low. Ullrey (1983) reported a mean calcium requirement for antler deposition of 0.5–1.0 g/d over the entire growth period for young white-tailed deer. For caribou the demand is nearly 15-fold higher at 15 g/d (Moen and Pastor, 1988), suggesting a relatively greater mineral requirement for antler growth in *Rangifer*. Requirement is clearly related to antler weight, and also to antler growth rate, with maximum demand in the final 20 percent of the growth period. For male caribou, this maximum requirement is approximately 24 g/d (Moen and Pastor, 1988); for white-tailed deer, it is approximately 2.5–3.0 g/d. However, given that marked seasonal storage and cyclical osteoporosis as skeletal calcium is used to support antler growth (Brown, 1990; Baxter et al., 1999), a more reasonable estimate of calcium requirement is probably that associated with the entire growing period.

Calcium concentration in newborn fetuses is estimated at 11.5 g/kg fetal weight (Pfeffer and Keunecke, 1986; Kessler, 1991; Pfeffer and Rodehutscord, 1998). Fetus and conceptus growth rate was calculated assuming the interspecies relation of birth weight and maternal body weight (Oftedal, 1985) and a fetal relative growth rate of 2.1 percent/d in the final trimester (Robbins and Moen, 1975).

For lactation, calcium requirements at a daily peak milk output are 1.5–2.0 (mean 1.75) percent of body weight (Oftedal, 1985) and a mean calcium content of 0.3 g/100 g milk (Jenness and Sloan, 1970; Luick et al., 1974).

In analyses of calcium requirements for maintenance, the effect of DMI on endogenous calcium loss was not estimated as it has been for other small ruminants. If it is assumed that endogenous calcium loss increases by ~ 0.25 g/kg increase in DMI, the following equation can be derived:

$$\text{Ca requirement for maintenance (g/d)} = (0.025 \times \text{BW} + 0.25 \times \text{DMI})/0.34$$

where BW is in kg, DMI in kg/d, 0.025 = endogenous Ca loss (g/kg BW), and 0.34 = Ca retained/Ca fed. This equation predicts a winter dietary requirement of 0.45–0.6 percent for white-tailed deer to elk/wapiti, but when voluntary daily DMI exceeds 100 g/kg$^{0.75}$ in summer, the high DMI results in a dietary requirement of 0.24–0.3 percent.

A summary of the net deposition of calcium in body gain, fetal growth, antler growth, and lactation is listed below and is based on equations from references listed in the discussion above.

Net Ca requirement for body weight gain was assumed to be 11 g/kg ADG.

Net Ca requirement of the fetus near term (g/d) = $11.5 \times 0.166 \times \text{kg BW}^{0.90} \times 0.021$

Net Ca requirement for antler growth (g/d) = $0.05 \times$ kg BW (except reindeer/caribou)

Net Ca requirement for antler growth (g/d) = $0.11 \times$ kg BW (male reindeer/caribou)

Net Ca requirement for antler growth (g/d) = $0.03 \times$ kg BW (female reindeer/caribou)

Net Ca requirement for peak lactation (g/d) = $0.0175 \times$ kg BW $\times$ 3.2

To calculate the total requirements for calcium it was assumed that net deposition of calcium was corrected for the efficiency in calcium retention, usually 0.39, and added to maintenance requirements, viz:

Ca requirement for growth = Ca for maintenance + (net Ca for growth/0.39)

Ca requirement for lactation = Ca for maintenance + (net Ca for peak milk/0.39)

Ca requirement for males = Ca for maintenance + (net Ca for growth + net Ca for antlers)/0.39

Ca requirement for reindeer females = Ca for maintenance + (net Ca for milk + net Ca for antlers)/0.39

Calcium Deficiencies

Calcium deficiency leads to rickets in young animals, osteomalacia in adults, and milk fever in lactating ewes and does. Rickets is also caused by phosphorus or vitamin D_3 deficiency. The bone is less resistant and may fracture, and teeth are soft with irregular wear (see also Chapter 13 for more information on hypocalcemia or milk fever). Cereals are very deficient in calcium; therefore, high-grain diets for growing animals are prone to cause rickets. It may be shown as knock-knees, bowed legs, or Z-form of legs. The Ca:phosphorus (P) ratio in cereals is < 1, which also may cause urolithiasis.

Calcium Toxicities

The maximum dietary calcium level is 1.5 percent of diet dry matter (NRC, 2005), which is lower than the previously accepted value of 2.0 percent (NRC, 1980). Calcium toxicity leads to hypercalcemia and soft tissue calcification (McDowell, 1989). It may arise from plants containing the active metabolite of vitamin D_3 (see the section on vitamin D_3 in Chapter 8).

Calcium Sources

Calcium is one of the least costly nutrients. Sources include calcium carbonate, limestone, calcium chloride, dicalcium phosphate, and soft rock. Legumes are particularly rich in calcium with a relatively high Ca:P ratio. Cereal grains are extremely deficient in calcium and rich in phosphorus. Therefore, mineral supplements for high-grain diets should have high calcium and low or nil phosphorus concentrations. The opposite applies to animals fed forages under most conditions, except where heavy and continuous phosphorus fertilization of crops is practiced.

PHOSPHORUS

Phosphorus (P) is one of the essential elements in the animal's diet that represents the most potential risk for environmental pollution. Therefore, its level in the diet should be accurate for optimum animal performance with minimum environmental impact. Phosphorus is a structural component of bone and teeth, in the form of hydroxyapatite, and an important component of many metabolically active compounds. Energy storage and release compounds (ATP/ADP), genetic material (nucleic acids), cell membranes (phospholipids), nerve tissue, and many coenzymes essential for metabolic activity contain phosphorus. Maintenance of acid-base balance depends on the ratio of HPO_4^{-2} and $H_2PO_4^{-1}$.

Normal range of phosphorus in plasma is 4–6 mg/100 mL in adults and 6–9 mg/100 mL in young domestic ruminants. Plasma concentrations outside these ranges affect animal performance. However, the normal range in cervids is higher at 5–13 mg/100 mL (Staaland et al., 1984; Grasman and Hellgren, 1993).

Phosphorus Utilization and Homeostasis

The main site of phosphorus absorption is the small intestine (Bravo et al., 2003a). Phosphorus homeostasis is achieved through secretion into the saliva, variable absorption, renal excretion, and bone mobilization and storage. The main route of endogenous phosphorus excretion is via feces (Bravo et al., 2003b). The fecal endogenous phosphorus represents 85 percent of total fecal phosphorus, mostly from saliva. Phosphorus excretion via urine may be important when dietary phosphorus is above 5 g/kg DMI (Bravo et al., 2003b; Dove and Charmley, 2004).

Phosphorus Requirements of Sheep

The maintenance requirement of phosphorus for sheep was estimated based on total endogenous loss and an absorption coefficient. ARC (1965) estimated this loss as 42.5 mg/kg BW, which later was reduced to 14 mg/kg BW (ARC, 1980). NRC (1985) calculated total endogenous loss as 20 mg/kg BW per day for sheep at maintenance, early gestation, and growing. However, for late gestation and during lactation, the total endogenous loss of phosphorus was increased to 30 mg/kg BW. AFRC (1991) ignored endogenous losses in urine and estimated total endogenous loss based on DMI of high-quality diets with the following equation:

$$P,\ g/d = 0.693 \times DMI - 0.06$$

For diets with up to 50 percent forages, AFRC (1991) applied a 1.6 factor to the equation given above to compensate for salivary flow of phosphorus, which is the main determinant of fecal endogenous phosphorus (Bravo et al., 2003b). NRC (2001) estimated fecal losses of dairy cattle as 1.0 g P/kg DMI for cows and 0.8 g P/kg DMI for growing animals. However, they added 0.002 g P/kg BW as estimator of endogenous urinary loss. The absorption coefficient used by NRC (1985) to estimate maintenance requirements was 0.60, the same coefficient suggested for mature sheep (ARC, 1980). AFRC (1991) used 0.64 and 0.70 as absorption coefficients for low- or high-quality diets, respectively. Bravo et al. (2003a) found a mean absorption coefficient of 0.72 for growing sheep. For pregnant and lactating ewes, the corresponding values were 0.56 and 0.71. Phosphorus absorption depends on intake (NRC, 2001; Bravo et al., 2003a) and type of feedstuffs. NRC (2001) used a value of 0.64 for forages and 0.70 for concentrates. In this publication, the phosphorus requirements for maintenance of sheep were calculated using the following formula:

$$P \text{ requirement for maintenance, g/d} = \frac{1.6 \times (0.603 \times DMI - 0.06)}{0.60}$$

Previous estimations of phosphorus requirements for growth considered 6 g phosphorus deposited/kg empty body gain (ARC, 1980; NRC, 1985). However, it was adopted to formulate the requirements considering sheep maturity, and the corresponding changes in phosphorus deposition in bone (AFRC, 1991). The following formula was used to estimate the phosphorus requirements of growing animals. This approach intends to minimize use of dietary phosphorus, environmental contamination, and urinary calculi incidence.

$$P \text{ requirement for growth, g/d} = \frac{(0.693 \times DMI - 0.06) + (ADG \times (1.2 + 3.188 \times MW^{0.28} \times BW^{-0.28}))}{0.72}$$

where DMI = dry matter intake, kg/d; ADG = average daily weight gain, kg; MW = mature weight, kg; and BW = actual body weight, kg.

The requirements of phosphorus for lactating sheep were estimated considering milk yield (MY, kg/d) and 1.3 g P/kg milk (ARC, 1980). The absorption coefficient used was 0.60 for yearling and mature ewes. The previous recommendation used 1.4 g P/kg milk and 0.70 as an absorption coefficient (NRC, 1985). The 1.6 factor to estimate maintenance requirements was included for mature ewes, but deleted for yearling ewes.

$$P \text{ requirement for lactation, g/d} = \frac{(1.6 \times (0.693 \times DMI - 0.06)) + (1.3 \times MY)}{0.60}$$

Phosphorus requirements for gestating ewes were calculated for the period 105–133 days, and the last 14 days of gestation. It was calculated from ARC (1980) that phosphorus deposited in the conceptus was 0.111 and 0.138 g/day for each kg of lamb born, respectively. The absorption coefficient used was 0.60. The previous recommendation (NRC,

1985) considered the same source of data for phosphorus deposition during gestation. However, requirements were calculated for the first 15 weeks and the last 4 weeks of gestation. Absorption coefficients used were 0.60 and 0.70, respectively. Most gestating ewes are fed forages with absorption coefficients lower than 0.70 (NRC, 2001). Therefore it was decided to use a 0.60 absorption coefficient.

$$\text{P requirement for gestation (105 to 133d), g/day} = \frac{(1.6 \times (0.693 \times \text{DMI} - 0.06)) + (0.111 \times \text{LBW})}{0.60}$$

$$\text{P requirement for gestation (133 to 147d), g/day} = \frac{(1.6 \times (0.693 \times \text{DMI} - 0.06)) + (0.138 \times \text{LBW})}{0.60}$$

where LBW = typical birth weight of the litter, kg.

In the case of gestating yearling ewes, an additional amount of phosphorus was added considering a growth rate of 75 g/day, and 75 percent maturity based on the estimation of phosphorus deposited in weight gain.

Phosphorus Requirements of Goats

Requirement for phosphorus in the diets of modern, higher-performing animals has increased as it has for calcium. Adequate supply of phosphorus to the animal depends on the chemical form of phosphorus, vitamin D_3 status of animal and diet, level of performance, and level of calcium in the diet. The total phosphorus required for maintenance, growth, pregnancy, and lactation was estimated by a factorial method (AFRC, 1997) using the latest collections of goat data where possible (Haenlein, 1992; AFRC, 1997; Meschy, 2000), and sheep and cattle data to make adjustments where necessary.

Maintenance requirements are estimated based on endogenous fecal and urinary losses of phosphorus. Based on 138 balance trials, Pfeffer (1989) estimated phosphorus requirement for maintenance in goats with the following equation: P (g/day) = 0.081 + 0.88 DMI, where DMI is in kg/day. This estimate was later confirmed by Deitert and Pfeffer (1993) and seems adequate but is lower than the phosphorus maintenance requirements for sheep and cattle adapted for goats by AFRC (1997). This difference has been explained by Meschy (2000) that goats have better phosphorus recycling through saliva than through urea (Tisserand and Alrhamoun, 1998). In addition, the difference was supported by higher phosphorus concentration of saliva from goats than other ruminants (Kessler, 1991). This estimate of the maintenance requirement for phosphorus is similar to an estimate based on live body weight (30 mg/kg BW: Kessler, 1991; Haenlein, 1992), but is more reflective of changing conditions.

The phosphorus requirement for gain adopted from sheep data ranges from 5.1–7.3 g/kg LW gain, decreasing with age. However, AFRC (1997) used requirements ranging from 6.3–8.8 g/kg LW gain as used for cattle. Although goats generally have a higher bone ratio in the body than sheep (AFRC, 1997), they probably recycle phosphorus better and have higher phosphorus concentrations in saliva. Therefore, the use of a lower value of 6.5 g P/kg LW gain for goats is recommended.

Phosphorus required for pregnancy depends on size and number of kids carried. This requirement is for the mineralization of fetuses and should be considered only during the last 50 days of pregnancy. The average phosphorus composition of newborn kids is 6.6 g/kg BW (Pfeffer and Keunecke, 1986; Kessler, 1991; Pfeffer and Rodehutscord, 1998). Therefore, the phosphorus requirement is calculated as 0.132 g/kg fetus per day for the last 50 days of pregnancy.

Phosphorus required for lactation depends on phosphorus concentration in milk and amount of milk produced. The phosphorus concentration of goat's milk decreases from early to late lactation and ranges from 0.92–1.06 g/kg milk with a median of 0.97 g/kg of milk (Guéguen, 1997; Schmidely et al., 2002). The recommendation here is 1 g P/kg of milk.

The true absorption coefficient (TAC) for phosphorus in goats is determined to be 65 percent, understanding that this value is higher than the 60 percent coefficient used for sheep and will vary depending on many factors. Total absorption coefficient for phosphorus seems to be higher in goats (Meschy, 2000). Values of 65 percent (Kessler, 1991), 75 percent (Pfeffer, 1989), and 64–70 percent (AFRC, 1997) have been used.

Phosphorus Requirements of Cervids

Estimates have been made of phosphorus requirements for maintenance based on interspecies comparisons of phosphorus balance at maintenance and when growing antlers in males (French et al., 1956; Ullrey et al., 1975; Grassman and Hellgren, 1993). These estimates were used as a basis for using the factorial approach to estimating net phosphorus deposited and dietary requirements. Daily DMI was not used as a determinant of requirements, as is recommended for sheep and goats. Net phosphorus requirements were expressed on BW or $BW^{0.75}$ basis.

In cervids, as in other ruminants, endogenous phosphorus loss originates as saliva, with most saliva phosphorus being reabsorbed by the small intestines (Staaland et al., 1984). Regression of fecal phosphorus loss against phosphorus intake yields a daily endogenous fecal loss of 12 mg/kg for white-tailed deer and reindeer (Staaland et al., 1984; Grasman and Hellgren, 1993); an estimate similar to that for sheep and goats. The daily endogenous urinary phosphorus loss is low compared with endogenous fecal loss at approximately 0.3 mg/kg BW (Muir et al., 1987). To apply the factorial approach to estimate dietary requirement, an estimate of the coefficient of absorption (A) is needed. Few determinations of

A are available; however in cervids as in other ruminants, A varies with phosphorus intake, and probably is higher during pregnancy and lactation (ARC, 1980). For two studies, A was 0.6 in reindeer in winter (Staaland et al., 1984) and 0.43 for white-tailed deer in summer (Grasman and Hellgren, 1993), but in both studies A became negative when phosphorus balance was negative. Using these estimates of daily endogenous losses and an A of 0.6, expected dietary phosphorus requirement for maintenance is 12/0.6, or 20 mg/kg BW. Phosphorus balance for maintenance in males after completion of antlerogenesis was achieved at a daily intake of 21 mg/kg BW (59 mg/kg $BW^{0.75}$; Grasman and Hellgren, 1993). Thus, for nonproductive males, agreement between the factorial and balance approaches is excellent.

Phosphorus requirements of male deer are related to antler weight and also to antler growth rate, with maximum demand in the final 20 percent of the growth period (approximately 49 days). Because antler size and growth increase hyperallometrically with BW (kg $BW^{1.33-1.63}$) (Grasman and Hellgren, 1993; Moen and Pastor, 1998), larger cervids have proportionally larger phosphorus requirements. For white-tailed deer growing antlers at 26 g DM/kg $BW^{0.75}$ (621 g/d), daily phosphorus intake to achieve balance is 35 mg/kg (94 mg/kg $BW^{0.75}$; Grasman and Hellgren, 1993). At a daily net phosphorus deposition in antlers of white-tailed deer (29 mg/kg $BW^{0.75}$, 10 mg/kg BW), the daily net requirement is 12 + 10, or 22 mg/kg BW and the daily dietary requirement is 22/0.6, or 37 mg/kg BW (103 mg/kg $BW^{0.75}$), which is only 10 percent greater than the phosphorus intake that achieves phosphorus balance in male white-tailed deer growing antlers (Grasman and Hellgren, 1993). For male caribou, the maximum phosphorus requirement is approximately 12 g/d from day 65 to 97 of antler growth (Moen and Pastor, 1988); for white-tailed deer, it is approximately 0.6 g/d. Thus, whereas the phosphorus requirements to produce antlers in white-tailed deer are less than those for pregnancy and lactation (Brown, 1990; Grasman and Hellgren, 1993), for caribou, a species that produces the largest antlers per unit BW, the total phosphorus requirement of large males (approximately 0.95 kg) exceeds that of the combined requirements for gestation, lactation, and antler growth in females (approximately 0.25 kg) (Moen and Pastor, 1998). Simulation analysis suggests that large male caribou may need to draw down as much as 50 percent of their phosphorus deposited in antlers from bones to meet antlerogenesis requirements, whereas no draw down may be necessary for small deer species (Grasman and Hellgren, 1993; Moen and Pastor, 1998).

The phosphorus requirement for body growth of 6.5 g P/kg BW gain for goats is recommended for cervids.

Phosphorus concentration in newborn fetuses is estimated at 6.6 g/kg fetal weight (Pfeffer and Keunecke, 1986; Kessler, 1991; Pfeffer and Rodehutscord, 1998) in the last 50 days of pregnancy. Fetus and conceptus growth rates were calculated assuming the interspecies relationship of birth weight and maternal body weight (Oftedal, 1985) and a fetal relative growth rate of 2.1 percent/d in the final trimester (Robbins and Moen, 1975).

For lactation, phosphorus requirement was estimated at a daily peak milk output of 1.5–2.0 (mean 1.75) percent of body weight (Oftedal, 1985), and a mean phosphorus content of 0.24 g/100 g milk for the first three weeks of lactation (Jenness and Sloan, 1970; Luick et al., 1974).

Using the factorial approach, the following equations were used to estimate net and dietary requirements for phosphorus:

$$\text{Dietary P requirement for maintenance (g/d)} = (12 + 0.3)\ \text{mg/kg BW/A}$$

Where 12 and 0.3 are, respectively, the endogenous fecal and urinary phosphorus losses (g/kg BW) and A is the coefficient of phosphorus absorption (0.4–0.6). A summary of the net deposition of phosphorus in body gain, fetal growth, antler growth, and lactation is listed below and is based on equations from references listed in the discussion above.

Net P requirement for body weight gain was assumed to be 6.5 g/kg ADG.

Net P requirements of the fetus near term (g/d) = $6.6 \times 0.166 \times \text{kg BW}^{0.90} \times 0.021$

Net P requirements for antler growth (g/d) = $0.029 \times$ kg BW (except reindeer/caribou)

To calculate the dietary requirements for phosphorus it was assumed that net deposition of phosphorus was corrected for A, usually 0.4–0.6, and added to maintenance requirements, viz:

P requirement for growth = P for maintenance + (net P for growth/A)

P requirement for lactation = P for maintenance + (net P for peak milk/A)

P requirement for males = P for maintenance + (net P for growth + net P for antlers)/A

P requirement for reindeer females = P for maintenance + (net P for milk + net P for antlers)/A

Phosphorus Deficiencies

A phosphorus deficiency causes reductions in feed intake and pica in ruminants. Other visible conditions and symptoms include reduced weight gain, poor bone mineralization leading to bone deformation (see the section above on calcium deficiencies), estrus suppression and poor conception rates, and lowered milk production (Underwood and Suttle, 1999). Phosphorus deficiencies may be found under range conditions because of low phosphorus and high calcium in the forages (Preston et al., 1977; Ramirez et al., 2001). Ruminant species that include greater proportions of leaves and legumes in their diets are less prone to the deficiency under grazing conditions, due to the higher phosphorus content in leaves and legumes in comparison with stems and grasses (Minson, 1990).

Phosphorus Excess

Cereals have excessive phosphorus in relation to calcium, which may lead to urinary calculi formation and skeletal softening. Maximum tolerable level of phosphorus in diet dry matter is 0.6 percent (NRC, 2005). The greatest concern with phosphorus may be related to the Ca:P ratio. The Ca:P ratio may affect absorption of calcium or phosphorus when either is > 7:1 or < 1:1 (ARC, 1980), although when phosphorus is deficient, a Ca:P ratio of 3.6 was detrimental for sheep (Wan Zahari et al., 1990). However, when phosphorus is adequate, a Ca:P ratio of 5.4 does not affect sheep performance (Rajaratne et al., 1990). Management practices of crops and manure distribution lead to phosphorus runoff and eutrophication (Sharpley et al., 2003). However, they may also decrease the Ca:P ratio in forages. This problem may be more important in regions with soil pH close to neutral, where phosphorus uptake by plants is highest.

Phosphorus Sources

Phosphorus is the most expensive component of mineral mixtures. Sources include dicalcium phosphate, soft rock, monosodic phosphate, monoammonium phosphate, and bone meal. One problem associated with some phosphorus sources may be their high content of fluorine (NRC, 1980). The risk of transmissible spongiform encephalopathies in bone meal prevents its use as a calcium and phosphorus source in several countries. Grains are rich in phytic acid, which depresses phosphorus availability (Bravo et al., 2003a); however, phytase activity of ruminal microorganisms renders most of the phosphorus available for absorption (Clark et al., 1986). Phytase activity in the rumen may be limited under some conditions (Godoy and Meschy, 2001).

SODIUM AND CHLORINE

Sodium (Na) and chlorine (Cl) are considered together because of their close ionic relationship and because they usually are provided to animals as common salt (NaCl). Salt is fed to provide sodium and chlorine, as an incentive for animals to consume other mineral elements or feeds, and as a limiter of feed consumption. However, in the body, sodium and chlorine function independently in many roles. The abundance, low cost, palatability, and low toxicity of common salt have encouraged liberal use of this mineral. However, energy cost to animals (Arieli et al., 1989) and environmental concerns necessitate determining the requirements more accurately.

Sodium is important for the absorption of chlorine, amino acids, glucose, and water and is associated with potassium in maintaining ionic balance in body fluids. Sodium is absorbed from the rumen, omasum, and intestines with a 91 percent apparent absorption (ARC, 1980). In some winter diets of cervids sodium absorption is less than 90 percent and can be negative for reindeer and caribou fed diets high in lichen (White et al., 1984). Sheep, goats, and deer absorb more sodium in the large intestines than cattle, which causes feces to have greater dry matter content than that of cattle. Under free grazing, sodium supply in plants varies seasonally (Staaland and White, 2001) and many species including cattle, sheep, goats, and deer may become sodium insufficient or deficient (Blair-West et al., 1968; Weeks and Kirkpatrick, 1976; Hyvärinen et al., 1977; Staaland et al., 1980; Åhman et al., 1986; Robbins 1993). These animals display an innate appetite for sodium (Denton and Sabine, 1961) and may visit regions rich in sodium either as aquatic vegetation or mineral licks (Weir, 1972; Fraser and Reardon, 1980; Calef and Lortie, 1975; Staaland et al., 1986; Staaland and White, 2001). Providing sodium as salt blocks can alleviate seasonal sodium deficiencies.

Sodium forms part of diverse transport systems such as Na/K pump, Na-H antiporter, Na-HCO_3-Cl co-transporter, Na-K-Cl co-transporter, Na-Ca exchanger, and Na^+ channel. These transporters are important in glucose and amino acid uptake by tissues, maintenance of body temperature, neuromuscular activation, and nerve function. Normal plasma values range from 3,200–3,500 mg Na/L (Kaneko, 1989).

Chlorine is vital in the digestion of protein, absorption of amino acids and minerals, regulation of osmotic pressure, and maintenance of acid-base balance (Underwood and Suttle, 1999). The body contains 0.10–0.11 percent chlorine, mainly in extracellular fluids. Normal plasma values for sheep are 3,367–3,652 mg/L (Puls, 1994). Chlorine is absorbed from the rumen in adults and from the small intestine in young and adult animals. Chlorine is secreted into the omasum in exchange for bicarbonate and as HCl into the abomasum, where it enhances digestion. The coefficient of absorption is approximately 85 percent, but can be as high as 98 percent of consumption (ARC, 1980; White et al., 1984). Of chlorine excreted, more than 90 percent of it is via urine.

Because estimates of chlorine requirements are not available for cervid species it is recommended that those for sheep and goats be used.

Sodium and Chlorine Requirements of Sheep and Goats

Sodium requirements were estimated for sheep and goats using a factorial approach considering maintenance, growth, pregnancy, and lactation. ARC (1980) estimated the sodium requirements for maintenance in sheep considering 5.8 mg fecal loss and 20.0 mg urinary loss per kg BW, and 0.91 absorption coefficient. However, the sodium requirements obtained with these calculations are higher than found under practical feeding conditions (NRC, 1985; Michell, 1995). Towers et al. (1984) found responses in ewes to sodium supplementation when the forage contained 0.07 percent sodium. Underwood and Suttle (1999) used 5 mg sodium as urinary loss to calculate maintenance requirement of sheep. The requirement of sodium for growth 1.1 g/kg LW gain considered the amount of sodium deposited in the weight gain (ARC, 1980) and average daily gain (ADG, kg), which is similar to that adopted by Underwood and Suttle (1999). The sodium requirements for gestating ewes were calculated for the period 105–133 days, and the last 14 days of gestation. It was calculated from ARC (1980) that sodium deposited in the conceptus was 0.021 and 0.013 g/day for each kg of lamb born. The yearling ewes require additional amounts of sodium, which are calculated based on their growth and the sodium deposited in weight gain given previously. The sodium content of milk given by NRC (1985) and also used by NRC (1980) is 0.4 g/kg milk.

Studies with goats are more limited. Schellner (1972/73) found 0.3 g Na/kg DM was inadequate to maintain growth, lactation, and reproduction in goats and 1.7 g Na/kg DM was sufficient. Many other authors have made recommendations for sodium or salt consumption as a percentage of DM, amount/head, or amount/kg milk (Eriksson et al., 1976; NRC, 1981; Kessler, 1991; Haenlein, 1992; AFRC, 1997; Meschy, 2000), based on observations or extended from data with other species. In order to estimate total daily sodium requirement, endogenous losses of sodium, sodium required for gain, late pregnancy, lactation, and true absorption coefficient should be estimated. These estimates were derived from data or recommendations reported by a number of researchers (Pfeffer and Keunecke, 1986; Kessler, 1991; Haenlein, 1992; Guéguen, 1997; Pfeffer and Rodehutscord, 1998; Stelwagen et al., 1999; Meschy, 2000).

Chlorine requirements for sheep and goats were determined from limited data and recommendations from various sources (ARC, 1980; NRC, 1985; Pfeffer and Keunecke, 1986; Guéguen et al., 1989; Kessler, 1991; Guéguen, 1997; Pfeffer and Rodehutscord, 1998; NRC, 2001).

Below are the equations used to estimate daily requirements for sodium and chlorine for sheep and goats with BW, ADG, LBW, and MY expressed in kg. Requirements for gestation in goats are estimated for the last 50 days of pregnancy.

Sodium and Chlorine Requirements of Sheep and Goats

Species and Class	Sodium	Chlorine
Sheep		
Maintenance, g/d	$(0.0108 \times BW)/0.91$	$= (0.0079 \times BW)/0.85$
Growth, g/d	$(1.1 \times ADG)/0.91$	$= (0.8 \times ADG)/0.85$
Gestation, g/d		
(105 to 133 d)	$(0.021 \times LBW)/0.91$	$= (0.015 \times LBW)/0.85$
(133 to 147 d)	$(0.013 \times LBW)/0.91$	$= (0.009 \times LBW)/0.85$
Lactation, g/d	$(0.4 \times MY)/0.91$	$= (1.1 \times MY)/0.85$
Goats		
Maintenance, g/d	$(0.015 \times BW)/0.80$	$= (0.022 \times BW)/0.80$
Growth, g/d	$(1.6 \times LWG)/0.80$	$= (1.0 \times LWG)/0.80$
Gestation, g/d	$(0.034 \times LBW)/0.80$	$= (0.024 \times LBW)/0.80$
Lactation, g/d	$(0.4 \times MY)/0.80$	$= (1.1 \times MY)/0.80$

Sodium Requirements of Cervids

The recommended daily sodium requirements for maintenance in wildlife species is 9.0 mg/kg BW (Robbins, 1993). The coefficient of absorption was very high at 0.98. However, it may be too high for reindeer and caribou. In a dietary study comparing a high-quality, high-sodium, diet (786 mg/100 g) with that based on lichens with low sodium content (6–18 mg/100 g), the deduced daily excretion rates for feces and urine were 2.2 and 1.0 mg/kg BW, respectively, which gives a daily dietary sodium requirement of 3.2/0.98, or 3.3 mg/kg BW (Staaland et al., 1984; White et al., 1984). Staaland and White (2001) conclude that if the daily maintenance sodium requirement is 9.0 mg/kg BW, then reindeer and caribou must select for aquatic plants high in sodium, visit mineral licks, or migrate to coastal tundra ranges in order to make use of the higher sodium environment and to make up a seasonal sodium deficiency. If the maintenance sodium requirement is in fact approximately three times lower than that recommended by Robbins (1993), then reindeer and caribou could more easily meet requirements and only the most productive animals might become insufficient in sodium reserves on a seasonal basis. Thus, for deer in general it is recommended to use a daily dietary maintenance requirement of 9.0 mg/kg BW, and for reindeer/caribou to use a daily value of 3.2 mg/kg BW.

A summary of the net deposition of sodium in body gain, fetal growth, antler growth, and lactation is given as:

Net Na requirement for body weight gain was assumed to be 1.1 g/kg ADG (from sheep and goats

Net Na requirements of the fetus near term (g/d) = $0.013 \times 0.166 \times$ kg $BW^{0.90} \times 0.021$ (0.013 is sodium retention in concepta g/kg gain)

Net Na requirements for antler growth (g/d) = 5(mg/g) × 26 g/kg $BW^{0.75}$ (except reindeer/caribou)

Net Na requirements for antler growth (g/d) = 5(mg/g) × 182 g/kg BW (male reindeer/caribou)

Net Na requirements for antler growth (g/d) = 5mg/g × 20 g/kg BW (female reindeer/caribou)

Net Na requirement for peak lactation (g/d) = 0.0175 × kg BW × 32 mg/L

To calculate the dietary requirements for sodium it was assumed that net deposition of sodium was corrected for the absorption coefficient, usually 0.98, and added to maintenance requirements, viz:

Na requirement for growth = Na for maintenance + (net Na for growth/A)

Na requirement for lactation = Na for maintenance + (net Na for peak milk/A)

Na requirement for males = Na for maintenance + (net Na for growth + net Na for antlers)/A

Na requirement for reindeer females = Na for maintenance + (net Na for milk + net Na for antlers)/A

Sodium and Chlorine Deficiencies

Sodium deficiency is widespread worldwide (McDowell, 1997), because all types of feeds are deficient, except some bushes from semiarid regions (e.g., *Atriplex* spp.). Deficiency signs include pica and reduced feed intake and growth. Short-term deficiencies of sodium can not be detected in plasma. It is recommended to measure the Na:K ratio in saliva. When the ratio is below 4:1, then an incipient sodium deficiency is present (McSweeney et al., 1988).

Chloride deficiency has not been shown. Low chlorine levels in plasma can arise from water excess or metabolic alkalosis. Chloride can be of concern when sodium bicarbonate is added to fattening diets and salt is removed from the diet.

Sodium and Chlorine Toxicities

According to the literature reviewed, salt toxicity is reached with 4 percent salt in the diet DM (NRC, 2005). This value is considerably lower than the previous value of 9 percent reported (NRC, 1980) based on work of Meyer et al. (1955). When an animal ingests salt, water intake and urine excretion increase to eliminate the excess sodium consumed. However, when the physiological capacity to increase water intake and excrete urine is reached, the animal decreases its intake of salt. Salt intake is increased when it is provided free choice in a loose form than when provided in a block form (Smith et al., 1953). The addition of salt to supplements for grazing animals is an option used to limit supplement intake. High chlorine levels in plasma may result from dehydration or metabolic acidosis.

POTASSIUM

Potassium (K) is the main intracellular cation, and its major function is to maintain the membrane potential of the cells. Intracellular concentration of potassium is about 150 mM, while extracellular concentration is 5 mM. These concentrations are maintained by the Na-K ATPase pump, which drives nerve conduction, synaptic transmission, muscle contraction, fluid transport, hormone release, and embryonic development (Petersen, 1997). Potassium is a cofactor for enzymes like pyruvate kinase and activation of Na-K ATPase. Potassium is absorbed from the ruminoreticulum, omasum, and intestines of adult ruminants and is carried in the blood at levels ranging from 150 to 200 mg/L of plasma (Kaneko, 1989). Hopson et al. (1997) confirmed the same range for deer during an 11-month study. Hypokalemia or hyperkalemia result when potassium levels in plasma are below or above the normal range, respectively. When potassium increases in plasma due to dietary intake or exercise, insulin or catecholamines stimulate the Na-K ATPase, to restore potassium levels (Petersen, 1997). Hyperkalemia has been documented in deer with post-capture myopathy and during the rut, which may be due to protein catabolism (Hopson et al., 1997) or red cell hemolysis (Kaneko, 1989). Red cell damage arises when antioxidant nutrients are deficient. The main excretory route of excess potassium is the kidney, under the control of aldosterone. This hormone increases sodium resorption by the kidney with concomitant excretion of potassium.

Potassium Requirements of Sheep and Goats

Potassium is not stored in the body and should be supplied daily, but, under natural conditions, diets contain adequate supplies of potassium. According to summarized research, previous potassium recommendations for sheep (NRC, 1985) ranged from 0.50 to 0.80 percent of diet DM for growing animals and lactating ewes, respectively. Environmental concerns of contamination with potassium require diminishing its content in manure. The factorial approach used to estimate potassium requirements in this revision increases the precision and minimizes overfeeding.

The potassium requirements for sheep were determined for maintenance, growth, mid- and late pregnancy, and lactation. A 0.90 absorption coefficient (NRC, 2001) was used in these calculations. The maintenance requirements of potassium were calculated from endogenous fecal and urinary excretions estimated to be 2.6 g/kg DMI (NRC, 2001) and 0.038 g/kg BW (ARC, 1980), respectively. The requirements for growth considered 1.8 g potassium deposited per kg ADG (ARC, 1980). Fetal growth for the period 105–133 days and the last 14 days of gestation deposited 0.029 and 0.023 g/day, respectively, of potassium for each kg of lamb born (LBW) (ARC, 1980). Potassium requirements for lactating ewes were calculated considering 1.4 g potassium per kg milk (ARC, 1980).

Goat requirements for potassium proposed by AFRC (1997) were 5 g/kg DM for kids and 8 g/kg DM for lactating goats. A higher potassium level (12 g/kg DM) was beneficial when fed to goats; however, its possible negative impact on magnesium absorption (Fontenot, 1979) must be considered to ensure animals receive the recommended level of dietary magnesium. In using the factorial approach, potassium requirements for maintenance, growth, pregnancy during the last 50 days of gestation, and lactation were considered using limited goat data, applicable cattle and sheep data, and recommendations from several sources (Pfeffer and Keunecke, 1986; Kessler, 1991; Haenlein, 1992; AFRC,

1997; Guéguen, 1997; Pfeffer and Rodehutscord, 1998; Meschy, 2000; Aganga et al., 2002). An absorption coefficient of 0.90 was used in all calculations.

Below are the equations used to estimate daily requirements for potassium for sheep and goats with BW, ADG, LBW, and MY expressed in kg. Requirements for gestation in goats are estimated for the last 50 days of pregnancy.

Potassium Requirements of Sheep and Goats

Species and Class		
Sheep		
Maintenance, g/d	=	(2.6 × DMI + 0.038 × BW)/0.90
Growth, g/d	=	(1.8 × ADG)/0.90
Gestation, g/d		
(105 to 133 d)	=	(0.029 × LBW)/0.90
(133 to 147 d)	=	(0.023 × LBW)/0.90
Lactation, g/d	=	(1.4 × MY)/0.90
Goats		
Maintenance, g/d	=	(2.6 × DMI + 0.05 × BW)/0.90
Growth, g/d	=	(2.4 × ADG)/0.90
Gestation, g/d	=	(0.042 × LBW)/0.90
Lactation, g/d	=	(2.0 × MY)/0.90

Potassium Requirements of Cervids

Values are not available. The values for goats are recommended.

Potassium Deficiencies

Potassium deficiency could arise when animals are fed diets high in grain and low in forages, because grains contain between 0.32 and 0.50 percent potassium (Underwood and Suttle, 1999). Mature forages grown under range conditions and in soils low in potassium also may be low in potassium. Deficiency signs (Puls, 1994) include reduced growth and feed intake, emaciation, stiffness and humped back, muscle paralysis, and rhabdomyolysis (muscle cell death with release of contractile proteins).

Potassium Excess

The maximum tolerable level of potassium is 2.0 percent of diet dry matter (NRC, 2005), although most temperate grasses require between 2.0 and 3.5 percent potassium in their dry matter to ensure maximum yield (Underwood and Suttle, 1999). Forages from soils heavily fertilized with potassium or with large amounts of wastes/slurry from confinement livestock operations have more than 3.0 percent potassium (Wilkinson and Stuedemann, 1979). Therefore, many cultivated forages from the temperate regions will exceed the theoretical maximum tolerable level but are unlikely to cause toxicity symptoms except under prolonged consumption. The potassium excess may induce hypomagnesemia (grass tetany) or hypocalcemia (milk fever). Molasses also has potassium concentrations between 3 and 5 percent (Underwood and Suttle, 1999).

Potassium Sources

Potassium sources such as potassium chloride, potassium carbonate, potassium sulfate, potassium acetate, potassium bicarbonate, dibasic potassium phosphate, and potassium phosphate monohydrate are readily available sources (NRC, 2001). Good quality forages or molasses can be included in the diet as potassium sources, particularly with stressed animals in the receiving diets.

MAGNESIUM

Magnesium (Mg) is found in bone (70 percent), inside cells (29 percent), and in extracellular fluids (1 percent) and is required in more than 300 metabolic reactions associated with functions of energy production, synthesis of essential molecules, structural formations, ion transport, cell signaling, and cell migration (Shils, 1997). Adenosine triphosphate forms a complex with magnesium to participate in almost all metabolic processes to provide energy. Magnesium is required for the synthesis of nucleic acids and glutathione and for activity of several enzymes that participate in the synthesis of carbohydrates and lipids. Cell membranes, chromosomes, and bone require magnesium as a structural component. The transport of potassium and calcium across membranes requires magnesium, which affects conduction of nerve impulses and muscle contraction. The complex Mg-ATP is needed for phosphorylation of protein involved in cell signaling and also in the formation of cyclic adenosine monophosphate.

The normal concentrations of magnesium in plasma range from 1.8–3.5 mg/100 mL. Hypomagnesemia occurs when magnesium levels in plasma are between 1.0 and 1.8 mg/100 mL. Further decrease is usually accompanied by tetany (Underwood and Suttle, 1999).

Magnesium Absorption

The small intestine and ruminoreticulum are the primary sites for absorption of magnesium in young and adult animals, respectively (Littledike and Cox, 1979). Absorbability of the magnesium is the most important dietary consideration. Absorption depends on concentration of soluble magnesium and a sodium-linked transport system. Solubility of magnesium is high with low ruminal pH (< 6.5), a condition more likely to occur with concentrate feeds in comparison with forage diets. Spring forages are low in magnesium and high in potassium and are associated with low magnesium status in animals (Mayland and Grunes, 1979). Irrigated pastures with high levels of potassium and nitrogen fertilization are prone to induce tetany. This effect may be due to interference with magnesium absorption (Fontenot, 1979). Unsaturated fatty acids from forages are known to form insoluble complexes with magnesium. Aluminum ingestion with soil also may interfere with magnesium absorption (Fontenot et al., 1989).

Magnesium Requirements of Sheep and Goats

Dietary magnesium requirements for sheep and goats can vary with age, growth rate, or production. Magnesium status of the animal also may affect requirements, but bone resorption is very limited. The estimates of magnesium requirements have increased over the years to overcome problems associated with hypomagnesemia at parturition and, particularly, in early lactation ewes (NRC, 2001). The requirement values of 0.04–0.08 percent of diet dry matter (NRC, 1975) were increased to 0.12, 0.15, and 0.18 percent of dry matter for growing lambs, ewes in late gestation, and ewes in early lactation, respectively (NRC, 1985). Additionally, it was recommended to increase the dietary magnesium to 0.20 percent for early lactation ewes grazing forages high in nitrogen and potassium content.

In this edition, requirements of magnesium were estimated by the factorial method using available data (Pfeffer and Keunecke, 1986; Kessler, 1991; Haenlein, 1992; Guéguen, 1997; Pfeffer and Rodehutscord, 1998; Meschy, 2000; Aganga et al., 2002) and recommendations (ARC, 1980; AFRC, 1997). Absorption coefficients of 0.17 for sheep (ARC, 1980) and 0.20 for goats (Kessler, 1991) provide margins of safety to avoid grass tetany. Magnesium requirements for gestating ewes were calculated for the period 105–133 days and the last 14 days of gestation. In goats, requirements for gestation were calculated for the last 50 days of pregnancy.

Magnesium Requirements of Sheep and Goats

Species and Class

Sheep

Maintenance, g/d	=	$(0.003 \times BW)/0.17$
Growth, g/d	=	$(0.41 \times ADG)/0.17$
Gestation		
(105 to 133 d), g/d	=	$(0.009 \times LBW)/0.17$
(133 to 147 d), g/d	=	$(0.013 \times LBW)/0.17$
Lactation, g/d	=	$(0.17 \times MY)/0.17$

Goats

Maintenance, g/d	=	$(0.0035 \times BW)/0.20$
Growth, g/d	=	$(0.40 \times ADG)/0.20$
Gestation, g/d	=	$(0.006 \times LBW)/0.20$
Lactation, g/d	=	$(0.14 \times MY)/0.20$

Magnesium Requirements of Cervids

Values are not available. The values for goats are recommended.

Magnesium Deficiencies

Magnesium deficiency causes tetany with convulsions. Outbreaks of tetany occur most frequently in nursing ewes shortly after they are turned out to pasture in the spring (grass tetany). It may also occur with lush growth of cereal forages during fall or winter. Incidence is highest with old ewes, during the first 4 or 5 weeks after lambing, when magnesium requirements for lactation are maximal (Littledike and Cox, 1979).

Magnesium Toxicities

Magnesium toxicosis is unlikely except by accidental feeding of high levels. Oral administration of 0.5 percent dietary magnesium to wethers did not produce toxicity, but administration of 0.8 percent or higher resulted in signs of toxicosis. In goats, high magnesium intake may cause urolithiasis (James and Chandron, 1975). Signs of magnesium toxicosis are lethargy, disturbance in locomotion, diarrhea, lower feed intake, lower levels of performance, and death (NRC, 1980). Maximum tolerable concentration of magnesium is 0.6 percent in the diet dry matter (NRC, 2005).

Magnesium Sources

Sources of supplemental magnesium include magnesium oxide, magnesium sulfate, magnesium chloride, and magnesium carbonate. Magnesium levels of forages can be increased by using dolomite or other magnesium-containing soil amendments (Minson, 1990).

SULFUR

Sulfur (S) is found in methionine, cysteine, cystine, homocysteine, cystathionine, taurine, biotin, thiamin, lipoic acid, coenzyme A, glutathione, fibrinogen, and heparin. Methionine is a contributor of sulphur for the synthesis of all of these compounds except biotin and thiamin (Underwood and Suttle, 1999). Biotin and thiamin are synthesized by rumen microorganism (Briggs et al., 1964; Breves et al., 1981). Chondroitin sulfate is found in cartilage, bones, tendons, and walls of blood vessels. The sulphur-containing amino acids provide a binding site for formation of disulfide bridges and binding of zinc within proteins. These cross bridges are largely responsible for the tertiary structure and zinc fingers of proteins. The sulfate anion participates in the acid-base balance of the animal.

Methionine, thiamin, and biotin cannot be synthesized at the tissue level. However, substantial amounts of these essential nutrients can be obtained by microbial synthesis in the rumen. If microbial synthesis cannot provide enough of these nutriments, they should be added to the diet.

The normal range of sulfate in plasma of sheep is 2–5 mg/100 mL.

Sulfur Requirements of Sheep and Goats

Wool in sheep has the greatest concentration of sulfur. This suggests that wool sheep may have higher requirements than hair sheep. The amount of sulfur in 2 kg of wool (approximately one-half annual growth for wool breeds) is approximately the same as the sulfur found in the rest of the body. The sulfur contents of proteins range from 0.3–1.6 percent, with an average of 1.0 percent. This approximates a nitrogen (N):S ratio of 16:1, which is generally the basis for suggesting sulfur requirements. However, wool and hair have high concentrations of sulfur-containing amino acids. Sulfur concentrations of wool and hair are around 4 to 5 percent, with a concomitant N:S ratio of 4:1. Therefore, for wool sheep an N:S ratio of 10:1 is suggested. For haired sheep, a ratio of 12:1 is recommended. When the diet contains low levels of protein and/or much of the dietary nitrogen is from nonprotein nitrogen, sulfur supplementation is obligatory.

Feeding trials with sheep, summarized and reviewed by ARC (1980), suggest that 0.18 percent dietary sulfur is adequate (ARC, 1980). In one trial, it was found that 0.47 percent sulfur was adequate. In this case, the sulfur source was elemental sulfur, which has low bioavailability (Henry and Ammerman, 1995).

Reports by Qi et al. (1992a,b, 1993, 1994a,b) have attempted to evaluate and set guidelines for sulfur requirements for different breeds of goats. They concluded that the sulfur requirement for lactating dairy goats during early lactation was > 0.16 percent and < 0.36 percent of DM. The optimal dietary sulfur level for maximum daily gain of Angora and Alpine kids was 0.22 percent of DM for a ratio of N:S of 10.4:1. Required sulfur for optimum gain (100 g/day) in kids is 2.3 g/day and for mohair production in adult goats is 3.1 g/day (Qi et al., 1993). These values encompass maintenance. Therefore, sulfur requirements were set as 0.22 percent of DM for maintenance, gestation, and growth of goats, and 0.26 percent of DM for lactating does.

Sulfur Deficiencies

Deficiency signs include reduced feed intake and production, wool loss, excessive salivation and lacrimation, emaciation, and death. Sulfur is a requirement for growth of microorganisms; therefore, a dietary sulfur deficiency will depress diet digestibility and utilization of lactate and will increase blood urea.

Sulfur Toxicities

The maximum tolerable dietary concentration of sulfur is 0.3 percent of dry matter when animals are fed concentrate diets, or 0.50 percent with high-forage diets (NRC, 2005). High levels of sulfur in the diet interfere with copper and selenium absorption and utilization. Ingestion of high levels of sulfur, due to dietary supplements or plants rich in sulfur, may induce polioencephalomalacia, especially with metabolizable energy-rich diets that reduce rumen pH and excessive production of rumen sulfide (Gould, 1998). Drinking water may contain high levels of sulfate to cause sulfur toxicosis in ruminants. Therefore, maximum concentration of sulfate in drinking water of ruminants fed high-concentrate diets should not exceed 600 mg sulfate/L (200 mg S/L) or 2,500 mg sulfate/L (834 mg S/L) when the diets contain at least 40 percent forage (NRC, 2005). Acute sulfur toxicity causes diarrhea, muscle tremors, hydrogen sulfide odor in breath, dispnea, and death.

Sulfur Sources

Bioavailability of sulfur sources for rumen microorganisms and sheep were reviewed by Henry and Ammerman (1995). In general, elemental sulfur is less available than organic and other inorganic sources for both rumen microorganisms and sheep. Inorganic sources such as sodium sulfite, sodium sulfate, calcium sulfate, ammonium sulfate, potassium sulfate, and magnesium sulfate can be good sources when nitrogen, phosphorus, and other nutrients are adequate for microbial growth. Methionine and cysteine are good sources of sulfur for the microorganisms. Protected methionine or its analogues can be appropriate to supply methionine for breeds of sheep or goats highly productive of wool or mohair (Underwood and Suttle, 1999).

CATION-ANION DIFFERENCE OR ACID-BASE BALANCE

Optimum production requires a balance in the acid:base of diet. Diets with positive acid:base balance have been associated with better growth and milk production. Therefore, acid:base (acidosis and alkalosis) balance of the diet is an important consideration when feeding lactating animals, as it may alleviate milk fever or udder edema (Tucker et al., 1992; Goff and Horst, 1997), or heat-stressed animals, where an imbalance causes respiratory alkalosis. In both of these conditions the animal loses considerable amounts of cation, and balance may be disturbed. Major elements contributing to acid:base balance are dietary cations (sodium and potassium, and to a lesser extent calcium and magnesium) and anions (chlorine and sodium, and to a lesser extent potassium). Acid:base balance is measured by cation and anion differences (CAD) and is expressed in terms of milliequivalents (mEq millimolecular weights divided by valences). Cation-anion difference is calculated as $((Na^+ + K^+) - (Cl^- + S^{-2}))$/kg DM (Ender et al., 1971). Acid:base balance may be referred to as dietary electrolyte balance (DEB) and calculated as $(Na^+ + K^+ - Cl^-)$ (Mongin, 1980). More recently, dietary CAD can be expressed as (Na + K + 0.15 Ca + 0.15 Mg) – (Cl + S + P) (Goff et al., 1997). The optimum DEB for cattle in response to milk production ranged from 200 to 375 mEq/kg DM (Tucker et al., 1988; West et al., 1991). Jackson et al. (1992) reported that feed intake and weight gain were higher for dairy calves receiving diets of 370 mEq/kg DM than those receiving 0.0 mEq and suggested that there may be an optimum dietary level of CAD for gain. Optimum CAD is defined at 300–500 mEq/kg DM for cattle. Forages have high CAD values (> 100 mEq/kg DM); cereal grain has low CAD values (< 20 mEq/kg DM), and protein supplements may have high (soybean) or low (fish meal) CAD (NRC, 1989).

Optimum CAD or DEB for goats is not defined. In lactating dairy goats (Qi et al., 1992b), levels of sulfur in the diet ranging from 0.16–0.36 percent of DM did not affect acid:base balance. However, dietary sulfur at 0.21 percent of DM is required for improved gain, and it reduced metabolic acidity in Alpine goat kids (Qi et al., 1994a).

COBALT

The mammalian tissues have no requirement for cobalt (Co) per se but require vitamin B_{12}, which is synthesized by ruminal microorganisms that require cobalt. Only 3–13 percent of available cobalt is incorporated into vitamin B_{12} (Smith and Marston, 1970). Dietary cobalt requirements were established as 0.1mg/kg diet dry matter in NRC (1975) and as 0.1–0.2 mg/kg dry matter in NRC (1985). The upper range in requirements reflects possible greater requirements when high-energy rations are fed (Smith and Marston, 1970; ARC, 1980). In goats, Haenlein (1992) recommended a range of 0.10–0.15 mg Co/kg DM, but Meschy (2000) suggested 0.10 because goats seem to be less sensitive to a cobalt deficiency (Clark et al., 1987). Rumen microorganisms require between 0.5 and 1.0 mg Co/kg diet dry matter for optimum growth (Durand and Kawashima, 1980). The ARC (1980) reviewed nine reports on cobalt requirements for sheep fed a semi synthetic or forage diets. Except in two cases, the requirements were between 0.08 and 0.11 mg cobalt per kg diet dry matter. Reports that higher amounts of cobalt (0.25–0.35 mg/kg DM) can enhance rumen digestion of forages (Lopez-Guisa and Satter, 1992) and increase the bacterial population in the rumen (Young, 1979) are not considered sufficient evidence to justify raising requirement estimates at this time. The committee recommends 0.11 mg Co/kg DM for goats and maintains the previous recommendation of 0.10–0.20 mg Co/kg diet dry matter for sheep.

Cobalt Deficiencies

Severe cobalt deficiencies in sheep and cattle are known as bush-sickness in New Zealand, coast disease in South Australia, wasting disease in Western Australia, salt disease in Florida, makuruitis in Kenya, pining in Great Britain, and Grand Traverse disease in Michigan (Underwood and Suttle, 1999). It is an enzootic marasmus or severe wasting condition affecting ruminants of all ages and types with high mortality. Minson (1990) reviewed 15 reports where weight gain was increased from 55–102 g/day when growing sheep were supplemented with either cobalt or vitamin B_{12}.

Ruminant animals are more sensitive to cobalt deficiency than nonruminants, and sheep are more susceptible than cattle and goats. Body store of cobalt is sufficient enough that an animal will not show signs of deficiency for several months; however, rumen microbes show the deficiency (rise in succinate in the rumen) within a few days when animals are placed on a cobalt-deficient diet (Kennedy et al., 1996).

Cobalt Toxicities

Early signs of toxicity include failure to grow, unthriftiness, and loss of weight (Smith, 1997). If continued, fatty degeneration of the liver and anemia will develop (Underwood and Suttle, 1999). There is a low likelihood of toxicity when feeding cobalt to ruminants; however, it has been suggested that cattle may be less tolerant to cobalt than sheep, and toxicity is unknown for goats. ARC (1980) established 30 mg/kg DM as the maximum tolerance level, but Guéguen et al. (1988) recommended that cobalt not exceed 10 mg/kg diet DM. The NRC (2005) suggested a maximum tolerable level of 25 mg Co/kg dry matter. This recommendation was based mainly on findings that lambs fed up to 40 mg cobalt/kg DM for 60 days were healthy without loss of performance (Henry et al., 1997).

Dietary Considerations for Cobalt

Sandy soils in the southeastern United States, Atlantic coast, and parts of Michigan, Wisconsin, Minnesota, Iowa, Missouri, and Nebraska are deficient in cobalt, and forages grown in these areas may lack sufficient cobalt to meet the requirements. Legumes tend to have more cobalt than grasses grown under the same conditions. Cobalt is low in high-pH soil (alkali soil) but high in plants grown in waterlogged areas. Grains are usually poor sources of cobalt. Cobalt supplementation may alleviate phalaris staggers, a neurological syndrome induced by alkaloids present in *Phalarus tuberosa* (Ulvund, 1985).

All sources of inorganic cobalt are suitable for supplementation; however, oxide forms are less available (Henry, 1995). Slow release (oxide form of cobalt) glass pellets placed in the rumen have been used successfully on pasture. Cobalt can be indirectly supplemented in cobalt-deficient areas as fertilizer to increase cobalt in soil and its uptake by plants (Minson, 1990). Cobalt can be incorporated continuously in the diet as cobalt salts or oxide or in drinking water. Intramuscular injection of vitamin B_{12} also has been suggested at the latter part of pregnancy and has improved performance in newborns. Oral drenching should be adequate if doses are provided frequently.

COPPER

Copper (Cu) is a very important element because of its roles in the actions of many crucial enzyme systems. Among these are cytochrome c oxidase, which creates the conditions required for the generation of ATP in the mitochondria (Harris, 1997); lysil oxidase, which is involved with collagen and elastin (Mäki, 2002); dopamine β-monooxygenase, which converts dopamine to norepinephrine; and monoamine oxidase, also required in the proper metabolism of dopamine, norepinephrine, epinephrine, and serotonin. Collagen forms the matrix required for calcium and phosphorus deposition and for bone formation, whereas elastin is an elastic protein found in arteries and major blood vessels, lungs, elastic ligaments, tendons, and skin. Ceruloplasmin is a blood protein that contains most of plasma copper (> 95 percent: Hellman and Gitlin, 2002). This protein converts iron stored in the liver from the ferrous to the ferric form for its incorporation into hemoglobin (Williams et al., 1983). Hephaestin is an analogous protein to ceruloplasmin, which does the same function in the intestines (Chen et al., 2004). The proper function of the central nervous system depends on available copper for the formation and maintenance of myelin, the insulating tissue of axons and nerve fibers. The most evident function of copper is the synthesis of melanins (pigments of hair, wool, and skin) via tyrosinase. Copper is involved in iron metabolism and insulin function (Wang et al., 1996), protection from oxidants (Saenko et al., 1994), development of central nervous system (Fell et al., 1965), normal function of immune system (Solaiman et al., 2004), and lipid metabolism (Engle et al., 2000). Copper at high levels (100 mg/day) stimulated growth and feed efficiency (Solaiman et al., 2005) and may be an alternative to anthelmintics to control nematode parasites in goats (Chartier et al., 2000).

Copper Homeostasis

Normal levels of copper in plasma are 0.8–1.5 mg Cu/L for all ruminants. Plasma copper in goats ranges from 0.9–1.39 mg/L (Galbraith et al., 1997; Solaiman et al., 2001). Copper absorption is more important than its concentration in the feed. Copper absorption estimated in sheep is relatively poor ranging from 1.4–12.8 percent (Underwood and Suttle, 1999) and can be influenced by type of diet and level of molybdenum, sulfur, iron, and, to a lesser extent, calcium and zinc (Davis and Mertz, 1987). However, young animals may absorb up to 90 percent of dietary copper (ARC, 1980). Absorption of copper is either through pinocytosis (young ruminant on fluid diet) or an active saturable and passive unsaturable (Davis and Mertz, 1987). Presence of rumen microorganisms, especially protozoa, adversely affects copper absorption through sulfide formation. A 70–75 percent absorption rate of copper in newborn ruminants can be reduced to < 10 percent in adults, and in the presence of antagonists, reduced to 1 percent (Price and Chesters, 1985). Copper level in plasma fluctuates only to a limited extent and is regulated by biliary and fecal excretion and level of liver copper storage as metallothionein complex. Deviations from the average are not detectable, even during a copper deficiency. Biliary secretion may enhance hepatic copper recycling through absorption. Urinary excretion of copper is small and relatively constant in all species.

Metallothionein is a protein found in the liver, small intestine, and several other tissues. This protein normally binds copper and zinc ions. Its synthesis is induced by metals (cadmium, zinc, copper, mercury, gold, and bismuth), steroids (glucocorticoids, estrogens, and progesterone), catecholamines, and interleukin-1 (Bremner and Beattie, 1990). Metallothionein functions to limit absorption of excess copper and zinc in the small intestine; to detoxify metals (cadmium, zinc, copper, mercury) by binding and storing them in the liver; and to mount an immune response by scavenging zinc from plasma and releasing copper from liver. The liver capacity to store metals within metallothionein is limited; therefore, when the liver contains around 1,000 mg Cu/kg DM (NRC, 2005) and there is a stressor agent, the copper is released into the blood and toxicosis ensues.

Copper Requirements of Sheep and Goats

The copper requirement for sheep was set as 5 mg/kg dry matter of diet (NRC, 1975) and later increased to 7–11 mg/kg dry matter (NRC, 1985). ARC (1980) estimated copper requirements from 1–8.6 mg/kg dry matter of diet, depending on the physiological state of the sheep. Underwood and Suttle (1999) estimated Cu requirements from 4.3–28.4 mg/kg dry matter. These latter estimates were based on absorption coefficients of 0.06, 0.03, and 0.015 for roughages plus concentrates, normal green pasture, and molybdenum-rich pastures, respectively.

In this edition, copper requirements are estimated with the factorial method for sheep. The following equations were developed from information obtained from ARC (1980) and Grace and Clark (1991). The great variation in absorption coefficients of copper combined with variable levels of absorption antagonists (molybdenum, sulfur, iron, cadmium, zinc) and metabolic interactions (molybdenum, zinc, cadmium, steroids, immune response) means that tabulated copper requirements give only an approximate measure of dietary need (Suttle, 2002). For the same reasons, determination of copper status of animals with biochemical indices is an enigma (Lee et al., 2002).

$$\text{Copper for growing lambs, mg/day} = \frac{0.004 \times \text{BW} + 0.0137 \times \text{WP} + 0.00106 \times \text{LWG}}{\text{AC}}$$

The copper requirements for gestating ewes considered a deposition of 0.2 mg/day for a 4-kg lamb. For yearling ewes, a growth component can be included; otherwise it may be eliminated from the equation.

$$\text{Copper for gestating ewes, mg/day} = \frac{0.004 \times BW + 0.0137 \times WP + 0.00106 \times LWG + 0.05 \times LBW}{0.06}$$

The copper requirement for lactating ewes considered that milk contains 0.2 mg Cu/kg.

$$\text{Copper for lactating ewes, mg/day} = \frac{0.004 \times BW + 0.0137 \times WP + 0.00106 \times LWG + 0.2 \times MP}{0.045}$$

where BW = bodyweight, kg; WP = typical or total annual wool production, kg; LWG = live weight gain, g/d; LBW = typical birth weight of lamb(s), kg; MP = milk production, kg/day; and AC = absorption coefficient for classes and weights of sheep (ARC, 1980).

Copper Requirements of Sheep

Class and Weight	Absorption Coefficient
Lamb, preweaning	
5 kg	0.90
10 kg	0.53
20 kg	0.20
Lamb, postweaning (pasture)	0.045
Lamb, postweaning (feedlot)	0.06
Ewe, gestation	0.06
Ewe, lactation	0.045

Data are not available to justify using the factorial method to set copper requirements for goats. Copper requirements for goats were established by Kessler (1991) and adopted by Meschy (2000) to be 8–10 mg/kg of diet DM. Higher levels of copper in commercial goat milk (0.39 mg/kg: Park, 2000) and Tswana goat milk (1.0–2.0 mg/kg: Aganga et al., 2002) have been reported that may increase requirements for lactating dairy goats. Haenlein (1992) proposed 10–23 mg/kg diet DM, which was similar to the 10–20 mg/kg proposed by AFRC (1997). Recent data reported by Solaiman et al. (2004, 2006) indicated that higher copper (100 mg/day fed with basal diet containing 13.8 mg Cu/kg DM; average daily feed intake (AFDI) = 1.1 kg) increased ADG and gain efficiency and enhanced immune responses in goats compared to basal diet alone. These data suggest that meat goats may require more copper for optimal growth. However, Luginbuhl et al. (2000) found no effect on feed intake, weight gain, feed efficiency, or carcass yield when wether kids were fed diets containing 6.2, 16.2, or 36.2 mg Cu/kg DM for 88 days. In that study, plasma and liver concentrations of copper increased linearly with dietary copper concentrations, but there were no signs of copper toxicity. Also, goats tolerated 60 mg added Cu/kg DM for 137 days with no sign of copper toxicity (Zervas et al., 1990). Therefore, the committee recommends increasing the copper requirement of lactating goats to 15 mg/kg DM, mature goats and bucks to 20 mg/kg DM, and growing goats to 25 mg/kg diet DM. Adjustments should be made for the level of molybdenum and sulfur in the diet.

Sulfur and molybdenum content of the diet affect absorption coefficient of copper. Presence of high dietary molybdenum and sulfur promote formation and absorption of thiomolybdate into the blood rendering copper unavailable; thus, liver and plasma copper may not accurately reflect copper status of the animal (Suttle, 1991). Within the normal dietary concentrations of sulfur (1.5–2.5 g/kg dry matter) and molybdenum (1–2 mg/kg dry matter), Table 7-1 was developed to estimate the absorption coefficient of copper. The mean absorption coefficient was 0.045 with a standard deviation of 0.005.

Copper Requirements of Cervids

Several studies point to the requirement for copper in wildlife systems (Hyvärinen et al., 1977; Barboza and Blake, 2001; O'Hara et al., 2001; Barboza et al., 2003). Recommendations for lactating and growing animals are reported (Rombach et al., 2002, 2003; Barboza et al., 2003). Otherwise, the committee recommends using data from sheep and goats until controlled studies to estimate requirements for cervid species have been completed.

Copper Deficiencies

Liver normally contains 200–300 mg Cu/kg DM (Underwood and Suttle, 1999). Copper concentrations of < 20 mg/kg liver DM (5 mg/kg wet weight) along with < 0.5 mg Cu/L in plasma indicate deficiency. Copper deficiency is manifested as hypochromic microcytic anemia in all species if copper inadequacy is severe and prolonged. Improper endochondral ossification and uneven bone growth can result

TABLE 7-1 Copper Absorption Based on Normal Molybdenum and Sulfur Content of the Diet[a]

Dietary Sulfur (g/kg)	Dietary Molybdenum (mg/kg)	Copper Absorption (percentage)
1.5	1.0	5.15
2.0	1.0	4.65
2.5	1.0	4.20
1.5	1.5	5.03
2.0	1.5	4.51
2.5	1.5	4.04
1.5	2.0	4.91
2.0	2.0	4.36
2.5	2.0	3.88
Mean copper absorption, percentage		4.53
Standard deviation		0.50

[a]Suttle and McLauchlin (1976).

in generalized osteoporosis and occasional bone fracture in grazing animals. Connective tissue disorder results in defects in articular cartilages (Thompson et al., 1994) by impaired collagen and elastin development. Cardiovascular disorders; depigmentation of skin, hair, and wool; defective keratinization of wool resulting in the loss of crimp and a harsh hairy appearance ("steely wool"); scouring; infertility; and increased susceptibility to diseases are all symptom of inadequate copper in the diet. Newborn lambs and kids from copper-deficient ewes and does during the third trimester of pregnancy manifest neonatal or congenital ataxia because of insufficient myelin synthesis in the fetal brain. A delayed ataxia also affects lambs and kids (Ivan et al., 1990), which can be found between 1 and 2 months after birth. This ataxia affects the rear quarter due to insufficient myelin synthesis, after birth, for proper development of spinal cord nerves.

Copper is the most common trace element deficient for deer in New Zealand, United States, China, and England (Wilson and Grace, 2002). The deficiency is manifested as enzootic ataxia and osteochondrosis (Wilson and Grace, 2002). For this reason, there are efforts to estimate requirements of copper (Grace and Wilson, 2002). In New Zealand, it was estimated that deer with adequate copper status had concentrations in serum or liver greater than 0.51 mg/L or 6.4 mg/kg fresh tissue, respectively (Grace and Wilson, 2002). Copper supplementation strategies include Cu-EDTA injections, Cu-oxide needles, copper fertilization of pastures, and novel forages rich in copper (Grace and Wilson, 2002; Barry et al., 2002).

Copper Toxicities

Chronic copper poisoning is characterized by two phases: (1) prehaemolytic, when copper accumulates in the liver to exceed 1,000 mg Cu/kg DM, and (2) haemolytic crises, when copper is released from liver in lysosomes and blood copper value rises followed by haemoglobinuria, haemoglobinaemia, and jaundice. Elevated levels of liver enzymes such as sorbitol dehydrogenase, gamma glutamyle transferase, and glutamic oxaloacetic transaminase are indicative of liver tissue damage and precede death (Solaiman et al., 2001). The prehaemolytic phase lasts from a few weeks to more than a year. The second phase lasts from hours to days (Fuentealba and Aburto, 2003).

Breed differences exist for both sheep and goats in susceptibility to toxicosis from copper. Texel lambs retained 9.5 percent of ingested copper in their livers, while Suffolk lambs retained only 1.3 percent (Suttle et al., 2002) when they were fed a diet with 6.1 mg Cu/kg dry matter. Another susceptible breed is North Ronaldsay sheep (Fuentealba and Aburto, 2003). Meat goats have tolerated 60 mg added Cu/kg DM for 137 days (Zervas et al., 1990), and goats receiving 100–300 mg Cu/day (average DMI was 1.00 kg/day) for 35 weeks did not show signs of copper toxicity (Solaiman et al., 2001). These reports clearly indicate that dairy (Nubian) and meat goats (Boer crosses) are more tolerant to copper toxicity than sheep. Also, young kids having higher absorption especially through liquid diet (60 percent) may be more susceptible to toxicity.

The maximum tolerable copper concentration for sheep is 15 mg/kg dry matter when their diets contain normal molybdenum (1–2 mg/kg DM) and sulfur (0.15–0.25 percent) concentrations (NRC, 2005). The maximum tolerable copper level for goats is not established (NRC, 2005). The committee suggests that goats, especially meat goats, have a higher tolerance than other ruminants but are reluctant to identify a toxic level. Until further research, a cautious approach would be to use the cattle level (40 mg/kg) in usual management.

Dietary Considerations for Copper

Copper, molybdenum, sulfur, and iron should be considered together in determining proper feeding management. The availability of copper is reduced in the presence of molybdenum, sulfur, and iron. Also, adding molybdenum to an otherwise toxic diet can reduce the toxicity of copper. Readers are referred to NRC (2005) for a full discussion. Fresh grasses are poor sources of copper, in comparison with cured hay, because of lower availability of copper in fresh grasses. Copper is lower in temperate grasses but higher in tropical grasses than in legumes. Acid soils increase copper and lower molybdenum in forages; however, molybdenum is higher in alkaline or high organic matter containing soil (also high in sulfur). Copper absorption by plants is also limited by an alkaline pH or high organic matter content. Liming can increase molybdenum in forage and disturb the Cu:Mo ratio. Cu:Mo ratios of at least 4:1 (Miller et al., 1988) are considered safe and will avoid copper deficiency.

Copper can be applied as copper-containing fertilizer to increase copper levels in plants or can be supplemented in the sulfate, carbonate, or oxide forms. Fertilization with poultry/swine waste from animals fed high levels (~ 250 ppm) of copper can improve copper in soils. In range condition, salt licks containing copper (0.5–1.9 percent) can prevent or alleviate deficiencies. Because of the distinct risk of copper toxicosis in sheep (and perhaps other species or breeds), mineral mixtures used as supplements should be designed specifically for the ruminant species to be supplemented.

IODINE

The major function of iodine (I) is in the synthesis of thyroid hormones, tetraiodothyronine or thyroxin (inactive T_4), and triiodothyronine (active T_3). The activation/deactivation of thyroid hormones requires the selenoenzymes iodothyronine deiodinases (Behne and Kyriakopoulos, 2001). Thyroid glands contain 80 percent of the iodine in the body. Thyroid hormones control oxidation rate and protein synthesis in all cells. They regulate fetus development, set basal metabolic rate and thermal regulation, and influence digestion, muscle function, immune system, and seasonality of reproduction.

Iodine Homeostasis

Iodine is efficiently absorbed at about 80–90 percent from the gastrointestinal tract allowing efficient recycling of iodine secreted into the abomasum. Long-term iodine study with goats has indicated that iodine content of the body is highly correlated with iodine concentration of feeds (Groppel et al., 1989). Plasma iodine is actively taken by thyroid glands, combined with tyrosine to form T_4 (an inactive transport form of hormone that can change to the active form, T_3) and stored as thyroglobulin. Depending on iodine status of the animal, 20–65 percent of dietary iodine may be taken by thyroid glands. These glands contain more than 80 percent of body iodine. Some is stored in muscle and liver, and a small portion exists as free iodine. Excess iodine is excreted through urine and/or secreted in milk. Raw soybeans contain a heat-labile substance that can impair iodine recycling (Hemken, 1960).

Iodine Requirements of Sheep, Goats, and Deer

In the previous editions, (NRC, 1975, 1985), it was recommended that sheep diets contain 0.10–0.80 mg I/kg dry matter. ARC (1980) recognized a range of 0.05–1.25 mg I/kg diet dry matter, suggesting 0.5 mg I/kg diet dry matter as the requirement, to be increased to 2.0 mg I/kg diet when significant amounts of goitrogens are present in the diet. The requirement suggested in this edition is 0.50 mg I/kg diet dry matter for growing animals, and up to 0.80 mg I/kg diet for lactating ewes. ARC (1980) recommendations were supported later by work of Guéguen et al. (1988) and Lamand (1981) in goats. Meschy (2000) claimed that iodine requirements of goats are higher than those for other ruminants. This statement was based on the fact that iodine levels considered as adequate for dairy cows (0.3 mg/kg DM) were insufficient to prevent goiter in kids (Lamand, 1981). There are no sufficient data to support a higher iodine requirement for goats than sheep. Therefore, requirements adopted for this edition are as follows:

Iodine Requirements of Sheep and Goats

Species and Class	mg/kg Diet
Sheep	
Growing and mature, nonlactating	0.5
Lactating ewes	0.8
Goats	
Growing and mature, nonlactating	0.5
Lactating does	0.8

Watkins et al. (1983) concluded that diets containing 0.26 mg I/kg DM were adequate for white-tailed deer in the United States. An iodine deficiency is manifested as goiter in fawns (Grace and Wilson, 2002).

Iodine Deficiencies

The clinical manifestation of iodine deficiency is an enlarged thyroid gland (goiter), a compensatory result of deficient thyroid hormones production either by action of goitrogens or iodine deficiency per se. An iodine deficiency can affect brain development in newborns and cause stillborn and hairless young. Other symptoms of iodine deficiencies include infertility or sterility and poor conception, increased susceptibility to cold stress, skin and hair disorders, and low milk production. Deficiencies can occur when iodine is not adequately present in the environment (iodine-deficient areas), when goitrogens interfere with thyroid gland activity (kale and rapeseed, cruciferous plants), if other trace elements such as selenium and iron interfere, or as a result of environmental factors such as cold stress (Underwood and Suttle, 1999). The main effect of iodine deficiency is lamb mortality that can range from 25–66 percent (Sargison and West, 1998). Correction of an iodine deficiency has increased lamb crop by 75 percent (Minson, 1990) and the twinning rate by 14 percent (Sargison and West, 1998).

Iodine Toxicity

Toxicity from iodine is unlikely in ruminants because of the large margin between the requirement (0.5 mg/kg DM) and the tolerable level (50 mg/kg DM) in their diets (NRC, 2005). However, horses are very sensitive to excess iodine (maximum tolerable level = 5 mg/kg DM: NRC, 2005). Toxicity symptoms can result from overconsumption of an iodine supplement causing an accumulation in the body and hypothyroidism. Visible symptoms include goiter, excessive nasal and ocular discharge, coughing, bronchopneumonia, hair loss, and dermatitis (Hillman and Cutis, 1980). Clinical changes include elevated metabolic rate, rise in body temperature, increased heart rate, elevated blood glucose and urea, and immunosuppression (Haggard et al., 1980).

Dietary Considerations for Iodine

Iodine is highly variable in forages but usually adequate except in the geographic regions known to be deficient. The Great Lakes regions and the northwestern United States are iodine-deficient areas. McDowell (1997) stated that iodine deficiency is worldwide. Cereal and oilseed meals are poor sources of iodine, whereas fish meal is a rich source. Concentration of iodine in water may reflect that of soil. Some plants such as kale, cabbage (thiocyanate), rapeseed (thiocyanate and goitrin), or cruciferous plants (thiouracil) are goitrogens that either reduce the uptake of iodine or interfere with T_4 to T_3 conversion. Plants with low levels of cyanide (sorghum-sudangrass) can cause iodine deficiency due to thiocyanate produced by hepatic cyanide detoxification. The iodide salts of sodium, potassium, and calcium or the more stable pentacalcium orthoperiodate or ethylenediamine dihydroiodate (EDDI) can be provided in salt licks or salt blocks to protect against or treat an iodine deficiency. The U.S. Food and Drug Administration (FDA) has set a limit on EDDI supplementation at 10 mg/d to limit iodine secretion in milk that may cause toxicity in humans. The limitation of animal protein sources for ruminant feeding and its replacement with vegetable sources, plus the development of forage varieties with high content of goitrogens (Sargison and West, 1998), requires more attention to iodine nutrition.

IRON

Iron (Fe) is the most abundant trace mineral of the body, and about 60 percent of it is in hemoglobin that is necessary for transporting oxygen and carbon dioxide to and from the tissues and lungs. Iron status in the body is controlled by absorption mainly from the duodenum. The absorption of iron depends on the need of the animal and is higher in iron-deficient animals or diets. Absorption can drop from 60 percent to 9 percent with diets containing 8 to 1,270 mg Fe/kg (Fairweather-Tait and Wright, 1984). Growing animals on a milk diet low in iron have higher absorption than those with adequate iron levels. Iron excretion is limited and is controlled by absorption. Iron is involved in energy metabolism via activation of succinate dehydrgenase in the Krebs cycle. Cytochromes a, b, and c are involved in electron transfer. Iron also activates hydroxylases, which affect connective tissue formation, and is contained in peroxidases that remove oxidants and improve resistance to disease.

Iron Requirements of Sheep and Goats

The dietary iron requirement for sheep was set at 30 mg Fe/kg dry matter in the previous edition (NRC, 1985) and by ARC (1980). NRC (2001) set the absorbed iron requirement for dairy cattle as 34 mg Fe/kg weight gain. For goats, AFRC (1997) adopted estimates of Lamand (1981) and ARC (1980) of 30 mg/kg DM diet. Haenlein (1987) justified higher requirements for goats because they are more often affected by internal parasites and suggested higher values ranging from 30–100 mg/kg diet DM, depending on the age and iron status of the animal. Feeding requirements were not set by NRC (1981) due to lack of data on goats.

In this edition, iron requirements for sheep were determined by the factorial method. For growing lambs, it was considered that endogenous losses were 14 μg/kg body weight, iron deposited in wool was 30 mg/kg clean wool, and iron deposited in weight gain was 55 mg/kg (Grace and Clark, 1991). The absorption coefficients employed were 0.50 and 0.19 for unweaned and weaned lambs, respectively (Grace and Clark, 1991). For gestating ewes, it was considered that during the last third of gestation, the iron deposited in the conceptus was 2.0 mg/d. For yearling ewes, the weight gain factor can be considered; otherwise, it may be deleted from the equation. The absorption coefficient was 0.10, similar to that used for dairy cows (NRC, 2001). For lactating ewes it was considered that milk contains 0.9 mg/kg produced. For goats, it was determined that the factorial approach to calculating iron requirements was not justified because of lack of data. In a study reported by Park and Attaie (1988), iron content of muscle (longissimus dorsi, biceps femoris) in goats (27–29 mg/kg) was more similar to cattle (23–26 mg/kg) than sheep (16–16.3 mg/kg). Considering data from NRC (2000), NRC (2001), House and Bell (1993), and Bremner and Dalgarno (1973) and recommendations by Haenlein (1987), liberal estimates of 95 mg/kg diet and 35 mg/kg diet are suggested for growing and mature goats, respectively. It is assumed that the requirement for older animals is lower because considerable recycling of iron occurs when red blood cells turn over (Underwood, 1977), and in older animals blood volume is not increasing as it is for younger animals. An additional 5 mg/kg diet is suggested to account for iron in mohair for Angora goats.

Iron Requirements of Sheep and Goats

Species and Class	Requirement or Equation
Sheep	
Maintenance	0.014 mg/kg BW/0.10
Growth	55 mg/kg LWG/AC
Pregnancy (last one-third)	0.5 mg/kg LBW/0.10
Lactation	0.9 mg/kg MY/0.10
Wool	30 mg/kg CFW/(365 × 0.10)
Goats	
Growing	95 mg/kg diet
Pregnant	35 mg/kg diet
Lactating	35 mg/kg diet
Mohair (Angora) goats	Add 5 mg/kg diet

where BW = body weight, kg; LWG = live weight gain, g/d; AC = absorption coefficient (lambs unweaned = 0.50, and lambs weaned = 0.19); LBW = litter birth weight, kg; MY = milk yield, kg/day; CFW = clean fleece weight, kg.

Iron Deficiencies

Iron deficiency may affect animals long before changes in the hemoglobin formation. Iron deficiency manifests itself as animals having loss of appetite, poor growth, lethargy, blanching of mucous membrane, increased respiration, and high mortality (Underwood and Suttle, 1999). Storage of iron in liver, kidney, and spleen are exhausted, and the animal exhibits hypochromic microcytic anemia. Early onset of iron deficiency anemia is different than late developing anemia by lack of cobalt and copper. Impaired thermoregulation and susceptibility to diseases links iron deficiency to hypothyroidism.

Iron Toxicities

Free iron is an oxidant and can cause peroxidative damage to lipid membranes, especially in the liver. The extent of the injury depends on vitamin E status of the animal. Vitamin E deficiency increases an animal's susceptibility to iron toxicity. Consumption of high levels of iron from soil along with unsaturated fat (polyunsaturated fatty acids) in the spring herbage may present hazardous conditions for grazing animals. High levels of iron in forages (549 to 990 mg Fe/kg dry matter) may cause copper deficiency in lambs and goats (Ivan et al., 1990). Maximum tolerable level of dietary iron is 500 mg/kg DM (NRC, 2005).

Dietary Considerations for Iron

Iron content of feeds depends on the plant species, type of soil, and degree of soil contamination. Soils with acid pH favor iron absorption into plant roots, particularly from red soils rich in iron. In this situation, forages can contain from 300–2,500 mg Fe/kg dry matter. Iron deficiency has not been demonstrated in grazing animals because of high iron content of forages and grasses. However, animals kept indoors and fed concentrate grain mixtures and milk-based diets containing limited iron may develop deficiencies. Also heavy parasite load in goats may impose iron deficiency. Most cereal grains are low in iron. However, oilseed meals are richer than cereal grain. It should be noted that phytate iron is readily available to ruminant animals in contrast to poultry.

Inorganic iron supplements vary little in availability to the animal. Ferrous sulfate and ferric citrate are more available than ferric oxide. Ferric oxide is a poor source and may interfere with copper absorption.

MANGANESE

Manganese (Mn) is involved in functions of several metaloenzymes, including glycosyl transferases, which are involved in the synthesis of mucopolysaccharides, formation of cartilage for proper bone development, and formation of prothrombin necessary for blood clotting. Pyruvate carboxylase, a manganese-dependent enzyme, is involved in glucose and lipid metabolism in both ruminants and nonruminants. Diets deficient in manganese result in reduced fat deposition and backfat thickness in goat kids (Anke et al., 1973); however, manganese-deficient diets may enhance copper uptake. Increased copper intake reduced backfat thickness in goats (Solaiman et al., 2006) as it did in cattle (Engle et al., 2000).

Manganese containing superoxide dismutase (as those containing copper and zinc) protects cells from peroxidative damage caused by high dietary levels of polyunsaturated fatty acids (Malecki and Greger, 1996). Manganese is required for normal estrus, conception, gestation, and healthy offspring (Doisey, 1973; Hurley and Keen, 1987).

Manganese Homeostasis

Manganese concentration in the body is low, ranging from 0.5–3.9 mg/kg DM in the carcasses of sheep and calves (Suttle, 1979; Grace, 1983) and regulated by absorption. Absorption rate was recorded as high as 40 percent in calves fed a milk replacer containing 0.7 mg Mn/kg (Kirchgessner and Neese, 1976), whereas absorption occurred at only 4.9 percent when a milk replacer containing 142 mg Mn/kg was fed (Suttle, 1979). Manganese absorption from solid diets is less than 5 percent. The endogenous pathway of excretion of manganese is through bile. As the level of manganese increases in the diet, higher amounts are excreted in the feces. There is no evidence of manganese storage in the body (liver or bone), and manganese accumulates in the liver or other tissues in direct proportion to dietary intake. This may be due to an impaired homeostasis rather than storage (Underwood and Suttle, 1999). Almost no manganese is excreted in the urine (NRC, 2000).

Manganese Requirements of Sheep and Goats

Previously, the dietary manganese requirement for sheep was set as 20 mg/kg dry matter (NRC, 1985). ARC (1980) suggested that 10 mg Mn/kg diet dry matter was adequate for growth and that 20–25 mg Mn/kg diet dry matter could be adequate for skeletal development of sheep, based on cattle data. Masters et al. (1988) found that 13 mg Mn/kg diet dry matter was adequate for growth, and 19 mg Mn/kg diet dry matter was adequate for testicular growth of lambs. Requirements suggested for goats include 20–25 (ARC, 1980), 20–40 (Haenlein, 1992), 40–50 (Meschy, 2000), 60–120 (Lamand, 1981), and 60 mg/kg diet DM (AFRC, 1997). The NRC (2001) used a factorial approach for dairy cattle and more closely estimated the requirements. Maintenance requirement was set at 0.002 mg/kg BW, for growth at 0.7 mg/kg ADG, for pregnancy at 0.3 mg/d, and for lactation at 0.03 mg/kg MY. The required manganese for pregnancy can be adjusted for goats to be 0.05 mg/day.

The requirements for both sheep and goats were estimated by the factorial method. Endogenous losses of 2 µg/kg BW were used to estimate maintenance requirements. Manganese deposited in wool and mohair was 2.5 mg/kg clean fiber. Manganese deposited in weight gain was 0.47 mg/kg (Grace and Clark, 1991) for lambs and 0.70 for kids

(Suttle, 1979). For pregnancy, 0.02 (Grace and Clark, 1991) and 0.025 (NRC, 2001) mg Mn/kg LBW were used for sheep and goats, respectively. The manganese secreted in milk was calculated as 0.055 mg/kg MY for sheep and 0.03 mg/kg MY for goats. A 0.0075 absorption coefficient for manganese was adopted for all calculations (NRC, 2001).

Manganese Requirements of Sheep and Goats

Species and Class	Requirement or Equation
Sheep	
Maintenance	0.002 mg/kg BW/0.0075
Growth	0.47 mg/kg LWG/0.0075
Pregnancy (last one-third)	0.02 mg/kg LBW/0.0075
Lactation	0.055 mg/kg MY/0.0075
Wool	2.5 mg/kg CFW/(365 × 0.0075)
Goats	
Maintenance	0.002 mg/kg BW/0.0075
Growing	0.7 mg/kg LWG/0.0075
Pregnant	0.025 mg/kg LBW/0.0075
Lactating	0.03 mg/kg MY/0.0075
Mohair (Angora) goats	2.5 mg/kg CFW/(365 × 0.0075)

where BW = bodyweight, kg; LWG = live weight gain, kg/d; LBW = litter birth weight, kg; MY = milk yield, kg/day; and CFW = clean fleece weight, kg.

Manganese Requirements of Cervids

The values for sheep and goats are recommended.

Manganese Deficiencies

Signs of manganese deficiency may vary depending on degree and duration of deprivation as well as age of the animal. In young animals decreased endochondral bone growth can cause severe skeletal abnormality. In goats, deficiency symptoms are expressed as tarsal joint excrescences, leg deformity, and ataxia (Anke et al., 1973). Depressed estrous and poor conception rates have been associated with manganese deficiency in goats (Anke et al., 1973).

Manganese Toxicity

Manganese is low in toxicity even at high levels. A mutual metabolic antagonism exists between manganese and iron. High levels of manganese may interfere with iron metabolism and reduce iron in heart and plasma (Grace, 1973). The minimum level of manganese that can reduce appetite and growth rate in weaned lambs was between 3,000 and 4,500 mg/kg DM (Wong-Valle et al., 1989). The maximum tolerable level given by NRC (2005) is 2,000 mg Mn/kg diet DM. This value is twice as high as the previous recommendation (NRC, 1980).

Dietary Considerations for Manganese

Manganese deficiencies have not been reported for grazing animals; however, animals fed corn silage and corn and barley as supplement may exhibit manganese deficiency. High levels of calcium, iron, phosphorus, and potassium may induce manganese deficiency (Lassiter et al., 1972). Pastures have a high level of manganese (86 mg/kg DM), whereas seeds and grains are low. Protein supplements of animal origin have low levels of manganese (0.2–20 mg/kg); however, plant protein concentrates are higher (35–55 mg/kg). Manganese sulfate has higher availability (10 percent) than manganese in feeds (3–4 percent). Manganese carbonate and manganese oxides are used as supplements and their availability is less than that of the sulfate salt by 30–35 percent less. Although manganese methionine was 1.2 times as available as manganese sulfate (Henry et al., 1992), it was not superior to the sulfate source when liver, kidney, and bone manganese levels were evaluated in lambs fed up to 2,000 mg Mn/kg DM (Henry et al., 1992).

MOLYBDENUM

Molybdenum (Mo) is an essential micromineral in the diets of livestock because of its roles in several oxidase enzymes (Johnson, 1997). Molybdenum absorption occurs from the small intestine through an active transport system that is shared with and inhibited by sulfate. In ruminants, sulfur seldom reaches the small intestine in the sulfate form (usually as sulfides or amino acids); therefore, the potential antagonism seldom occurs. Free ionic molybdate is transported in plasma and stored in tissues as molybdoprotein bound to enzymes. Excess absorbed molybdenum is excreted through urine and competes with sulfate for sites of re-absorption (similar for ruminant and nonruminants). Differences in sulfur metabolism in the gut underlie susceptibility for toxicity and tolerability of molybdenum in different species (Underwood and Suttle, 1999).

Molybdenum Requirements of Sheep and Goats

There is a significant variation in molybdenum requirements for different species. According to the collected information in NRC (2001) for dairy cattle, NRC (2000) for beef cattle, and literature on sheep, there is no report on requirements for molybdenum in the diet. However, a requirement of 0.5 mg Mo/kg diet dry matter was set for sheep (NRC, 1975, 1985). Kessler (1991) and Haenlein (1992) set the requirements at 0.1 mg/kg diet DM for goats and added that goats are more susceptible to molybdenum deficiency than other ruminants. However, there are no data to support this. The AFRC (1997) did not set molybdenum requirements for goats. Molybdenum fed in semipurified diets at 1 mg/kg DM to goat kids improved intake and growth, whereas diets containing 0.06 mg/kg diet DM failed to optimize intake and growth (Anke et al., 1978). Low dietary levels of molybdenum (< 1 mg/kg DM) increase copper absorption and thus can put sheep at higher risk of copper toxicity (NRC, 1975). General recommendations of 0.5 mg/kg diet for sheep and 0.1 to 1 mg/kg diet for goats are accepted for this edition.

Molybdenum Deficiencies

Goat kids fed diets containing low molybdenum (0.06 mg/kg DM) had reduced intake (by 29 percent), poor growth, reproductive failure, and mortality when compared to those fed 1 mg Mo/kg diet DM (Anke et al., 1978). Therefore, signs of deficiency include loss of appetite, growth depression, reproductive failure, and mortality (Anke and Risch, 1989). Loss of appetite may be caused by inefficient cellulolytic fermentation and may reflect the need for molybdenum by rumen microbes (Sharrif et al., 1990). Molybdoenzymes may be important in triggering inflammatory response to trauma caused by invasion of internal parasites of grazing livestock.

Molybdenum Toxicities

The toxic levels of molybdenum in diets depend on the species, chemical form of molybdenum, type of diet, concentration of sulfur in the diet, and copper status of the animal. Goats fed alfalfa hay harvested from pastures fertilized with 200 kg Mo/hectare (molybdenum content approximately 200 mg/kg DM) had elevated liver, serum, and kidney molybdenum and normal feces with no toxic effects for 4 weeks; however, sheep fed similarly had severe diarrhea. Goats tolerated 1,000 mg/kg diet DM with no visible signs of toxicity, but semen quality decreased (Falke and Anke, 1987). Symptoms in cattle, which are more affected than sheep, are severe diarrhea, weight loss, anorexia, and reproductive failure (Thomas and Moss, 1952). Sheep display diarrhea and joint and bone abnormalities (Suttle and Field, 1968). Increased molybdenum in the diet may increase copper-thiomolybdates formation in the rumen (reduced copper absorption) or formation of trichloroacetic acid-insoluble copper complexes in plasma (reduced copper uptake by tissues) and cause copper deficiency in ruminants. Cattle affected by molybdenum toxicity respond positively to treatment with copper sulfate. Treatment with sulfur (sulfate) is effective in nonruminants; however, in sheep, increased sulfur intake shifts the route of molybdenum excretion from urine to feces while increasing molybdenum retention (Grace and Suttle, 1979). Maximum tolerable level of molybdenum for sheep is 5 mg/kg diet DM (NRC, 2005).

Dietary Considerations for Molybdenum

Soil concentrations of molybdenum vary (1–20 mg/kg DM) with sandy soils having the lower amounts and soils from marine origin having the higher concentrations. Neutral and alkaline soils, along with high moisture and organic matter, enhance molybdenum uptake by forages (McDowell, 1992). Cereals have low molybdenum concentrations (1.1 mg/kg), and forages may range from 0.9–2.6 mg/kg DM. Corn silage contains molybdenum at the low range with legumes and grasses containing about 1.8–2.0 mg/kg DM. Most livestock feeds have sufficient amounts of molybdenum; however, both deficiencies and toxicities can occur because of impacts of copper and sulfur.

SELENIUM

Selenium (Se) is a structural component of specific proteins called selenoproteins. They are grouped in five glutathione peroxidases (GPx), three deiodinases, three thioredoxin reductases, selenophosphate synthetase, selenoprotein P, selenoprotein W, 15kDa-selenoprotein, and 18kDa-selenoprotein (Köhrle, 2000; Behne and Kyriakopulos, 2001).

The peroxidases enzymes function to protect cells from oxidant damage and to ensure membrane integrity. Membranes particularly at risk include those in mitochondrial, red blood, and gastrointestinal cells (Behne and Kyriakopulos, 2001). The deiodinases control the availability of T_3 and its share on growth, development, differentiation, and metabolism of animals (Köhrle, 2000). The reductases function as antioxidants, cell growth factors, inhibitors of apoptosis, recycling of ascorbic acid, DNA synthesis, and gene transcription (Mustacich and Powis, 2000). Selenophosphate synthetase is the enzyme required to convert selenide into selenophosphate that donates its selenium during the synthesis of selenocysteine. All selenium sources need to be transformed into selenide for their incorporation into the specific selenoproteins (Behne and Kyriakopulos, 2001).

Selenoprotein P contains about 50 percent of the selenium in plasma and probably functions as selenium transporter and antioxidant (Saito and Takahashi, 2000). Selenoprotein W concentration is highest in skeletal and heart muscles of sheep (Yeh et al., 1997). The concentrations of selenoproteins P and W in tissues are related to selenium ingestion (Yeh et al., 1997; Saito and Takahashi, 2000).

This wide array of involvement of selenoproteins in the various metabolic pathways explains the breadth and magnitude of some of the effects of selenium status on growth, reproduction, immunity, and mortality of animals.

Selenium Homeostasis

Selenium absorption occurs mainly from the intestines in ruminants (Koenig et al., 1997) and is lower than in nonruminants (34 vs. 85 percent, respectively: Wright and Bell,

1966). Absorption is lower with forage-based diets compared with concentrate-based diets (Koenig et al., 1997). Absorption of selenium from sodium selenite or selenomethionine (or yeast) is similar in lambs (Ehlig et al., 1967; Koenig et al., 1997) and goats (Aspila, 1991). However, urinary excretion of selenium is higher when sodium selenite is fed to lambs (Ehlig et al., 1967) or goats (Aspila, 1991) compared to selenenomethionine. Diets containing 0.24 percent or 0.40 percent sulfur decrease the concentration of selenium in sheep tissues (Pope et al., 1979; van Ryssen et al., 1998). Sodium selenite and sodium selenate were equally effective as selenium sources for lambs based on concentrations of selenium in serum, muscle, liver, and activity of glutathione peroxidase (Podoll et al., 1992). The major selenium compound in cereal grains, forages, plant proteins, and selenized yeast is selenomethionine (Whanger, 2002), which can be incorporated nonspecifically into body proteins. The selenomethionine will be incorporated into organs with high rates of protein synthesis such as skeletal muscles, erythrocytes, pancreas, liver, kidney, and gastrointestinal mucosa (Schrauzer, 2000). The selenium stored in tissues as selenomethionine is utilized for selenoprotein synthesis and provides a buffer during critical periods (Schrauzer, 2000), thereby providing a better nutrition than inorganic selenium sources. The nonspecific incorporation of natural selenomethionine in muscle tissues have provided a tool to produce beef and lamb meat with high selenium content for human consumption (Lawler et al., 2004; Taylor, 2005) with feeds from seleniferous areas. This implies that dietary selenium levels are higher than the requirement (2.9 vs. 0.3 mg Se/kg DM), which are named supranutritional. The increase in the selenium content of tissues related to its dietary content partially explains the differences in ruminant products between countries such New Zealand (Grace and Clark, 1991) and the United States (Ullrey, 1987), which may help explain the differences in selenium requirements (Figure 7-1).

Selenium Requirements of Sheep, Goats, and New World Camelids

Selenium requirements were estimated by the factorial method for both sheep and goats. Previous calculations of sheep requirements by this method (ARC, 1980) were adopted by Grace (1994) and Underwood and Suttle (1999). For goats, values for sheep (ARC, 1980; NRC, 1985) and cattle (NRC, 2001) and recommendations by Haenlein (1992), based on data from Anke et al. (1987b,c), and by Meschy (2000) were used to estimate selenium requirements.

Requirements for selenium for maintenance, growth, pregnancy, lactation, and fiber growth (wool or mohair) were estimated. The endogenous loss of selenium was estimated as 0.25 μg/kg live weight (Grace and Clark, 1991) and is the basis of the calculation of maintenance. The requirements for growth and wool were determined as 0.50 mg/kg weight gain and 0.38 mg/kg clean wool, which are selected values from an array of reported values and estimates (NRC, 1985; Ullrey, 1987; Grace and Clark, 1991; Ellison, 1992; Schrauzer, 2000; Taylor, 2005). The requirement for gestating ewes was calculated with 0.010 mg accumulated daily (Grace and Clark, 1991). The amount of selenium in milk from ewes was given as 0.006 mg/kg with a range from 0.002–0.020 mg/kg (Grace and Clark, 1991). However, Puls (1994) gave an optimum range from 0.025–0.250 mg Se/kg milk. A value of 0.14 mg Se/kg milk was adopted.

Values used for goats were taken from cattle and sheep requirements with adjustments where possible. Endogenous losses in feces (0.015 mg/kg diet) and urine (0.083 mg/d) adjusted from cattle data (NRC, 2001) were used to calculate maintenance requirements. Deposits of selenium in the fetus during late gestation (last 50 days) were determined as 0.0021 mg/kg LBW. Estimates of composition of gain and milk were 0.5 mg/kg LWG and 0.1 mg/kg MY.

Herdt (1995) determined the concentration of selenium in plasma of pregnant and lactating llamas and their crias from 29 herds. Herds were from either high or low selenium areas of the United States. Mean selenium supplementation was 0.74 mg/d (range: 0 to 5.4), which is equivalent to 0.19 mg Se/kg dry matter. Herdt (1995) predicted that llamas with > 160 ng Se/mL of serum and crias with > 85 ng Se/mL serum will be in adequate selenium status.

Selenium Requirements of Sheep, Goats, and New World Camelids

Species and Class	Requirement or Equation
Sheep	
Maintenance	0.00025 mg/kg BW/AC
Growth	0.50 mg/kg LWG/AC
Pregnancy	
(last one-third)	0.0025 mg/kg LBW/AC
Lactation	0.14 mg/kg MY/AC
Wool	0.38 mg/kg CFW/AC
Goat	
Maintenance	0.015 mg/kg DMI + 0.083 mg/AC
Growth	0.5 mg/kg LWG/AC
Pregnancy	
(last one-third)	0.0021 mg/kg LBW/AC
Lactation	0.10 mg/kg MY/AC
Mohair	0.38 mg/kg CFW/AC
NWC (supplementation level)	0.74 mg/d

where BW = bodyweight, kg; AC = absorption coefficient (forages = 0.3l; and concentrates = 0.60); LWG = live weight gain, kg/d; LBW = litter birth weight, kg; MY = milk yield, kg/day; CFW = clean fleece weight, kg.

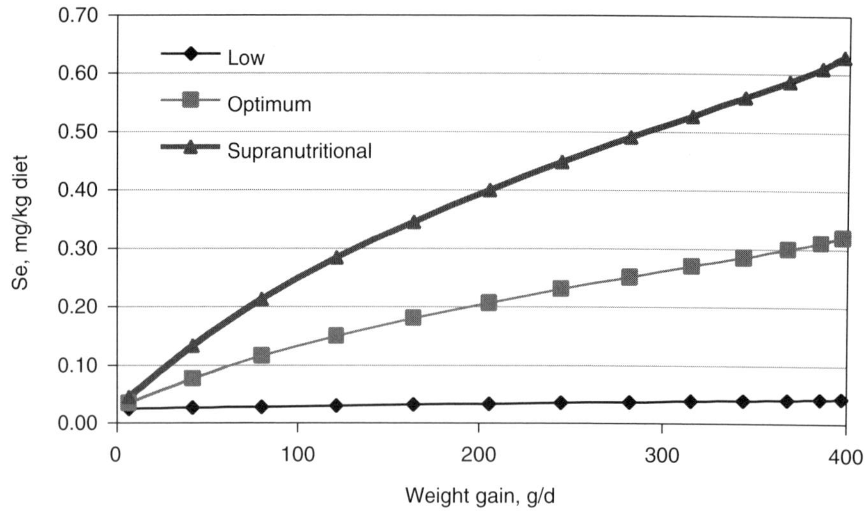

FIGURE 7-1 Selenium requirements of growing lambs based on performance and selenium content of carcass.

The maintenance requirement and absorption coefficients of 30 and 60 percent for forages and concentrates, respectively (NRC, 2001), were used to estimate selenium requirements of growing sheep and goats. However, the factorial method allows estimates of requirements applicable to other conditions (Figure 7-1).

The selenium requirements that can be calculated with the above equations need to comply with current FDA regulations (FDA, 2004). Selenium can be added to sheep diets from sodium selenite or sodium selenate in the following forms:

- In complete feeds at a level not to exceed 0.3 parts per million;
- In feed supplements for limit feeding at a level not to exceed an intake of 0.7 milligrams per head per day;
- In salt-mineral mixture for free-choice up to 90 parts per million in the mixture at a rate not to exceed an intake of 0.7 milligrams per head per day;
- Into each ton of complete feed by adding no less than 1 pound of a premix containing no more than 272.4 milligrams of added selenium per pound.

An update from the FDA (2005) allows use of selenium yeast in complete feed for goats and sheep at levels not to exceed 0.3 parts per million added selenium.

Selenium Requirements of Cervids

The values for sheep and goats are recommended.

Selenium Deficiencies

The main manifestation of selenium deficiency is white muscle disease. It may be congenital or delayed. Sheep are more susceptible than cattle to selenium deficiency (Muth, 1963; Grace, 1994). Lamb mortality may reach 65 percent under extreme conditions (NRC, 1983). However, goats are more susceptible than lambs or calves to white muscle disease (Rammel et al., 1989). The deaths of 66 percent of goat kids in the Mexican plateau are due to white muscle disease (Ramírez-Bribiesca et al., 2001). Lamb mortality was reduced 17 percent in 4 experiments, and growth rate of survivors was increased 45 percent in 19 experiments reviewed by Minson (1990). Besides white muscle disease in young deer, conception is also decreased in yearlings at the beginning of the breeding season when selenium is deficient (Grace and Wilson, 2002). Within forages, legumes promote greater incidence of white muscle disease than grasses (Whanger et al., 1972), which may be due to higher sulfur contents of legumes and the presence of cyanogenic glycosides. Sulfur supplementation of pregnant ewes increases the incidence of white muscle disease in their lambs (Hintz and Hogue, 1964). White clover may contain high levels of cyanogenic glycosides that increase the incidence of white muscle disease in lambs (Gutzwiller, 1993). Menzies et al. (2003) found 3.3 percent of cull ewes and 42.6 percent of market lambs with marginal selenium concentrations in their livers. Vitamin E was also marginal in 10 and 90 percent of cull ewes and market lambs, respectively. Low dietary vitamin E may have increased the amount of selenium required in the diet to prevent white muscle disease (Miller et al., 1988).

Regions that are selenium deficient (less than 0.5 mg Se/kg of soil) include New England, New York, New Jersey, Delaware, Pennsylvania, Maryland, West Virginia, Florida, Ohio, Indiana, Illinois, Michigan, Wisconsin, Washington State, Oregon, and the coastal regions of Virginia, the Carolinas, and Georgia (NRC, 1983). Most countries of Latin

America, Northern Europe, New Zealand, Australia, Indonesia, Kenya, Philippines, South Africa, Sudan, Swaziland, Uganda, and China have regions with selenium deficiency (McDowell, 1997; Underwood and Suttle, 1999).

Selenium Toxicities

Although selenium toxicity under natural conditions was considered a great problem in Wyoming, Raisbeck et al. (1993) did not find any confirmed selenosis from 1947 to 1987 in the Wyoming State Veterinary Laboratory records. During the 3-year period 1988–1991, four horses with selenosis were confirmed, but none in sheep or cattle. Hoff et al. (1998) found only four documented cases of selenium toxicosis out of 887 cases of metal toxicosis in wild birds and domestic livestock from Ontario, Canada, during 1990–1995. The main problems with excess selenium are due to mixing errors or overdosing with injectable preparations. In these cases, the toxicity is acute and is manifested as poor growth, high selenium content in tissues, abnormal gait, vomiting, dispnea, tetanic spasms, labored respiration, and death (NRC, 2005). Until recently, a set of symptoms described as "blind staggers" was considered to be caused by chronic (or subacute) selenium poisoning. However, recent research (O'Toole and Raisbeck, 1995) has discounted this concept, and blind staggers is believed to be caused by the consumption of high-sulfate alkali water (Merck, 2006). Chronic selenosis or alkali disease causes wool losses and death of sheep.

Regions with high selenium concentrations in soils are South Dakota, Wyoming, Montana, North Dakota, Nebraska, Kansas, Colorado, Utah, Arizona, and New Mexico in the United States, and Alberta, Saskatchewan, and Manitoba in Canada (NRC, 1983). McDowell (1997) listed 21 countries from Latin America, Africa, and Asia with selenium toxicity.

The maximum tolerable level of selenium was increased from 2.0 (NRC, 1980) to 5.0 mg/kg DM (NRC, 2005). The latter value was set considering animal health. However, it was stated that lower values are necessary to avoid excessive accumulation in edible tissues (NRC, 2005). Linseed meal was used to protect animals from selenium toxicity, due to its content of linustatin and neolinustatin (Smith et al., 1980).

Selenium Sources

Selenium sources allowed for livestock are sodium selenite, sodium selenate, and yeast (FDA, 2004). Selenium supplementation can be provided through direct injection or oral drenching with sodium selenite (0.1 mg/kg LW) at 1 to 3-month intervals in grazing animals (Meneses et al., 1994); increasing selenium intake in the diet by using selenium-rich ingredients or providing selenized mineral supplements (11.8 mg Se/kg); providing soluble glass boluses as slow release selenium; and treating forages and pastures with selenium solution. Application of less soluble forms of $BaSeO_4$ at 10 g Se/hectare in granular form is effective for 3 years (Whelan et al., 1994).

Camelids and cervids are not considered among the animals that may be supplemented with selenium (FDA, 2004, 2005). An option to solve the problems with these animals is to use forages grown in the seleniferous regions.

ZINC

Zinc (Zn) plays a major role in growth and health of all animals. It is involved in numerous metalloenzymes and is linked to vitamin A synthesis, CO_2 transport, protein metabolism, degradation of collagen fibrils, carbohydrate metabolism, destruction of free radicals, erythrocyte membrane stability, and essential fatty acid metabolism (Underwood and Suttle, 1999). Perhaps more important are its functions in gene expression and appetite. Zinc, along with cysteine and histidine, creates zinc finger domains in DNA-binding protein (Berg, 1990) that influences transcription and cell replication (Chesters, 1992). Therefore, the vital role that zinc plays in the body metabolism may relate to this function. Zinc may be involved in gene expression of cholecystokinin (an appetite-regulating hormone) in the intestine, which clearly associates zinc deficiency to anorexia (Cousins, 1997). Zinc, as a part of thymosin, regulates cell-mediated immunity (NRC, 2001). Supplementation with Zn-methionine improved udder resistance to stress and milk quality in goats (Salama et al., 2003).

Zinc Homeostasis

Plasma zinc values range from 0.8–1.2 mg Zn/L in sheep (Puls, 1994) and from 1.12–2.56 mg/L in Nubian goats (Ahmed et al., 2001). Zinc, like a few other elements, is absorbed mainly in the small intestine (Flagstad, 1976) by active and saturable processes according to the needs of the animal (Suttle et al., 1982). Therefore, true absorbability is difficult to determine. In general, the level of zinc absorption is 60–70 percent in ruminants. Absorption can be limited by binding to metallothionein and can be affected by the presence of calcium, selenium, copper, and cadmium. Zinc is transported in plasma bound to albumin macroglobulin and metallothionein. Zinc is removed by the liver as Zn-metallothionein. This process can be enhanced by glucocorticoids and cytokines to reduce plasma zinc concentration (Cousins, 1996). Metallothionein has high affinity to cadmium and copper, resulting in observed interactions between these elements. Wool (100–200 mg Zn/kg DM) is a major source of zinc, and in the bloodstream, 80 percent of zinc is in erythrocytes, mostly as carbonic anhydrase. The major route of zinc excretion is through the pancreas and feces with little excreted in the urine. The importance of endogenous loss to zinc homeostasis is minimal, and there is no evidence of zinc storage in animals. However, in case of a deficiency, redistribution from muscle and bone may delay deficiency symptoms (Underwood and Suttle, 1999).

Zinc Requirements of Sheep and Goats

The dietary requirements of zinc for sheep were set as 20 mg/kg dry matter for growing animals, and 33 mg/kg dry matter for optimum reproductive performance of males and females, and for lactating ewes (NRC, 1985). Factorial estimation of dietary requirements for growing sheep ranged from 24–51 mg Zn/kg dry matter (ARC, 1980). The requirement for adults and gestating and lactating ewes ranged from 20–39 mg Zn/kg dry matter. The requirements set by the factorial method are within the range found by several researchers looking at semisynthetic diets or under most field conditions.

The zinc requirements in this edition were estimated by the factorial method. It was considered that daily endogenous loss of zinc was 0.076 mg Zn/kg BW, zinc deposited in weight gain was 24 mg/kg, and wool contains 115 mg Zn/kg (ARC, 1980). For gestating ewes it was considered that the amount of zinc deposited daily was 1.5 mg during the last one-third of gestation for a 4 kg lamb (ARC, 1980). For lactating ewes, it was considered that milk contains 7.4 mg Zn/kg (Grace and Clark, 1991). Absorption coefficients are variable, according to the weight of the animal.

Zinc requirement for growth in goats is less than those required for growth of sex organs, milk production, and pregnancy. NRC (1981) recommended 10 mg Zn/kg diet DM to be adequate for growth, production, and reproduction. For sheep, NRC (1985) differentiated the requirements at 20 mg/kg diet DM for growing animals and 33 mg/kg diet DM for reproduction. AFRC (1997) set the requirements at 50 mg Zn/kg diet DM and up to 80 mg/kg diet DM for breeding herds in the presence of antagonists. In this edition, zinc requirements for goats were calculated using the factorial method based on data from dairy cattle (NRC, 2001) and adjusted where possible based on other estimates (Haenlein, 1992; AFRC, 1997; Meschy, 2000) and available data with goats. Endogenous fecal losses were determined at 0.033 mg Zn/kg BW and obligatory urine losses at 0.012 mg Zn/kg BW; therefore, the total maintenance requirement was set at 0.045 mg Zn/kg BW (Hansard et al., 1968). Average body weight gain requires 16–31 mg Zn/kg (Miller, 1970; Kirchgessner and Neese, 1976). A total gestation requirement for zinc was estimated at 2 mg/day, based on House and Bell (1993) data, adjusted for goats (1:6 cow:goat ratio). Goat milk contains 3–8 mg Zn/kg (Park, 2000; Aganga et al., 2002), depending on breed, diet, and level of production. Dietary requirements depend on availability or absorbability of zinc in the diet. ARC (1980) proposed an absorption coefficient of 50 percent for preruminants on milk diet, 30 percent for growing ruminants, and 20 percent for adult ruminants. However, NRC (2001) suggested a more conservative value of 15 percent for more practical cases.

Zinc Requirements of Sheep and Goats

Species and Class	Requirement or Equation
Sheep	
Maintenance	0.076 mg/kg BW
Growth	0.024 g/kg LWG/AC
Pregnancy (last one-third)	0.375 mg/kg LBW/AC
Lactation	7.4 mg/kg MY/AC
Wool	115 mg/kg CFW/(365 × AC)
Goats	
Maintenance	0.045 mg/kg BW/AC
Growth	0.025 g/kg LWG/AC
Pregnancy (last one-third)	0.5 mg/kg LBW/AC
Lactation	5.5 mg/kg MY/AC
Mohair	115 mg/kg CFW/(365 × AC)

where BW = bodyweight, kg; LWG = live weight gain, g/d; AC = absorption coefficient (lamb with 5 to 10 kg BW = 0.55, lamb with 20 kg BW = 0.30, lamb with > 40 kg BW = 0.20, adult sheep = 0.15, preweaned kid = 0.50, weaned kid = 0.30, and adult goat = 0.15); LBW = litter birth weight, kg; MY = milk yield, kg/day; CFW = clean fleece weight, kg.

Zinc Requirements of Cervids

The values for sheep and goats are recommended.

Zinc Deficiencies

A zinc deficiency caused low concentrations of Zn in the sex organs of rams and goats but not in calves (Miller et al., 1967). Young goats had low plasma vitamin A values with zinc-deficient diets with adequate levels of vitamin A in the diet (Chhabra and Arora, 1993). Symptoms associated with zinc-deprived animals include anorexia, skeletal and reproductive disorders, impairment of the immune system, and abnormalities in skin and wool.

Zinc Toxicities

Ruminants have less tolerance to high zinc intake than nonruminant animals. Lambs receiving diets containing 1–1.7 g Zn/kg DM as zinc oxide exhibited reduced weight gain and feed efficiency, depressed feed intake, and eventually pica. At higher levels, rumen fermentation was disturbed, and rumen volatile fatty acid production and acetate to propionate ratio were reduced (Ott et al., 1966). The maximum tolerable level for sheep is 300 mg Zn/kg diet DM (NRC, 2005).

Dietary Considerations for Zinc

Zinc concentrations fall between 25–50 mg Zn/kg DM for most forage pastures, 13–25 mg/kg for hays, and 12–45 mg/kg for corn silage. Cereal grains contain 30–40 mg/kg DM with higher amounts concentrated on the outer layer similar to that observed in manganese. Protein sources have higher concentrations ranging from 50–70 mg/kg DM in plant sources to 80–120 mg/kg DM in animal sources (Underwood, 1962).

Zinc can be provided through fertilizers, thereby increasing the zinc content of forage, or in salt licks (containing 1–2 percent zinc) for grazing animals. Oral drenching with zinc sulfate and intraruminal pellets with slow-release zinc has been effective in supplying sufficient zinc to overcome deficiencies. Zinc provided in organic forms (Zn-amino acids chelates) was not better than inorganic sources such as oxides and sulfates (Swinkels et al., 1996; Campbell et al., 1999). Zinc absorption, retention, and tissue deposition are similar for zinc-methionine and zinc sulfate (Nockels et al., 1993; Rojas et al., 1995). In other studies, growth performance was similar with both sources (Galyean et al., 1995; Berrie et al., 1995). However, zinc-lysine had greater bioavailability than zinc oxide and zinc sulfate based on concentrations of zinc and metallothionein in kidney, liver, and pancreas (Rojas et al., 1995).

OTHER POTENTIALLY ESSENTIAL OR TOXIC ELEMENTS

Aluminum is not considered an essential element but can be toxic at levels above 1,000 mg/kg of diet (NRC, 2005) and may affect reproduction and the newborn (Angelow et al., 1993). Possible links of aluminum with silicon (Carlisle and Curran, 1993) and magnesium (Allen et al., 1984) have been noted.

Arsenic was known as a poisonous element for years and was used as a pesticide or toxin to other pathogens. Goats, and perhaps other ruminants, may require arsenic at a low level (50 μg/kg of diet: Anke et al., 1991), but with a low maximum tolerable level of 30 mg/kg of diet (NRC, 2005). Arsenic is more correctly classified as a toxic element. The liver, kidney, and skin are deposit sites for arsenic (Selby et al., 1977). Beneficial pharmacological effects of arsenic may confuse determinations of its essentiality.

Boron (B) is an essential nutrient for plants, but its essentiality for goats or other animals is questionable. Small et al. (1997) reported an association between low serum boron and poor conception rate in cattle, but no cause and effect was determined. Boron varies in composition in soils and plants (Kabata-Pendias and Pendias, 1992) and was shown to be absorbed and excreted in cattle (Green and Weeth, 1977; Weeth et al., 1981) and in sheep (Brown et al., 1989). At 300 mg/kg DM, animals exhibited depressed appetite and retarded growth (Green and Weeth, 1977). The maximum tolerable level in sheep diets was estimated as 150 mg B/kg diet DM (NRC, 2005).

Cadmium (Cd) is contained in most feeds and forages at < 0.5 mg Cd/kg, far below the maximum tolerable concentration of cadmium of 10 mg/kg diet DM (NRC, 2005). The minimum cadmium requirement for goats is set at 300 μg Cd/kg DM. At less than 15 μg Cd/kg DM, goats exhibited impaired growth, myasthenia, reduced milk production, and shortened life span and produced unthrifty kids when compared to goats supplemented with cadmium at 250 μg/kg diet DM (Anke et al., 1991). Cadmium occurs in the soil at safe levels (Archer and Hodgson, 1987; Phillip et al., 2004); however, superphosphate fertilizers and sewage sludge are major source of cadmium that can contaminate soil, water, and plants and increase cadmium uptake by humans. Zinc smelting and zinc plating operations also have been sources of contamination. In the unlikely case of toxicity, cadmium can interfere with the absorption of copper, zinc, and iron. Cadmium is poorly absorbed but can accumulate in the muscle and can disturb the balance of other minerals in the body (Phillip et al., 2004).

Chromium is considered a required element, but neither a deficiency nor a toxicity is likely to occur under normal conditions. Dietary requirements for chromium are not defined, but they appear to increase under stress conditions such as exercise, transportation, and infections when urinary losses of chromium are increased (Anderson, 1987). Roles, functions, and effects that have been described for chromium include enhancement of sensitivity of cells to insulin, involvement in glucose metabolism and the immune response (Burton, et al., 1993), and improvement of energy status and milk production in dairy cows (Besong et al., 1996; Yang et al., 1996). Chromium appears in soil at 1–121 mg/kg DM (Archer and Hodgson, 1987) and in feeds at 0.01–4.2 mg/kg DM, cereals having the lower content and legumes higher in the range. Chromium in the small intestine is absorbed poorly in its inorganic forms but at a higher level in organic forms (Olsen et al., 1996). NRC (2005) established 3,000 (oxide) and 100 (chloride) mg/kg as maximum tolerable levels for chromium. Chromium in its trivalent form is essentially nontoxic. Hexavalent chromium was reported to disturb mitochondrial oxygen consumption (Ryberg and Alexander, 1990).

Fluorine (F) is generally regarded as a toxin and not a nutrient, although small quantities of fluorine can strengthen bones and teeth. Anke and Groppel (1989) and Anke et al. (1997b) induced fluorine deficiencies in goats by feeding a semi-synthetic diet containing < 0.3 mg F/kg diet DM for 10 generations. Lesions and symptoms that developed included retarded growth, higher mortality, and shorter lifespan compared with control animals. They estimated the requirement at 1–2 mg/kg DM. Feeds and forages contain 1–6 mg/kg DM. The maximum tolerable level is 60 mg/kg diet for sheep and 40 mg/kg diet DM for cattle (NRC, 2005). Water can be an important source of fluorine that may cause dental fluorosis (> 2 mg/L) or skeletal fluorosis (> 4 mg/L) in animals and humans (NRC, 1974, 2006). In the states of Colorado, Oklahoma, New Mexico, Idaho, Virginia, Texas, South Carolina, and California, some water sources may cause fluorosis (NRC, 2005, 2006). The minimum acceptable P:F ratio is 100 in the United States (Thompson, 1980). Absorbed fluorine is deposited in the bone but the percent deposited decreases as intake increases (Shupe, 1980). Placental and mammary barriers limit its transfer to the fetus and milk (Forsyth et al., 1972; Wheeler et al., 1985; Underwood and Suttle, 1999). Fluorine is an accumulative poison and signs of toxicity may be delayed. Signs of chronic toxicity include irreversible skeletal abnormalities and dental lesions. A total metabolic breakdown and death occur with acute poisoning (Underwood and Suttle, 1999).

Lead (Pb) is the leading cause of poisoning in farm animals (Neathery and Miller, 1975). It is an accumulative poison present in appreciable amount in soil (mining areas), sewage sludge, automotive exhaust fumes (leaded gasoline), discarded batteries, and, in the past, in paint. Lead is absorbed poorly by ruminants (3–10 percent: Fick et al., 1976) and absorption can be hindered further by the presence of high sulfur, iron, calcium, phosphorus, zinc, fat, and protein (Morrison et al., 1977; White et al., 1985). Lead accumulates in the bone (Schroeder and Tipton, 1968), blood, liver, and kidney. Accumulations reach plateaus in the blood and liver but increase linearly in the kidney at higher levels of intake (Fick et al., 1976). Increased levels of lead in newborns and milk suggests placental and mammary transport (Carson et al., 1974; Suttle et al., 1997). Retarded growth, disturbed iron metabolism, anemia, and impaired lipid metabolism were observed in animals fed diets containing < 200 μg Pb/kg DM (Kirchgessner et al., 1991; Nielson, 1996) suggesting lead as an essential element. The maximum tolerable level for sheep and cattle was set at 100 mg/kg diet DM (NRC, 2005). Chronic lead toxicity is associated with osteoporosis and may cause hydronephrosis in young lambs (Butler et al., 1957; Quarterman et al., 1977). In acute cases, impaired neurological functions, blindness, gastrointestinal hemorrhages, anemia, and liver necrosis may prevail (Radostits et al., 1994). Calcium and phosphorus supplementation may reduce lead poisoning by capturing and diluting lead in newly formed bone (Underwood and Suttle, 1999).

Lithium (Li) is abundant in soil, so a deficiency in grazing animals is very unlikely. Lithium, like sodium, may be readily absorbed and excreted with minimum retention in tissues. The levels of sodium and potassium in the diet may affect absorption. Plasma concentrations of lithium are low (< 0.02 mg/L) and linearly related to intake, thereby allowing the use of lithium salts as markers for intake of feed supplement on pastures (Vipond et al., 1995). Anke et al. (1983) reported retarded growth, impaired fertility, low birth weights, and shorter lifespans in goats on a lithium-deficient diet (3.3 μg/kg diet DM). Clinical indicators of a lithium deficiency in goats were reduced serum dehydrogenases and aldolases and liver monoamine oxidase (Szilagyi et al., 1989). The requirement for lithium was set at more than 2 μg/kg diet DM by Haenlein (1992) for goats. The actual required level and environmental factors that may impact the requirement are unknown. Toxicity is rarely encountered in farm animals. However, animals can exhibit depression, diarrhea, ataxia, and death after consuming 500–700 mg Li/kg LW as LiCl (Johnson et al., 1980). The maximum tolerable level was set as 25 mg Li/kg diet DM for sheep and cattle (NRC, 2005).

Mercury has no demonstrated nutritional value for any species. Mercury exists at low levels in soils (0.09 mg/kg DM) and plants (< 0.1 mg/kg DM); however, industrial discharges of inorganic mercury can contaminate water and enhance its conversion into more potent organic form (methylated mercury) through marine organisms. Mercury is a poisonous heavy metal that is poorly absorbed (1–15 percent) in its inorganic form and highly absorbable (59 percent as methyl mercury chloride and 90 percent as phenyl derivatives) in its organic forms in the body (Kostial et al., 1978; Clarkson, 1987). The majority of mercury absorbed in its organic form is found in muscle with small amounts in urine and milk (1.1 percent and 0.17 percent, respectively: Neathery et al., 1974). Organic mercury compounds are lipid-soluble and tend to cross the blood-brain barrier easier and cause neurological problems. Mercury has affinity for sulfhydryl groups and cysteine-rich molecules such as metallothionein, from which it can interact with zinc and cadmium metabolism. Addition of selenium or vitamin E to the diet provides some protection against mercury toxicity. Mercury creates an oxidative stress at the cell membrane level (Underwood and Suttle, 1999). Fish meal contains high levels of both organic mercury and selenium. Fungicides used for coating seed grains (Radostits et al., 1994) or treating wounds with mercury may also cause threat of mercury poisoning. Signs of inorganic mercury poisoning are acute hemorrhagic gastroenteritis. In lower doses, it can cause depression, anorexia, stiff legged gait, and paresis. Lesions and symptoms seen in later stages include loss of hair, intense itching, scabby lesions around the anus and vulva, shedding teeth, diarrhea, acute renal failure, and death (Bulger and Siegel, 1975; Radostits et al., 1994). Organic mercury poisoning causes incoordination, blindness, and convulsions, symptoms similar to those that develop with thiamine deficiencies such as polioencephalomalacia (Oliver and Platonow, 1960; Davis et al., 1965; Herigstad et al., 1972). Maximum tolerable level was set at 2 mg/kg DM (NRC, 2005).

Nickel (Ni) is present at very low levels in soils (23.7 mg/kg DM: Archer and Hodgson, 1987) and crops (0.13–2.7 mg/kg DM: Kabata-Pendias and Pendias, 1992) and is poorly absorbed (1–5 percent) by animals. The concentration of nickel in plasma is low (< 0.017 μmol/kg) but higher (0.77 μmol/kg) in the liver and much higher (2.7 μmol/kg) in the kidney (Stangl and Kirchgessner, 1996). Main route of excretion is in feces. Nickel may be needed for rumen microorganisms as its supplementation has increased ruminal urease activity, growth rate, and feed efficiency of lambs and steers (Spears, 1984). Anke et al. (1991) reported that goats fed a diet deficient in nickel (< 100 µg/kg diet DM) had decreased hemoglobin, produced offspring having lower liver zinc, and exhibited parakeratosis-like changes in the skin and hair. Nickel at 1 mg/kg diet can alleviate the deficiencies. More recently, Adeloye and Yousouf (2001) reported increased feed intake, nitrogen retention, and body weight gain in goats receiving adequate (10 mg/kg DM) compared with inadequate (0.3 mg/kg DM) nickel. A nickel deficiency in grazing livestock is unlikely, and only animals on cereal-based diets may encounter deficiencies. Haenlein (1992) suggested a dietary requirement for goats of 300–350 µg Ni/kg DM. Maximum tolerable level is set at 100 mg/kg in cattle and sheep (NRC, 2005).

Rubidium was reported by Anke et al. (1997a) to be necessary for normal reproduction in goats. Goats on a rubidium-deficient diet (0.28 mg/kg DM) had higher incidences of abortion, lower birth weights, lower weaning weights, and increased mortality when compared to the control goats. These results, though interesting, have not been corroborated, and the designation of rubidium as a required element is not justified at this time. The NRC (2005) did not include a maximum tolerable level for rubidium in diets for farm animals.

Silicon is abundant in soils, in and on plant tissue (20–80 mg/kg DM), and inside the gastrointestinal tracts of grazing animals. Small amounts are absorbed (< 1 percent) from the small intestine, transported in blood as monosilicic acid, and distributed within the soft tissues (Carlisle, 1986). Most animal products are low in silicon (3 mg/kg DM) and milk is marginal (1 mg/L). Silicon has been shown to be essential only in chicks fed diets containing 1 mg Si/kg DM vs. 250 mg Si/kg DM. Chicks on the deficient diet had retarded growth and impaired bone and cartilage development (Carlisle, 1986). Excess intake of silicon may decrease DM digestibility (Van Soest and Jones, 1968). Urinary calculi in male ruminants contain silica (combination of silicon and oxygen). The maximum tolerable level was set at 0.2 percent of the diet primarily to guard against the negative impact of silicon on digestibility (NRC, 2005).

Tin (Sn) is present at low levels in the soil (0.9–1.7 mg/kg DM: Kabata-Pendias and Pendias, 1992) and is low in feeds and forages. Tin is poorly absorbed and retained in tissues (< 1 mg/kg DM). Rats showed retarded growth on diets containing 0.5 mg Sn/kg DM compared to those fed 1–2 mg/kg DM. Tin may be involved in the tertiary structure of proteins and oxidation-reduction reactions (Underwood and Suttle, 1999). The maximum tolerable level of tin was set tentatively as 100 mg/kg diet DM (NRC, 2005).

Vanadium is abundant in soil and is considered for its pharmacological and toxicological properties. The level of vanadium in pastures and crops is low; therefore, soil ingestion is a major source of vanadium intake. Also, certain phosphate supplements are rich in vanadium that may be consumed collaterally (Sell et al., 1982; Davison et al., 1997). Animals absorb very little vanadium (1.6 percent in sheep: Paterson et al., 1986). Once absorbed, it is readily transported across membranes and binds to protein (transferrin and lactoferrin), and, substituting for phosphate, it can mimic cyclic adenosine monophosphate. As peroxovanadate, it can influence free radical generation and mimics insulin (Nielson, 1996). Anke et al. (1989) fed female goats a diet deficient in vanadium (< 10 µg/kg DM) and recorded reduced intake, reduced milk production, bone abnormality, impaired reproduction, small litter size, and high mortality in kids and does when compared to control animals. The requirements for goats were set at 10–25 µg/kg DM, a level that is far lower than would be expected under normal conditions. Vanadium toxicosis inhibits Na-K ATP'ases (Cantly et al., 1977). Toxicity can cause irreversible damage to the liver and kidney. High levels (400–800 mg/day) fed to lamb caused diarrhea and anorexia (Hansard et al., 1978). The maximum tolerable level is set at 50 mg/kg diet (NRC, 2005). Rock phosphates have high vanadium concentrations (6,000 mg/kg) and potentially could be a toxic source.

REFERENCES

Adeloye, A. A., and M. B. Yousouf. 2001. Influence of nickel supplementation from nickel sulphate hexhydrate and nickel-sodium monofluorophosphate on the performance of the West African dwarf kids. Small Ruminant Res. 39:195–198.

AFRC (Agricultural and Food Research Council). 1991. Technical Committee on Responses to Nutrients, Report 6. A reappraisal of the calcium and phosphorus requirements of sheep and cattle. Nutrition Abstracts and Reviews (Series B) 61:573–612.

AFRC. 1997. Technical Committee on Responses to Nutrients, Report 10. The nutrition of goats. Nutrition Abstracts and Reviews (Series B) 67: 806–815.

Aganga, A. A., I. O. Amarteifio, and N. Nkile, N. 2002. Effect of stage of lactation on nutrient composition of Tswana sheep and goat's milk. J. Food Compos. Anal. 15:533–543.

Åhman, B., A. Rydberg, and G. Åhman. 1986. Macrominerals in free-ranging Swedish reindeer during winter. Rangifer Spec. Iss. No. 1:31–38.

Ahmed, M. M. M., T. F. M. Hamed, and M. E. S. Barri. 2001. Variation of zinc and copper concentrations in the plasma of Nubian goats according to physiological state. Small Ruminant Res. 39(2):189–193.

Allaway, W. H. 1986. Soil-plant-animal and human interrelationships in trace element nutrition. Pp. 465–487 in Trace Elements in Human and Animal Nutrition, 5th ed.,vol. 2, W. Mertz, ed. Orlando, FL: Academic Press.

Allen, V. G., D. L. Robinson, and F. Hemby. 1984. Effect of ingested aluminum sulphate on serum magnesium and the possible relationship to hypomagnesaemic tetany. Nutr. Rep. Int. 29:107–115.

Anderson, R. A. 1987. Chromium. Pp. 225–244 in Trace Elements in Human and Animal Nutrition, 5th ed., vol. 1, W. Mertz, ed. San Diego: Academic Press.

Angelow, L., M. Anke, B. Groppel, M. Glei, and M. Muller. 1993. Aluminum: An essential element for goats. Pp. 699–704 in Proc. 8th Inter. Symp. on Trace Elements in Animals and Man, M. Anke, D. Meissner, and C. F. Mills, eds. Dresden: Verlag Media Touristic, Gersdorf.

Anke, M., and B. Groppel. 1989. Fluorine deficiency symptoms in the goat. P. 346 in Proc. Macro- and Trace Element Seminar, University Leipzig-Jena, Germany, Dec. 19–20.

Anke, M., and M. A. Risch. 1989. Importance of molybdenum in animal and man. P. 303 in Proc. 6th Inter. Trace Element Symp., University Leipzig-Jena, Germany.

Anke, M., B. Groppel, W. Reisseg, H. Ludke, M. Grun, and G. Dittrich. 1973. Manganmangel bein Wiederkauer. 3. Manganmangelbedingte Fortpflanzungs Skelett- und Nervenstorungen bei weiblichen Weiderkauern und ihren Nachkommen. Archive fur Tlerernabrung 23:197–211.

Anke, M., M. Green, M. Partschefeld, and B. Groppel. 1978. Molybdenum deficiency in ruminants. Pp. 230–233 in Proc. 3rd Inter. Symp. Trace Element Metabolism in Man and Animals, M. Kirchgessener, ed., Arbeitskreis for Tieremahrungsforschung, Weihenstephan.

Anke, M., B. Groppel, H. Kronemann, and M. Gruen. 1983. Evidence for the essentiality of lithium in goats. P. 58 in Proc. 4th Inter. Trace Element Symp., University Leipzig-Jena, Germany.

Anke, M., B. Groppel, and A. Schmidt. 1987a. New results on the essentiality of cadmium in ruminants. P. 556 in Proc. Symp. Trace Subst. in Environm. Health XXI, Univ. Missouri, Columbia.

Anke, M., L. Angelow, B. Groppel, and W. Arnhold. 1987b. Effect of selenium deficiency upon reproduction and milk production of goats. P. 440 in Proc. Macro- and Trace Element Seminar, University Leipzig-Jena, Germany, Dec. 21–22.

Anke, M., L. Angelow, B. Groppel, T. Kosla, and M. Langer. 1987c. Effect of selenium deficiency upon feed consumption and growth of goats. P. 431 in Proc. Macro- and Trace Element Seminar, University Leipzig-Jena, Germany, Dec. 21–22.

Anke, M., B. Groppel, K. Grun, M. Langer, and W. Arnhold. 1989. The essentiality of vanadium for animals. Pp. 17–27 in Proc. 6th Inter. Trace Element Symp., vol. 1. Friedrich Schiller University, Jena.

Anke, M., B. Groppel, and V. Krause. 1991. The essentiality of the toxic elements cadmium, arsenic and nickel. Pp. 11-6–11-8 in Proc. 7th Inter. Symp. on Trace Elements in Man and Animals (TEMA 7), B. Momcilovic, ed., Dubrovnik, IMI, Zagreb.

Anke, M., H. Gurtler, L. Angelow, J. Gottschalk, C. Drobner, S. Anke, H. Illingunther, M. Muller, W. Arnold, and V. Shafter. 1997a. Rubidium—an essential element for animals and humans. Pp. 189–191 in Proc. 9th Symp. on Trace Elements in Man and Animals, P. W. F. Fischer, M. R. L'Abbe, K. A. Cockell, and R. S. Gilson, eds. Ottawa: NRC Research Press.

Anke, M., H. Gurtler, H. Neubert, M. Glei, S. Anke, M. Jaritz, H. Freytag, and V. Shafter. 1997b. Effect of fluorine-poor diets in generations of goats. Pp. 192–194 in Proc. 9th Symp. on Trace Elements in Man and Animals, P. W. F. Fischer, M. R. L'Abbe, K. A. Cockell, and R. S. Gilson, eds. Ottawa: NRC Research Press.

ARC (Agricultural Research Council). 1965. Nutrient Requirements of Farm Livestock. 2. Ruminant. London: ARC.

ARC. 1980. The Nutrient Requirements of Ruminant Livestock. Slough, UK: Commonwealth Agricultural Bureaux.

Archer, F. C., and J. H. Hodgson. 1987. Total and extractable trace elements content of soils in England and Wales. J. Soil Sci. 38:421–431.

Arieli, A., E. Naim, R. W. Benjamin, and D. Pastemark. 1989. The effect of feeding saltbush and sodium chloride on energy metabolism in sheep. Animal Prod. 49:451–457.

Aspila, P. 1991. Metabolism of selenite, selenomethionine and feed-incorporated selenium in lactating goats and dairy cows. J. Agric. Sci. Finland 63:9–74.

Barboza, P., and J. Blake. 2001. Ceruloplasmin as an indicator of copper reserves in wild ruminants at high latitude. J. Wildl. Diseases 37:324–331.

Barboza, P. S., E. J. Rombach, J. E. Blake, and J. A Nagy. 2003. Copper status of muskoxen: A comparison of wild and captive populations. J. Wildl. Diseases 39:610–619.

Barry, T. N., S. O. Hoskin, and P. R. Wilson. 2002. Novel forages for growth and health in farmed deer. New Zealand Vet. J. 50:244–251.

Baxter, B. J., R. N. Andrews, and G. K. Barrell. 1999. Bone turnover with antler growth in red deer (*Cervus elaphus*). Anat. Record 256:14–19.

Behne, D., and A. Kyriakopulos. 2001. Mammalian selenium-containing proteins. Annu. Rev. Nutr. 21:453–473.

Berg, J. M. 1990. Zinc fingers and other metal binding domains: Elements for interactions between molecules. J. Biol. Chem. 256:6513–6518.

Bergerud, A. T. 1976. The annual antler cycle in Newfoundland caribou. Can. Field-Nat. 90:449–463.

Berrie, R. A., D. M. Hallford, and M. L. Galyean. 1995. Effects of zinc source and level on performance, carcass characteristics, and metabolic hormone concentrations of growing and finishing lambs. Prof. Anim. Sci. 11:149–156.

Besong, S., J. Jackson, S. Trammel, and D. Amaral-Phillips. 1996. Effect of supplemental chromium picolinate on liver triglycerides, blood metabolites, milk yield and milk composition in early-lactation cows. J. Dairy Sci. 79 (Suppl. 1):97.

Blair-West, J. R., J. P. Coghlan, D. A. Denton, J. F. Nelson, E. Orchard, B. A. Scoggins, R. D. Wright, K. Myers, and C. L. Junqueira. 1968. Physiological, morphological and behavioural adaptation to a sodium deficient environment by wild native Australian and introduced species of animals. Nature (London) 217:922–928.

Braithwaite, G. D. 1983. Calcium and phosphorus requirements of the ewe during pregnancy and lactation. 1. Calcium. Br. J. Nutr. 50:711–722.

Bravo, D., D. Sauvant, C. Bogaert, and F. Meschy. 2003a. II. Quantitative aspects of phosphorus absorption in ruminants. Reprod. Nutr. Dev. 43:271–284.

Bravo, D., D. Sauvant, C. Bogaert, and F. Meschy. 2003b. III. Quantitative aspects of phosphorus excretion in ruminants. Reprod. Nutr. Dev. 43:285–300.

Bremner, I., and J. H. Beattie. 1990. Metallothionein and the trace minerals. Annu. Rev. Nutr. 10:63–83.

Bremner, I., and A. C. Dalgarno. 1973. Iron metabolism in the veal calf. 2. Iron requirements and the effect of copper supplementation. Br. J. Nutr. 30:61–76.

Breves, G., M. Brandt, H. Hoeller, and K. Rohr. 1981. Flow of thiamin to the duodenum in dairy cows fed different rations. J. Agric. Sci. Cambridge 96:587–591.

Briggs, M. H., T. W. Heard, A. Whitcroft, and M. L. Hogg. 1964. Studies on urea-fed cattle. 2. Rumen levels of B vitamins and related coenzymes. Life Sci. 3:11–14.

Bronner, F. 1997. Calcium. Pp. 13–61 in Handbook of Nutritionally Essential Mineral Elements, D. L. O'Dell and R. E. Sunde, eds. New York: Marcel Dekker.

Brown, R. D. 1990. Nutrition and antler development. Pp. 426–441 in Horns, Pronghorns and Antlers, G. A. Bubenik and A. B. Bubenik, eds. New York: Springer-Verlag.

Brown, T. F., M. E. McCormick, D. R. Morris, and L. K. Zerinque. 1989. Effect of boron on mineral balance in sheep. Nutr. Res. 9:503–512.

Bubenik, G. A., R. G. White, and L. Bartoš. 2000. Antler growth in male and female reindeer and its relationship to seasonal blood levels of alkaline phosphatase. Folia Zool. 49:161–166.

Bulger, R. E., and F. L. Siegel. 1975. Alterations of the renal papilla during mercuric chloride induced acute tubular necrosis. Lab. Invest. 33:712–719.

Burton, J. L., B. A. Mallard, and D. N. Mowat. 1993. Effects of supplemental chromium on immune responses of peri-parturient and early lactation dairy cows. J. Anim. Sci. 71:1532–1539.

Butler, E. J., D. I. Nisbet, and J. M. Robertson. 1957. Osteoporosis in lambs in a lead mining area. 1. A study of the naturally occuring disease. J. Comparative Path. 67:378–398.

Calef, G. W., and G. M. Lortie. 1975. A mineral lick of the barren-ground caribou. J. Mammol. 56:240–242.

Campbell, M. H., J. K. Miller, and F. N. Schrick. 1999. Effect of additional cobalt, copper, manganese, and zinc on reproduction and milk yield of lactating dairy cows receiving bovine somatotropin. J. Dairy Sci. 82:1019–1025.

Cantly, L. C., Jr., L. Josephson, R. Warner, M. Yanagisawa, C. Lechene, and G. Guidotti. 1977. Vanadate is a potent (Na, K)-ATPase inhibitor found in ATP derived from muscle. J. Biol. Chem. 252:7421–7423.

Carlisle, E. M. 1986. Silicon. Pp. 373–390 in Trace Elements in Human and Animal Nutrition, 5th ed., vol. 2, W. Mertz, ed. Orlando, FL: Academic Press.

Carlisle, E. M., and M. J. Curran. 1993. Aluminum: An essential element for the chick. Pp. 695–698 in Proc. 8th Inter. Symp. on Trace Elements in Man and Animals, M. Anke, D. Meissner, and C. F. Mills, eds. Gersdorf: Verlag Media Touristik.

Carson, T. L., G. A. Van Gelder, G. C. Karas, and W. B. Buck. 1974. Slowed learning in lambs prenatally exposed to lead. Arch. of Environ. Health 29:154–156.

Chartier, C., E. Etter, H. Hoste, I. Pors, C. Koch, and B. Dellac. 2000. Efficacy of copper oxide needles for the control of nematode parasites in dairy goats. Vet. Res. Commum. 24:389–399.

Chen, H., Z. K. Attieh, T. Su, B. A. Syed, H. Gao, R. M. Alaeddine, T. C. Fox, J. Usta, C. E. Naylor, R. W. Evans, A. T. McKie, G. J. Anderson, and C. D. Vulpe. 2004. Hephaestin is a ferroxidase that maintains partial activity in sex-linked anemia mice. Blood 103:3933–3939.

Chesters, J. K. 1992. Trace elements–gene interactions. Nutr. Rev. 50: 217–223.

Chhabra, A., and S. P. Arora. 1993. Effect of vitamin A and zinc supplement on alcohol dehydrogenase and superoxide didmutase activities of goat tissues. Indian J. Anim. Sci. 63:334–338.

Chrisp, J. S., A. R. Sykes, and N. D. Grace. 1989. Kinetic aspects of calcium metabolism in lactating sheep offered herbage with different calcium concentrations and the effect of protein supplementation. Br. J. Nutr. 61:45–58.

Clark, R. G., L. Mantleman, and G. A. Verkerk. 1987. Failure to obtain a weight response to vitamin B_{12} treatment in young goats grazing pasture that was cobalt deficient for sheep. New Zealand Vet. J. 35:38–39.

Clark, W. D., Jr., J. E. Wohlt, R. L. Gilbreath, and P. K. Zajac. 1986. Phytate phosphorus intake and disappearance in the gastrointestinal tract of high producing dairy cows. J. Dairy Sci. 69:3151–3155.

Clarkson, T. W. 1987. Mercury. Pp. 417 in Trace Elements in Human and Animal Nutrition, vol. 7, W. Mertz, ed. New York: Academic Press.

Cousins, R. B. 1996. Zinc. In Present Knowledge in Nutrition, 7th ed., I. J. Filer and E. E. Ziegler, eds. Washington, DC: International Life Science Institute, Nutrition Foundation.

Cousins, R. B. 1997. Differential mRNA display, competitive polymerase chain reaction and transgenic approaches to investigate zinc-responsive genes in animals and man. Pp 849–852 in Proc. 9th Symp. on Trace Elements in Man and Animals, P. W. F. Fischer, M. R. L'Abbe, K. A. Cockell, and R. S. Gibson, eds. Ottawa: NRC Research Press.

Cowan, I. McT., and V. C. Brink. 1949. Natural game licks in the Rocky Mountain National Parks of Canada. J. Mammol. 30:379–387.

Davis, E. T., A. H. Phill, D. F. Collings, J. A. J. Venn, and G. D. Bridges. 1965. Cerebrocortical necrosis in calves. Vet. Res. 77:90–96.

Davis, G. K., and W. Mertz. 1987. Copper. Pp. 301–364 in Trace Elements in Human and Animal Nutrition, 5th ed., vol. 1, W. Mertz, ed. San Diego: Academic Press.

Davison, A., L. Kowalski, Y. Xuefeng, and T. Siu-Sing. 1997. Vanadium as a modulator of cellular regulation-the role of redox reactivity. Pp. 229–233 in Proc. 9th Symp. on Trace Elements in Man and Animals, P. W. F. Fischer, M. R. L'Abbe, K. A. Cockell, and R. S. Gibson, eds. Ottawa: NRC Research Press.

Deitert, C., and E. Pfeffer. 1993. Effects of reduced P supply in combination with adequate or high Ca intake on performances and mineral balances in dairy goats during pregnancy and lactation. J. Anim. Phys. Anim. Nutr. 69:12–21.

Denton, D. A., and J. R. Sabine. 1961. The selective appetite for Na^+ shown by Na^+ deficient sheep. J. Physiol. 167:97–116.

Doisey, E. A., Jr. 1973. Micronutrient controls on biosynthesis of clotting proteins and cholesterol. P. 193 in Trace Substances in Environmental Health, D. D. Hemphill, ed. Columbia: University of Missouri.

Dove, H., and E. Charmley. 2004. Relationships between phosphorus intake, plasma phosphorus and faecal and urinary phosphorus excretion in young sheep. Anim. Prod. Aust. 25:37–40.

Durand, M., and R. Kawashima. 1980. Influence of minerals in rumen digestion. Pp. 375–408 in Digestive Physiology and Metabolism in the Ruminant, Proc. V Inter. Symp. on Ruminant Physiology, Y. Ruckebusch and P. Thivend, eds. Lancaster, UK: MTP Press.

Ehlig, C. F., D. E. Hogue, W. H. Allaway, and D. J. Hamm. 1967. Fate of selenium from selenite or selenomethionine, with or without vitamin E, in lambs. J. Nutr. 92:121–126.

Eiben, B., S. Scharla, K. Fischer, and H. Schmidt-Gayk. 1984. Seasonal variation of serum 1,25-dihydroxyvitamin D_3 and alkaline phosphatase in relation to antler formation in the fallow deer (*Dama dama* L.). Acta Endocrinol. 107:141–144.

Ellison, R. S. 1992. A review of copper and selenium reference ranges in cattle and sheep. Pp. 3–26 in Trace Elements in Ruminants. Wellington, NZ: Foundation for Continuing Education of the N. Z. Veterinary Association.

Ender, F., I. W. Dishington, and A. Helgebostad. 1971. Calcium balance studies in dairy cows under experimental induction and prevention of hypocalcaemic paresis puerperalis. The solution of the aetiology and the prevention of milk fever by dietary means. Z. Tierphysiol. 28: 233–256.

Engle, T. E., J. W. Spears, T. A. Armstrong, C. L. Wright, and J. Odle. 2000. Effects of dietary copper source and concentration on carcass characteristics and lipid and cholesterol metabolism in growing and finishing steers. J. Anim. Sci. 78:1053–1059.

Eriksson, S., S. Sanne, and S. Thomke. 1976. Fodermedelstabeller och Utfodringsre kommendationer, 2nd ed. Stockholm: LTS Forlag.

Fairweather-Tait, S. J., and A. J. A. Wright. 1984. The influence of previous iron intake on the estimation of bioavailability of Fe from a test meal given to rats. Br. J. Nutr. 51:185–191.

Falke, H., and M. Anke. 1987. The reaction of goats to molybdenum loads. P. 448 in Proc. of Macro- and Trace Element Seminar, University Leipzig-Jena, Germany, Dec. 21–22.

FDA (U. S. Food and Drug Administration). 2004. Title 21. Food and Drugs: Food additives permitted in feed and drinking water of animals. Available at http://a257.g.akamaitech.net/7/257/2422/04nov200 31500/ edocket.access.gpo.gov/cfr_2001/aprqtr/pdf/21cfr573.920.pdf. Accessed April 10, 2005.

FDA. 2005. CVM update. FDA permits the use of selenium yeast in sheep and goat feed. Available at http://www.fda.gov/cvm/CVM_Updates/ SEsheep.htm. Accessed April 10, 2005.

Fell, B. F., C. F. Mills, and R. Boyn. 1965. Cytochrome oxidase deficiency in the motor neurones of copper deficient lambs: A histochemical study. Res. Vet. Sci. 6:170–177.

Fick, K. R., C. B. Ammerman, S. M. Miller, C. F. Simpson, and P. E. Loggins. 1976. Effect of dietary lead on performance, tissue mineral composition and lead absorption in sheep. J. Anim. Sci. 42:515–523.

Flagstad, T. 1976. Lethal trait A 46 in cattle intestinal zinc absorption. Nord. Vet. Med. 28:160–169.

Fontenot, J. P. 1979. Animal nutrition aspects of grass tetany. Pp. 51–62 in Grass Tetany, Special Publication Number 35, M. Stelly, V. V. Rendig, and D. L. Grunes, eds. Madison: American Society of Agronomy.

Fontenot, J. P., V. G. Allen, G. E. Bunce, and J. P. Goff. 1989. Factors influencing magnesium absorption and metabolism in ruminants. J. Anim. Sci. 67:3445–3455.

Forsyth, D. M., W. G. Pond, and I. Krook. 1972. Dietary calcium and fluoride interactions in swine: In utero and neonatal effects. J. Nutr. 102: 1639–1646.

Fraser, D., and E. Reardon. 1980. Attraction of wild ungulates to mineral-rich springs in central Canada. Holarctic Ecol. 3:36–40.

French, C. E., L. E. McEwan, N. D. Magruder, R. H. Ingram, and R. W. Swift. 1956. Nutrient requirements for growth and antler development in the white-tailed deer. J. Wildl. Manage. 20:221–232.

Fuentealba, C., and E. M. Aburto. 2003. Animal models of copper-associated liver disease. Comp. Hepatology 2:5.

Galbraith H., W. Chigwada, J. R. Scaife, and W. R. Humphries. 1997. The effect of dietary molybdenum supplementation on tissue copper concentrations, mohair fibre and carcass characteristics of growing Angora goats. Anim. Feed Sci. Technol. 67:83–90.

Galyean, M. L., K. J. Malcoim-Callis, S. A Gunter, and R. A. Berrie. 1995. Effect of zinc source and level and added copper lysine in the receiving diet on performance by growing and finishing steers. Prof. Anim. Sci. 11:139–148.

Godoy, S., and F. Meschy. 2001. Utilization of phytate phosphorus by rumen bacteria in a semi-continuous culture system (Rusitec) in lactating goats fed on different forage to concentrate ratios. Reprod. Nutr. Dev. 41:259–265.

Goff, J. P., and R. L. Horst. 1997. Effect of addition of potassium or sodium, but not calcium, to prepartum ration on milk fever in dairy cows. J. Dairy Sci. 80:176–186.

Goff, J. P., R. Ruiz, and R. L. Horst. 1997. Relative acidogenic activity of commonly used anionic salts—re-thinking the dietary cation-anion difference equations. J. Dairy Sci. 80 (Suppl. 1):169.

Gould, D. H. 1998. Polioencephalomalacia. J. Anim. Sci. 76:309–314.

Grace, N. D. 1973. Effect of high dietary Mn level on the growth rate and the level of mineral elements in the plasma and soft tissues of sheep. NZ J. Agric. Res. 16:177–180.

Grace, N. D. 1983. Amounts and distribution of mineral elements associated with fleece-free empty body weight gains in grazing sheep. NZ J. Agric. Res. 26:59–70.

Grace, N. 1994. Managing Trace Element Deficiencies. Ruakura, NZ: New Zealand Pastoral Agriculture Research Institute Ltd. 70 p.

Grace, N. D., and R. G. Clark. 1991. Trace element requirements, diagnosis and prevention of deficiencies in sheep and cattle. Pp. 321–346 in Physiological Aspects of Digestion and Metabolism in Ruminants, T. Tsuda, Y. Sasaki, and R. Kawashima, eds. San Diego: Academic Press.

Grace, N. D., and N. F. Suttle. 1979. Some effects of sulphur intake on molybdenum metabolism in sheep. Br. J. Nutr. 41:125–136.

Grace, N. D., and P. R. Wilson. 2002. Trace element metabolism, dietary requirements, diagnosis and prevention of deficiencies in deer. New Zealand Vet. J. 50:252–259.

Grasman, B. T., and E. C. Hellgren. 1993. Phosphorus nutrition in white-tailed deer: Nutrient balance, physiological responses, and antler growth. Ecology 74:2279–2296.

Green, G. H., and H. J. Weeth. 1977. Responses of heifers to boron in water. J. Anim. Sci. 46:812–818.

Groppel, B., M. Anke, E. Scholz, and B. Koehler. 1989. Supply and status of iodine in ruminants. XII. Influence of iodine supply upon iodine contents of thyroid in goats and sheep. Pp. 295–301 in Proc. Macro- and Trace Element Seminar, University Leipzig-Jena, Germany.

Guéguen, L. 1997. La valeur nutritionnelle minérale du lait de chèvre. Pp. 67–80 in Intérêts Nutritionnels et Diététique du Lait de Chevre, G. Freund, ed. Niort: INRA.

Guéguen, L., M. Lamand, and F. Meschy. 1988. Nutrition mineral. Pp. 95–111 in Alimentation des Bovins, Ovins and Caprins, R. Jarrige, ed. Paris: INRA.

Guéguen, L., M. Lamand, and F. Meschy. 1989. Mineral Requirements. Pp. 49–56 in Ruminant Nutrition: Recommended Allowance and Feed Tables, R. Jarrige, ed. Paris: INRA.

Gutzwiller, A. 1993. The effect of a diet containing cyanogenetic glycosides on the selenium status and the thyroid function of sheep. Anim. Prod. 57:415–419.

Haenlein, G. F. W. 1987. Mineral and vitamin requirements and deficiencies. Pp. 1249–1266 in Proc. IV Inter. Conference on Goats, vol. 2, O. P. Santana, A. G. da Silvaand, and W. C. Foote, eds. Brasilia, Brazil.

Haenlein, G. F. W. 1992. Advances in the nutrition of macro and micro elements in goats. Pp. 933–950 in Proc. V Inter. Conference on Goats, New Delhi, India.

Haggard, D. L., H. D. Stowe, G. H. Coner, and D. W. Johnson. 1980. Immunological effects of experimental iodine toxicosis in young cattle. Am. J. Vet. Res. 41:539–543.

Haigh, J. C., and R. J. Hudson. 1993. Farming Wapiti and Red Deer. St. Louis, MO: Mosby-Year Book, Inc.

Hansard, S. L., A. S. Mohammed, and J. W. Turner. 1968. Gestation age effects upon maternal-fetal zinc utilization in the bovine. J. Anim. Sci. 27:1097–1102.

Hansard, S. L., C. B. Ammerman, K. R. Fick, and S. M. Miller. 1978. Performance and vanadium content of tissues in sheep as influenced by dietary vanadium. J. Anim. Sci. 46:1091–1095.

Harris, E. D. 1997. Copper. Pp. 231–274 in Handbook of Nutritionally Essential Mineral Elements, B. L. O'Dell and R. A. Sunde, eds. New York: Marcel Dekker.

Hellman, N. E., and J. D. Gitlin. 2002. Ceruloplasmin metabolism and function. Annu. Rev. Nutr. 22:439–458.

Hemken, R. W. 1960. Iodine. J. Dairy Sci. 53:1138–1143.

Henry, P. R. 1995. Cobalt bioavailability. Pp. 119–126 in Bioavailability of Nutrients for Animals: Amino Acids, Minerals, and Vitamins, C. B. Ammerman, D. H. Baker, and A. J. Lewis, eds. San Diego: Academic Press.

Henry, P. R., and C. B. Ammerman. 1995. Sulfur bioavailability. Pp. 349–366 in Bioavailability of Nutrients for Animals: Amino Acids, Minerals, and Vitamins, C. B. Ammerman, D. H. Baker, and A. J. Lewis, eds. San Diego: Academic Press.

Henry, P. R., C. B. Ammerman, and R. C. Little. 1992. Relative bioavailability of manganese from a manganese methionine complex and inorganic sources for ruminants. J. Dairy Sci. 75:3473–3478.

Henry, P. R., R. C. Littell, and C. B. Ammerman. 1997. Bioavailability of cobalt sources for ruminants. 1. Effects of time and dietary cobalt concentration on tissue cobalt concentration. Nutr. Res. 17:947–955.

Herdt, T. H. 1995. Blood serum concentrations of selenium in female llamas (Lama glama) in relationships to feeding practices, region of United States, reproductive stage, and health of offspring. J. Anim. Sci. 73:337–344.

Herigstad, R. R., C. K. Whitehair, N. Beyer, O. Mickelson, and M. J. Zabik. 1972. Chronic methylmercury toxicosis in calves. JAVMA 160: 173–182.

Hillman, D., and A. R. Cutis. 1980. Chronic iodine toxicity in dairy cattle: Blood chemistry, leucocytes and milk iodine. J. Dairy Sci. 63:55–63.

Hintz, H. F., and D. E. Hogue. 1964. Effect of selenium, sulfur, and sulfur amino acids on nutritional muscular dystrophy in the lamb. J. Nutr. 82:495–502.

Hoff, B., H. J. Boermans, and J. D. Baird. 1998. Retrospective study of toxic metal analyses requested at a veterinary diagnostic toxicology laboratory in Ontario (1990–1995). Can. Vet. J. 39:39–43.

Hopson, N. B., P. F. Fennessy, and J. M. Thompson. 1997. Plasma potassium—An indicator of protein catabolism in deer? Proc. New Zealand Soc. Anim. Prod. 57:144–146.

House, W. A., and A. W. Bell. 1993. Mineral accretion in the fetus and adnexa during late gestation in Holstein Cows. J. Dairy Sci. 76: 2999–3010.

Hove, K., H. Staaland, and R. G. White. 1986. Calcium absorption in reindeer: Effect of diet and vitamin D. Rangifer Spec. Iss. No.1:361–362.

Høymork, A., and E. Reimers. 2002. Antler development in reindeer in relation to age and sex. Rangifer 22:75–82.

Hurley, L. S., and C. L. Keen. 1987. Manganese. Pp. 185–223 in Trace Elements in Human and Animal Nutrition. 5th ed., vol. 1, W. Mertz, ed. San Diego: Academic Press.

Hyvärinen, H., R. N. B. Kay, and W. J. Hamilton. 1977. Variation in the weight, specific gravity, and composition of the antlers of red deer (*Cervus elaphus* L.). Br. J. Nutr. 28:301–311.

Hyvärinen, H., T. Helle, M. Niemenen, P. Vayrynen, and R. Vayrynen. 1977. The influence of nutrition and seasonal conditions on mineral status in the reindeer. Can. J. Zool. 55:648–655.

INRA (Institut National de la Recherche Agronomique). 1988. Alimentation des Bovins, Ovins et Caprins. Paris: INRA.

Ivan, M., M. Hidiroglou, S. L. Al-Ismaily, H. S. Al-Sumry, and R. B. Harper. 1990. Copper deficiency and posterior paralysis (Shalal) in small ruminants in the Sultanate of Oman. Trop. Anim. Hlth. Prod. 22:217–225.

Jackson, J. A., D. M. Hopkins, Z. Xin, and R. W. Hemken. 1992. Influence of cation-anion balance on feed intake, body weight gain, and humoral response of dairy calves. J. Dairy Sci. 75:1281–1286.

James, C. S., and K. Chandron. 1975. Enquiry into the role of minerals in experimental urolithiasis in goats. Indian Vet. J. 52:251–258.

Jenness, R., and R. E. Sloan. 1970. The composition of milk of various species: A review. Dairy Sci. Abstr. 32:599–612.

Johnson, J. H., H. R. Crookshank, and H. E. Smally. 1980. Lithium toxicity in cattle. Vet. Hum. Toxicol. 22:248–251.

Johnson, J. L. 1997. Molybdenum. Pp. 413–438 in Handbook of Nutritionally Essential Mineral Elements, B. I. O'Dell and R. A. Sunde, eds. New York: Marcel Dekker.

Kabata-Pendias, A., and H. Pendias. 1992. Trace Elements in Soils and Plants, 2nd ed. Boca Raton, FL: CRC Press.

Kaneko, J. J. 1989. Clinical Biochemistry of Domestic Animals, 3rd ed. New York: Academic Press.

Kelsall, J. P. 1968. The Caribou. Ottawa: Queen's Printer.

Kennedy, D.G., S. Kennedy, and P. B. Young. 1996. Effects of low concentrations of dietary cobalt on rumen succinate concentrations in sheep. Int. J. Vitamin a Nutr. Res. 66:86–92.

Kessler, J. 1991. Mineral nutrition of goats. Goat Nutr. 46:104–119.

Kirchgessner, M., and K. R. Neese. 1976. [Copper, manganese, and zinc contents in the whole body and in individual parts of veal calves at different weights (author's transl.)]. Z. Lebensm. Unfers. Forsch. 161:1–6.

Kirchgessner, M., D. L. Plass, and A. M. Reichlmayr-Lais. 1991. Lead deficiency in swine. Pp. 11-20–11-21 in Proc. 7th Inter. Symp. on Trace Elements in Man and Animals, B. Momcilovic, ed. Dubrovnik, IMI, Zagreb.

Koenig, K. M., L. M. Rode, R. D. H. Cohen, and W. T. Buckley. 1997. Effects of diet and chemical form of selenium on selenium metabolism in sheep. J. Anim. Sci. 75:817–827.

Köhrle, J. 2000. The deiodinase family: Selenoenzymes regulating thyroid hormone availability and action. Cell. Mol. Life Sci. 57:1853–1863.

Kostial, K., S. Jugo, I. Rabar, and T. Maljkovic. 1978. Influence of age on metal metabolism and toxicity. Environ. Health Persp. 25:81–86.

Låg, J. 1963. Plant nutrition and precipitation in Norway. Res. Norwegian Agric. 14:553–563.

Lamand, M. 1981. Metabolisemeet besoins en oligo-elements. Pp. 210–217 in Nutrition and Systems for Goat Feeding, vol. 1, P. Morand-Fehr, A. Bourbouze, and M. de Simiance, eds. Tours, France: Symposium Proceedings of ITOVIC-INRA International Nutrition Systems Goat Feeding Internacion.

Lassiter, J. W., W. J. Miller, F. M. Pate, and R. P. Gentry. 1972. Effect of dietary calcium and phosphorus on Mn Metabolism following single tracer intraperitoneal and oral doses in rats. Proc. Soc. Exp. Biol. Med. 139:345–348.

Lawler, T. L., J. B. Taylor, J. W. Finely, and J. S. Caton. 2004. Effect of supranutritional and organically bound selenium on performance, carcass characteristics, and selenium distribution in finishing beef steers. J. Anim. Sci. 82:1488–1493.

Lee, J., S. O. Knowles, and D. M. West. 2002. Predicting copper status of cattle remains an enigma. Proc. New Zealand Soc. Anim. Prod. 62: 319–324.

Lincoln, G. A. 1971. Puberty in a seasonally breeding male; the red deer stag (*Cervus elaphus* L.). J. Reprod. Fert. 25:41–54

Littledike, E. T., and P. S. Cox. 1979. Clinical, mineral, and endocrine interrelationships in hypomagnesemic tetany. Pp. 1–50 in Grass Tetany, Special Publication Number 35, M. Stelly, V. V. Rendig, and D. L. Grunes, eds. Madison, WI: American Society of Agronomy.

Long, T. A., R. L. Cowan, C. W. Wolfe, T. Rader, and R. W. Swift. 1959. Effect of seasonal feed restriction on antler development of white-tailed deer. Penn. Agr. Exp. Sta. Progress Report 209.

Lopez-Guisa, J. M., and L. D. Satter. 1992. Effect of copper and cobalt addition on digestion and growth in heifers fed diets containing alfalfa silage and corn crop residues. J. Dairy Sci. 75:247–256.

Luick, J. R., R. G. White, A. M. Gau, and R. Jenness. 1974. Compositional changes in the milk secreted by grazing reindeer. I. Gross composition and ash. J. Dairy Sci. 57:1325–1333.

Luginbuhl, J. M., M. H. Poore, J. W. Spears, and T. T. Brown. 2000. Effect of dietary copper level on performance and copper status of growing meat goats. Sheep Goat Res. J. 16:65–71.

Mäki, J. 2002. Lysyl oxidases. Cloning and characterization of the fourth and the fifth human lysyl oxidase isoenzymes, and the consequences of a targeted inactivation of the first described lysyl oxidase isoenzyme in mice. University of Oulu, Finland. 73 pp.

Malecki, E. A., and J. L. Greger. 1996. Manganese protects against heart mitochondrial lipid peroxidation in rats fed high levels of polyunsaturated fatty acids. J. Nutr. 126:27–33.

Masters, D. G., D. I. Paynter, J. Briegel, S. K. Baker, and D. B. Purser. 1988. Influence of manganese intake on body, wool and testicular growth of young rams and on the concentration of manganese and activity of manganese enzymes in tissues. Aust. J. Agric. Res. 39:517–524.

Mayland, H. F., and D. L. Grunes. 1979. Soil-climate-plant relationships in the ethiology of grass tetany. Pp. 123–175 in Grass Tetany, Special Publication Number 35, M. Stelly, V. V. Rendig, and D. L. Grunes, eds. Madison, WI: American Society of Agronomy.

McDowell, L. R. 1989. Vitamins in Animal Nutrition: Comparative Aspects to Human Nutrition. San Diego: Academic Press.

McDowell, L. R. 1992. Minerals in Animal and Human Nutrition. New York: Academic Press.

McDowell, L. R. 1997. Minerals for Grazing Ruminants in Tropical Regions. 3rd ed. Bulletin. Gainesville: University of Florida. 81 p.

McSweeney, C. S., R. B. Cross, B. T. Wholohan, and M. R. Murphy. 1988. Diagnosis of sodium status in small ruminants. Aust. J. Agric. Res. 39:935–942.

Meneses, A., T. R. Batra, and M. Hidiroglou. 1994. Vitamin E and selenium in milk of ewes. Can. J. Anim. Sci. 71:567–569.

Menzies, P. I., H. Boermans, B. Hoff, T. Durzi, and L. Langs. 2003. Survey of the status of copper, interacting minerals, and vitamin E levels in the livers of sheep in Ontario. Can. Vet. J. 44(11):898–906.

Merck. 2006. The Merck Veterinary Manual. Whitehouse Station, NJ: Merck & Co. Available at: http://www.merckvetmanual.com/mvm/index.jsp.

Meschy, F. 2000. Recent progress in the assessment of mineral requirements of goats. Liv. Prod. Sci. 64:9–14.

Meyer, J. H., W. C. Weir, N. R. Ittner, and J. D. Smith. 1955. The influence of high sodium chloride intake by fattening sheep and cattle. J. Anim. Sci. 14:412–418.

Michell, A. R. 1995. Physiological roles for sodium in mammals. Pp. 91–106 in Sodium in Agriculture, C. J. C. Phillips and P. C. Chiy, eds. Canterbury, UK: Chalcombe Publications.

Miller, J. K., N. Ramsey, and F. C. Madsen. 1988. The trace elements. Pp. 343–400 in The Ruminant Animal; Digestive Physiology and Nutrition, D. C. Church, ed. Englewood Cliffs, NJ: Prentice-Hall.

Miller, W. J. 1970. Zinc nutrition of cattle: A review. J. Dairy Sci. 53: 1123–1135.

Miller, W. J., D. M. Blackmon, J. M. Hiers, Jr., P. R. Fowler, C. M. Clifton, and R. P. Gentry. 1967. Effects of adding two forms of supplemental zinc to a practical diet on skin regeneration in Holstein heifers and evaluation of a procedure for determining rate of wound healing. J. Dairy Sci. 50:715–721.

Minson, D. J. 1990. Forage in Ruminant Nutrition. San Diego: Academic Press.

Moen, R., and J. Pastor. 1998. Simulating antler growth and energy, nitrogen, calcium and phosphorus metabolism in caribou. Rangifer Spec. Iss. No. 10:85–97.

Mongin, P. 1980. Electrolytes in nutrition: Review of basic principles and practical application in poultry and swine. Pp. 1–15 in Proc. Inter. Mineral Conference, Orlando, FL.

Morrison, J. N., J. Quarterman, and W. R. Humphries. 1977. The effect of dietary calcium and phosphate on lead poisoning in lambs. J. Comp. Pathology 87:417–429.

Muir, P. D., A. R. Sykes, and G. K. Barrell. 1987. Growth and mineralization of antlers in red deer (Cervus elaphus). NZ J. Agric. Res. 30:305–315.

Mustacich, D., and G. Powis. 2000. Thioredoxin reductase. Biochem. J. 346:1–8.

Muth, O. R. 1963. White muscle disease, a selenium-responsive myopathy J. Am. Med. Assoc. 142:272–277.

NRC (National Research Council). 1974. Nutrients and Toxic Substances in Water for Livestock and Poultry. Washington, DC: National Academy Press.

NRC. 1975. Nutrient Requirements of Sheep. Washington, DC: National Academy Press.

NRC. 1980. Mineral Tolerance of Domestic Animals. Washington, DC: National Academy Press.

NRC. 1981. Nutrient Requirements of Goats: Angora, Dairy, and Meat Goats in Temperate and Tropical Countries. Washington, DC: National Academy Press.

NRC. 1983. Selenium in Nutrition. Washington, DC: National Academy Press.

NRC. 1984. Nutrient Requirements of Beef Cattle, 6th rev. ed. Washington, DC: National Academy Press.

NRC. 1985. Nutrient Requirements of Sheep, 6th rev. ed. Washington, DC: National Academy Press.

NRC. 1989. Nutrient Requirements of Dairy Cattle, 6th rev. ed. Washington, DC: National Academy Press.

NRC. 2000. Nutrient Requirements of Beef Cattle, 7th rev. ed. Washington, DC: National Academy Press.

NRC. 2001. Nutrient Requirements of Dairy Cattle, 7th rev. ed. Washington, DC: National Academy Press.

NRC. 2005. Mineral Tolerance of Animals, 2nd rev. ed. Washington, DC: The National Academies Press.

NRC. 2006. Fluoride in Drinking Water: A Scientific Review of EPA's Standards. Washington, DC: The National Academies Press.

Neathery, M. W., and W. J. Miller. 1975. Metabolism and toxicity of cadmium, mercury, and lead in animals: A review. J. Dairy Sci. 58: 1767–1781.

Neathery, M. W., W. J. Miller, R. P. Gentry, P. E. Stake, and D. M. Blackmon. 1974. Cadmium-109 and methyl mercury-203 metabolism, tissue distribution, and secretion into milk of cows. J. Dairy Sci. 57: 1177–1183.

Nielson, F. H. 1996. Other trace elements. Pp. 109–119 in Present Knowledge in Nutrition, 7th ed., L. J. Filer and E. E. Ziegler, eds. Washington, DC: International Life Science Institute, Nutrition Foundation.

Nockels, C. F., J. DeBonis, and J. Torrent. 1993. Stress induction affects copper and zinc balance in calves fed organic and inorganic copper and zinc sources. J. Anim. Sci. 71:2539–2545.

Oftedal, O. T. 1985. Pregnancy and lactation. Pp. 215–238 in Bioenergetics of Wild Herbivores, R. J. Hudson and R. G. White, eds. Boca Raton, FL: CRC Press.

O'Hara, T. M., G. Carroll, P. Barboza, K. Mueller, J. Blake, V. Woshner, and C. Willetto. 2001. Mineral and heavy metal status as related to a mortality event and poor recruitment in a moose population in Alaska. J. Wildl. Diseases 37:509–522.

O'Toole, M., and M. F. Raisbeck. 1995. Pathology of experimentally induced chronic selenosis (alkali disease) in yearling cattle. J. Vet. Diagn. Invest. 7:364–373.

Oliver, W. T., and N. Platonow. 1960. Studies on the pharmacology of the N-(ethyl mercuri)-p-toluenesulfonanilide. Am. J. Vet. Res. 21:906–916.

Olsen, Q. R., D. C. Rule, R. A. Field, G. D. Snowder, and C. Y. Hu. 1996. Dietary chromium picolinate does not influence growth or carcass composition in feedlot lambs. Sheep and Goat Res. J. 12:22–24.

Ott, E. A., W. H. Smith, R. B. Harrington, and W. M. Beeson. 1966. Zinc toxicity in ruminants. II. Effect of high levels of dietary zinc on gains, feed consumption and feed efficiency of beef cattle. J. Anim. Sci. 25: 419–423.

Park, Y. W. 2000. Comparison of mineral and cholesterol composition of different commercial goat milk products manufactured in USA. Small Ruminant Res. 37:115–124.

Park, Y. W., and R. Attaie.1988. Iron contents of muscle meat and liver in Alpine and Nubian goats. Small Ruminant Res. 1:387–395.

Paterson, B. W., S. L. Hansard, C. B. Ammerman, P. R. Henry, L. A. Zech, and W. R. Fisher. 1986. Kinetic model for whole body vanadium metabolism: Studies in sheep. Amer. J. Physiology 251:R325–R332.

Peek, J. M., K. T. Schmidt, M. J. Dorrance, and B. L. Smith. 2002. Supplemental feeding and farming of elk. Pp. 614–647 in North American Elk: Ecology and Management, D. E. Toweill and J. W. Thomas, eds. Washington, DC; London: Smithsonian Institution Press.

Petersen, L. N. 1997. Potassium in nutrition. Pp. 153–183 in Handbook of Nutritionally Essential Mineral Elements, B. L. O'Dell and R. A. Sunde, eds. New York: Marcel Dekker.

Pfeffer, E. 1989. Phosphorus requirements in goats. Pp. 42–46 in Proc. Inter. Meeting on Mineral Nutrition and Mineral Requirements in Ruminants, Kyoto, Japan, 1989. Kyoto: Showado Insatsu.

Pfeffer, E., and R. Keunecke. 1986. Untersuchungen über die Gehalte an Protein, Fett und Mineralstoffen im Körper wachsender Ziegen. J. Anim. Phys. Anim. Nutr. 54:166–171.

Pfeffer, E., and M. Rodehutscord. 1998. Body chemical composition and utilization of dietary energy by male Saanen kids fed either milk to satiation or solid complete feeds with two proportions of straw. J. Agric. Sci., Cambridge 131:487–495.

Pfeffer, E., M. Rodehutscord, and G. Breves. 1995. Effects of reducing dietary calcium and/or phosphorus on performance and body composition in male kids. J. Anim. Phys. Anim. Nutr.—Zeitschrift für Tierphysiologie Tierernarhrung und Futtermittelkunde 74:243–252.

Phillip, C. J. C., P. C. Chiy, and H. M. Omed. 2004. The effects of cadmium in feed, and its amelioration with zinc, on element balances in sheep. J. Anim. Sci. 82:2489–2502.

Podoll, K. L., J. B. Bernard, D. E. Ullrey, S. R. DeBar, P. K. Ku, and W. T. Magee. 1992. Dietary selenate versus selenite for cattle, sheep, and horses. J. Anim. Sci. 70:1965–1970.

Pope, A. L., R. J. Moir, M. Somers, E. J. Underwood, and C. L. White. 1979. The effect of sulphur on ^{75}Se absorption and retention in sheep. J. Nutr. 109:1448–1455.

Preston, R. L., N. L. Jacobson, K. D. Wiggers, M. H. Wiggers, and G. N. Jacobson. 1977. Phosphorus in Ruminant Nutrition. West Des Moines, IA: National Feed Ingredients Association.

Price, J., and J. K. Chesters. 1985. A new bioassay for assessment of copper bioavailability and its application in a study of the effect of molybdenum on the distribution of available copper in ruminant digesta. Br. J. Nutr. 53:323–336.

Puls, R. 1994. Mineral Levels in Animal Health: Diagnostic Data. Clearbrook, British Columbia: Sherpa Int.

Qi, K., C. D. Lu, F. N. Owens, and C. F. Lupton. 1992a. Sulphate supplementation of Angora goats—metabolic and mohair responses. J. Anim. Sci. 70:2828–2837.

Qi, K., C. D. Lu, and F. N. Owens. 1992b. Sulfate supplementation of Alpine goats—effects on milk yield and composition, metabolites, nutrient digestibilities, and acid-base balance. J. Anim. Sci. 70: 3541–3550.

Qi, K., C. D. Lu, and F. N. Owens. 1993. Sulfate supplementation of growing goats—effects on performance, acid-base balance, and nutrient digestibilities. J. Anim. Sci. 71:1579–1587.

Qi, K., C. D. Lu, and F. N. Owens. 1994a. Effects of sulfate supplementation on performance, acid-base balance, and nutrient metabolism in Alpine kids. Small Ruminant Res. 15:9–18.

Qi, K., C. D. Lu, F. N. Owens, and C. J. Lupton. 1994b. Effects of sulfate supplementation on performance, acid-base balance, and nutrient metabolism in Angora kids. Small Ruminant Res. 15:19–29.

Quarterman, J., J. N. Morrison, W. R. Humphries, and C. F. Mills. 1977. The effect of dietary sulphur and of castration on lead poisoning in lambs. J. Comparative Path. 87:405–416.

Radostits, O., D. Blood, and C. Gay. 1994. Veterinary Medicine, 8th ed. London: Bailliere Tindall.

Raisbeck, M. F., E. R. Dahl, D. A. Sanchez, E. L. Belden, and D. O'Toole. 1993. Naturally occurring selenosis in Wyoming. J. Vet. Diagn. Invest. 5:84–87.

Rajaratne, A. A. J., D. Scott, J. K. Thompson, W. Buchan, K. Pennic. 1990. The effect of variation in dietary calcium supply on the phosphorus requirements of growing lambs. Anim. Prod. 51:135–142.

Ramírez, R. Q., G. F. W. Haenlein, and M. A. Nuñez González. 2001. Seasonal variation of macro and trace mineral contents in 14 browse species that grow in northeastern Mexico. Small Ruminant Res. 39: 153–159.

Ramírez-Bribiesca, J. E., J. L. Tórtora, L. M. Hernández, and M. Huerta. 2001. Main causes of mortalities in dairy goat kids from the Mexican plateau. Small Ruminant Res. 41:77–80.

Rammell, C. G., K. G. Thompson, G. R. Bentley, and M. W. Gibbons. 1989. Selenium, vitamin E and polyunsaturated fatty acid concentrations in goat kids with and without nutritional myodegeneration. New Zealand Vet. J. 37:4–6.

Rees, M. C., D. J. Minson, and F. W. Smith. 1974. The effect of supplementary and fertilizer sulphur on voluntary intake, digestibility, retention time in the rumen, and site of digestion of pangola grass in sheep. J. Agric. Sci., Cambridge 82:419–422.

Robbins, C. T. 1993. Wildlife Feeding and Nutrition. New York: Academic Press.

Robbins C.T., and A.N. Moen. 1975. Uterine composition and growth in pregnant white-tailed deer. J. Wildl. Manage. 39: 684–691.

Rojas, L. X., L. R. McDowell, R. J. Cousins, F. G. Martin, N. S. Wilkinson, A. B. Johnson, and J. B. Velazquez. 1995. Relative bioavailability of two organic and two inorganic zinc sources fed to sheep. J. Anim. Sci. 73:1202–1207.

Rombach, E. P., P. S. Barboza, and J. E. Blake. 2002. Utilization of copper during lactation and neonatal development in muskoxen. Can. J. Zool. 80:1460–1469.

Rombach, E. P., P. S. Barboza, and J. E. Blake. 2003. Costs of gestation in an Arctic ruminant: Copper reserves in muskoxen. Comp. Biochem. Physiol. 134C:157–168.

Ryberg, D., and J. Alexander. 1990. Mechanism of chromium toxicity in mitochondria. Chemic-Biol. Interact. 75:141–151.

Saenko, E. L., A. I. Yaroplov, and E. D. Harris. 1994. Biological functions of caeruloplasmin expressed through copper-binding sites. J. Trace Elements in Experimental Med. 7:69–88.

Saito, Y., and K. Takahashi. 2000. Selenoprotein P: Its structure and functions. J. Health Sci. 46:409–413.

Salama, A. A. K., G. Caja, E. Albanell, X. Such, R. Casals, and J. Plaixats. 2003. Effects of dietary supplements of zinc-methionine on milk production, udder health and zinc metabolism in dairy goats. J. Dairy Res. 70: 9–17.

Sargison, N. D., and D. M. West. 1998. Iodine deficiency: An emerging problem in New Zealand sheep flocks? Proc. New Zealand Soc. Anim. Prod. 58:202–204.

Schellner, G. 1972/73. Die Wirkung von Natriummangel und Natriumbeifutterung auf Wachstum, Milch- und Milchfettleistung und Fruchtbarkeit bei Ziegen. Jabrbuch fur Tierernabrung und Futterung 8:246–259.

Schmidely, P., F. Meschy, J. Tessier, and D. Sauvant. 2002. Lactation response and nitrogen, calcium, and phosphorus utilization of dairy goats differing by the genotype for alpha S1-casein in milk, and fed diets varying in crude protein concentration. J. Dairy Sci. 85:2299–2307.

Schrauzer, G. N. 2000. Selenomethionine: A review of its nutritional significance, metabolism and toxicity. J. Nutr. 130:1653–1656.

Schroeder, H. A., and I. H. Tipton. 1968. The human body burden of lead. Arch. Environ. Health. 17:965–978.

Selby, L. A., A. A. Case, G. D. Osweiler, and H. M. Mays. 1977. Epidemiology and toxicology of arsenic poisoning in domestic animals. Environ. Health Perspectives 19:183–189.

Sell, J. L., J. A. Arthur, and L. L. Williams. 1982. Adverse effects of dietary vanadium, contributed by dicalcium phosphate on albumen quality. Poultry Sci. 61:2112–2116.

Sharpley, A. N., T. Daniel, T. Sims, J. Lemunyon, R. Stevens, and R. Parry. 2003. Agricultural Phosphorus and Eutrophication, 2nd ed. U.S. Department of Agriculture, Agricultural Research Service, ARS–149. 44 pp.

Sharrif, M. A., R. J. Boila, and K. M. Wittenberg. 1990. Effect of dietary molybdenum on rumen dry matter disappearance in cattle. Can. J. Anim. Sci. 70:319–323.

Shils, M. E. 1997. Magnesium. Pp. 117–152 in Handbook of Nutritionally Essential Minerals, B. L. O'Dell and R. A. Sunde, eds. New York: Marcel Dekker.

Shupe, J. L. 1980. Clinicopathologic features of fluoride toxicosis in cattle. J. Anim. Sci. 51:746–757.

Sim, J. S., and R. J. Hudson. 1991. Chemical characteristics and processing technology of Alberta wapiti antlers. Proc. Intern. Wildl. Ranch. Symp. 2:533–535.

Small, J. A., E. Charmley, A. V. Rodd, and A. H. Freeden. 1997. Serum mineral concentrations in relation to estrus and conception in beef heifers and cows fed conserved forage. Can. J. Anim. Sci. 77:55–62.

Smith, C. R., Jr., D. Weisleder, R. Miller, I. S. Palmer, and O. E. Olson. 1980. Linustatin and neolinustatin: Cyanogenic glycosides of linseed meal that protect animals against selenium toxicity. J. Org. Chem. 45:507–510.

Smith, R. M. 1997. Cobalt. Pp. 357–388 in Handbook of Nutritionally Essential Mineral Elements, D. L. O'Dell and R. E. Sunde, eds. New York: Marcel Dekker.

Smith, R. M., and H. R. Marston. 1970. Production, absorption, distribution and excretion of vitamin B_{12} in sheep. Br. J. Nutr. 24:857–877.

Smith, S. E., F. W. Lengemann, and J. T. Reid. 1953. Block vs. loose salt consumption by dairy cattle. J. Dairy Sci. 36:762–765.

Solaiman, S. G., M. A. Maloney, M. A. Qureshi, G. Davis, and G. D'Andrea. 2001. Effects of high copper supplements on performance, health, plasma copper and enzymes in goats. Small Ruminant Res. 41: 127–139.

Solaiman, S. G., T. Craig Jr., G. Reddy, C. E. Shoemaker, and G. F. W. Haenlein. 2004. Effects of supra-nutritional Cu levels on growth, rumen fermentation and immune responses of goat kids. Pp. 136–144 in Macro- and Trace Elements Mengen- und Spurenelemente, vol. 1, M. Anke, G. Flachowsky, K. Kisters, U. Schafer, H. Schenkel, M. Seifert, and M. Stoeppler, eds. Jena, Germany: Friedrich Schiller University.

Solaiman, S. G., C. E. Shoemaker, and G. H. D'Andrea. 2005. The effect of supra-nutritional level of Cu on vital signs, growth performance and Cu status in goat kids. Pp. 97–106 in Proc. Tennessee Nutrition Conf.

Solaiman, S. G, C. E. Shoemaker, W. R. Jones, and C. R. Kerth. 2006. The effect of high level of Cu on serum lipid profile and carcass characteristics in goat kids. J. Anim. Sci. 84:171–177.

Spears, J. 1984. Nickel as a "new trace element" in the nutrition of domestic animals. J. Anim. Sci. 59:823–835.

Staaland, H., and K. Hove. 2000. Seasonal changes in sodium metabolism in reindeer (*Rangifer tarandus*) in an inland area of Norway. Arctic Antarc. Alpine Res. 32:286–294.

Staaland, H., and R. G. White. 2001. Regional variation in mineral content of plants and its significance for migration by arctic reindeer and caribou. Alces 37:479–509.

Staaland, H., R. G. White, J. R. Luick, and D. F. Holleman. 1980. Dietary influences on sodium and potassium metabolism of reindeer. Can. J. Zool. 58:1728–1734.

Staaland, H., E. Jacobsen, and R.G. White. 1984. The effect of mineral supplements on nutrient concentrations and pool sizes in the alimentary tract of reindeer fed lichens or concentrates during winter. Can. J. Zool. 62:1232–1241.

Staaland, H., K. Hove, and R. G. White. 1986. Mineral absorption in relation to nutritional ecology of reindeer. Rangifer Spec. Iss. No. 1:279–287.

Stangl, G. I., and M. Kirchgessner. 1996. Effect of nickel deficiency on various metabolic parameters of rats. Anim. Physiol. Anim. Nutr. 75:164–174.

Stelwagen, K., V. C. Farr, and H. A. McFadden. 1999. Alteration of the sodium to potassium ratio in milk and the effect on milk secretion in goats. J. Dairy Sci. 82:52–59.

Stephenson, D. C., and R. D. Brown. 1984. Calcium kinetics in male white-tailed deer. J. Nutr. 114:1014–1024.

Suttle, N. F. 1979. Copper, iron, manganese and zinc concentrations in the carcasses of lambs and calves and the relationship to trace elements required for growth. Br. J. Nutr. 42:89–96.

Suttle, N. F. 1991. The interactions between copper, molybdenum and sulfur in ruminant nutrition. Ann. Rev. of Nutr. 11:121–140.

Suttle, N. F. 2002. Meeting the copper requirements of ruminants. Pp. 221–236 in Recent Developments in Ruminant Nutrition 4, J. Wiseman and P. C. Garnsworthy, eds. Nottingham, UK: Nottingham University Press.

Suttle, N. F., and A. C. Field. 1968. Effect of intake of copper, molybdenum and sulphate on copper metabolism in sheep. 1. Clinical condition and distribution of copper in blood of the pregnant ewes. J. Comparative Pathol. 93:379–389.

Suttle, N. F., and M. McLauchlin. 1976. Predicting the effects of dietary molybdenum and sulphur on the availability of copper to ruminants. Proc. Nutr. Soc. 35:22A–23A.

Suttle, N. F., H. Lioyed–Davies and A. C. Field. 1982. A model for zinc metabolism in sheep given a diet of hay. Br. J. Nutr. 47:105–112.

Suttle, N. F., J. Brebner, B. Stark, N. Sweet, and J. W. Hall. 1997. Placental and mammary transfer of lead and cadmium by ewes exposed to lead and cadmium enriched, sewage sludge treated soils. Pp. 168–170 in Proc. 9th Symp. on Trace Elements in Man and Animals, P. W. F. Fischer, M. R. L'Abbe, K. A. Cockell, and R. S. Gibson, eds. Ottawa: NRC Research Press.

Suttle, N. F., R. M. Lewis, and J. N. W. Small. 2002. Effects of breed and family on rate of copper accretion in the liver of purebred Charolais, Suffolk and Texel lambs. Anim. Sci.75:295–302.

Swinkels, J. W. G. M., E. T. Kornegay, W. Zhou, M. D. Lindemann, K. E. Webb, and M. W. A. Verstegen. 1996. Effectiveness of a zinc amino acid chelate and zinc sulphate in restoring serum and soft tissue zinc concentration when fed to zinc depleted pigs. J. Anim. Sci. 74:2420–2430.

Szilagyi, M., Anke, M., Balogh, I., Regius-Mocsenyi, A. and Suri, A. 1989. Lithium status and animal metabolism. Proc. 6th Intern. Trace Element Symposium, University Leipzig-Jena, Germany, 1249.

Taylor, J. B. 2005. Time-dependent influence of supranutritional organically bound selenium on selenium accumulation in growing wether lambs. J. Anim. Sci. 83:1186–1193.

Thomas, J. W., and S. Moss. 1952. The effect of orally administered molybdenum on growth, spermatogenesis and testis histology of young dairy bulls. J. Dairy Sci. 34:929–934.

Thompson, D. J. 1980. Industrial considerations related to fluoride toxicity. J. Anim. Sci. 51:767–772.

Thompson, K. G., L. Audige, D. G. Arthur, A. F. Juhan, M. B. Orr, K. D. McSporran, and P. R. Wilson. 1994. Osteochondrosis associated with copper deficiency in young farmed red deer and wapiti × red deer hybrids. New Zealand Vet. J. 42:137–143.

Tisserand, J. L., and W. Alrhamoun. 1998. Comparisons du recyclage de l'uree sanguine chez les ovins et les caprins. Renc. Rech. Ruminants 5:221.

Tomlinson, D. J. 2002. Effect of organic and inorganic trace mineral supplementation on beef and dairy production. Presentation at XXX Reunión Anual de la Asociación Mexicana de Producción Animal, October 13–15, Guadalajara, Jal.

Towers, N. R., P. W. Young, and D. C. Smeaton. 1984. Sodium requirements of grazing ruminants. Proc. New Zealand Soc. Anim. Prod. 44: 155–157.

Tucker, W. B., G. A. Harrison, and R. W. Hemken. 1988. Influence of dietary cation-anion balance on milk, blood, urine, and rumen fluid in lactating dairy cattle. J. Dairy Sci. 71:346–354.

Tucker, W. B., J. F. Hogue, G. D. Adams, M. Aslam, I. S. Shin, and G. Morgan. 1992. Influence of dietary cation-anion balance during the dry period on the occurrence of parturient puresis in cows fed excess calcium. J. Anim. Sci. 70:1238–1250.

Ullrey, D. E. 1983. Nutrition and antler development in white-tailed deer. Pp. 49–59 in Antler Development in Cervidae, R. D. Brown, ed. Kingsville, TX: Caesar Kleberg Wildl. Res. Inst.

Ullrey, D. E. 1987. Biochemical and physiological indicators of selenium status in animals. J. Anim. Sci. 65:1712–1726.

Ullrey, D. E., W. G. Youatt, H. E. Johnson, L. D. Fay, B. L. Schoepke, W. T. Magee, and K. K. Keahey. 1973. Calcium requirements of weaned white-tailed deer fawns. J. Wildl. Manage. 37:187–194.

Ullrey, D. E., W. G. Youatt, H. E. Johnson, A. B. Cowan, L. D. Fay, R. L. Covert, W. T. Magee, and K. K. Keahey. 1975. Phosphorus requirements of weaned white-tailed deer fawns. J. Wildl. Manage. 39:590–595.

Ulvund, M. J. 1985. Chronic poisoning in a lamb grazing Phalaris arundinacea. Acta Vet. Scand. 26:286–288.

Underwood, E. J. 1962. A preliminary investigation of sources of zinc in Australian poultry diets. Pp. 216–218 in Proc. 12th World Poultry Congress, Sydney, Australia.

Underwood, E. J. 1977. Trace Elements in Human and Animal Nutrition, 4th ed. New York: Academic Press.

Underwood, E. J., and N. Suttle. 1999. The Mineral Nutrition of Livestock, 3rd ed. New York: CAB International.

van Ryssen, J. B. J., P. S. M. van Malsen, and F. Hartmann. 1998. Contribution of dietary sulfur to the interaction between selenium and copper in sheep. J. Agric. Sci. Camb. 130:107–114.

Van Soest, P. J., and L. H. P. Jones. 1968. Effect of silica in forages upon digestibility. J. Dairy Sci. 51:1644–1649.

Vipond, J. E., G. Horgan, and D. Anderson. 1995. Estimation of food intake in sheep by blood assay for lithium content following ingestion of lithium-labelled food. Anim. Sci. 60:513A.

Wan Zahari, M., J. K. Thompson, D. Scott, and W. Buchan. 1990. The dietary requirements of calcium and phosphorus for growing lambs. Anim. Prod. 50:301–308.

Wang, Y. R., J. Y. J. Wu, S. K. Reaves, and K. Y. Lei. 1996. Enhanced expression of hepatic genes in copper deficient rats detected by the messenger RNA differential display method. J. Nutr. 126:1772–1781.

Watkins, B. E., D. E. Ullrey, R. F. Nachreiner, S. M. Schmidt. 1983. Effects of supplemented iodine and season on thyroid activity of white-tailed deer. J. Wildlife Manage. 47:47–58.

Watson, A. 1971. Climate and antler shedding and performance of red deer in North East Scotland. J. Appl. Ecol. 8:53–67.

Weeks, H. P. Jr., and C. M. Kirkpatrick. 1976. Adaptations of whitetailed deer to naturally occurring sodium deficiencies. J. Wildl. Manage. 40:610–625.

Weeth, H. J., C. F. Speth, and D. R. Hanks. 1981. Boron content of plasma and urine as indicators of boron intake in cattle. Am. J. Vet Res. 42:474–477.

Weir, J. S. 1972. Spatial distribution of elephants in an African National Park in relation to environmental sodium. Oikos 23:1–13.

West, J. W., B. G. Mullinix, and T. G. Sandifer. 1991. Changing dietary electrolyte balance for dairy cows in cool and hot environments. J. Dairy Sci. 74:1662–1674.

Whanger, P. D. 2002. Selenocompounds in plants and animals and their biological significance. J. Am. Col. Nutr. 21:223–232.

Whanger, P. D., P. H. Weswig, J. E. Oldfield, P. R. Cheeke, and O. H. Muth. 1972. Factors influencing selenium and white muscle disease: Forage types, salts, amino acids and dimethyl sulfoxide. Nutr. Rep. Int. 6:21–37.

Wheeler, S. M., T. B. Brock, and D. Teasdale. 1985. Effect of adding 30 mg fluoride/l drinking water given to pregnant ewes and their lambs upon physiology and wool growth. J. Anim. Sci., Cambridge 105:715–726.

Whelan, B. R., N. J. Barrow, and D. W. Peters. 1994. Selenium fertilization for pastures grazed by sheep. I. Selenium concentration in whole blood and plasma. Aust. J. Agr. Res. 45:863–875.

White, R.G., E. Jacobsen and H. Staaland. 1984. Secretion and absorption of nutrients in the alimentary tract of reindeer fed lichens or concentrates during the winter. Can. J. Zool. 62:2364–2376.

White, F., M. W. Neathery, R. P. Gentry, W. J. Miller, K. R. Logner, and D. M. Blackmon. 1985. The effects of different levels of dietary lead on zinc metabolism in dairy calves. J. Dairy Sci. 68:1215–1225.

White, R.G., F. L. Bunnell, E. Gaare, T. Skogland and B. Hubert. 1981. Ungulates on Arctic ranges. Pp. 397–483 in Tundra Ecosystems: A Comparative Analysis, IBP Vol. 25, L. C. Bliss, O. W. Heal, and J. J. Moore, eds. Cambridge: Cambridge Univ. Press.

Whitehead, D. C. 2000. Nutrient Elements in Grassland: Soil-Plant-Animal Relationships. New York: CABI Publishing.

Whiteman, P. C., L. R. Humphreys, and N. H. Montheith. 1974. A Course Manual in Tropical Pasture Science. Brisbane, Australia: A. A. U. C. S.

Widdowson, E. M., and J. W. T. Dickerson. 1964. Chemical composition of the body. Pp. 1–247 in Mineral metabolism, vol. II, part A, C. L. Comar and F. Bronner, eds. New York: Academic Press.

Wilkinson, S. R., and J. A. Stuedemann. 1979. Tetany hazard of grass as affected by fertilization with nitrogen, potassium, or poultry litter and methods of grass tetany prevention. Pp. 93–122 in Grass Tetany, Special Publication Number 35, M. Stelly, V. V. Rendig, and D. L. Grunes, eds. Madison, WI: American Society of Agronomy.

Wilson P. R., and N. D. Grace. 2002. Practical considerations for diagnosis and management of Cu status of deer. Proc. New Zealand Soc. Anim. Prod. 62:315–318.

Williams, D. M., F. S. Kennedy, and B. G. Green. 1983. Hepatic iron accumulation in iron-deficient rats. Br. J. Nutr. 50:653–660.

Wolfe G. J. 1983. The relationship between age and antler development in wapiti. Pp. 29–36 in Antler Development in Cervidae, R. D. Robert, ed. Kingsville, TX: Caesar Kleberg Wildl. Res. Inst.

Wong-Valle, J., P. R. Henry, C. B. Ammerman, and P. V. Rao. 1989. Estimation of the relative bioavailability of manganese sources for sheep. J. Anim. Sci. 67:2409–2414.

Wright, P. L., and M. C. Bell. 1966. Comparative metabolism of selenium and tellurium in sheep and swine. Am. J. Physiol. 211:6–10.

Yang, W. Z., D. N. Mowat, A. Subiyanto, and R. M. Liptrap. 1996. Effect of chromium supplementation on early lactation performance of Holstein cows. Can. J. Anim. Sci. 76:221–230.

Yeh, J. J., Q. P. Gu, M. A. Beilstein, N. E. Forsberg, and P. D. Whanger. 1997. Selenium influences tissue levels of selenoprotein W in sheep. J. Nutr. 127:394–402.

Young, R. S. 1979. Cobalt in Biology and Biochemistry (pp. 50–86). New York: Academic Press.

Zervas, G., E. Nikolau, and A. Mantzios. 1990. Comparative study of chronic copper poisoning in lambs and young goats. Anim. Prod. 50: 497–506.

8

Vitamins

INTRODUCTION

Vitamins are a group of complex organic compounds that are essential for multiple metabolic and physiologic processes. Unlike other organic nutrients, vitamins typically are required in minute amounts (micrograms to milligrams per day). Vitamins are classified as either fat-soluble or water-soluble. The fat-soluble vitamins A, D, E, and K consist only of carbon, hydrogen, and oxygen, whereas some of the water-soluble vitamins also contain nitrogen, sulfur, or cobalt. A clinical deficiency of a vitamin will produce specific deficiency signs and symptoms. The more common subclinical deficiencies may occur in which clinical signs are not evident but animal performance or overall health may be less than optimal.

FAT-SOLUBLE VITAMINS

Small ruminants require all of the fat-soluble vitamins. Only vitamins A and E commonly are required in the diet because vitamins D and K are often synthesized in amounts sufficient to satisfy requirements. Vitamin D is synthesized by ultraviolet radiation of the skin, whereas vitamin K is synthesized by indigenous bacteria of the digestive tract. Supplemental sources of vitamins D or K may be necessary when animals are deprived of exposure to ultraviolet radiation or consume a vitamin K antagonist.

Vitamin A

Vitamin A is a nearly colorless, fat-soluble, long-chain, unsaturated alcohol with five double bonds. The vitamin is made up of isoprene units with alternate double bonds, starting with one in the β-ionone ring that is conjugated with those in the side chain. The terminal end of the side chain may contain an alcohol (retinol), aldehyde (retinal or retinaldehyde), or carboxyl group (retinoic acid). The primary form of vitamin A in animal tissues and milk exists as esters of retinol, retinyl esters. Of the 16 possible isomers, all-*trans* retinol is the parent substance of vitamin A. The retinal involved in the vision cycle is derived from metabolism of retinol, and the retinoic acid involved with tissue differentiation is derived from retinol that is subsequently oxidized via retinal to retinoic acid (Olson, 1991). Thus, vitamin A is a generic term used to describe all β-ionone derivatives, other than carotenoids, that exhibit the biological activity of all-*trans* retinol (Anonymous, 1987).

Plant material contains the vitamin's precursor in several forms known as carotenoids. Of over 500 carotenoids that have been isolated from nature, only about 60 possess biological activity (Olson, 1991). These carotenoid compounds commonly are referred to as provitamin A because the body can transform them into the active vitamin; however, carotenoids typically must contain at least one non-hydroxylated β-ionone to become biologically active. The carotenoids are orange-yellow pigments that occur mainly in green leaves and to a lesser extent in yellow corn. The four carotenoids of particular nutritional importance for small ruminants include α-carotene, β-carotene, γ-carotene, and cryptoxanthine (the main carotenoid of yellow corn). The most active and quantitatively the most important of these provitamins is all-*trans* β-carotene.

A number of factors influence the bioavailability of carotene and vitamin A. Digestion and absorption from the digestive tract are the first determinants of vitamin A activity. Wing (1969) reported that apparent digestibility of carotene averaged 78 percent, which was influenced by season of forage harvest, type of forage, plant species, and plant dry matter. Studies reviewed by Ullrey (1972) indicated that appreciable amounts (40–70 percent) of carotene and vitamin A were degraded in the forestomach of ruminants, but pre-intestinal absorption could not be ruled out at that time. More recent evidence from studies conducted in vitro suggests that ruminal degradation of vitamin A is associated with activity of the ruminal microbes. Disappearance of vitamin A during a 24-hour (h) in vitro ruminal fermentation system was 16 and 19 percent when donor steers were fed hay and straw, respectively (Rode et al., 1990). Weiss et al. (1995) demonstrated that 80 percent of added retinol was recovered after a 24 h incubation period in fluid collected from ruminally cannulated cows consuming an 80 percent forage diet, but recovery of added retinol dropped to 28 percent when cows were fed 50 percent concentrate. In vitro disappearance of retinol increased to approximately 80 percent when ruminal fluid was collected from steers fed 70 percent concentrate (Rode et al., 1990). Lower ruminal pH associated with feeding concentrates may enhance disappearance of vitamin A. Low pH caused isomerization of all-*trans* retinol and deesterification of retinyl esters to more labile retinol (DeRitter, 1976). Upon release from other molecules within feedstuffs via enzymatic action in the stomach and upper duodenum, vitamin A and the provitamin carotenoids are absorbed mainly in the upper half of the intestine (Olson, 1991).

Retinol and the carotenoids pass into the mucosal cells where the carotenoids are cleaved by 15,15′-carotenoid dioxygenase to retinal. Retinaldehyde reductase then reduces retinal to retinol. Almost all the absorbed carotene is cleaved in the intestine of the sheep and goat (McDowell, 1989). Retinol may then be esterified to long-chain fatty acids within the mucosal cells before being transported through the lymphatic system to the liver, where it may be stored until being mobilized to fulfill a metabolic requirement. The enzymatic conversion of β-carotene by the intestinal mucosa reflected retinol content in the liver (Yang and Tume, 1993). This subcommittee presumed this relationship to be true for cervids because white-tail deer, like sheep and goats, have virtually colorless body fat (Ullrey, 1972).

Previous NRC committees elected to express vitamin A activity in terms of international units (IU). Based upon rat data, an IU of vitamin A = 0.3 μg of retinol, 0.344 μg of retinyl acetate, or 0.55 μg of retinyl palmitate. Vitamin A may also be expressed as retinol equivalents (RE). Because RE is generally accepted throughout the world (Bieri and McKenna, 1981), RE has been used to describe vitamin A activity (Scott and Rodriquez-Amaya, 2000): 1 RE was defined as 1 μg of all-*trans* retinol; 6 μg of all-*trans* β-carotene; or 12 μg of other provitamin A carotenoids (NRC, 1989).

In the previous version of Nutrient Requirements of Goats (NRC, 1981), 1 mg of β-carotene = 400 IU of vitamin A, which was originally based on values obtained from lambs fed corn silage (Martin et al., 1968). However, corn silage may only be about 66 percent as effective as β-carotene for maintaining liver stores of vitamin A (Miller et al., 1969; Rumsey, 1975). Based upon the prevention of elevated cerebrospinal fluid (CSF) pressure, the previous revision of Nutrient Requirements of Sheep (NRC, 1985) proposed that the vitamin A equivalence for β-carotene was 681 IU of vitamin A/mg of β-carotene. Using the value 0.24 mg of all-*trans*-retinyl palmitate/mg of carotene (436 IU vitamin A/mg of carotene) reported by Martin et al. (1968) and average relative efficiency by which corn silage carotene is used to support liver stores of vitamin A (Miller et al., 1969; Rumsey, 1975), the vitamin A equivalence for β-carotene equates to 0.3636 mg of all-*trans*-retinyl palmitate/mg of β-carotene. Converted to IU (661 IU of vitamin A/mg of β-carotene), this value is remarkably close to that which NRC (1985) recommended applies to all-*trans* β-carotene (681 IU/mg of all-*trans* β-carotene). Although the activity of 15,15′ β-carotene dioxygenase was 2.5 to 4.8 times greater in goats than cattle (Mora et al., 2000), estimates of V_{max} for enzymatic conversion of β-carotene by the intestinal mucosa were 0.21 versus 0.27 nmol substrate split/mg protein/h for sheep versus goats (Yang and Tume, 1993). Vitamin A transport in the goat (Sreekrishna and Cama, 1979) is comparable to that of sheep (Donoghue et al., 1983b), and tolerance to low-carotene diets is similar for adult sheep and goats (NRC, 1981). Thus, this subcommittee recommends 671 IU of vitamin A/mg of β-carotene and 436 IU of vitamin A/mg of other common carotenoids for both sheep and goats. Using the conversion of 1 IU = 0.3 μg of retinol, 201.3 μg of retinol is obtained from 1 mg of β-carotene and 130.8 μg of retinol is obtained from 1 mg of other common carotenoids. In terms of biopotency, 1 RE = 1 μg of all-*trans* retinol, 5.0 μg of all-*trans* β-carotene, or 7.6 μg of other carotenoids. The efficiency of carotenoid conversion into vitamin A by other small ruminants is unknown.

Previous requirements for vitamin A have been established based on the amount of the active vitamin required to prevent clinical signs of deficiency. The NRC (1985) suggested that the minimum vitamin A requirements were based on elevated CSF pressure because this measurement was a more sensitive indicator of poor vitamin A status than night blindness. Based upon the prevention of increased CSF pressure in calves (Eaton, 1969), the minimum requirement for vitamin A should be between 66 to 73 μg of β-carotene or 14.1 RE/kg live weight per day. This particular recommendation is consistent with the concept of the FAO/WHO (1988) basal daily intake, which is the intake level that prevents signs of deficiency. According to FAO/WHO (1988), a safe level of intake provides a suitable body reserve of vitamin A to satisfy requirements during periods of low intake. Liver vitamin A concentrations of 20 μg/g should provide ample reserves to maintain satisfactory plasma retinol for 4 months of low vitamin A intake in humans (Olson, 1987). Daily intake of 434 μg of β-carotene/kg of live weight (86.8 RE/kg) would be necessary to maintain 20 μg of retinol/g of liver in lambs (Faruque and Walker, 1970).

Results of vitamin A depletion studies have indicated that plasma vitamin A concentrations are maintained by mobilizing liver vitamin A reserves (Rousseau et al., 1954; Wright and Hall, 1979). Growing lambs were able to maintain adequate plasma vitamin A levels after 10 weeks of consuming a carotene-deficient diet, but levels of plasma vitamin A were deficient within 13 weeks after consuming the carotene-deficient diet (Ghanem and Farid, 1982). A period of about 4 months was required to create deficient levels of plasma vitamin A in adult goats fed a diet formulated to deplete liver stores (Frier et al., 1974). Based on estimates of efficiency of vitamin A transfer from the intestine to plasma (Donoghue et al., 1983a), subsequent retinol homeostasis (Donoghue et al., 1983b), and relationships published by May et al. (1987), daily intake of 31.4 RE/kg of body weight (BW) would be required to maintain liver reserves at a level sufficient to prevent deficient plasma vitamin A concentrations when stored vitamin A is mobilized over a 10-week period. This new recommendation (104.7 IU/kg of BW) is comparable to that recommended (110 IU/kg of BW) in the newest revision of Nutrient Requirements of Dairy Cattle (NRC, 2001).

The requirement for growing small ruminants was increased to 100 RE/kg of BW (Donoghue et al., 1983a,b). The previous Nutrient Requirements of Sheep (NRC, 1985) recommended a 1.8- and 2.1-fold increase in requirements for animals in late gestation and during lactation, respectively. Requirements for gestation would conceivably vary according to day of pregnancy and number of developing fetuses. The committee on Nutrient Requirements of Small Ruminants recommends 45.5 RE/kg for small ruminants in late gestation. The premise for this recommendation was to satisfy the requirements of the growing conceptus and to account for increased maintenance requirements of animals during late pregnancy. For example, a 70 kg mature ewe producing 10 kg of conceptus would require 1,000 RE for the growing conceptus in addition to 2,637.6 RE for the ewe, which accounted for a 20 percent increase in maintenance requirements of the ewe during late gestation. Expressed as a proportion of ewe BW, the requirement would be 45.5 RE/kg. In the absence of more recent definitive information, the vitamin A requirement for lactation was set at 17.6 percent above that for late gestation (NRC, 1985). Thus, the new vitamin A requirement for lactation becomes 53.5 RE/kg of BW. This committee recognized that level of milk production and secretion of vitamin A into milk may influence vitamin A requirements during lactation. Specific recommendations were not possible, however, due to obvious differences in milk production among the small ruminants as well as breed (Sawaya et al., 1984) and diet (Fedele et al., 2004) influences on vitamin A concentration in the milk.

Definitive information on vitamin A requirements for New World camelids (NWC) has not been published. Van Saun (2006) predicted that 3,000 to 3,600 IU of vitamin A/kg of diet dry matter was necessary to satisfy the minimum requirements of vitamin A for NWC consuming dry matter at 1.25 to 1.5 percent of BW. This recommendation was lower than the 6,600 to 11,000 IU/kg values suggested by Johnson (1989) for llamas. Based on extrapolations of requirements for beef and sheep, Van Saun (2006) also indicated that the minimal vitamin A requirement for llamas and alpacas was 13.5 RE/kg of BW. However, using 1.6 kg as the average amount of hay dry matter necessary to meet daily maintenance energy requirements of a 150 kg llama (Johnson, 1994) and suggested requirements of Johnson (1989), the animal's vitamin A requirement for maintenance would be from 21.1 to 35.2 RE/kg of BW. This committee recommends that vitamin A requirements are similar between New World camelids and other small ruminants considered in this publication.

Cervids may require additional retinoic acid to enhance growth and development of antlers (Price and Allen, 2004). Injecting 10 mg of retinoic acid into the lateral portion of the growing pedicle of fallow bucks resulted in accelerated growth of the cranial appendage (Kierdorf and Kierdorf, 1998) and increased first antler volume (Kierdorf and Bartos, 1999). Bucks experience normal antler growth without supplemental retinoic acid. Therefore, routine supplementation of retinoic acid is only necessary if the goal is to achieve greater than normal antler growth.

Carotenoids are the principal source of vitamin A for small ruminants. The green parts of plants are typically rich in carotene. The likelihood of a deficiency is minimal if small ruminants have access to modest amounts of green foliage. Alternatively, low carotene intake by grazing livestock is common in geographical locations that experience prolonged dry seasons and under conditions of winter feeding or protracted drought when access to green foliage may not occur for more than 3 to 4 months. The circumstances most conducive to vitamin deficiencies are extended periods of drought, diets primarily composed of grain-based concentrates and no green foliage, feeding mainly corn silage and a concentrate mixture low in retinol equivalents, neonatal animals consuming milk from mothers on a low intake of vitamin A, and when grains containing low carotene content are substituted for yellow corn (McDowell, 1989).

Deficiency symptoms associated with avitaminosis A in lambs were thoroughly described by Ghanem and Farid (1982). The first stage was marked by the development of xerophthalmia, which started with corneal opacity followed by ulceration of the cornea and ended with shrinking of the eyeball. Blindness occurred with the onset of corneal ulceration. The second stage of deficiency was associated with a variety of symptoms, starting with abnormal fluctuations in BW followed by growth retardation and weight loss. At about the same time, weakness and incoordination of movements developed. Paralysis of the hind quarters occurred in some animals. Thereafter, convulsions were followed by death. Although clinical signs of deficiency were not observed in a long-term vitamin A depletion study, Frier et al. (1974) noted that symptoms of hypovitaminosis A in adult goats were partially in accord with those of the calf. The hypovitaminotic A adult goat exhibited an increase in resistance to CSF absorption and a higher incidence of squamous metaplasia of the parotid duct and gland. Goats experiencing vitamin A deficiency had reduced feed intake and lost

BW after 25 weeks. Furthermore, some deterioration in the physical properties of wool is to be expected with rations deficient in vitamin A (Franklin et al., 1955; Farid and Ghanem, 1982). Vitamin A deficiency has also resulted in decreased sperm quality (Lindley et al., 1949) and increased sperm abnormalities (Abdulkareem et al., 2005) in rams. If a vitamin A deficiency occurs in pregnant ruminants, they may either abort or produce blind, dead, or weak offspring that will not survive (McDowell, 1989). Retained placenta may also be encountered with vitamin A deficiency (NRC, 1985).

Typical diets contain adequate carotene to prevent vitamin A deficiency. Free-ranging small ruminants with access to green foliage will consume enough carotene to allow for sufficient vitamin A storage in the liver to prevent deficiencies during periods of low intake; however, supplemental vitamin A is necessary when ruminants experience conditions most conducive to complete depletion of liver reserves. Although marginal deficiency adversely affecting performance by a few percentage points is not easily detected (Miller, 1979), it is often beneficial to supplement grazing livestock with vitamin A in the middle to late dry season (McDowell, 1989) or before liver reserves are completely depleted. A single megadose of supplemental vitamin A has been demonstrated to be as effective as lower doses supplemented more frequently (Franklin et al., 1955; Ghanem and Farid, 1982).

Caution must be exercised with provision of vitamin A to small ruminants because overzealous use of highly potent forms of vitamin A (i.e., retinol, retinyl acetate, and retinyl palmitate) can result in toxicity. NRC (1987) presumed the upper safe level for goats and sheep is 13,500 RE/kg of diet DM, which was based on the results of Frier et al. (1974). Those authors demonstrated that mature goats consuming retinyl acetate to provide 17,640 μg of retinol/kg of live weight had decreased daily feed consumption after 7 weeks and decreased BW by 8 weeks. Hypervitaminosis A in goats manifested as mild hyperemia of the perinealinguinal skin, hyperhidrosis and seborrhea of the ventral abdominal and inguinal skin, and lameness. Goats necropsied after 16 weeks of hypervitaminosis A had epidermal hyperplasia of the skin, thinner than normal radius bones, and marked osteolysis of individual ulnas bones.

Blood concentrations persistently greater than 100 μg of retinol/dL is indicative of toxicity (Eaton, 1969). Average weekly plasma retinol concentrations were 187.5 or 150.7 μg/dL in mature ewes fed 6,000 or 18,000 μg of retinol/kg of BW for 6 weeks (Donoghue et al., 1979). Donoghue et al. (1979) noted that average daily feed consumption by mature ewes over the 6-week period decreased by 29.8 and 52.4 percent when daily retinol intake was 6,000 and 18,000/kg BW, and serum activity of glutamic-oxalacetic transaminase increased in ewes with hypervitaminosis A.

This subcommittee recommends that intake of vitamin A from retinol or retinyl esters should not exceed 6,000 μg of retinol/kg of live weight. Vitamin A toxicity is normally not a practical problem unless unreasonably high levels of retinol or retinyl esters are administered or fed for greater than 4 weeks. However, high intake of carotenoids from natural feedstuffs does not produce vitamin A toxicity (NRC, 1987). The efficiency of carotene conversion to vitamin A declines progressively with increased intake, which may be a natural homeostatic control mechanism that protects ruminants from harmful effects due to excessive consumption of provitamin A (Miller, 1979). Percentage transfer of retinol from the digestive tract also decreased precipitously as supplemental dietary levels increased (Donoghue et al., 1983a). The irreversible conversion of retinol to retinoic acid may provide a metabolic outlet for retinol and retinal (Vitamin Nutrition Compendium, 2000).

Vitamin D

Vitamin D is a pro-hormone formed by ultraviolet irradiation of plant material or the animal's skin to form ergocalciferol (vitamin D_2) or cholecalciferol (vitamin D_3). A general scheme of vitamin D metabolism and the factors that influence vitamin D activity were presented by Littledike and Goff (1987). Vitamin D enters the blood from the digestive tract or the skin (as the precursor, 7-dehydrocholesterol) and rapidly accumulates in the liver and adipose tissue. In the liver, vitamin D precursors are converted to 25-hydroxyvitamin D [25-(OH)D]. This metabolite is the major form of vitamin D in circulation under normal conditions and serves as the precursor of the other vitamin D metabolites (Horst and Littledike, 1982). Once 25-(OH)D reaches the kidney, it is converted to the most biologically active form, 1,25-$(OH)_2$D. The primary role of 1,25-$(OH)_2$D is to maintain normal blood calcium (Ca) and phosphorus (P) concentrations by facilitating Ca and P transport across the intestinal brush border (Wasserman and Taylor, 1976) and enhancing bone resorption (DeLuca, 1984).

Vitamin D activity is measured in international units, where 1 IU is equivalent to the antirachitic activity of 0.025 μg of crystalline vitamin D_3 (Collins and Norman, 1991). Due to insufficient data published to the contrary, the vitamin D requirements for all classifications of domesticated small ruminants are comparable to previous recommendations (ARC, 1980; NRC, 1981, 1985). The vitamin D requirement for maintenance and early pregnancy is 5.6 IU/kg BW. Neonates are provided with enough vitamin D from their dams to prevent early rickets if their dams have received sufficient vitamin D (NRC, 1981, 1985). In addition to placental transmission (Hidiroglou and Williams, 1981), indirect supplementation of the suckling ruminant with vitamin D_3 may be achieved through maternal injection and subsequent mammary transfer (Hidiroglou and Knipfel, 1984). Additional vitamin D requirements are 213 IU/d for late pregnancy and 760 IU/kg milk production for lactation. For growing and developing small ruminants, an additional 54

IU/d vitamin D is required for every 50 g daily weight gain. Vitamin D requirements are 20 percent greater for animals less than 4 months of age that have been weaned early. Vitamin D requirements of growing New World camelids are not known, but vitamin D deficiency has been implicated in a hypophosphatemic rickets syndrome of young growing crias (Van Saun et al., 1996). Vitamin D supplementation greater than levels needed to maintain minimal serum vitamin D concentrations suggested for ruminants may be necessary to minimize potential problems with vitamin D-responsive rickets (Smith and Van Saun, 1996). Therefore, 30 IU of vitamin D/kg BW has been suggested for maintenance, pregnancy, and lactation (Van Saun, 2006). Vitamin D requirements may also increase when Ca, and perhaps P, requirements (refer to Chapter 7) are not satisfied (Scott and McLean, 1981). Moreover, Miller et al. (1993) hypothesized that nutrients required for antioxidant defense may be essential for in vivo production of 1,25-$(OH)_2$D. A deficiency in nutrients involved in inactivation of reactive oxygen metabolites could contribute to a vitamin D deficiency.

It has been suggested that natural feedstuffs containing vitamin D_2 supply the majority of vitamin D to wool-bearing ruminants because wool and lanolin cover decrease the efficiency of photochemical conversion of vitamin D_3 (Horst et al., 1981). Vitamin D status was two to three times greater in shorn sheep than unshorn animals, and blood levels of vitamin D decreased to pre-shearing values as new fleece grew (Zintzen and Boyazoglou, 1973). Wallis et al. (1949) reported that vitamin D_2 content of 66 forages collected throughout the United States ranged from 26.7 to 638 IU/kg. Despite lower concentrations of vitamin D_2 in certain forages, small ruminants housed outside are not expected to be deficient in vitamin D. In vivo synthesis made a considerable contribution to the vitamin D status of sheep with heavy and extreme wool covering (Andrews and Cunningham, 1945).

Small ruminants that are deprived of exposure to ultraviolet (UV) irradiation are susceptible to vitamin D deficiency. The physiological half-life of 25-(OH)D is only about 16 d for animals exposed to UV radiation (Hidiroglou, 1987), whereas the half-life may only be about 8 d for animals receiving vitamin D orally (Hidiroglou and Karpinski, 1989). Osteodystrophy has been reported in animals experiencing prolonged periods of cloudy weather (Crowley, 1961) and in animals reared indoors without access to sunlight or artificial lighting that provides UV radiation (Hidiroglou et al., 1979).

In all but the extreme northern latitudes, however, sunlight stimulates sufficient endogenous production of vitamin D_3 (Littledike and Goff, 1987). Smith and Wright (1984) concluded that the synthesis of the vitamin D_3 in the skin plays a dominant role in vitamin D status of grazing animals. Others (Hidiroglou et al., 1985; Hidiroglou, 1987) demonstrated a significant increase in plasma vitamin D_3 and 25-(OH)D concentrations following exposure to UV irradiation. Vitamin D status was improved more effectively by 10 h exposure to the natural sunlight spectrum than by supplementing sheep with 2,000 IU/d vitamin D_3 (Hidiroglou and Karpinski, 1989).

Prolonged exposure to UV does not significantly increase the previtamin D_3 concentration above about 15 percent of the initial provitamin concentration (Holick, 1987). Steady-state levels of 25-(OH)D in circulation are reached within 4 weeks of continuous exposure to UV radiation (Hidiroglou, 1987; Hidiroglou and Karpinski, 1989). Although the length of time required to achieve steady-state levels is over twice as long as UV exposure, circulating levels of 25-(OH)D also plateau after continuous intake of vitamin D_3 (Hines et al., 1986; Hidiroglou and Karpinski, 1989). Nevertheless, development of atherosclerosis is possible when small ruminants consume excessive amounts of vitamin D (Hines et al., 1985). Appreciable amounts of vitamin D_3 were recorded in a variety of tissues for up to 4 months following an intramuscular injection of vitamin D_3 (Hidiroglou and Williams, 1984). However, vitamin D homeostasis may be maintained as long as daily vitamin D intake is below 100 IU/kg BW (Smith et al., 1985). Therefore, small ruminants experiencing normal conditions would not be expected to exhibit vitamin D intoxification unless overzealous use of dietary supplements or injectable preparations is common practice.

The maximum tolerable levels of vitamin D_3 are 25,000 IU/kg of diet if the diet is consumed for less than 60 days, whereas small ruminants can only tolerate 2,200 IU/kg of diet DM if the diet is consumed for greater than 60 d (NRC, 1987). Consumption of calcinogenic plants that contain a glycoside of 1,25$(OH)_2$D, such as *Cestrum diurnum*, *Nierembergia veitchii*, *Solanum esuriale*, *Solanum malacoxylon*, *Solanum torvum*, *Solanum verbascifolium*, and *Trisetum flavescens* may cause rapid hypercalcemia and widespread metastatic calcification (Mello, 2003). Although not all calcinogenic plants are equally potent (Mello and Habermehl, 1992), as little as 50 mg of air-dried *Solanum malacoxylon* leaves three times weekly caused bone mineralization defects in sheep (Woodard et al., 1994).

Vitamin E

Vitamin E is a generic term used for all tocol and tocotrienol derivatives that exhibit the activity of α-tocopherol. The IU established for vitamin E is based on the biological potency of 1 mg of the fully racemic form of *dl*-α-tocopheryl acetate; the naturally occurring form, *d*-α-tocopherol, has a biopotency of 1.49 IU/mg, whereas chemical esterification with acetate to produce *d*-α-tocopheryl acetate has a biopotency of 1.36 IU/mg (NRC, 1987). Natural tocopherols and tocotrienols are distributed widely in plants occurring mainly as free alcohols in lipid fractions of green leaves and seeds. In a review of 455 published articles, Dicks (1965) reported that the majority of tocopherol in forage matter was α-tocopherol. Regardless of the presence of other isomers (β, γ, and δ) in feeds, only α-tocopherol appears in significant levels in blood and tissues of animals (Hidiroglou et al., 1992a). Isomers of β, γ, and δ-tocopherol have some, but very low, biological activity (NRC, 1987). Therefore, vitamin E and α-tocopherol will be used interchangeably throughout the remainder of this section.

The principal metabolic function of vitamin E is closely linked to the selenium-containing enzyme glutathione peroxidase. Both glutathione peroxidase and vitamin E function to protect biological membranes from oxidative damage. Vitamin E is known primarily for its action as an antioxidative component of cell membranes that prevents peroxidative damage to the cell membrane and membranes of subcellular organelles by free radicals (Burton and Ingold, 1989). The antioxidative role becomes very important during the immune response when macrophages and neutrophils produce large quantities of superoxide and hydrogen peroxide from molecular oxygen to destroy foreign organisms (Ross, 1977; Badwey and Karnovsky, 1980). Additional immune responses attributed to vitamin E include enhanced humoral immunity via elevated immunoglobulin G (IgG), enhanced phagocytosis by polymorphonuclear cells, and enhanced cell-mediated immunity by increased stimulation of lymphocytes to mitogens and antigens (Tengerdy, 1990b). The antioxidant effect of vitamin E also modulates the biosynthesis and activity of important cell regulators, prostaglandins, thromboxane, and leukotrienes (Tengerdy, 1989, 1990a). Protection by vitamin E against peroxidative inactivation of steroidogenic enzymes (Miller et al., 1993) and prostaglandin $F_{2\alpha}$ effects on corpora luteal regression (Vierk et al., 1998) may also impact reproduction. Therefore, proper α-tocopherol status is important in protecting ruminants from nutritional muscular dystrophy and promoting increased productivity by enhancing immune (McDowell et al., 1996) and reproductive (Hemingway, 2003) functions.

Previous vitamin E requirements seemed to be established by determining the level necessary to prevent signs of nutritional muscular dystrophy (ARC, 1980; NRC, 1985). Similarly, Van Saun (2006) based vitamin E requirements for New World camelids on recommendations for beef (NRC, 1996) and sheep (NRC, 1985). Although the previous committee on Nutrient Requirements for Goats (NRC, 1981) indicated that evidence of spontaneous vitamin E deficiency signs in goats was lacking, Ross et al. (1989) noted that nutritional myopathy in goats has been reported worldwide. Nutritional myopathy associated with vitamin E deficiency also has been reported for free-ranging white-tailed deer (Tramontin et al., 1983) and wapiti (David and Winterbottom, 1996). Vitamin E requirements recommended hereafter shall be for all small ruminants, although data available in the literature are limited primarily to sheep.

Determination of vitamin E requirements in isolation is exceptionally difficult because of the interrelationships with other dietary factors. Minimum requirements for dietary vitamin E of growing and pregnant sheep were 10.0 and 15.0 mg/kg of dry matter (DM), but 15 to 30 mg of vitamin E/kg DM may be inadequate if dietary selenium is deficient (ARC, 1980). Thus, the previous NRC (1985) recommendations of 20 IU of vitamin E/kg DM for lambs less than 20 kg and 15 IU of vitamin E/kg DM for other classes of sheep assumed adequate dietary selenium. Vitamin E deficiency in the face of adequate selenium has also been presented as nutritional myodegeneration (Maas et al., 1984) and subcapsular liver rupture (Green et al., 1995). In a survey of vitamin E levels in the livers of sheep in Ontario, Menzies et al. (2003) reported that 90 percent of market lambs had low to deficient vitamin E status. Moreover, myopathy and hepatic lipidosis were observed in weaned lambs consuming diets that were adequate to meet NRC (1985) requirements (Menzies et al., 2004). In light of these findings and more recent evidence demonstrating the benefits of supplementing vitamin E above previously established minimums, this subcommittee recommended that vitamin E requirements should be increased.

Plasma or serum concentrations of vitamin E commonly have been used to assess nutritional status of vitamin E (Hidiroglou et al., 1992a). Clinical lesions of white muscle disease were associated with < 1.0 to 1.5 μg of α-tocopherol/mL in serum (McMurray and Rice, 1982). Values of < 2.0 μg/mL have been considered deficient (McMurray and Rice, 1982; Maas et al., 1984). Many tissues may store vitamin E but the liver is the major storage organ for α-tocopherol (Hidiroglou et al., 1970a), and plasma α-tocopherol levels are maintained by mobilizing hepatic reserves during short-term inadequate intake of vitamin E (Karpinski and Hidiroglou, 1990; Fry et al., 1993). Serum concentration of α-tocopherol exceeds 2.0 μg/mL in about 1 week's time when sheep are fed supplemental *dl*-α-tocopheryl acetate daily (Hidiroglou et al., 1992b). Plasma α-tocopherol concentrations also return to baseline levels within 1 week following a single intraruminal bolus of vitamin E (Hidiroglou and Charmley, 1991). Mild subclinical myopathy may occur within 2 to 8 weeks in sheep consuming a diet devoid of vitamin E (Fry et al., 1993). Four weeks was sufficient to decrease serum α-tocopherol ≤ 1 μg/mL in lambs consuming a diet deficient in vitamin E (Njeru et al., 1994a).

This subcommittee recognized that there is inconsistency regarding the adequacy of relying solely on serum or plasma α-tocopherol concentrations as an index of vitamin E status. No direct relationship was found between vitamin E and plasma α-tocopherol content in sheep fed graded levels of *dl*-α-tocopheryl acetate (Hidiroglou and Charmley, 1990). Circulating vitamin E may be influenced by blood lipids making serum α-tocopherol an unreliable index of vitamin E status (Charmley et al., 1992). Weiss et al. (1994) concluded that when concentrations of plasma lipids are different because of diet, concentrations of α-tocopherol in the plasma should be expressed on a lipid basis. However, expressing serum α-tocopherol relative to blood lipids did not improve the relationship between serum α-tocopherol and vitamin E intake in sheep (Njeru et al., 1994a). For this reason and the paucity of data on differing expressions of plasma or serum α-tocopherol concentrations, this subcommittee elected to use plasma or serum α-tocopherol concentrations to indicate vitamin E status of small ruminants.

The NRC (1985) recommendation of 20 IU of vitamin E/kg of feed for early-weaned lambs with rapid growth potential was based on the observations of Sharman (1973). For a 20 kg lamb consuming 1.2 kg DM, this is equivalent to 1.2 mg of *dl*-α-tocopherol/kg BW. This is comparable to the weekly dose of 11.0 mg of *dl*-α-tocopherol/kg of live weight reported by Ewan et al. (1968) to prevent deaths due to white muscle disease. However, 42 to 60 kg lambs consuming a diet fortified to meet NRC (1985) recommendations (15 IU/kg DM) plus supplementary vitamin E provided at 30 IU/d were unable to maintain serum α-tocopherol > 2.0 μg/mL (Njeru et al., 1994a). Likewise, white-tailed deer fed a basal diet containing 5.5 mg/kg of vitamin E and fortified with 45 IU of vitamin E/kg were unable to maintain plasma α-tocopherol > 2.0 μg/mL throughout a 24-month period (Brady et al., 1978).

Dierenfeld (1994) suggested that the vitamin E requirements of cervids reared in captivity were 5- to 10-fold greater than dietary vitamin E recommendations for livestock. For a 50 kg lamb consuming 1.5 kg of DM (NRC, 1985) and the diet described by Njeru et al. (1994a), daily intake of vitamin E greater than 1.1 IU/kg of live weight would be necessary to maintain circulating concentration of vitamin E ≥ 2.0 μg/mL. Results of pharmacokinetic studies indicate that the vitamin E dose required to maintain plasma concentration of α-tocopherol ≥ 2.0 μg/mL would be 1.7, 3.0, and 3.3 mg of α-tocopherol/kg of live weight when administered intravenously (Hidiroglou and Karpinski, 1988), intramuscularly (Hidiroglou and Karpinski, 1991), and intraperitoneally (Toutain et al., 1995). Plasma vitamin E concentrations were 1.6 times greater in sheep given a single intraperitoneal bolus of *dl*-α-tocopheryl acetate compared with the same dose administered intraruminally (Hidiroglou and Charmley, 1991). Thus, 5.3 mg of dietary vitamin E/kg of live BW would be required to maintain blood α-tocopherol concentrations above the aforementioned critical minimum level. Total vitamin E intake required for a 50 kg sheep would be 265 IU/d. This value compares well with results of Hidiroglou and Charmley (1990), who reported that plasma α-tocopherol concentrations averaged 2.1 μg/mL in 45 to 55 kg lambs fed supplemental *dl*-α-tocopheryl acetate at 200 mg/d and a basal diet containing 25 to 32 mg total tocopherol/kg DM. Although 42 to 60 kg lambs fed a diet containing 15.4 IU/kg DM and 60 IU/d of supplemental *dl*-α-tocopheryl acetate had serum vitamin E concentrations of 3.18 μg/mL after 60 d (Njeru et al., 1994a), this concentration should be considered a minimum based on guidelines established from limited data (Hidiroglou et al., 1992a). Hidiroglou et al. (1992b) noted that serum tocopherol concentrations of 35 kg lambs fed 325 IU/d of vitamin E peaked between 15 and 21 d, then exhibited a plateau within the minimal range suggested by Hidiroglou et al. (1992a). Therefore, the newly suggested minimum daily requirement of 5.3 IU of vitamin E/kg of live BW seems reasonably appropriate for most lamb production situations.

Vitamin E requirements increase if the goal is to enhance immune response or extend the storage case life of lamb meat. Dietary vitamin E at 20 times previously established requirements (NRC, 1985) was shown to boost immunocompetence of sheep experimentally exposed to recurrent infections in the endemic area (Tengerdy, 1989, 1990b). This would be equivalent to 9 IU of vitamin E/kg BW for a 50 kg lamb consuming a diet based on previous NRC (1985) recommendations. Vitamin E is the major lipid-soluble antioxidant in animal tissues which acts post-mortem to delay oxidative deterioration of meat (Wood and Enser, 1997). Daily supplementation of vitamin E at 8.6 times greater than previously established requirements (500 IU of vitamin E/d) to feedlot lambs slaughtered at 52.9 kg extended the storage case life of retail lamb cuts, but 1,000 IU for lambs finished at 49.7 kg did little to improve storage attributes of lamb cuts beyond that achieved by feeding 500 IU/d (Wulf et al., 1995). Likewise, Turner et al. (2002) predicted that maximum concentrations of α-tocopherol in the longissimus muscle occurred at an intake of 584 IU of vitamin E/d for lambs averaging 53.1 kg at slaughter. This subcommittee recommends 10 IU of vitamin E/kg of BW as an aid to protect small ruminants from infectious disease and to extend the storage life of lamb meat. Dietary strategies designed to increase polyunsaturated fatty acid content of small ruminant animal food products may further increase vitamin E requirements (Demirel et al., 2004), but data are currently too scant to provide recommendations for these dietary situations.

Neonatal ruminants are particularly susceptible to low vitamin E status. Lambs are born with low levels of vitamin E because placental transfer of vitamin E to the fetus in utero is very limited (Hidiroglou et al., 1970b; Pehrson et al., 1990; Njeru et al., 1994b). The severity or incidence of vitamin E-responsive diseases seems to be influenced by placental and mammary gland transfer of α-tocopherol (Hidiroglou et al., 1972). Although supplemental vitamin E given to the lamb at birth will increase lamb serum α-tocopherol levels, this practice in most cases is not effective in reducing lamb mortality or increasing lamb performance (Hatfield et al., 2000). Providing colostrum rich in vitamin E is necessary to meet the requirement of the newborn (McDowell et al., 1996). Based on results of Pehrson et al. (1990) and Njeru et al. (1994b), minimal vitamin E requirements established for growing lambs also should be considered minimum requirements for late gestational (3 to 4 weeks prepartum) ewes to maintain vitamin E status of newborn lambs through mammary transfer of tocopherol into colostrum. Providing supplemental vitamin E to the ewe during late gestation has often decreased lamb mortality and improved lamb productivity (Hatfield et al., 2000). Lamb serum IgG, BW gain, and ultimately weaning weight were greater for lambs reared by ewes treated with vitamin E (Gentry et al., 1992). Supplementing ewes with 330 IU of vitamin E/d for approximately 21 days during late pregnancy reduced lamb mortality, which contributed to a 2.6 kg increase in total lamb production per ewe (Kott et al., 1998). Provision of dietary vitamin E to pregnant ewes at approximately 5.6 IU/kg BW for 32 days prepartum increased 3-day-old lamb serum α-tocopherol concentrations but not serum IgG or antiters to parainfluenza 3 in offspring from ewes challenged with parainfluenza type 3 prepartum (Daniels et al., 2000). Thus, vitamin E supplementation of the late gestational ewe above the minimum recommended levels may be necessary to enhance immunocompetence of neonatal small ruminants. Offspring mortality from white muscle disease was 25–31.25 percent less for white-tailed does consuming a diet fortified with vitamin E than for does consuming a diet not fortified with vitamin E throughout their life cycle (Brady et al., 1978). Additional vitamin E may need to be administered directly to the nursing offspring because of a precipitous drop in vitamin E transfer across the mammary gland with the onset of copious milk production (Pehrson et al., 1990; Njeru et al., 1994b). Weekly intramuscular injections of 1,000 IU of *dl*-α-tocopherol may protect membranes of the musculo-skeletal system from oxidation during growth (Maiorano et al., 1999). For suckling lambs weighing 15.9 kg at 33 d (Maiorano et al., 1999), this would be equivalent to 9.0 IU of vitamin E/kg BW if administered daily ((1,000 IU/wk)/(7 d/wk^{-1}))/15.9 kg). This value would need to be 12 IU of vitamin E/kg BW if consumed in a creep feed because intramuscular injections are 3.0 times more effective at maintaining plasma concentration of α-tocopherol ≥ 2.0 μg/mL than oral doses of the vitamin (Hidiroglou and Karpinski, 1991). Additional research is needed to determine the effectiveness of providing additional vitamin E in creep feed offered to small ruminants.

The minimum recommendation of 5.3 IU vitamin E/kg BW also applies to dairy breeds of small ruminants. Parenteral administration of 0.1 mg of selenium and 5 IU vitamin E/kg BW at 2-week intervals about 1 month before parturition reduced somatic cell count and improved some indicators of natural immune responses during early lactation (Morgante et al., 1999). Supplemental vitamin E at 1.67 IU/kg BW above NRC (1975) recommendations also decreased apparent oxidative stress associated with mammary involution during the dry-off period (Colitti et al., 2000). Although the transfer efficiency of vitamin E across the mammary gland is low, maintaining adequate vitamin E may prevent milk fat oxidation (Chilliard and Ferlay, 2004), which would help maintain freshness (McDowell et al., 1996).

Tissue concentrations of α-tocopherol are governed by the actual absorbed dose (Toutain et al., 1995). Vitamin E is not expected to be metabolized or oxidized as extensively as vitamin A in the rumen of ruminants. Using radiolabeled α-tocopherol, Astrup et al. (1974) reported no significant degradation after a 24-hour in vitro incubation with ruminal contents from a fasted sheep fed a 50 percent alfalfa chaff and 50 percent oats diet. More recent publications indicate also that ruminal metabolism of vitamin E is negligible for all forage (McDiarmid et al., 1994), 50 percent forage (Weiss et al., 1995), and high concentrate (Leedle et al., 1993) diets. Although preintestinal disappearance of vitamin E averaged 8.4, 22.2, 25.0, and 42.4 percent for diets containing 20, 40, 60, and 80 percent corn (Alderson et al., 1971), duodenal recovery of vitamin E of 79.0–92.0 percent in sheep fed diets based on dried grass may be related to methodological inadequacies or incomplete extraction of tocopherols because there is no known mechanism by which vitamin E is degraded in the rumen (Chikunya et al., 2004). Absorption of tocopherols takes place in the small intestine primarily through the lymphatic system, and transport occurs via a lipoprotein complex (Machlin, 1990). Emulsification preceding absorption is requisite for esterified α-tocopherol because plasma concentrations of α-tocopherol were less when vitamin E was administered directly into the duodenum of sheep (Hidiroglou et al., 1991) and cattle (Roquet et al., 1992) compared with intraruminal administration. Moreover, feeding diets supplemented with fat, which would enhance emulsification capacity, increased plasma concentrations of α-tocopherol (Weiss et al., 1994; Weiss and Wyatt, 2003).

Small ruminants at pasture, or those receiving adequate green feeds, should normally be of adequate vitamin E status (Hemingway, 2003). However, the level of α-tocopherol in forage crops generally decreases as plants approach phenological maturity. In their review of the literature, Kivimae and Carpena (1973) found that concentrations of α-tocopherol in alfalfa and in timothy (*Phleum* spp.) declined 20–65 percent depending on whether the crop was harvested in the late-vegetative or full-flowering stage of development. Brown (1953) reported extraordinarily large differences in α-tocopherol concentrations of vegetative vs. fully mature grasses. Concentrations of vegetative grass samples ranged from 22.1 to 30.3 ppm, collectively. Upon maturity, α-tocopherol levels dropped 79, 89, 87, and 90 percent for meadow fescue (*Festuca pratensis*), orchard grass (*Dactylis glomerata*), timothy (*Phleum pratense*), and perennial rye grass (*Lolium perenne*), respectively. Leaves were also shown to contain three to four times more α-tocopherol than the stems (Brown, 1953; Dicks, 1965). Although as little as 33–37 percent loss in vitamin E can be expected from green-up to maturity for certain forages, such as sudan grass and wheat grass (Dicks, 1965), long-term curing may decrease α-tocopherol levels even further.

The concentration of vitamin E is much greater in fresh grass than in harvested and processed forages. Concentrations of α-tocopherol in first-cutting alfalfa/timothy declined from 70 ppm to 35 ppm and 15 ppm from the time of harvest for silage and hay, respectively (M. Hidiroglou et al., 1994). The studies reviewed by Kivimae and Carpena (1973) indicated that high moisture content and prolonged exposure to heat resulted in significant losses of α-tocopherol. Losses were heightened as storage duration increased. Thus, provision of supplemental vitamin E may be warranted for small ruminants consuming low-quality range or harvested forages.

A number of vitamin E products are available for bolstering the vitamin E status of small ruminants. The acetate ester of *dl*-α-tocopherol is the most widely available supplemental source of vitamin E; *dl*-α-tocopheryl acetate is very stable, readily hydrolyzed in the digestive tract, and potent as an in vivo antioxidant (McDowell et al., 1996). In addition to the aforementioned effects of route of administration, biopotency is influenced by chemical formulation/carrier of vitamin E supplements. Biological potencies of *d*-α-tocopherol, *dl*-α-tocopherol, and *dl*-α-tocopheryl acetate presented in NRC (1987) seem appropriate (Hidiroglou et al., 1989; M. Hidiroglou et al., 1992b, 1994; Ochoa et al., 1992). Whereas esterification of tocopherol with nicotinate (Hidiroglou and Charmley, 1991) and succinate (Hidiroglou and Singh, 1991) have reduced biopotency, the bioavailability of acetylated α-tocopherol can be increased when combined with *d*-α-tocopherol polyethylene glycol succinate (Hidiroglou et al., 1992b). The form in which vitamin E was supplemented orally had no effect on the ratio of tissue to plasma α-tocopherol levels (N. Hidiroglou et al., 1994). Thus, supplementation with any of the commercially available vitamin E products will improve vitamin E status. Although hypervitaminosis E has not been documented in ruminants, 75 IU/kg of BW daily is a tentative presumed safe level (NRC, 1987).

Vitamin K

Vitamin K is a generic term used to describe a group of quinone compounds that exhibit antihemorrhagic effects. The three most common isomers of vitamin K are the plant form phylloquinone (vitamin K_1), bacterial form menaquinone (vitamin K_2), and synthetic form menadione (vitamin K_3). Vitamin K_3 and its derivatives are the forms used in feed supplements (Combs, 1992).

The ruminal microorganisms generally synthesize and supply vitamin K in amounts sufficient to meet the ruminant animal's requirements. Supplemental vitamin K is usually only justified when small ruminants are suspected to have consumed sufficient quantities of vitamin K antagonists. For example, sweet vernal grass (*Anthoxanthum odoratum*) and yellow-flowered (*Melilotus officinalis*) and white-flowered (*Melilotus alba*) sweetclover emit a distinct, vanilla-like odor due to the presence of coumarin in the plants. Metabolism of coumarin by fungi during the molding process produces the vitamin K inhibitor dicumarol. Because dicumarol antagonizes vitamin K, an essential component of the blood-clotting process, feeding moldy sweet vernal grass or sweetclover to small ruminants may cause hemorrhage and uncontrollable bleeding. Successful treatment of dicumarol intoxification has been demonstrated with injectable vitamin K_1 (Alstad et al., 1985) and K_3 (Radostits et al., 1980). However, responses to vitamin K therapy have been somewhat dependent on differences in dicumarol source and dosages. Therefore, prevention by avoiding feedstuffs containing dicumarol may be a better alternative to treatment. In addition to dicumoral, other vitamin K antagonists include sulfonamide antibiotics, mycotoxins (T-2 toxin), warfarin (Vitamin Nutrition Compendium, 2000), and 4-hydroxycoumarins isolated from *Ferula communis* L (Lamnaouer, 1999). If vitamin K therapy is necessary, vitamin K_3 or its derivatives have an LD_{50} in the range of a few hundred mg/kg BW (NRC, 1987).

WATER-SOLUBLE VITAMINS

In general, water-soluble vitamin requirements of small ruminants can be met by escape of dietary sources from ruminal metabolism and through endogenous synthesis. Microbial synthesis of the B vitamins in the rumen is thought to satisfy the ruminant's requirements. Self-sufficiency exhibited by ruminants due to the synthesis of the B vitamins by ruminal microorganisms has been established for over 50 years (Agrawala et al., 1953). Likewise, ruminants are capable of synthesizing their own vitamin C (ascorbic acid) because they have the enzyme L-gulanolactone oxidase responsible for the conversion of gulonic acid to gulanolactone in ascorbic acid synthesis (Bender, 1992). Despite early indications of self-sufficiency for the water-soluble vitamins, many subsequent inquiries have been made regarding the adequacy of water-soluble vitamins in ruminants.

Establishing Requirements for Water-Soluble Vitamins

In comparing extrapolated potential requirements from swine requirements (NRC, 1998) and average concentrations in milk with estimated supply based on limited research, the Nutrient Requirements of Dairy Cattle (NRC, 2001) noted that only folic acid and pantothenic acid may be limiting. Although several studies have demonstrated production and/or health benefits when diets have been supplemented with water-soluble vitamins, the levels of the vitamins given to induce such responses are usually for specialized production situations and may not necessarily reflect requirements for normal growth or reproduction (Huber, 1988). NRC (2001) was not able to provide recommendations for water-soluble vitamin requirements because almost no research was available on requirements for various stages of dairy production. Likewise, information is not generally sufficient to establish recommendations for water-soluble vitamin requirements for small ruminants.

The ability to provide dietary recommendations for the water-soluble vitamins is complicated because of extensive metabolism of the vitamins that occurs by the rumen microorganisms. The ruminal microorganisms' requirements for the B vitamins have been discussed briefly (Wolin et al., 1997). Those authors indicated that most of the major species of rumen microorganisms require one or more of the B vitamins, but their individual requirements differ, and not all of the microorganisms in the rumen synthesize all of the B vitamins. Many B vitamins are of importance to the rumen bacteria because they participate in many biochemical reactions in ruminal microbial metabolism (Nagaraja et al., 1997). Van Gylswyk et al. (1992) concluded that dietary supply of certain B vitamins may sometimes be too low to allow optimal growth of some bacterial species. Consequently, the production responses resulting from dietary supplementation of B vitamins may be related to factors occurring in the rumen.

Biotin

The ruminant's ability to satisfy requirements via ruminal synthesis of biotin has been questioned (Frigg et al., 1993). Biotin is a required nutrient for several species of ruminal cellulolytic and saccarolytic bacteria (Baldwin and Allison, 1983). Diets based on grains, which often reduce ruminal pH, seem to alter rumen microbial synthesis and utilization of biotin. Results of in vitro studies suggest that disruption in the growth of cellulolytic bacteria due to reduced ruminal pH decreases microbial production (Abel et al., 2001) or utilization (Rosendo et al., 2003) of biotin. Little synthesis of biotin occurred in the rumen, but considerable synthesis appeared to occur in the small and large intestine of steers fed 85.5 percent grain diets (Miller et al., 1986). Nevertheless, serum biotin concentrations were not affected in wethers fed diets ranging from 5–91 percent concentrate (Peterson et al., 2004). Supplemental feeding of biotin has increased serum biotin concentrations and improved measures of hoof health in dairy cattle (NRC, 2001), but such data are not available for small ruminants.

Choline

The choline requirement has not been firmly established for ruminants. Huber (1988) suggested 21 mg/kg BW as the choline requirements for ruminants. Thus, the traditional definition of a vitamin would exclude choline because it is required in gram rather than milligram amounts.

Both naturally occurring choline in feeds and dietary choline from supplements are degraded extensively in the rumen (Neil et al., 1979; Sharma and Erdman, 1989). Dietary supplementation with unprotected choline is presumed to be useless because the methyl groups of the compound are converted to methane in the rumen (Neil et al., 1978). Choline, however, may be synthesized from ethanolamine with the donation of methyl groups from *S*-adenosylmethionine ultimately derived from methionine (Neil et al., 1979). In lactating dairy goats, 28 percent of methionine methyl groups were transferred to choline (Emmanuel and Kennelly, 1984). Additionally, sheep recycle choline very efficiently (Dawson et al., 1981). Significant amounts of choline are synthesized in extrahepatic tissues and choline is extensively re-circulated between the intestine and liver (Robinson et al., 1984, 1987). It is not known if other small ruminants have the same ability as sheep to recycle choline, but responses to rumen-protected choline or betaine are comparable between sheep and goats.

Betaine, an oxidative product of choline, is also extensively degraded in the rumen but nearly 100 percent of radiolabeled betaine carbons were recovered in the body tissues of sheep (Mitchell et al., 1979). Betaine can substitute for *S*-adenosylmethionine as a methyl donor for the direct methylation of phosphatidylethanolamine to affect phosphatidylcholine and phosphatidylethanolamine concentrations (Sugiyama et al., 1998). Betaine also actively participates in methionine metabolism by donating methyl groups for the remethylation of homocysteine to methionine.

Given the interrelationships between choline, betaine, and methionine in the regulation of methylation processes and that methionine is usually one of the most limiting amino acids (Chapter 5), researchers have explored the use of choline or betaine to spare methionine. Intravenous infusion of choline and carnitine reduced the irreversible loss of methionine by 18–25 percent in sheep (Lobley et al., 1996). Reduced entry into the transulfuration pathway because of a repression in methionine adenosyltransferase activity occurs when methionine in blood plasma increases in sheep (Radcliffe and Egan, 1978). Intravenous injections of betaine have increased plasma methionine in kid goats (Puchala et al., 1995). Increased methionine availability for protein synthesis may increase production of milk (Erdman and Sharma, 1991), meat (Fernández-Figares et al., 2002), and wool (Reis et al., 1990). Responses to supplemental betaine are greater when goats consume a diet low in protein (Puchala et al., 2000; Banskalieva et al., 2005), which supports the methionine sparing concept.

Another possible effect of choline and betaine involves lipid metabolism. Choline and betaine may increase the synthesis of carnitine, which may in turn alter body fat distribution (Bryant et al., 1999) to reduce carcass fat (Fernández et al., 1998). The extra demand for methyl groups for the secretion of methyl compounds in the milk is facilitated by enhancing the rate of de novo methyl group synthesis (Xue and Snoswell, 1985). Consequently, milk fat percentage may be increased upon supplementing betaine (D. Fernández et al., 2004).

Current evidence suggests that small ruminants may experience a choline deficiency and production may be increased with supplementation. Hsu et al. (1991) demonstrated that choline disappearing from the small intestine of wether lambs was 87 percent of requirements suggested by Huber (1988). Feeding rumen-protected choline or rumen-protected betaine has increased live weight gain by 10

(Bryant et al., 1999) to 60 percent (Puchala et al., 2000). Incorporating betaine in the diet of goats has increased milk yield by 12 (C. Fernández et al., 2004) to 36 percent (D. Fernández et al., 2004). However, production responses to supplemental choline or betaine have been inconsistent. Live weight gain of growing lambs was not affected by feeding nonprotected betaine at 0.2 percent of the diet (Fernández et al., 1998) or rumen-protected choline to provide less than 2 grams of choline per day (Bryant et al., 1999). Feeding either rumen-protected betaine or rumen-protected choline did not affect live weight gain of growing goats fed a high-protein diet (Puchala et al., 2000). Incorporating betaine in the diet at 0.2 percent of the diet of lactating goats tended to increase milk production (Fernández et al., 2000), but 0.4 percent dietary betaine did not improve milk production of goats experiencing a subclinical intramammary infection (Sánchez et al., 2001). Milk yield also did not increase during the first two months of lactation when lactating dairy goats were fed a diet with 0.4 percent betaine (D. Fernández et al., 2004). Responses are often greater for betaine than choline, which may result from dissimilar metabolic fates (Banskalieva et al., 2005). Further research is required before recommendations for choline requirements can be established for small ruminants.

Cyanocobalamin (Vitamin B_{12})

Cyanocobalamin is a generic term used to describe 5,6-dimethylbenzimidazole cobamide cyanide, which is also known as true vitamin B_{12}. Vitamin B_{12} has several metabolic functions, the most important of which includes functioning as an essential component in propionate and methionine metabolism. Underwood (1977) suggested that small ruminant requirements for vitamin B_{12} are of the same order as those for nonruminants but higher than those for humans. The classical research conducted by Marston (1970) established that sheep with fully functional reticulo-rumens require about 11 µg of vitamin B_{12} daily. Cobalt is incorporated into the structure of vitamin B_{12} by ruminal microorganisms (Smith and Marston, 1970). Adequate intake of cobalt is required for the rumen microorganisms to synthesize sufficient amounts of vitamin B_{12} to satisfy the host animal's metabolic requirement, and it has been assumed that ruminant requirements for vitamin B_{12} are equal to ruminal bacteria requirements for cobalt (Girard, 2000), because one atom of cobalt is part of the vitamin B_{12} molecule. Goats are suspected to be more resistant to cobalt deficiency than sheep (Clark et al., 1986b; Mburu et al., 1993), but it has generally been assumed that the minimum requirements of cobalt for sheep are adequate for goats (Lee and Marston, 1969). More recent evidence indicates that the goat's requirement for vitamin B_{12} is comparable to that of the sheep (Kadim et al., 2003, 2004; Johnson et al., 2004). Although no reference range exists for cervids' vitamin B_{12} concentrations (Clark et al., 1986a), values regarded sufficient for sheep have been used to indicate adequacy of vitamin B_{12} in red deer (Peet and Hepworth, 1993; Audigé et al., 1999). Likewise, plasma vitamin B_{12} levels of clinically normal guanacos appeared to be similar to those of domestic ruminants (Hastings and Gascoyne, 1992). Therefore, this subcommittee suggests that vitamin B_{12} requirements are the same for sheep, goats, cervids, and New World camelids.

In a summarization of three experiments in which a total of 61 estimates of duodenal flow of vitamin B_{12} were determined in sheep, Bigger et al. (1976) noted that daily production of vitamin B_{12} averaged 1,729 µg or 2.84 µg/g of digestible DM intake for diets with 0.5 to 1.0 ppm cobalt. Earlier publications indicated that values for daily ruminal production of vitamin B_{12} ranged from 400 µg (Smith and Marston, 1970) to 2,240 µg (Elliot et al., 1971), and sheep fed high-concentrate diets produced 0.9 µg/g of digestible DM intake in the rumen (Sutton and Elliot, 1972). Sutton and Elliot (1972) noted that vitamin B_{12} disappearance ranged from 1 to 35 percent of duodenal flow. Smith and Marston (1970) proposed an apparent absorption efficiency of approximately 5 percent for vitamin B_{12}, which was slightly less than values for sheep fed high-concentrate (8.4–9.5 percent) or high-roughage (22.0–37.9 percent) diets (Rickard and Elliot, 1978). The highest absorption coefficient reported by Rickard and Elliot (1978) was noted for animals that had the lowest ruminal production of vitamin B_{12}. Regression analysis of 34 data points revealed that intestinal absorption of vitamin B_{12} averaged 21 percent (Hedrich et al., 1973). Roughage-based diets were fed to 80 percent of the sheep in studies summarized by Bigger et al. (1976). Ruminal production data reported by Bigger et al. (1976) and average intestinal disappearance reported by Hedrich et al. (1973) suggest that sheep consuming roughage-based diets with adequate cobalt are not expected to experience vitamin B_{12} deficiency. For sheep fed high-concentrate diets with adequate cobalt, a minimum of 110 g of digestible DM would be necessary for the animal to meet its vitamin B_{12} requirement. Based on ruminal production and the lowest intestinal absorption data of Sutton and Elliot (1972), however, sheep would need to consume 1,222 grams of digestible DM along with sufficient cobalt to satisfy their requirement for vitamin B_{12}. Although it seems as if vitamin B_{12} requirements of the small ruminant will often be satisfied if the animal consumes adequate cobalt, there may be instances where supplemental vitamin B_{12} could be warranted.

Vitamin B_{12} synthesized in the rumen may be utilized by the ruminal microorganisms before the vitamin is available for absorption by the animal. In vitro studies indicated that survival and growth of ciliated protozoa were enhanced with the addition of vitamin B_{12} (Bonhomme et al., 1982). Vitamin B_{12} dependence has also been demonstrated in batch and continuous cultures of propionate-producing bacteria (Strobel, 1992). Vitamin B_{12} serves as a cofactor for methyl malonyl-CoA isomerase, which catalyzes the conversion of methyl malonyl-CoA to succinyl-CoA during the production of propionate.

It is not known whether vitamin B_{12} supplementation of ruminant diets enhances ruminal production of propionate (Nagaraja et al., 1997), but feeding propionic acid or sodium propionate decreased ruminal production of vitamin B_{12} (Roussev et al., 1975). Moreover, daily production of true vitamin B_{12} only represented 42 percent of the total B_{12} compounds (Bigger et al., 1976). Total activity of vitamin B_{12} in ruminal fluid of sheep decreased from 63 to 35 percent when dietary cobalt was 0.04 to 0.34 ppm (Gawthorne, 1970). Disproportional production of vitamin B_{12} analogs relative to true B_{12} may saturate cellular transport of the active vitamin (Ørskov, 1994) and decrease liver storage of true B_{12} (Walker and Elliot, 1972), which has been suggested to create a vitamin B_{12} deficiency (Ørskov, 1994). Furthermore, increased ruminal production of propionate has been associated with increased proportions of vitamin B_{12} analogs relative to true B_{12} (Ørskov, 1994). Feeding high-concentrate, low-roughage diets decreased ruminal synthesis of true B_{12} and increased synthesis of B_{12} analogs that do not perform the coenzyme function of true B_{12} in mammals (Sutton and Elliot, 1972). Garton et al. (1972) attributed unusually high proportions of odd-numbered and branched-chain fatty acids in adipose tissue from sheep fed diets rich in readily fermentable carbohydrate to an overloading of the vitamin B_{12}-dependent enzyme system methyl malonyl-CoA mutase. Methylmalonate competes with malonic acid in the donation of two-carbon units for fatty acid synthesis leading to increased proportion of odd- and branched-chain fatty acids in subcutaneous fat (Duncan et al., 1974). This condition is exacerbated when vitamin B_{12} deficiency occurs as a result of insufficient consumption of cobalt (Kennedy et al., 1994).

Deficiency of cobalt in ruminants is, in effect, deficiency of vitamin B_{12} with pathological features including neurological and muscular lesions that may be the consequence of hepatic damage (Fell, 1981). Reduced tissue activities of the vitamin B_{12}-dependent enzymes, methyl malonyl-CoA mutase and methionine synthase contribute to the development of fatty degeneration of the liver (Kennedy et al., 1990, 1992, 1994). Tissue activity of methyl malonyl-CoA mutase is limited by vitamin B_{12} functioning as a coenzyme rather than the enzyme per se (Peters and Elliot, 1984). Although it may be impossible to separate the effects of cobalt deficiency-induced vitamin B_{12} deficiency from the effects caused by decreased feed intake (Kennedy et al., 1997), Rice et al. (1989) noted that the defect in methyl malonyl-CoA mutase preceded the onset of loss of production and clinical signs of disease. In addition to inappetance, poor production, and the aforementioned pathological conditions, vitamin B_{12} deficiency may cause ill-thriftiness (Pearson, 1987; Black et al., 1988), serous ocular discharge and photosensitivity (Ulvund and Pestalozzi, 1990), compromised immune function (Vellema et al., 1996), increased susceptibility to certain parasitic infestations (Ferguson et al., 1989; Vellema et al., 1996), and enteric bacterial infections (Al-Zadjali et al., 2004), with anemia occurring rather late in the course of the deficiency (Fell, 1981). Cardiovascular lesions likely result from a lack of transmethylation of homocysteine to methionine in the vitamin B_{12}-deficient sheep (Mohammed and Lamand, 1986).

Vitamin B_{12} deficiency has been characterized as a slow-developing energy deficiency (Underwood, 1977), which results in impaired thyroid function (Mgongo et al., 1981). Perturbations along the hypothalamo-pituitary axis are associated with irregular estrous cycles in vitamin B_{12}-deficient goats (Mgongo et al., 1984). Lower conception rates have been observed in yearling red deer hinds with poor vitamin B_{12} status (Audigé et al., 1999). Vitamin B_{12} deficiency in sheep was not associated with lower conception rate, but rather with lower lamb survival (Fisher and MacPherson, 1991). Pregnant ewes experiencing a vitamin B_{12} deficiency had increased incidence of stillbirths and perinatal mortality of lambs (Duncan et al., 1981; Fisher and MacPherson, 1991).

Production responses to supplemental vitamin B_{12} have been inconsistent. Although measurable physiological differences in propionate metabolism are associated with differences in liver B_{12} status, these are not reflected in feed intake or growth rate (Rickard and Elliot, 1982). Impairment of propionate metabolism, though significant, may not be severe enough to explain suboptimal weight gain (Kennedy et al., 1991). Factors other than vitamin B_{12} status also may influence hepatic propionate uptake and utilization when propionate entry rate is increased within the physiological range (Peters et al., 1983). Peters and Elliot (1983) demonstrated 60 percent greater hepatic conversion of propionate to glucose with vitamin B_{12} enhancement of cobalt-depleted lactating ewes consuming the same amount of feed as cobalt-depleted ewes, but this effect was not sufficient to elicit an increase in milk production. Likewise, there was no advantage to providing supplemental vitamin B_{12} to lambs fed monensin-supplemented, high-concentrate diets containing adequate cobalt (Daugherty et al., 1986). More recent studies conducted with much larger numbers of animals, however, indicated that elevation of serum vitamin B_{12} concentrations and reduction of serum methylmalonic acid was associated with at least a 25 percent improvement in live weight gain (Gruner et al., 2004). Clearly, additional research is needed to elucidate production responses to vitamin B_{12} supplementation under a variety of conditions before recommendations can be firmly established.

Provision of supplemental vitamin B_{12} to the neonatal small ruminant is not necessary if maternal vitamin B_{12} status is adequate. Colostrum is a rich source of vitamin B_{12} (Ramos et al., 1994), and although the vitamin B_{12} concentration of milk declines considerably during the first 2 (Ramos et al., 1994) to 3 (Marca et al., 1996) weeks of lactation, supplementing nursing lambs with vitamin B_{12} did not affect average daily weight gain (Marca et al., 1996; Gruner et al., 2004). It seems possible that the preruminant animal requires less vitamin B_{12} than a fully functional ruminant because it can obtain glucose directly from consumption of milk (Quirk and Norton, 1987).

Folic Acid

Folic acid is a generic term for different forms of this vitamin, which is an essential coenzyme for one-carbon transfer reactions required in numerous metabolic pathways involved in nucleic acid, protein, and amino acid synthesis. Folic acid participates in the synthesis of methionine from homocysteine and carbon donors such as serine or formate. The vitamin exists in nature primarily as reduced one-carbon substituted forms of pteroylpolyglutamates (Bailey, 1988). Folic acid is also an important cofactor in the metabolism of certain ruminal bacteria (Nagaraja et al., 1997), and rumen microbial degradation of dietary and supplementary folic acid can be greater than 97 percent (Zinn et al., 1987).

Due to transformation and synthesis by the rumen microorganisms, an actual dietary requirement of folic acid for small ruminants has not been established. Huber (1988) recommended 3.3 mg of folic acid/100 kg BW should be available for absorption, which was 65 percent less than the requirement suggested by NRC (2001) for dairy cows. Zinn et al. (1987) reported that intestinal supply of folic acid was only about 10 percent of estimated requirements for feedlot calves. Estimates of folic acid requirements for the bovine were based on extrapolation of requirements for swine. Ford et al. (1972) based a "guesstimate" requirement for lactating goats on nutrient allowances for humans. However, extremely large interspecies differences in transport and serum concentrations of folate indicate that the metabolic role of folic acid may not be comparable among sheep and nonruminant animals (Branda, 1981). Based on serum folate concentrations and transport kinetics by erythrocytes published by Branda (1981), requirements of folic acid for adult sheep would be 3–5 percent that of swine and 10–20 percent that of humans. NRC (1989) recommends 3 μg/kg BW for adults. Thus, folic acid requirements of sheep with functional rumens would be expected to range from a low of 0.3 μg/kg BW to a high of 2.5 μg/kg BW. Published values for concentration of folic acid in the blood are similar between adult sheep and goats. Although values for blood folate in other small ruminants are not known, this subcommittee recommends that requirements for folic acid are the same among sheep, goats, cervids, and New World camelids.

A paucity of data is available to assess folic acid status of small ruminants. Folate is both actively and passively transported across the placenta during late gestation, and the vitamin is stored primarily in the liver of the developing fetus (Narkewicz et al., 2002). Folate status of the newborn kid is relatively low (Ford et al., 1972). Content of folic acid is greatest in the colostrum and declines precipitously with the onset of copious milk production (Ford et al., 1972; Girard et al., 1996). Folate balance of the kid may be more precarious than that of lambs because concentration of folic acid in goat's milk is at least five times less than that of ewe's milk. Increased folate binding capacity mediated by milk folate binding protein, however, may assist the neonatal kid build folate reserves for when milk folate intake is very low (Salter and Blakeborough, 1988). Rumen microbial synthesis of folic acid begins with the onset of a functional rumen (Poe et al., 1972). Using the net microbial synthesis of 0.42 mg/kg of total tract digestible organic matter published by Zinn et al. (1987), small ruminants would not be expected to experience a folic acid deficiency if the animals consume enough feed to satisfy their energy requirements. The only reports of folic acid deficiency in small ruminants are with sheep experiencing a vitamin-B_{12} deficiency severe enough to decrease voluntary intake to less than 200 g/d (Smith and Osborne-White, 1973; Gawthorne and Smith, 1974; Smith et al., 1974).

Niacin

Niacin is a generic term for pyridine 3-carboxylic acids and their derivatives that demonstrate activity similar to nicotinamide. Nicotinamide is a constituent of the coenzymes nicotinamide adenine dinucleotide (NAD) and nicotinamide adenine dinucleotide phosphate (NADP). These coenzymes are essential to mitochondrial respiration and the metabolism of carbohydrates, amino acids, and lipids.

Niacin requirements for small ruminants are not known. It has generally been accepted that rumen microbial synthesis of niacin is adequate to meet the requirements of the host animal; however, niacin supply to high-performing ruminants may be suboptimal (Harmeyer and Kollenkirchen, 1989). In a review of three studies conducted with growing lambs, Brent and Bartley (1984) noted that supplemental niacin at 100 ppm or 500 ppm improved overall performance. Supplemental niacin has also been advocated as a prophylactic agent for the prevention of ketosis (Herdt and Emery, 1992). The anti-ketogenic effects of niacin have been attributed to the vitamin's antilipolytic action (Herdt and Emery, 1992) and hyperglycemic action associated with decreased glucose utilization and insulin resistance (Thornton and Schultz, 1980).

Some of the benefits provided by supplemental niacin may be a combination of ruminal and systemic effects. Improvements in animal performance resulting from supplemental niacin may be related to effects occurring in the rumen (Brent and Bartley, 1984). Ruminal responses to supplemental niacin, however, have been equivocal. Many researchers (Schussler et al., 1978; Bartley et al., 1979; Riddell et al., 1980, 1981; Shields et al., 1983) have reported an increase in microbial protein synthesis, whereas others (Schaetzel and Johnson, 1981; Abdouli and Schaefer, 1986a,b) reported that supplemental niacin did not increase production of microbial protein. There appears to be an optimum ruminal niacin concentration below which synthesis will occur and above which there is no net synthesis (Byers, 1981). The optimal ruminal concentration theory is highly probable because only a few ruminal bacterial species are known to require niacin or niacinamide (Abdouli and Schaefer, 1985). Additionally, ruminal fluid niacin concentrations are normally much higher than the concentrations required for maximum growth rates of niacin-requiring species (Abdouli and Schaefer, 1986b). Increased blood glucose sometimes noted in ruminants fed supplemental niacin (Herdt and Emery, 1992) may be related to an increase in ruminal molar proportion of propionate in response to niacin supplementation (Riddell et al., 1980; Flachowsky et al., 1988). However, the effect of niacin supplementation on ruminal propionate is inconsistent (Nagaraja et al., 1997). Inconsistent responses in growth performance (Flachowsky et al., 1988) and lactation performance (NRC, 2001) to supplemental niacin are not surprising considering the vast inconsistencies in ruminal responses to supplemental niacin. Increasing daily duodenal flow of niacin had no influence on nicotinamide concentration of whole blood in sheep (Kollenkirchen et al., 1992). Collectively, available data do not support the routine use of supplemental niacin in diets of small ruminants.

Pantothenic Acid

Pantothenic acid is a constituent of the cofactors coenzyme A and acyl carrier protein and is therefore essential for metabolism of carbohydrates, lipids, and to some extent amino acids. The vitamin also participates in the synthesis of heme, cholesterol, and acetylcholine. Evidence that pantothenic acid synthesis occurs in the rumen of sheep was provided initially by McElroy and Goss (1939). Rumen microbial synthesis of pantothenic acid in bovine appears to be 20 to 30 times more than dietary amounts (NRC, 2001). Sheep fed an artificial diet devoid of pantothenic acid for 3 weeks had 29 mg of pantothenic acid entering the duodenum (Finlayson and Seeley, 1983). The amount of pantothenic acid entering the duodenum was the same as the amount provided by the diet to over four times greater than dietary supply in sheep fed typical diets (Finlayson and Seeley, 1983). Pantothenic acid requirements of small ruminants have not been established, but extrapolating requirements of growing pigs (NRC, 1998) to the growing lamb would indicate that a 45 to 50 kg lamb requires 14.84 mg of pantothenic acid daily. Calculation of intestinal disappearance from data of Finlayson and Seeley (1983) indicated that only three of nine diets would satisfy theoretical requirements of a 45 to 50 kg lamb. Such data are not available for other small ruminant animals or for small ruminants in various stages of production. However, the potential for growing lambs to experience a pantothenic acid deficiency corroborates the observations made by the subcommittee working on requirements for dairy cattle (NRC, 2001). NRC (2001) adopted net microbial synthesis of 2.2 mg of pantothenic acid/kg of total tract digestible organic matter estimated by Zinn et al. (1987). Clearly, additional research is necessary to assess pantothenic acid status of small ruminants.

Pyridoxine (Vitamin B_6)

Vitamin B_6 is a generic term for 2-methylpyridine derivatives that have the biological activity of pyridoxine. The predominant dietary form of this vitamin is pyridoxine, which is converted to its active forms pyridoxal and pyridoxamine by microbial cells and animal tissue. Phosphorylation of the pyridoxal and pyridoxamine confers biological activity by producing the coenzymes pyridoxal phosphate and pyridoxalamine phosphate. Pyridoxal phosphate is of particular importance as it is involved in most reactions of amino acid metabolism, has roles in the biosynthesis of porphyrins and in the catabolism of glycogen, and may be involved in lipid metabolism (NRC, 1987). Like the other B vitamins, it has generally been thought that synthesis of vitamin B_6 by ruminal microorganisms was sufficient to satisfy the ruminant animal's requirement and dietary additions of vitamin B_6 were not necessary. Consequently, requirements of vitamin B_6 have not been established.

Addition of vitamin B_6 to the diet of ruminants has often been deemed unnecessary despite evidence demonstrating that vitamin B_6 effectively stimulated cellulose digestion by washed suspensions of mixed rumen bacteria (MacLeod and Murray, 1956). Many cellulolytic bacteria require pyridoxine (Wolin et al., 1997). Therefore, improved cellulose digestion is likely attributed to enhanced growth of the pyridoxine-requiring microorganisms. In vitro studies conducted with microbial isolates collected from the rumen of goats also demonstrated that vitamin B_6 additions enhanced production of lysine by mixed rumen protozoa, mixed rumen bacteria, as well as their mixture (El-Waziry and Onodera, 1997). In addition to lysine being one of the most limiting amino acids for milk production (NRC, 2001), lysine supply may be a major limitation to wool, and perhaps mohair, growth (Reis and Sahlu, 1994). Pyridoxine along with folic acid is also needed for wool growth (Reis, 1989). Pyridoxal kinase activity was greater in goat mammary tissue than in the liver (Coburn et al., 1992a), suggesting that requirements for vitamin B_6 may increase during lactation. Based on apparent similarities in pyridoxal metabolism between lactating goats and pigs (Coburn et al., 1992b), vitamin B_6 requirements for small ruminants are expected to be similar to those of swine. Vitamin B_6 requirements of growing pigs weighing 50 to 80 kg average 0.10 mg/$BW^{0.75}$, which is comparable to the requirements for lactating pigs (NRC, 1998). Based on net microbial synthesis of 5.6 mg of vitamin B_6/kg of total tract digestible organic matter (Zinn et al., 1987), a 70 kg small ruminant consuming 1 kg of digestible organic matter would receive nearly twice its theoretical requirement of vitamin B_6. Requirements of vitamin

B_6 for small ruminants are typically expected to be satisfied, but the potential to improve lysine supply to the small ruminant through the provision of supplemental vitamin B_6 deserves investigation.

Riboflavin (Vitamin B_2)

Riboflavin functions as a component of the coenzymes flavin mononucleotide and flavin adenine dinucleotide, which are involved in the intermediary transfer of electrons in metabolic oxidation-reduction reactions. Degradation of dietary riboflavin by rumen microorganisms (Owen and West, 1970; West and Owen, 1973) has complicated the ability to establish a dietary requirement of this vitamin for small ruminants. Requirements of the functional ruminant are expected to be satisfied as ruminal synthesis was nearly 1.5 times greater than intake regardless of diet type (Miller et al., 1986). Moreover, lactating goats fed a riboflavin-deficient diet excreted similar amounts of riboflavin in their urine and milk and maintained similar levels of milk production as goats supplemented with riboflavin (Crossland et al., 1958). Requirements of the neonatal small ruminants are also expected to be satisfied through normal consumption of colostrum and milk, but milk replacers must be fortified with riboflavin (Luecke et al., 1950).

Thiamin (Vitamin B_1)

Thiamin is a component of coenzymes that assist in the transfer of an activated aldehyde unit in several energy metabolism pathways. The vitamin also has a role, although not well defined, in nerve and brain function (Combs, 1992). Due to net microbial synthesis, a dietary requirement for thiamin has not been established for healthy animals with a functional rumen. Average daily flow of thiamin to the duodenum of sheep was 10 to 22 times the quantity of ingested thiamin, and thiamin disappearance from the small intestines was approximately equal to thiamin net synthesis in the reticulorumen (Breves et al., 1980). Average dry matter consumption by sheep in the study of Breves et al. (1980) was comparable to that required by small ruminants weighing 10 kg. Growing pigs of this size require 0.50 mg of thiamin daily (NRC, 1998). Average daily intestinal disappearance of thiamin reported by Breves et al. (1980) was 2.05 mg. Thus, sheep are typically expected to meet their requirements for thiamin through net microbial synthesis in the rumen. Thiamin balance studies conducted with other small ruminants are either meager or lacking, but disorders associated with thiamin deficiency commonly observed in sheep (Pierson and Jensen, 1975) have been reported also in goats (Smith, 1979; Thomas et al., 1987), deer (Edwin and Jackman, 1982), and New World camelids (Pugh, 1993; Beck et al., 1996).

Much interest in thiamin for ruminants has involved polioencephalomalacia. Polioencephalomalacia, also known as cerebrocortical necrosis, is a common nervous system disorder in which animals show clinical signs of dullness, blindness, muscle tremors, nystagmus, opisthotonus, head pressing, recumbency, and death. There is a large body of literature regarding the relationship between altered thiamin metabolism and polioencephalomalacia (Gould, 1998). Deficiencies of thiamin have been found when thiaminases associated with either feeds or produced from altered ruminal fermentation destroy thiamin or produce a thiamin analog that interferes with thiamin-requiring metabolic reactions (Brent and Bartley, 1984). Induction of ruminal acidosis seems to predispose animals to spontaneous outbreaks of polioencephalomalacia (Vestweber et al., 1974). The sudden drop in ruminal pH associated with acidosis had no deleterious effects on microbial production of thiamin (Alves de Oliveira et al., 1996), but this condition appears to allow for proliferation of thiaminase-producing bacteria in the animals inflicted with the disease (Morgan and Lawson, 1974; Boyd and Walton, 1977; Thomas et al., 1987). Other conditions that have linked thiamin deficiency to polioencephalomalacia include pre-embarkation feedlot preparation during transport across seas (Thomas et al., 1990), feeding corn silage (Candau and Massengo, 1982), grazing a fresh pasture produced in very wet conditions after heavy rain (Ben Said et al., 1986), the administration of the anthelmintics levamisole hydrochloride and thiabendazole (Linklater et al., 1977), and the administration of the coccidiostat amprolium (Thornber et al., 1981; Brent and Bartley, 1984; Lonkar and Prasad, 1993, 1994). Consumption of feedstuffs with naturally occurring thiaminase factors will also predispose small ruminants to polioencephalomalacia. Bracken fern (Evans, 1975), Italian ryegrass (*Lolium multiflorum*), and fresh fescue (*Festuca arundinacea*) contain various levels of thiaminase (Ramos et al., 2003). Polioencephalomalacia may also be induced in ruminants consuming excess dietary sulfur. Although excessive ruminal sulfide production is the primary cause of polioencephalomalacia in ruminants consuming high amounts of sulfur (Gould, 1998), supplementation with thiamin at 243 mg/kg of diet prevented development of clinical signs of the disease but did not prevent development of microscopic brain lesions (Olkowski et al., 1992). Oral supplementation with 1 g of thiamin may be sufficient to repress subclinical thiamin deficiency (Thomas, 1986) whereas parenterally administered thiamin restores tissue thiamin levels (Spicer and Horton, 1981) and is an effective treatment of thiamin deficiency (Ken Scarrat, 1981). Thiamin up to 1,000 times the requirement is presumed to be safe (NRC, 1987).

Vitamin C (Ascorbic Acid)

There is little definitive information concerning vitamin C requirements of small ruminants. It has generally been accepted that adult ruminants do not require dietary supplementation because they possess the enzymatic capacity to synthesize sufficient ascorbic acid to satisfy normal vitamin

C requirements. It seems possible that, like the bovine (Cummins and Brunner, 1991), nursing small ruminants do not synthesize endogenous vitamin C until approximately 3 weeks of age. Ascorbate levels in milk are expected to be adequate for nursing small ruminants consuming normal consumption amounts of milk (Richetti, 1987). Heightened exposure to environmental stress (Hidiroglou et al., 1977; Bouda et al., 1980; Cummins and Brunner, 1991) and diseases (Jagos et al., 1977; Hemingway, 1991) are expected to increase requirements for vitamin C. Oral administration of ascorbic acid increased blood plasma concentrations in 1- and 2-week-old lambs (Kolb et al., 1993), but rumen-protected forms of vitamin C must be fed to functional ruminants to exert the same effect (Hidiroglou et al., 1997). Injectable forms of ascorbic acid may also be used to increase blood levels of vitamin C, with the intramuscular route being more effective than the intravenous route (Black and Hidiroglou, 1996). Available literature is not adequate to determine therapeutic or desirable levels of ascorbic acid in the plasma of small ruminants.

REFERENCES

Abdouli, H., and D. M. Schaefer. 1985. Niacin saturation constants for *Lactobacillus plantarum* and *Treponema bryantii*. J. Dairy Sci. 68: 2372–2376.

Abdouli, H., and D. M. Schaefer. 1986a. Impact of niacin and length of incubation on protein synthesis, soluble to total protein ratio and fermentative activity of ruminal microorganisms. J. Anim. Sci. 62:244–253.

Abdouli, H., and D. M. Schaefer. 1986b. Effects of two dietary niacin concentrations on ruminal fluid free niacin concentration, and of supplemental niacin and source of inoculum on in vitro microbial growth, fermentative activity and nicotinamide adenine dinucleotide pool size. J. Anim. Sci. 62:254–262.

Abdulkareem, T. A., A. H. Al-Haboby, S. M. AL-Mjamei, and A. A. Hobi. 2005. Sperm abnormalities associated with vitamin A deficiency in rams. Small Ruminant Res. 57:67–71

Abel, H. J., I. Immig, C. Da Costa Gomez, and W. Steinberg. 2001. Effect of increasing dietary concentrate levels on microbial biotin metabolism in the artificial rumen simulation system (RUSITEC). Arch. Anim. Nutr. 55:371–376.

Agrawala, I. P., C. F. Huffman, R. W. Luecke, and C. W. Duncan. 1953. A quantitative study of rumen synthesis in the bovine and natural and purified diets. III. Riboflavin, pantothenic acid and niacin. J. Nutr. 49:631–638.

Alderson, N. E., G. E. Mitchell, Jr., C. O. Little, R. E. Warner, and R. E. Tucker. 1971. Preintestinal disappearance of vitamin E in ruminants. J. Nutr. 101:655–660.

Alstad, A. D., H. H. Casper, and L. J. Johnson. 1985. Vitamin K treatment of sweet clover poisoning in calves. J. Am. Vet. Med. Assoc. 187: 729–731.

Alves de Oliveira, L., C. Jean-Blain, A. Durix, S. Komisarczuk-Bony, and C. Durier. 1996. Use of a semi-continuous culture system (RUSITEC) to study the effect of pH on microbial metabolism of thiamin (Vitamin B_1). Arch. Anim. Nutr. 49:193–202.

Al-Zadjali, A., E. H. Johnson, and A. Srikandakumar. 2004. Serum vitamin B_{12} levels in Omani goats. Trop. Anim. Health Prod. 36:473–482.

Andrews, E. D., and I. J. Cunningham. 1945. The vitamin D requirement of sheep. NZ J. Sci. Technol. 27:223.

Anonymous. 1987. Nomenclature policy: Generic descriptors and trivial names for vitamins and related compounds. J. Nutr. 117:7–14.

ARC (Agricultural Research Council). 1980. The Nutrient Requirements of Ruminant Livestock. Slough, UK: Commonwealth Agricultural Bureaux.

Astrup, H. N., S. C. Mills, L. J. Cook, and T. W. Scott. 1974. Stability of α-tocopherol in rumen liquor of sheep. Acta. Vet. Scand. 15:451–453.

Audigé, L., P. Wilson, and R. S. Morris. 1999. Reproductive performance of farmed red deer (*Cervus elaphus*) in New Zealand IV. Biological markers as risk factors for yearling and adult hind conception. Anim. Reprod. Sci. 55:239–254.

Badwey, J. A., and M. L. Karnovsky. 1980. Active oxygen species and the functions of phagocytic leukocytes. Annu. Rev. Biochem. 49:695–726.

Bailey, L. B. 1988. Factors affecting folate bioavailability. Food Technol. 10:206–213.

Baldwin, R. L., and M. J. Allison. 1983. Rumen metabolism. J. Anim. Sci. 57:461–477.

Banskalieva, V., R. Puchala, A. L. Goetsch, J. Luo, and T. Sahlu. 2005. Effects of ruminally protected betaine and choline on net flux of nutrients across the portal-drained viscera and liver of meat goat wethers consuming diets differing in protein concentration. Small Ruminant Res. 57:193–202.

Bartley, E. E., E. L. Herod, R. N. Bechtle, D. A. Sapienza, and B. E. Brent. 1979. Effect of monensin or lasalocid with and without niacin or amicloral on rumen fermentation and feed efficiency. J. Anim. Sci. 49: 1066–1075.

Beck, C., A. J. Dart, M. B. Collins, D. R. Hodgson, and J. Parbery. 1996. Polioencephalomalacia in two alpacas. Aust. Vet. J. 74:350–352.

Ben Said, M. S., M. Zrelli, and J. Tournut. 1986. La nécrose du cortex cerebral: Une enzootic dans un troupeau d'ovino en Tunsie. Rev. Méd. Vét. 137:573–576.

Bender, D. A. 1992. Ascorbic acid (vitamin C). Pp. 360–393 in Nutritional Biochemistry of the Vitamin, D. A. Bender, ed. New York: Cambridge University Press.

Bieri, J. G., and M. C. McKenna. 1981. Expressing dietary values for fat-soluble vitamins: Changes in concepts and terminology. Am. J. Clin. Nutr. 34:289–295.

Bigger, G. W., J. M. Elliot, and T. R. Rickard. 1976. Estimated ruminal production of pseudovitamin B_{12}, factor A and factor B in sheep. J. Anim. Sci. 43:1077–1081.

Black, H., J. B. Hutton, R. J. Sutherland, and M. P. James. 1988. Failure to obtain a weight gain response to vitamin B12 treatment in young goats grazing pasture that was cobalt deficient for sheep. New Zealand Vet. J. 35:38–39.

Black, W. D., and M. Hidiroglou. 1996. Pharmacokinetic study of ascorbic acid in sheep. Can. J. Vet. Res. 60:216–221.

Bonhomme, A., M. Durand, C. Quintana, and S. Halpern. 1982. Influence du cobalt et de la vitamine B_{12} sur la croissance et la survie des ciliés du rumen *in vitro*, en function de la population bactérienne. Reprod. Nutr. Dev. 22:107–122.

Bouda, J., P. Jagos, R. Dvorak, and J. Ondrova. 1980. Vitamin E and C in the blood plasma of cows and their calves fed from buckets. Acta. Vet. Brno. 49:53–58.

Boyd, J. W., and J. R. Walton. 1977. Cerebrocortical necrosis in ruminants: An attempt to identify the source of thiaminase in affected animals. J. Comp. Pathol. 87:581–589.

Brady, P. S., L. J. Brady, P. A. Whetter, D. E. Ullrey, and L. D. Fay. 1978. The effect of dietary selenium and vitamin E on biochemical parameters and survival of young among white-tailed deer (*Odocoileus virginianus*). J. Nutr. 108:1439–1448.

Branda, R. F. 1981. Transport of 5-methyltetrahydrofolic acid in erythrocytes from various mammalian species. J. Nutr. 111:618–623.

Brent, B. E., and E. E. Bartley. 1984. Thiamin and niacin in the rumen. J. Anim. Sci. 59:813–822.

Breves G, H. Hoeller, J. Harmeyer, and H. Martens. 1980. Thiamin balance in the gastrointestinal tract of sheep. J. Anim. Sci. 51:1177–1181.

Brown, F. 1953. The tocopherol content of farm feeding-stuffs. J. Sci. Food Agric. 4:161–165.

Bryant, T. C., J. D. Rivera, M. L. Galyean, G. C. Duff, D. M. Hallford, and T. H. Montgomery. 1999. Effects of dietary level ruminally protected choline on performance and carcass characteristics of finishing beef steers and on growth and serum metabolites in lambs. J. Anim. Sci. 77:2893–2903.

Burton, G. W., and K. U. Ingold. 1989. Vitamin E as an in vitro and in vivo antioxidant. Ann. N. Y. Acad. Sci. 570:7–22.

Byers, F. M. 1981. Another look at niacin. Anim. Nutr. Health 36:36–42.

Candau, M., and J. Massengo. 1982. Evidence of a thiamine deficiency in sheep fed maize silage. Ann. Rech. Vét. 13:329–340.

Charmley, E., N. Hidiroglou, L. Ochoa, L. R. McDowell, and M. Hidiroglou. 1992. Plasma and hepatic α-tocopherol in cattle following oral or intramuscular supplementation. J. Dairy Sci. 75:804–810.

Chikunya, S., G. Demirel, M. Enser, J. D. Wood, R. G. Wilkinson, and L. A. Sinclair. 2004. Biohydrogenation of dietary *n*-3 PUFA and stability of ingested vitamin E in the rumen, and their effects on microbial activity in sheep. Br. J. Nutr. 91:539–550.

Chilliard, Y., and A. Ferlay. 2004. Dietary lipids and forages interactions on cows and goat milk fatty acid composition and sensory properties. Reprod. Nutr. Dev. 44:467–492.

Clark, R. G., J. Burbage, P. M. Marshall, T. Valler, and D. Wallace. 1986a. Absence of a vitamin B_{12} weight gain response in two trials with growing red deer (*Cervus elaphus*). New Zealand Vet. J. 34:199–200.

Clark, R. G., L. Mantelman, and G. A. Verkerk. 1986b. Failure to obtain a weight gain response to vitamin B_{12} treatment in young goats grazing pasture that was cobalt deficient for sheep. New Zealand Vet. J. 35:38–39.

Coburn, S. P., J. D. Mahuren, M. S. Kennedy, W. E. Schaltenbrand, and D. W. Townsend. 1992a. Metabolism of [^{14}C]- and [^{32}P]pyridoxal 5'-phosphate and [^{3}H]pyridoxal administered intravenously to pigs and goats. J. Nutr. 122:393–401.

Coburn, S. P., J. D. Mahuren, T. A. Pauly, K. L. Ericson, and D. W. Townsend. 1992b. Alkaline phosphatase activity and pyridoxal phosphate concentrations in the milk of various species. J. Nutr. 122: 2348–2353.

Colitti, M., G. Stradaioli, and B. Stefanon. 2000. Effect of α-tocopherol deprivation on the involution of mammary gland in sheep. J. Dairy Sci. 83:345–350.

Collins, E. D., and A. W. Norman. 1991. Vitamin D. Pp. 59–99 in Handbook of Vitamins, 2nd ed., revised and expanded, L. J. Machlin, ed. New York: Marcel Dekker.

Combs, Jr., G. F. 1992. The Vitamins: Fundamental Aspects in Nutrition and Health. Washington, DC: Academic Press.

Crossland, A., E. C. Owen, and R. Proudfoot. 1958. Riboflavin metabolism of cows and goats and rate of biosynthesis of riboflavin by the lactating goat. Br. J. Nutr. 12:312–329.

Crowley, J. P. 1961. Rickets in November-born lambs. Vet. Rec. 73: 295–297.

Cummins, K. A., and C. J. Brunner. 1991. Effect of calf housing on plasma ascorbate and endocrine and immune function. J. Dairy Sci. 74: 1582–1588.

Daniels, J. T., P. G. Hatfield, D. E. Burgess, R. W. Kott, and J. G. P. Bowman. 2000. Evaluation of ewe and lamb immune response when ewes were supplemented with vitamin E. J. Anim. Sci. 78:2731–2736.

Daugherty, M. S., M. L. Gaylean, D. M. Hallford, and J. H. Hageman. 1986. Vitamin B_{12} and monensin effects on performance, liver and serum vitamin B_{12} concentrations and activity of propionate metabolizing hepatic enzymes in feedlot lambs. J. Anim. Sci. 62:452–463.

David, G. P., and A. J. Winterbottom. 1996. Flying scapula in a red deer (*Cervus elaphus*). Vet. Rec. 139:20.

Dawson, R. M. C., D. W. Grime, and D. B. Lindsay. 1981. On the insensitivity of sheep to the almost complete microbial destruction of dietary choline before alimentary-tract absorption. Biochem. J. 196:499–504.

DeLuca, H. F. 1984. The metabolism, physiology and function of vitamin D. Pp.1–68 in Vitamin D: Basic and Clinical Aspects, R. Kumar, ed. Boston, MA: Martinus Nijhoff Publishing.

Demirel, G., A. M. Wachira, L. A. Sinclair, R. G. Wilkinson, J. D. Wood, and M. Enser. 2004. Effects of dietary *n*-3 polyunsaturated fatty acids, breed and dietary vitamin E on the fatty acids of lamb muscle, liver, and adipose tissue. Br. J. Nutr. 91:551–565.

DeRitter, E. 1976. Stability characteristics of vitamins in processed foods. Food Technol. 30:48–54.

Dicks, M. W. 1965. Vitamin E content of foods and feeds for human and animal consumption. Agric. Exp. Stat. Bull. 435, Univ. Wyoming, Laramie.

Dierenfeld, E. S. 1994. Vitamin E in exotics: Effects, evaluation and ecology. J. Nutr. 124:2579S–2581S.

Donoghue, S., D. S. Kronfeld, and C. F. Ramberg Jr. 1979. Plasma retinol transport and clearance in hypervitaminosis Am. J. Dairy Sci. 62:326–332.

Donoghue, S., W. Donawick, and D. S. Kronfeld. 1983a. Transfer of vitamin A from intestine to plasma in lambs fed low and high intakes of vitamin Am. J. Nutr. 113:2197–2204.

Donoghue, S., D. S. Kronfeld, and D. Sklan. 1983b. Retinol homeostasis in lambs given low and high intakes of vitamin A. Br. J. Nutr. 50:235–248.

Duncan, W. R. H., E. R. Ørskov, C. Fraser, and G. A. Garton. 1974. Effect of processing of dietary barley and of supplementary cobalt and cyanocobalamine on the fatty acid composition of lamb triglyceride with special reference to branched chain fatty acids. Br. J. Nutr. 32:71–75.

Duncan, W. R. H., E. Rona Morrison, and G. A. Garton. 1981. Effects of cobalt deficiency in pregnant and post-parturient ewes and their lambs. Br. J. Nutr. 46:337–344.

Eaton, H. D. 1969. Chronic bovine hypo- and hypervitaminosis A and cerebrospinal fluid pressure. Am. J. Clin. Nutr. 22:1070–1080.

Edwin E. E., and R. Jackman. 1982. Ruminant thiamine requirement in perspective. Vet. Res. Commun. 5:237–250.

Elliot, J. M., R. N. B. Kay, and E. D. Goodall. 1971. Production and absorption of vitamin B_{12} in the sheep – A preliminary study. Life Sci. 10:647–647.

El-Waziry, A. M., and R. Onodera. 1997. Effects of salinomycin and vitamin B_6 on the in vitro synthesis of lysine from the stereoisomers of 2,6-diaminopimelic acid by mixed rumen protozoa, bacteria, and their mixture. J. Gen. Appl. Microbiol. 43:109–114.

Emmanuel, B., and J. J. Kennelly. 1984. Kinetics of methionine and choline and their incorporation into plasma lipids and milk components in lactating goats. J. Dairy Sci. 67:1912–1919.

Erdman, R. A., and B. K. Sharma. 1991. Effect of dietary rumen-protected choline in lactating dairy cows. J. Dairy Sci. 74:1641–1647.

Evans, W. C. 1975. Thiaminases and their effects on animals. Vitam. Horm. 33:467–504.

Ewan, R. C., C. A. Baumann, and A. L. Pope. 1968. Effects of selenium and vitamin E on nutritional muscular dystrophy in lambs. J. Anim. Sci. 27:751–756.

FAO/WHO (Food and Agriculture Organization/World Health Organization). 1988. Requirements of vitamin A, iron, folate and vitamin B12. Report of a joint Food and Agriculture Organization/World Health Organization expert committee. FAO Food and Nutr. Series, Report No. 23.

Farid, M. F. A., and Y. S. Ghanem. 1982. Vitamin A deficiency and supplementation in desert sheep. II. Wool characteristics. World Rev. Anim. Prod. XVII:75–77.

Faruque, O., and D. M. Walker. 1970. The relative biological potencies of retinyl palmitate and β-carotene for the milk-fed lamb. Br. J. Nutr. 24: 23–28.

Fedele, V., R. Rubino, S. Claps, P. Manzi, S. Marconi, and L. Pizzoferrato. 2004. Seasonal variation in retinol concentration of goat milk associated with grazing compared to indoor feeding. S. Afr. J. Anim. Sci. 34(Suppl. 1):148–150.

Fell, B. F. 1981. Pathological consequences of copper deficiency and cobalt deficiency. Philosoph. Trans. Royal Soc. London. Series B, Biol. Sci. 294:153–168.

Ferguson, E. G. W., G. B. B. Mitchell, and A. MacPherson. 1989. Cobalt deficiency and *Ostertagi circumcincta* infection in lambs. Vet. Rec. 124:20.

Fernández, C., L. Gallego, and C. J. Lopez-Bote. 1998. Effect of betaine on fat content in growing lambs. Anim. Feed Sci. Technol. 73:329–338.

Fernández, C., J. R. Díaz, C. Garcés, X. Rubert-Aleman, J. J. Pascual, and R. Muelas. 2000. Influence of betaine added to the diet on milk composition in Murciana-Granadina lactating goats. Proc. 7th Inter. Conf. Goats. Tours, France, May 15–21.

Fernández, C., J. Fontecha, M. A. Latorre, C. Garcés, M. Soler, and J. M. de la Fuente. 2004. Influence of betaine on goat milk production and composition. S. Afr. J. Anim. Sci. 34(Suppl. 1):165–168.

Fernández, D., P. Sánchez-Seiquer, A. Sánchez, A. Contreras, and J. M. de la Fuente. 2004. Influence of betaine on milk yield and composition in primiparous lactating dairy goats. Small Ruminant Res. 52:37–43.

Fernández-Figares, I., D. Wray-Cahen, N. C. Steele, R. G. Campbell, D. D. Hall, E. Virtanen, and T. J. Caperna. 2002. Effect of dietary betaine on nutrient utilization and partitioning in the young growing feed-restricted pig. J. Anim. Sci. 80:421–428.

Finlayson, H. J., and R. C. Seeley. 1983. The synthesis and absorption of pantothenic acid in the gastrointestinal tract of the adult sheep. J. Sci. Food Agric. 34:427–432.

Fisher, G. E. J., and A. McPherson. 1991. Effect of cobalt deficiency in the pregnant ewe on reproductive performance and lamb viability. Res. Vet. Sci. 50:319–327.

Flachowsky, G., M. Matthey, and W. I. Ochrimenko. 1988. Influence of dietary niacin on volatile fatty acids in rumen liquid of sheep and rumen dry matter degradability of untreated and ammonia-treated wheat straw. Arch. Anim. Nutr. Berlin 38:99–108.

Ford, J. E., G. S. Knaggs, D. N. Salter, and K. J. Scott. 1972. Folate nutrition in the kid. Br. J. Nutr. 27:571–583.

Franklin, M. C., G. L. McClymont, P. K. Briggs, and B. L. Cambell. 1955. Maintenance rations for Merino sheep. II. The performance of weaners fed daily and weekly on rations of wheat and wheaten chaff at maintenance levels and the effect thereon of vitamin A supplements. Aust. J. Agric. Res. 6:324–342.

Frier, H. I., E. J. Gorgacz, R. C. Hall, A. M. Gallina, J. E. Roussen, H. D. Eaton, and S. W. Nielsen. 1974. Formation and absorption of cerebrospinal fluid in adult goats with hypo- and hypervitaminosis A. Am. J. Vet. Res. 35:45–55.

Frigg, M., D. Hartmann, and O. C. Straub. 1993. Biotin kinetics in serum of cattle after intravenous and oral dosing. Int. J. Vitam. Nutr. Res. 63:36–40.

Fry, J. M., G. M. Smith, M. C. McGrath, E. J. Speijers, and J. G. Allen. 1993. Plasma and tissue concentrations of α-tocopherol during vitamin E depletion in sheep. Br. J. Nutr. 69:225–232.

Garton, G. A., F. D. DeB. Hovell, and W. R. H. Duncan. 1972. Influence of dietary volatile fatty acids on the fatty-acid composition of lamb triglycerides, with special reference to the effect of propionate on the presence of branched-chain components. Br. J. Nutr. 28:409–416.

Gawthorne, J. M. 1970. The effect of cobalt intake on the cobamide and cobinamide composition of the rumen contents and blood plasma of sheep. Aust. J. Exp. Biol. Med. Sci. 48:285–292.

Gawthorne, J. M., and R. M. Smith. 1974. Folic acid metabolism in vitamin B_{12}-deficient sheep. Effects of injected methionine on methotrexate transport and the activity of enzymes associated with folate metabolism in liver. Biochem. J. 142:119–126.

Gentry, P. C., T. T. Ross, B. C. Oetting, and K. D. Birch. 1992. Effects of supplemental d-α-tocopherol on preweaning lamb performance, serum and colostrums tocopherol levels and immunoglobulin G titers. Sheep Res. J. 8:95–100.

Ghanem, Y. S., and M. F. A. Farid. 1982. Vitamin A deficiency and supplementation in desert sheep. I. Deficiency symptoms, plasma concentrations and body growth. World Rev. Anim. Prod. XVII:69–74.

Girard, C. L. 2000. A new look at the requirements of high-producing dairy cows for B-complex vitamins. In Recent Advances in Animal Nutrition, P. C. Garnsworthy and J. Wiseman, eds. Nottingham, UK: Nottingham University Press.

Girard, C. L., F. Castonguay, M. H. Fahmy, and J. J. Matte. 1996. Serum and milk folates during the first two gestations and lactations in Romanov, Finnsheep, and Suffolk ewes. J. Anim. Sci. 74:1711–1715.

Gould, D. H. 1998. Polioencephalomalacia. J. Anim. Sci. 76:309–314.

Green, L. E., K. Hovers, N. P. French, S. Jore, S. Taylor, and K. L. Morgan. 1995. Subcapsular liver rupture in young lambs associated with vitamin E deficiency. Vet. Record 136:197–198.

Gruner, T. M., J. R. Sedcole, J. M. Furlong, and A. R. Sykes. 2004. A critical evaluation of serum methylmalonic acid and vitamin B_{12} for the assessment of cobalt deficiency of growing lambs in New Zealand. New Zealand Vet. J. 52:137–144.

Harmeyer, J., and U. Kollenkirchen. 1989. Thiamin and niacin in ruminant nutrition. Nutr. Res. Rev. 2:201–225.

Hastings, B. E., and S. C. Gascoyne. 1992. Trace mineral levels in the guanaco (*Lama guanicoe*). Vet. Record 131:14–15.

Hatfield, P. G., J. T. Daniels, R. W. Kott, D. E. Burgess, and T. J. Evans. 2000. Role of supplemental vitamin E in lamb survival and production: A review. Proc. Am. Soc. Anim. Sci., 1999. Available at http://www.asas.org/symposia/proceedings/E24. Accessed December 16, 2002.

Hedrich, M. F., J. M. Elliot, and J. E. Lowe. 1973. Response in vitamin B_{12} production and absorption to increasing cobalt intake in the sheep. J. Nutr. 103:1646–1651.

Hemingway, D. C. 1991. Vitamin C in the prevention of neonatal calf diarrhea. Can. Vet. J. 32:184.

Hemingway, R. G. 2003. The influences of dietary intakes and supplementation with selenium and vitamin E on reproduction diseases and reproductive efficiency in cattle and sheep. Vet. Res. Commun. 27:159–174.

Herdt, T. H., and R. S. Emery. 1992. Therapy of disease of ruminant intermediary metabolism. Vet. Clinics N. Am. Food Anim. Pract. 8:91–107.

Hidiroglou, M. 1987. Kinetics of intravenously administered 25-hydroxyvitamin D_3 in sheep and the effects of exposure to ultraviolet irradiation. J. Anim. Sci. 65:808–814.

Hidiroglou, M., and E. Charmley. 1990. Response of plasma and tissue D-α-tocopherol in sheep to graded dietary levels of dl-α-tocopheryl acetate. Res. Vet. Sci. 49:122–124.

Hidiroglou, M., and E. Charmley. 1991. Comparative studies on bioavailability and tissue uptake of two intraruminally or intraperitoneally administered esters of α-tocopherol in sheep. Am. J. Vet. Res. 52:640–642.

Hidiroglou, M., and K. Karpinski. 1988. Pharmacokinetic disposition in sheep of various vitamin E preparations given orally or intravenously. Br. J. Nutr. 59:509–518.

Hidiroglou, M., and K. Karpinski. 1989. Providing vitamin D to confined sheep by oral supplementation vs ultraviolet irradiation. J. Anim. Sci. 67:794–802.

Hidiroglou, M., and K. Karpinski. 1991. Disposition kinetics and dosage regimen of vitamin E administered intramuscularly to sheep. Br. J. Nutr. 65:465–473.

Hidiroglou, M., and J. E. Knipfel. 1984. Plasma and milk concentrations of vitamin D_3 and 25-hydroxyvitamin D_3 following intravenous injection of vitamin D_3 or 25-hydroxy vitamin D_3. Can. J. Comp. Med. 48: 78–80.

Hidiroglou, M., and K. Singh. 1991. Plasma a-tocopherol profiles in sheep after oral administration of *dl*-α-tocopheryl acetate and *d*-α-tocopheryl succinate. J. Dairy Sci. 74:2718–2723.

Hidiroglou, M., and C. J. Williams. 1981. Transfer of tritium-labeled vitamin D_3 and 25 hydroxyvitamin D_3 in ovine placenta. Am. J. Vet. Res. 42:140–141.

Hidiroglou, M., and C. J. Williams. 1984. Vitamin D_3 levels in certain sheep tissues at various times after the intramuscular administration of vitamin D_3. Int. J. Vitamin Nutr. Res. 54:17–23.

Hidiroglou, M., K. J. Jenkins, J. R. Lessard, and E. Browsky. 1970a. Effect of feeding cod liver oil on the fate of radiotocopherol in sheep. Can. J. Physiol. Pharmacol. 48:751–757.

Hidiroglou, M., K. J. Jenkins, J. R. Lessard, and R. B. Carson. 1970b. Metabolism of vitamin E in sheep. Br. J. Nutr. 24:917–928.

Hidiroglou, M., K. J. Jenkins, and A. H. Corner. 1972. Control of nutritional muscular dystrophy in lambs by vitamin E implantations. Can. J. Anim. Sci. 52:511–516.

Hidiroglou, M., M. Ivan, and J. R. Lessard. 1977. Effects of ration and inside versus outside housing on plasma levels of ascorbic acid, lactic acid, glucose and cholesterol in Hereford steers wintered under practical conditions. Can. J. Anim. Sci. 57:51–59.

Hidiroglou, M., C. J. Williams, and M. Ivan. 1979. Pharmacokinetics and amounts of 25-hydroxycholecalciferol in sheep affected by osteodystrophy. J. Dairy Sci. 62:567–571.

Hidiroglou, M., C. J. Williams, and J. G. Proulx. 1985. Plasma vitamin D_3 response in cattle and sheep exposed to ultraviolet radiation. Int. J. Vit. Nutr. Res. 5:41–46.

Hidiroglou, M., G. Butler, and M. Ivan. 1991. Plasma vitamin E response in sheep dosed intraruminally or intraduodenally with various atocopherol compounds. Int. J. Vitam. Nutr. Res. 60:331–337.

Hidiroglou, M., T. R. Batra, and G. L. Roy. 1994. Changes in plasma α-tocopherol and selenium of gestating cows fed hay or silage. J. Dairy Sci. 77:190–195.

Hidiroglou, M., T. R. Batra, and X. Zhao. 1997. Comparison of vitamin C bioavailability after multiple or single oral dosing of different formulations in sheep. Reprod. Nutr. Dev. 37:443–448.

Hidiroglou, N., L. R. McDowell, and O. Balbuena. 1989. Plasma tocopherol in sheep and cattle after ingesting free or acetylated tocopherol. J. Dairy Sci. 72:1793–1799.

Hidiroglou, N., N. Cave, A. S. Atwal, E. R. Farnworth, and L. R. McDowell. 1992a. Comparative vitamin E requirements and metabolism in livestock. Ann. Rech. Vet. 23:337–359.

Hidiroglou, N., L. R. McDowell, A. M. Papas, M. Antapli, and N. S. Wilkinson. 1992b. Bioavailability of vitamin E compounds in lambs. J. Anim. Sci. 70:2556–2561.

Hidiroglou, N., L. R. McDowell, T. R. Batra, and A. M. Papas. 1994. Tissue α-tocopherol concentrations following supplementation with various forms of vitamin E in sheep. Reprod. Nutr. Dev. 34:273–278.

Hines, T. G., N. L. Jacobson, D. C. Beitz, and E. T. Littledike. 1985. Dietary calcium and vitamin D: Risk factors in the development of atherosclerosis in young goats. J. Nutr. 115:167–178.

Hines, T. G., R. L. Horst, E. T. Littledike, D. C. Beitz, and N. L. Jacobson. 1986. Vitamin D_3 and D_3 metabolites in young goats fed varying amounts of calcium and vitamin D_3. J. Dairy Sci. 69:385–391.

Holick, M. F. 1987. Photosynthesis of vitamin D in the skin: Effects of environmental and lifestyle variables. Fed. Proc. 46:1876–1882.

Horst, R. L., and E. T. Littledike. 1982. Comparison of plasma concentrations of vitamin D and its metabolites in young and aged domestic animals. Comp. Biochem. Physiol. 73B:485–489.

Horst, R. L., E. T. Littledike, J. L. Riley, and J. L. Napoli. 1981. Quantitation of vitamin D and its metabolites and their plasma concentrations in five species of animals. Anal. Biochem. 116:189–203.

Hsu, J. T., G. C. Fahey, Jr., J. H. Clark, L. L. Berger, and N. R. Merchen. 1991. Effects of urea and sodium bicarbonate supplementation of a high-fiber diet on nutrient digestion and ruminal characteristics of defaunated sheep. J. Anim. Sci. 69:1300–1311.

Huber, J. T. 1988. Vitamins in ruminant nutrition. Pp. 313–325 in The Ruminant Animal Digestive Physiology and Nutrition, D. C. Church, ed. Long Grove, IL: Waveland Press.

Jagos, P. L., J. Bouda, and R. Dvorak. 1977. The ascorbic acid levels in a case of bronchopneumonia in calves. Vet. Med. Praha. 22:133–136.

Johnson, E. H., K. Al-Habsi, E. Kaplan, A. Srikandakumar, I. T. Kadim, K. Annamalai, R. Al-Busaidy, and O. Mahgoub. 2004. Caprine hepatic lipidosis induced through the intake of low levels of dietary cobalt. Vet. J. 168:174–179.

Johnson, L. W. 1989. Nutrition. Vet. Clin. N. Am. Llama Med. 5:37–54.

Johnson, L. W. 1994. Llama nutrition. Vet. Clin. N. Am. Food Anim. Pract. 10:187–201.

Kadim, I. T., E. H. Johnson, O. Mahgoub, A. Srikandakumar, D. Al-Ajmi, A. Ritchie, K. Annamalai, and A. S. Al-Halhali. 2003. Effect of low levels of dietary cobalt on apparent nutrient digestibility in Omani goats. Anim. Feed Sci. Technol. 109:209–216.

Kadim, I. T., O. Mahgoub, A. Srikandakumar, D. S. Al-Ajmi, R. S. Al-Maqbaly, N. M. Al-Saqri, and E. H. Johnson. 2004. Comparative effect of low levels of dietary cobalt and parenteral injection of vitamin B_{12} on carcass and meat quality characteristics in Omani goats. Meat Sci. 66:837–844.

Karpinski, K., and M. Hidiroglou. 1990. Monitoring vitamin E pools in sheep tissue and plasma after intravenous dosing of radiotocopherol. Br. J. Nutr. 63:375–386.

Ken Scarratt, W. 1981. Polioencephalomalacia (cerebrocorticonecrosis). Pp. 1084–1085 in Current Veterinary Therapy, Food Animal Practice, J. L. Howard, ed. Philadelphia: W. B. Saunders.

Kennedy, D. G., A. Cannavan, A. Molloy, F. O' Harte, S. M. Taylor, S. Kennedy, and W. J. Blanchflower. 1990. Methylmalonyl-CoA mutase (*EC* 5.4.99.2) and methionine synthetase (*EC* 2.1.1.13) in tissues of cobalt-vitamin B_{12} deficient sheep. Br. J. Nutr. 64:721–732.

Kennedy, D. G., F. P. M. O'Harte, W. J. Blanchflower, and D. A. Rice. 1991. Sequential changes in propionate metabolism during the development of cobalt/vitamin B_{12} deficiency in sheep. Biol. Trace Elem. Res. 28:233–241.

Kennedy, D. G., W. J. Blanchflower, J. M. Scott, D. G. Weir, A. M. Molloy, S. Kennedy, and P. B. Young. 1992. Cobalt-vitamin B-12 deficiency decreases methionine synthase activity and phospholipids methylation in sheep. J. Nutr. 122:1384–1390.

Kennedy, D. G., S. Kennedy, W. J. Blanchflower, J. M. Scott, D. G. Weir, A. M. Molloy, and P. B. Young. 1994. Cobalt-vitamin B_{12} deficiency causes lipid accumulation of odd-numbered, branch chain fatty acids in the tissues of sheep. Br. J. Nutr. 71:67–76.

Kennedy, S., S. McConnell, H. Anderson, D. G. Kennedy, P. B. Young, and W. J. Blanchflower. 1997. Histopathologic and ultrastructural alterations of white liver disease in sheep experimentally depleted of cobalt. Vet. Pathol. 34:575–584.

Kierdorf, U., and L. Bartos. 1999. Treatment of the growing pedicle with retinoic acid increased the size of the first antlers in fallow deer (*Dama dama* L.). Comp. Biochem. Physiol. C Pharmacol. Toxicol. Endocrinol. 124:7–9.

Kierdorf, U., and H. Kierdorf. 1998. Effects of retinoic acid on pedicle and first antler growth in a fallow buck (*Dama dama* L.). Ann. Anat. 180:373–375.

Kivimae, A., and C. Carpena. 1973. The level of vitamin E content in some conventional feeding stuffs and the effects of genetic variety; harvesting; processing and storage. Acta. Agric. Scand. Suppl. 19:161–168.

Kolb, E., T. Kramer, M. Kuba, M. Leo, J. Linke, and M. Wahren. 1993. Concentration of ascorbic acid in the blood plasma of lambs and dogs before and after oral administration of ascorbic acid and ascorbic acid phosphate compounds and concentration in the urine of dogs over an 8-hour period afterwards. Mh. Vet. Med. 48:395–403.

Kollenkirchen, U., C. Kuhnigk, G. Breves, and J. Harmeyer. 1992. Effect of niacin supplementation on the concentration of niacin in rumen and duodenal digesta and in whole blood of sheep. Zentralbl. Veterinarmed. A 39:696–673.

Kott, R. W., V. M. Thomas, P. G. Hatfield, T. Evans, and K. C. Davis. 1998. Effects of dietary vitamin E supplementation during late pregnancy on lamb mortality and ewe productivity. J. Am. Vet. Med. Assoc. 212: 997–1000.

Lamnaouer, D. 1999. Anticoagulant activity of coumarins from Ferula communis L. Therapie 54:747–751.

Lee, H. J., and H. R. Marston. 1969. The requirement for cobalt of sheep grazed on cobalt-deficient pastures. Aust. J. Agric. Res. 20:905–918.

Leedle, R. A., J. A. Z. Leedle, and M. D. Butine. 1993. Vitamin E is not degraded by ruminal micro-organisms: Assessment with ruminal contents from a steer fed a high concentrate diet. J. Anim. Sci. 71:3442–3450.

Lindley, C. E., H. H. Brugman, T. J. Cunha, and E. J. Warwich. 1949. The effect of vitamin A deficiency on semen quality and the effect of testosterone and pregnant mare serum on vitamin A deficient rams. J. Anim. Sci. 8:590–602.

Linklater, K. A., D. A. Dyson, and K. T. Morgan. 1977. Faecal thiaminase in clinically normal sheep associated with outbreaks of polioencephalomalacia. Res. Vet. Sci. 22:308–312.

Littledike, E. T., and J. Goff. 1987. Interactions of calcium, phosphorus, magnesium, and vitamin D that influence their status in domestic meat animals. J. Anim. Sci. 65:1727–1743.

Lobley, G. E., A. Connell, and D. Revell. 1996. The importance of transmethylation reactions to methionine metabolism in sheep: Effects of supplementation with creatine and choline. Br. J. Nutr. 75:47–56.

Lonkar, P. S., and M. C. Prasad. 1993. Induced cerbrocortical necrosis in goats: Biochemical studies. Ind. J. Anim. Sci. 16:1128–1131.

Lonkar, P. S., and M. C. Prasad. 1994. Pathology of amprolium-induced cerebrocortical necrosis in goats. Small Ruminant Res. 13:85–92.

Luecke, R. W., R. Culik, F. Thorp Jr., L. H. Blakeslee, and R. H. Nelson. 1950. Riboflavin deficiency in the lamb. J. Anim. Sci. 9:420–425.

Maas, J., M. S. Bulgin, B. C. Anderson, and T. M. Frye. 1984. Nutritional myodegeneration associated with vitamin E deficiency and normal selenium status in lambs. J. Am. Vet. Med. Assoc. 184:201–204.

Machlin, L. J. 1990. Vitamin E. Pp. 100–144 in Handbook of Vitamins, 2nd ed., revised and expanded, L. J. Machlin, ed. New York: Marcel Dekker.

MacLeod, R. A., and J. F. Murray. 1956. Some factors affecting cellulose digestion by rumen microorganisms in vitro. J. Nutr. 60:245–259.

Maiorano, G., A. Manchisi, G. Salvatori, F. Filetti, and G. Oriani. 1999. Influence of multiple injections of vitamin E on intramuscular collagen and bone characteristics in suckling lambs. J. Anim. Sci. 77:2452–2457.

Marca, M. C., J. J. Ramos, T. Sáez, M. C. Sanz, M. T. Verde, and A. Fernández. 1996. Vitamin B_{12} supplementation of lambs. Small Rumin. Nutr. 20:9–14.

Marston, H. R. 1970. The requirement of sheep for cobalt or for vitamin B_{12}. Br. J. Nutr. 24:615–633.

Martin, F. H., D. E. Ullrey, H. W. Newland, and E. R. Miller. 1968. Vitamin A activity of carotenes in corn silage fed to lambs. J. Nutr. 96:269–274.

May, B. J., M. C. Calhoun, and G. R. Engdahl. 1987. A re-evaluation of the minimum vitamin A requirement of growing-finishing lambs. J. Anim. Sci. 65:1626–1632.

Mburu, J. N., J. M. Z. Kamau, and M. S. Badamana. 1993. Changes in serum levels of vitamin B_{12}, feed, live weight and haematological parameters in cobalt deficient small East African goats. Int. J. Vit. Nutr. Res. 63:135–139.

McDiarmid, R. E., W. Majak, and K. J. Cheng. 1994. Procedure for analysis of α-tocopherol acetate in bovine ruminal fluid. Can. J. Anim. Sci. 74:391–392.

McDowell, L. R. 1989. Vitamins in Animal Nutrition: Comparative Aspects to Human Nutrition. San Diego, CA: Academic Press.

McDowell, L. R., S. N. Williams, N. Hidiroglou, C. A. Njeru, G. M. Hill, L. Ochoa, and N. S. Wilkinson. 1996. Vitamin E supplementation for the ruminant. Anim. Feed Sci. Technol. 60:273–296.

McElroy, L. W., and H. A. Goss. 1939. Report on four members of the vitamin B complex synthesised in the rumen of the sheep. J. Biochem. 130:437–438.

McMurray, C. H., and D. A. Rice. 1982. Vitamin E and selenium deficiency diseases. Ir. Vet. J. 36:57–65.

Mello, J. R. B. 2003. Calcinosis—calcinogenic plants. Toxicon. 41:1–12.

Mello, J. R., and G. C. Habermehl. 1992. Calcinogenic plants and the incubation effect of rumen fluid. Dtsch. Tierärztl. Wochenschr. 99: 371–376.

Menzies, P., I. H. Boermans, B. Hoff, T. Durzi, and L. Langs. 2003. Survey of the status of copper, interacting minerals, and vitamin E levels in the livers of sheep in Ontario. Can. Vet. J. 44:898–906.

Menzies, P., L. Langs, H. Boermans, J. Martin, and J. McNally. 2004. Myopathy and hepatic lipidosis in weaned lambs due to vitamin E deficiency. Can. Vet. J. 45:244–247.

Mgongo, F. O. K., S. Gombe, and J. S. Ogaa. 1981. Thyroid status in cobalt and vitamin B_{12} deficiency in goats. Vet. Rec. 109:51–53.

Mgongo, F. O. K., S. Gombe, and J. S. Ogaa. 1984. The influence of cobalt/vitamin B_{12} deficiency as a «stressor» affecting adrenal cortex and ovarian activities in goats. Reprod. Nutr. Dev. 24:845–854.

Miller, B. L., J. C. Meiske, and R. D. Goodrich. 1986. Effects of grain source and concentrate level on B-vitamin production and absorption in steers. J. Anim. Sci. 62:473–483.

Miller, J. K., E. Brzezinska-Slebodzinska, and F. C. Madsen. 1993. Oxidative stress, antioxidants, and animal function. J. Dairy Sci. 76: 2812–2823.

Miller, R. W., R. W. Hemken, D. R. Waldo, and L. A. Moore. 1969. Effect of ethyl alcohol on the vitamin A status of Holstein heifers. J. Dairy Sci. 52:1998–2000.

Miller, W. J. 1979. Dairy Cattle Feeding and Nutrition. New York: Academic Press.

Mitchell, A. D., A. Chappell, and K. L. Knox. 1979. Metabolism of betaine in the ruminant. J. Anim. Sci. 49:764–774.

Mohammed, R., and M. Lamand. 1986. Cardiovascular lesions in cobalt-vitamin B_{12} deficient sheep. Ann. Rech. Vet. 17:447–450.

Mora, O., J. L. Romano, E. Gonzalez, F. Ruiz, and A. Shimada. 2000. Low cleavage activity of 15,15' dioxygenase to convert β-carotene to retinal in cattle compared with goats, is associated with yellow pigmentation of adipose tissue. Int. J. Vitam. Nutr. Res. 70:199–205.

Morgan, K. T., and G. H. Lawson. 1974. Thiaminase type 1-producing bacilli and ovine polioencephalomalacia. Vet. Rec. 95:361–363.

Morgante, M., D. Beghelli, M. Pauselli, P. Dall'ara, M. Capuccella, and S. Ranucci. 1999. Effect of administration of vitamin E and selenium during the dry period on mammary health and milk cell counts in dairy ewes. J. Dairy Sci. 82:623–631.

Nagaraja, T. G., C. J. Newbold, C. J. Van Nevel, and D. I. Demeyer. 1997. Manipulation of ruminal fermentation. Pp. 523–632 in The Rumen Microbial Ecosystem, 2nd ed., P. N. Hobson and C. S. Stewart, eds. London: Blackie Academic & Professional, an imprint of Chapman and Hall.

Narkewicz, M. R., G. Jones, H. Thompson, F. Kolhouse, and P. V. Fennessey. 2002. Folate cofactors regulate serine metabolism in fetal ovine hepatocytes. Pediatr. Res. 52:589–594.

Neil, A. R., D. W. Grime, and R. M. C. Dawson. 1978. Conversion of choline methyl groups through trimethyl amine into methane in the rumen. Biochem. J. 170:529–535.

Neil, A. R., D. W. Grime, A. M. Snoswell, A. J. Northrop, D. B. Lindsay, and R. M. C. Dawson. 1979. The low availability of dietary choline for the nutrition of the sheep. Biochem. J. 180:559–565.

Njeru, C. A., L. R. McDowell, N. S. Wilkinson, and S. N. Williams. 1994a. Assessment of vitamin E nutritional status in sheep. J. Anim. Sci. 72:3207–3212.

Njeru, C. A., L. R. McDowell, N. S. Wilkinson, S. B. Linda, and S. N. Williams. 1994b. Pre- and postpartum supplemental DL-α-tocopheryl acetate effects on placental and mammary vitamin E transfer in sheep. J. Anim. Sci. 72:1636–1640.

NRC (National Research Council). 1975. Nutrient Requirements of Sheep, 5th rev. ed. Washington, DC: National Academy Press.

NRC. 1981. Nutrient Requirements of Goats: Angora, Dairy, and Meat Goats in Temperate and Tropical Countries. Washington, DC: National Academy Press.

NRC. 1985. Nutrient Requirements of Sheep, 6th rev. ed. Washington, DC: National Academy Press.

NRC. 1987. Vitamin Tolerance of Animals. Washington, DC: National Academy Press.

NRC. 1989. Recommended Dietary Allowances, 10th ed. Washington, DC: National Academy Press.

NRC. 1996. Nutrient Requirements of Beef Cattle, 7th rev. ed. Washington, DC: National Academy Press.

NRC. 1998. Nutrient Requirements of Swine, 10th rev. ed. Washington, DC: National Academy Press.

NRC. 2001. Nutrient Requirements of Dairy Cattle, 7th ed. Washington, DC: National Academy Press.

Ochoa, L., L. R. McDowell, S. N. Williams, N. Wilkinson, J. Boucher, and E. L. Lentz. 1992. alpha-Tocopherol concentrations in serum and tissues of sheep fed different sources of vitamin E. J. Anim. Sci. 70:2568–2573.

Olkowski, A. A., S. R. Gooneratne, C. G. Rousseaux, and D. A. Christensen. 1992. Role of thiamine status in sulphur induced polioencephalomalacia in sheep. Res. Vet. Sci. 52:78–85.

Olson, J. A. 1987. Recommended dietary intakes (RDI) of vitamin A in humans. Am. J. Clin. Nutr. 45:704–716.

Olson, J. A. 1991. Vitamin A. Pp. 1–57 in Handbook of Vitamins, 2nd ed., revised and expanded, L. J. Machlin, ed. New York: Marcel Dekker.

Ørskov, E. R. 1994. Recent advances in understanding of microbial transformation in ruminants. Livest. Prod. Sci. 39:53–60.

Owen, E. C., and D. W. West. 1970. Metabolites of riboflavine in milk, urine and tissues of animals in relation to alimentary symbiotic bacteria. Br. J. Nutr. 24:45–60.

Pearson, A. B. 1987. White liver disease and pestivirus infection in goat kids. Surveillance N. Z. 14:21.

Peet, R. L., and K. Hepworth. 1993. Enzootic ataxia in red deer, *Cervus elaphus*. Aust. Vet. J. 70:395–396.

Pehrson, B., J. Hakkarainen, and L. Blomgren. 1990. Vitamin E status in newborn lambs with special reference to the effect of dl-α-tocopheryl acetate supplementation in late gestation. Acta. Vet. Scand. 31:359–367.

Peters, J. P., and J. M. Elliot. 1983. Effect of vitamin B_{12} status on performance of the lactating ewe and gluconeogenesis from propionate. J. Dairy Sci. 66:1917–1925.

Peters, J. P., and J. M. Elliot. 1984. Effects of cobalt or hydroxycobalamin supplementation on vitamin B-12 content and (*S*)-methylmalonyl-CoA mutase activity of tissue from cobalt-depleted sheep. J. Nutr. 114:660–670.

Peters, J. P., E. N. Bergman, and J. M. Elliot. 1983. Influence of vitamin B-12 status on hepatic propionic acid uptake in sheep. J. Nutr. 113:1221–1228.

Peterson, T. E., L. R. McDowell, R. J. McMahon, N. S. Wilkinson, O. Rosendo, W. M. Seymour, P. R. Henry, F. G. Martins, and J. K. Shearer. 2004. Balance and serum concentration of biotin in sheep fed alfalfa meal-based diets with increasing level of concentrate. J. Anim. Sci. 82:1165–1169.

Pierson R. E., and R. Jensen. 1975. Polioencephalomalacia in feedlot lambs. J. Am. Vet. Med. Assoc. 166:257–259.

Poe, S. E., G. E. Mitchell Jr., and D. G. Ely. 1972. Rumen development in lambs. III. Microbial B-vitamin synthesis. J. Anim. Sci. 34:826–829.

Price, J., and S. Allen. 2004. Exploring the mechanisms regulating regeneration of deer antlers. Phil. Trans. R. Soc. Lond. B 359:809–822.

Puchala, R., T. Sahlu, M. J. Herselman, and J. J. Davis. 1995. Influence of betaine on blood metabolites of Alpine and Angora kids. Small Ruminant Res. 18:137–143.

Puchala, R., V. Banskalieva, A. L. Goetsch, T. Sahlu, and I. Prieto. 2000. Effect of ruminally protected choline and betaine on productivity of Angora doelings. Proc. 7th Inter. Conf. Goats. Tours, France, May 15–21.

Pugh, D. G. 1993. Polioencephalomalcia in a llama herd. Equine Practice 15:24–26.

Quirk, M. F., and B. W. Norton. 1987. The relationship between the cobalt nutrition of ewes and the vitamin B_{12} status of ewes and their lambs. Aust. J. Agric. Res. 38:1071–1082.

Radcliffe, B. C., and A. R. Egan. 1978. The effect of diet and of methionine loading on activity of enzymes in the transulfuration pathway in sheep. Aust. J. Biol. Sci. 31:105–114.

Radostits, O. M., G. P. Searcy, and K. G. Mitchall. 1980. Moldy sweet clover poisoning in cattle. Can. Vet. J. 21:153–158.

Ramos, J. J., T. Saez, J. P. Bueso, M. C. Sanz, and A. Fernandez. 1994. Vitamin B_{12} levels in ewe colostrums and milk and in lamb serum. Vet. Res. 25:405–409.

Ramos J. J., C. Marca, A. Loste, J. A. Garcia de Jalón, A. Fernández, and T. Cubel. 2003. Biochemical changes in apparently normal sheep from flocks affected by polioencephalomalacia. Vet. Res. Commun. 27:111–124.

Reis, P. J. 1989. The influence of absorbed nutrients on wool growth. P. 185 in The Biology of Wool and Hair, G. E. Rogers, P. J. Reis, K. A. Ward, and R. C. Marshall, eds. London: Chapman and Hall.

Reis, P. J., and T. Sahlu. 1994. The nutritional control of the growth and properties of mohair and wool fibers: A comparative review. J. Anim. Sci. 72:1899–1907.

Reis, P. J., D. A. Tunks, and S. G. Munro. 1990. Effects of the infusion of amino acids into the abomasum of sheep, with emphasis on the relative value of methionine, cysteine and homocysteine for wool growth. J. Agric. Sci., Cambridge 114:59–68.

Rice, D. A., M. McLoughlin, W. J. Blanchflower, C. H. McMurray, and E. A. Goodall. 1989. Sequential changes in plasma methylmalonic acid and vitamin B_{12} in sheep eating cobalt-deficient grass. Biol. Trace Elem. Res. 22:153–164.

Richetti, F. 1987. Free and blood-bound ascorbic acid in milk producing cows, sheep and goats. First results. Acta. Med. Vet. 33:9–15.

Rickard, T. R., and J. M. Elliot. 1978. Absorption of vitamin B_{12} and factor B from the intestine of sheep. J. Anim. Sci. 46:304–308.

Rickard, T. R., and J. M. Elliot. 1982. Effect of factor B on vitamin B_{12} status and propionate metabolism in sheep. J. Anim. Sci. 55:168–173.

Riddell, D. O., E. E. Bartley, and A. D. Dayton. 1980. Effect of nicotinic acid on rumen fermentation in vitro and in vivo. J. Dairy Sci. 63:1429–1436.

Riddell, D. O., E. E. Bartley, and A. D. Dayton. 1981. Effect of nicotinic acid on microbial protein synthesis in vitro and on dairy cattle growth and milk production. J. Dairy Sci. 64:782–791.

Robinson, B. S., A. M. Snoswell, W. B. Runciman, and R. N. Upton. 1984. Uptake and output of various forms of choline by organs of the conscious chronically catheterized sheep. Biochem. J. 217:399–408.

Robinson, B. S., A. M. Snoswell, and B. P. Setchell. 1987. The enterohep-tatic recycling of bile choline in sheep. Comp. Biochem. Physiol. 88A:283–289.

Rode, L. M., T. A. McAllister, and K. J. Cheng. 1990. Microbial degradation of vitamin A in rumen fluid from steers fed concentrate, hay or straw diets. Can. J. Anim. Sci. 70:227–233.

Roquet, J., C. F. Nockels, and A. M. Papas. 1992. Cattle blood plasma and red blood cell α-tocopherol levels in response to different chemical forms and routes of administration of vitamin E. J. Anim. Sci. 70: 2542–2550.

Rosendo, O., D. B. Bates, L. R. McDowell, C. R. Staples, R. McMahon, and N. S. Wilkinson. 2003. Availability and ability of biotin for promoting forage fiber in vitro ruminal digestibility. J. Anim. Vet. Adv. 2:350–357.

Ross, A. D., C. G. Gee, A. R. B. Jackson, E. Hall, and P. L. Greentree. 1989. Nutritional myopathy in goats. Aust. Vet. J. 66:361–363.

Ross, D. 1977. Oxidative killing of microorganism by phagocytic cells. Trends Biochem. Sci. 2:61–64.

Rousseau, J. E., Jr., C. M. Dembiczak, K. L. Dolge, and H. D. Eaton. 1954. Relationship between plasma vitamin A and liver vitamin A in calves fed a vitamin depletion ration and calves fed minimum levels of vitamin A or carotene. J. Dairy Sci. 37:1376–1382.

Roussev, V., G. Ganev, and K. S. Zan. 1975. Vitamin B_{12} content in the complex stomach of small ruminants receiving propionic acid and sodium propionate in the food. Agressologie 16C:37–41.

Rumsey, T. S. 1975. Vitamin requirements for ruminants. Feedstuffs 47:30.

Salter, D. N., and P. Blakeborough. 1988. Influence of goat's-milk folate-binding protein on transport of 5-methyltetrahydrofolate in neonatal-goat small intestinal brush-border-membrane vesicles. Br. J. Nutr. 59:497–507.

Sánchez, P., R. Mueles, A. Sánchez, J. Rubert, J. Montanel, C. Luengo, A. Contreras, and C. Fernández. 2001. Influence of betaine on somatic cell count and goat milk composition. Ann. Meeting of Eur. Assoc. Anim. Prod. Budapest, Hungary.

Sawaya, W. N., J. K. Khalil, and A. F. Al-Shalhat. 1984. Mineral and vitamin content of goat's milk. J. Am. Dietetic Assoc. 84:433–435.

Schaetzel, W. P., and D. E. Johnson. 1981. Nicotinic acid and dilution rate effects on in vitro fermentation efficiency. J. Anim. Sci. 53:1104–1108.

Schussler, S. L., G. C. Fahey, Jr., J. B. Robinson, S. S. Masters, S. C. Loerch, and J. W. Spears. 1978. The effect of nicotinic acid on in vitro cellulose digestion and protein synthesis. Int. J. Vit. Nutr. Res. 48:359–367.

Scott, D., and A. F. McLean. 1981. Control of mineral absorption in ruminants. Proc. Nutr. Soc. 40:257–266.

Scott, K. J., and D. Rodriquez-Amaya. 2000. Pro-vitamin A carotenoid conversion factors: Retinol equivalents—fact or fiction? Food Chem. 69:125–127.

Sharma, B. K., and R. A. Erdman. 1989. In vitro degradation of choline from selected feedstuffs and choline supplements. J. Dairy Sci. 72: 2772–2776.

Sharman, G. A. M., 1973. Deficiencies of vitamin E and selenium as factors limiting the intensification of sheep production. Acta. Agric. Scand. Suppl. 19:181.

Shields, D. R., D. M. Schaefer, and T. W. Perry. 1983. Influence of niacin supplementation and nitrogen source on rumen microbial fermentation. J. Anim. Sci. 57:1576–1583.

Smith, B. B., and R. J. Van Saun. 1996. Hypophosphatemic rickets in South American camelids: Interaction of calcium, phosphorus, and vitamin D. Pp. 79–94 in Proc. Second European Symp. South American Camelids, M. Gerken and C. Renieri, ed. Univ. Degli Studi Di Camerino, Italy.

Smith, B. S. W., and H. Wright. 1984. Relative contributions of diet and sunshine to the overall vitamin D status of the grazing ewe. Vet. Rec. 115:537–538.

Smith, B. S. W., H. Wright, G. U. Aitchison, and J. A. Spence. 1985. Effects in sheep of high dietary levels of vitamin D_3 as measured by circulating concentrations of some vitamin D metabolites and skeletal examination. Res. Vet. Sci. 18:317–321.

Smith, M. C. 1979. Polioencephalomalacia in goats. J. Am. Vet. Med. Assoc. 174:1328–1332.

Smith, R. M., and H. R. Marston. 1970. Production, absorption, distribution and excretion of vitamin B_{12} in sheep. Br. J. Nutr. 24:857–877.

Smith, R. M., and W. S. Osborne-White. 1973. Folic acid metabolism in vitamin B_{12}-deficient sheep. Depletion of liver folates. Biochem. J. 136: 279–293.

Smith, R. M., W. S. Osborne-White, and J. M. Gawthorne. 1974. Folic acid metabolism in vitamin B_{12}-deficient sheep. Effects of injected methionine on liver constituents associated with folate metabolism. Biochem. J. 142:105–117.

Spicer, E. M., and B. J. Horton. 1981. Biochemistry of natural and amprolium-induced polioencephalomalacia in sheep. Aust. Vet. J. 57: 230–235.

Sreekrishna, K., and H. R. Cama. 1979. Characterization of vitamin A transport system from goat plasma. Biochim. Biophys. Acta. 581:136–141.

Strobel, H. J. 1992. Vitamin B_{12}-dependent propionate production by the ruminal bacterium *Prevotella ruminicola* 23. Appl. Environ. Microbiol. 58:2331–2333.

Sugiyama, K., A. Kumazawa, H. Zhou, and S. Saeki. 1998. Dietary methionine level affects linoleic acid metabolism through phosphatidylethanolamine *N*-methylation in rats. Lipids 33:325–242.

Sutton, A. L., and J. M. Elliot. 1972. Effect of ratio of roughage to concentrate and level of feed intake on ovine ruminal vitamin B_{12} production. J. Nutr. 102:1341–1346.

Tendgerdy, R. P. 1989. Vitamin E, immune response, and disease resistance. Ann. N. Y. Acad. Sci. 570:335–344.

Tengerdy, R. P. 1990a. Immunity and disease resistance in farm animals fed vitamin E supplement. Adv. Exp. Med. Biol. 262:103–110.

Tengerdy, R. P. 1990b. The role of vitamin E in immune response and disease resistance. Ann. N. Y. Acad. Sci. 587:24–33.

Thomas, K. W. 1986. Oral treatment of polioencephalomalacia and subclinical thiamine deficiency with thiamine propyl disulphide and thiamine hydrochloride. J. Vet. Pharmacol. Therap. 9:402–411.

Thomas, K. W., D. L. Turner, and E. M. Spicer. 1987. Thiamine, thiaminase and transketolase levels in goats with and without polioencephalomalacia. Aust. Vet. J. 64:126–127.

Thomas, K. W., A. P. Kelly, P. T. Beers, and R. G. Brennan. 1990. Thiamine deficiency in sheep exported live by sea. Aust. Vet. J. 67:215–218.

Thornber, E. J., R. H. Dunlop, J. M. Gawthorne, and C. R. Huxtable. 1981. Induced thiamin deficiency in lambs. Aust. Vet. J. 57:21–26.

Thornton, J. H., and L. H. Schultz. 1980. Effects of administration of nicotinic acid on glucose, insulin, and glucose tolerance in ruminants. J. Dairy Sci. 58:262–268.

Toutain, P. L., M. Hidiroglou, and E. Charmley. 1995. Pharmacokinetics and tissue uptake of D-α-tocopherol in sheep following a single intraperitoneal injection. J. Dairy Sci. 78:1561–1566.

Tramontin, R. R., R. C. Giles Jr., C. B. Hong, and L. E. Newman. 1983. Myodegeneration in Kentucky white-tailed deer. J. Am. Vet. Med. Assoc. 183:1263–1265.

Turner, K. E., K. E. McClure, W. P. Weiss, R. J. Borton, and J. G. Foster. 2002. Alpha-tocopherol concentrations and case life of lamb muscle as influenced by concentrate or pasture finishing. J. Anim. Sci. 80:2513–2521.

Ullrey, D. E. 1972. Biological availability of fat-soluble vitamins: Vitamin A and carotene. J. Anim. Sci. 35:648–657.

Ulvund, M. J., and M. Pestalozzi. 1990. Ovine white-liver disease (OWLD) in Norway: Clinical symptoms and preventative measures. Acta Vet. Scand. 31:53–62.

Underwood, E. J. 1977. Cobalt. Pp. 132–158 in Trace Elements in Humans and Animal Nutrition, 4th ed., E. J. Underwood, ed. New York: Academic Press.

Van Gylswyk, N. O., K. Wejdemar, and K. Kulander. 1992. Comparative growth rates of various rumen bacteria in clarified rumen fluid from cows and sheep fed different diets. Appl. Environ. Microbiol. 58:99–105.

Van Saun, R. J. 2006. Nutrient requirements of South American camelids: A factorial approach. Small Ruminant Res. 61.165–186.

Van Saun, R. J., B. B. Smith, and B. J. Watrous. 1996. Evaluation of vitamin D status of llamas and alpacas with hypophosphatemic rickets. J. Am. Vet. Med. Assoc. 209:1128–1133.

Vellema, P., V. P. M. G. Rutten, A. Hoek, L. Moll, and G. H. Wentink. 1996. The effect of cobalt supplementation on the immune response in vitamin B_{12} deficient Texel lambs. Vet. Immunol. Immunopathol. 55:151–161.

Vestweber J. G., H. W. Leipold, and J. E. Smith. 1974. Ovine ruminal acidosis: Clinical studies. Am. J. Vet. Res. 35:1587–1590.

Vierk, J. E., T. R. Hansen, K. J. Austin, E. A. Van Kirk, B. W. Hess, and W. J. Murdoch. 1998. Inhibition by tocopherol of prostaglandin-induced apoptosis in ovine corpora lutea. Prostaglandins Lipid Mediators 56:265–267.

Vitamin Nutrition Compendium. 2000. Parsippany, NJ: Roche Vitamins Inc.

Walker, C. K., and J. M. Elliot. 1972. Lactational trends in vitamin B_{12} status on conventional and restricted roughage rations. J. Dairy Sci. 55: 474–479.

Wallis, G. C., C. A. Smith, and R. H. Fishman. 1949. The vitamin D content of roughages. J. Dairy Sci. 32:715.

Wasserman, R. H., and A. N. Taylor. 1976. Gastrointestinal absorption of calcium and phosphorus. Pp. 137–155 in Handbook of Physiology, Sect. 7: Endocrinology Vol. VIII, Parathyroid Gland, G. D. Aurbach, ed. Washington, DC: American Physiological Society.

Weiss, W. P., and D. J. Wyatt. 2003. Effect of dietary fat and vitamin E on α-tocopherol in milk from dairy cows. J. Dairy Sci. 86:3582–3591.

Weiss, W. P., J. S. Hogan, K. L. Smith, and S. N. Williams. 1994. Effect of dietary fat and vitamin E on α-tocopherol and β-carotene in blood of peripartum cows. J. Dairy Sci. 77:1422–1429.

Weiss, W. P., K. L. Smith, J. S. Hogan, and T. E. Steiner. 1995. Effect of forage to concentrate ratio on disappearance of vitamins A and E during in vitro ruminal fermentation. J. Dairy Sci. 78:1837–1842.

West, D. W., and E. C. Owen. 1973. Degradation of riboflavin by alimentary bacteria of the ruminant and man: Production of 7,8-dimethyl-10-carboxymethylisoalloxazine. Br. J. Nutr. 29:33–41.

Wing, J. M. 1969. Effect of source and season on apparent digestibility of carotene in forage by cattle. J. Dairy Sci. 52:479–483.

Wolin, M. J., T. L. Miller, and C. S. Stewart. 1997. Microbe-microbe interactions. Pp. 467–491 in The Rumen Microbial Ecosystem, 2nd ed., P. N. Hobson and C. S. Stewart, eds. London: Blackie Academic & Professional, an imprint of Chapman and Hall.

Wood, J. D., and M. Enser. 1997. Factors influencing fatty acids in meat and the role of antioxidants in improving meat quality. Br. J. Nutr. 78 (Suppl. 1):S49–S60.

Woodard, J. C., G. Berra, B. Ruksan, B. Carrillo, and G. Erdos. 1994. Toxic effects of solanum malacoxylon on sheep bone. Bone 14:787–797.

Wright, K. E., and R. C. Hall, Jr. 1979. Association between plasma and liver vitamin A levels in the calf; Weanling pig, rabbit and rat; and adult goat fed fixed intakes of vitamin Am. J. Nutr. 109:1063–1072.

Wulf, D. M., J. B. Morgan, S. K. Sanders, J. D. Tatum, G. C. Smith, and S. Williams. 1995. Effects of dietary supplementation of vitamin E on storage and caselife properties of lamb retail cuts. J. Anim. Sci. 73: 399–405.

Xue, G. P., and A. M. Snoswell. 1985. Regulation of methyl group metabolism in lactating ewes. Biochem. Int. 11:381–385.

Yang, A., and R. K. Tume. 1993. A comparison of β-carotene-splitting activity isolated from intestinal mucosa of pasture-grazed sheep, goats, and cattle. Biochem. Molec. Biol. Int. 30:209–217.

Zinn, R. A., F. N. Owens, R. L. Stuart, J. R. Dunbar, and B. B. Norman. 1987. B-vitamin supplementation of diets for feedlot calves. J. Anim. Sci. 65:267–277.

Zintzen, H., and P. A. Boyazoglou. 1973. Vitamin D and its relation to calcium-phosphorus metabolism in ruminants. S. Afr. Vet. Med. Assoc. 44:25–36.

9

Water

INTRODUCTION

Water is considered an important nutrient because it is the universal solvent of life, comprising 99 percent of all molecules in the animal (Macfarlane and Howard, 1972) and between 50 and 81 percent of body mass (Robbins, 1993; NRC, 2001). The intracellular fluid pool of body water is a medium for chemical (hydrolytic) and other metabolic reactions within cells. Water in the extracellular fluid pool, and including transcellular water in the alimentary (digestive) tract (gut), is a transporter of heat, hormones, ions, nutrients, and metabolites and is a medium for elimination of metabolic end products. As a "buffer" with respect to heat balance, water dissipates heat through physiological body pools from a point of intracellular oxidation to the skin surface, where it can be lost by conductive, convective, radiative, and evaporative processes (Moen, 1973; Parker and Robbins, 1985b; NRC, 2003). Vaporization of water is a powerful means of losing heat from the body to achieve thermoregulation in the thermoneutral range (TNR), and especially when ambient temperatures increase above the upper critical temperature (T_{uc}) (Blaxter et al., 1959a,b; Parker and Robbins, 1985a). The water pool is the fluid source for the fetus and for the nursing offspring. For forestomach fermentors, the rumen-reticulum (R-R) and C1-C3 chambers of New World camelids (NWC) also serve as reservoirs that provide water for other physiological pools during temporarily induced shortage (Hecker et al., 1964; Shkolnik et al., 1980). Movement of ions and water molecules through the cell wall achieves regulation of intracellular volume and ion balance, thus concentrations of many ions in the extracellular fluid can vary as the animal achieves osmotic regulation and extracellular Na homeostasis under the influence of feeding events, water restriction, and other environmental effects (Robinson, 1957; Macfarlane and Howard, 1972; Kleiber, 1975; NRC, 1981, 1985, 2001, 2003). With such a large array of interrelations between physiological and biochemical processes, it is not surprising that animals have evolved excellent behavioral mechanisms to balance water losses by drinking. Thus, water use and requirements have been assessed from measurements of voluntary water intake by drinking. Although drinking usually dominates as the source of water intake in ruminants, also important are water intake in feed, termed preformed water, and water produced by metabolic reactions, termed metabolic water. The potential of preformed and metabolic water to meet water requirements of free-ranging animals is exemplified by the study by Lynch et al. (1972), who showed that sheep can graze year-round with no access to drinking water under some pasture systems. In both laboratory and field studies, assessment of water use is often measured as water turnover using water markers (Macfarlane, 1964; Longhurst et al., 1970; Macfarlane and Howard, 1972; Dove and Freer, 1979; Holleman et al., 1982; Nagy and Peterson, 1988). These studies show that the major integration of physiological and biochemical interactions result in water use being highly related to the vital processes of energy turnover and thermoregulation.

Under both controlled and field conditions, water turnover and daily energy expenditure (DEE) are correlated (Lifson and McClintock, 1966; Macfarlane and Howard, 1972; Nagy and Peterson, 1988). Some components contributing to water turnover are under genetic regulation as judged by the close similarities of identical twins (Macfarlane and Howard, 1966, 1972). Selection for wool production in the Merino sheep results in an increase in energy metabolism (Graham, 1968) that also is accompanied by an increase in water turnover (Macfarlane and Howard, 1966, 1970). A further linkage between water and energy metabolism is the nasal countercurrent system that is capable of recovering up to 80 percent of water, thus minimizing evaporative water and heat losses (Withers et al., 1979; Blix and Johnsen, 1983; Blix et al., 1983a,b). With such a set of regulated responses, one might expect water turnover in tissues to be tightly controlled. However, under variable environmental extremes, behavioral responses, and productivity (growth, gestation, and lactation), the turnover time of water in the body water pool (turnover time = 1/k [where k = $0.693/t_{1/2}$ and $t_{1/2}$ is the biological half-life of water]) ranges 20-fold from 2 to 41 d, because $t_{1/2}$ ranges from 1.4 to 28 d (Macfarlane, 1964; Longhurst et al., 1970; Macfarlane and Howard, 1972; Cameron et al., 1975; Larsen and Blix, 1985; Dove, 1988; Haggarty et al., 1998; Gotaas et al., 2000a; Williams et al., 2001). Under less severe environmental extremes, the $t_{1/2}$ of confined sheep, goats, and deer is 2.0 to 8.5 d (Knox et al., 1969; Longhurst et al., 1970; Church, 1971; NRC, 1981; Parker et al., 1993b; Midwood et al., 1994).

BODY WATER DISTRIBUTION AND CONTENT

Water is distributed throughout the physiological body pools of the animal. The total amount is termed total body water (TBW) and is determined by gravimetric analysis at slaughter. An estimate of TBW can be made by dilution of water markers in vivo after appropriate correction factors are applied. The physiological pools through which TBW is distributed include (1) the extracellular fluid (ECF), amounting to 31–38 percent of TBW, and (2) the intracellular fluid (ICF), amounting to 62–69 percent of TBW (Macfarlane et al., 1956; Purohit et al., 1972; NRC, 2001, 2003). Water, plus K^+ and other inorganic ions, and proteins within the different types of cell types of the body constitute the ICF pool. Measurement of ICF-water can be made by bioelectrical impedance spectroscopy, or as the difference between an estimation of nonalimentary water and the ECF water space using thiocyanate as a marker (Gad and Preston, 1990). The ECF includes blood plasma (25 percent of extracellular water) plus interstitial fluid (75 percent of extracellular water). Measurements of ECF sometimes include transcellular water in the gut. The ICF pool is highly regulated in volume. This is achieved by alterations in the ECF, which in turn is regulated to maintain a constant concentration of Na. Volume sensors, hormones, and water transfer mechanisms involving the hepatic-portal system, heart, and kidneys (Macfarlane and Howard, 1972) evolved to perform the regulatory functions. Understanding the mechanisms that control the shift in water between these pools is of interest for managing free-ranging and wild animals (Macfarlane, 1964; Macfarlane and Howard, 1972; Cameron and Luick, 1972; King, 1982). Shifts in water between the various pools are also important during dehydration and rehydration in desert and Mediterranean environments (Macfarlane et al., 1956; Macfarlane and Howard, 1972; Purohit et al., 1972; Shkolnik et al., 1975; Degen, 1977a; Shkolnik et al., 1980), during long-term undernutrition involving drought-feeding (Morris et al., 1962; McGregor, 2003), and during gestation (Cameron at al., 1975) and lactation (Degen 1977b; Woodford et al., 1984; Odwongo et al., 1985).

Control of Water in the Forestomachs and Gut

Water content of the gut, and particularly in the forestomachs of ruminants and NWC, is highly variable and constitutes 7–35 percent of BW (Hecker et al., 1964; Macfarlane 1964; Shkolnik et al., 1980). Rumen fill in concentrate selector–browser species (~ 9 percent: Nagy and Regelin, 1975; Hobson et al., 1976; Kay et al., 1980) is less than in grazers (13 percent: Kay et al., 1980; Clauss et al., 2003). Physiological condition also affects water content of the gut (Macfarlane, 1964), which can be 12–15 percent of BW in late gestation and winter in reindeer/caribou (Cameron et al., 1975; Gerhart et. al., 1996a) and 16–19 percent in sheep in late gestation (Faichney et al., 2004); 15 percent during lactation in the dairy cow (Andrew et al., 1995); 17–21 percent in young animals in winter (Staaland et al., 1984); and 15 percent in males (Peltier et al., 2003).

Although water content of the R-R varies between 12 and 25 g/100 g wet weight (WW), R-R water contributes a fairly constant 81–88 percent of the water content of the entire gut (Church, 1971; Staaland et al., 1984), except for pregnant sheep (42–52 percent: Faichney et al., 2004). Thus R-R water is 10–30 percent of the TBW pool of ruminants (Hecker et al., 1964; Shkolnik et al., 1980); that in C1-C3 of NWC appears similar given the data of Engelhardt et al. (1979). Variation in forestomach water is brought about by inflow of dry matter, mineral, free-water, and saliva; osmotically created fluxes; digestion and volatile fatty acid (VFA) production and absorption; and outflow dynamics of digesta (Engelhardt et al., 1979; Faichney and Boston, 1985; Argyle and Baldwin, 1988). A constant supply of saliva prevents complete emptying of the R-R under food deprivation (Hecker et al., 1964). Thus, residence time of water in the R-R is ~ 61 min. in wethers (Faichney and Boston, 1985) and 39–52 min. in pregnant ewes (Faichney et al., 2004). The R-R performs a critical role as a water reservoir during initial stages of water and food deprivation by maintaining and even increasing the plasma pool size during the first 2 days (Hecker et al., 1964), before a decrease in the plasma pool and ECF ensues in ruminants and NWC (Rosenmann and Morrison, 1963; Purohit et al., 1972). This effect may differ in desert-adapted species (Shkolnik et al., 1980). The initial water shift between physiological pools is the mechanism that resists dehydration and protects the ICF. Under intermittent hydration nondesert-adapted sheep and goat breeds drink to 15–20 percent of dehydrated BW, whereas desert-adapted breeds, as exemplified by the Bedouin goat and gazelle, can drink a volume equal to 25–30 percent of dehydrated BW (Shkolnik et al., 1975; Choshniak and Shkolnik, 1977; Shkolnik et al., 1980). The R-R becomes the major temporary water reservoir, holding water until physiological pools become rehydrated (Choshniak and Shkolnik, 1977; Shkolnik et al., 1980). When severely dehydrated domestic livestock consume water to approximately 30 percent of dehydrated BW, toxicity can occur (Church, 1971).

The response of the R-R long-term undernutrition is equivocal (Tyler et al., 1999), possibly due to an interaction with diet digestibility. An increase in R-R weight and water content occurs in association with an increase in ECF where diet quality is poor (sheep: Morris et al., 1962; caribou: Adamczewski et al., 1987). However, when diet digestibility is high, a decrease in feed and water intake is associated with a decrease in R-R fill and water content (caribou and reindeer: Staaland et al., 1984; White et al., 1984a; Ouellet et al., 1997).

Because gut fill can exert an important influence on BW, standardization of weighing procedures by withholding feed and water for 20–24 hours to give a measure of "shrunk" BW is used to minimize these effects (Sahlu et al., 2004). Measurements of BW in animals taken from extant condition are then termed "unshrunk" BW. Alternatively, species-specific estimates of total gut fill, and the water content of the fill, have been used to determine the water content of the "empty" body, also termed ingesta-free BW (Kay et al., 1981; Reimers et al., 1982; Parker et al., 1993b; Gerhart et al., 1996a; Ouellet et al., 1997; Peltier and Barboza, 2003).

BODY WATER AND ESTIMATION OF IN VIVO BODY COMPOSITION

Although BW is the common factor used to determine energy and nutrient requirements, an estimate of body condition improves precision and may change the goals of the management program (see Chapter 4, Energy; Chapter 5, Proteins). Body condition estimates can be made by determination of body condition score (Russel et al., 1969; Gerhart et al., 1996b), but the estimation of body lean and fat are determined more precisely by estimation of TBW using one or more body water markers, provided correction factors are applied (Sheng and Huggins, 1979; Russel et al., 1982). The most preferred markers are antipyrene, deuterated water (DOH), tritiated water (TOH) (Panaretto and Till, 1963; English, 1966; Reid et al., 1968; Holleman et al., 1982), oxygen-18 water (Haggarty, 1991), and urea (Bartle et al., 1988; Gad and Preston, 1990). The inverse relation between TBW/BW and body fat (Pace and Rathbun, 1945; Longhurst et al., 1970; Robbins, 1993) is used to derive prediction equations based on slaughter. The reader is referred to prediction equations developed for sheep (Panaretto, 1963, 1968; Foot and Greenhalgh, 1970a,b; Searle, 1970a,b; Donnelly and Freer, 1974; Searle and Hilmi, 1977; Russel et al., 1982) and goats (Panaretto and Till, 1963). The TBW pool varies between 51–81 percent BW (Staaland et al., 1982; Torbit et al., 1985; NRC 2001, 2003; Peltier and Barboza, 2003) and when gut water is removed, water content of the ingesta-free BW is 55–68 percent (Gerhart et al., 1996a). Variability in TBW content of the ingesta-free BW is largely associated with the quantity of fat because fat is water-free, and the water content of fat-free body mass in adult animals is relatively constant at ~ 73 percent (Pace and Rathbun, 1945; Robbins, 1993), although the reported range is 68–76 percent (Reid et al., 1968; Robbins et al., 1974: Ringberg et al., 1981; Reimers et al., 1982; DelGiudice et al., 1990; Gerhart et al., 1996a). Of the fat-free, water-free mass, 80–82 percent is protein and 18–20 percent is ash (Reid et al., 1968; Robbins, 1993). Water content of the fat-free body mass of immature ruminants exceeds that of adults, decreasing with age from 85 percent in the newborn, with the rate of decrease depending on the rate of fat deposition (Jagusch et al., 1970; Robbins et al., 1974; Ringberg et. al., 1981; Robbins, 1993; Gerhart et al., 1996a). Chemical maturity is defined as the age at which the ratio of water:protein:mineral becomes constant (Widdowson and Dickerson, 1960). Independent of species, from birth to maturity, water, protein, and ash are deposited at respectively 0.654–0.690, 0.239–0.264, and 0.071–0.100 kg/kg of fat-free, ingesta-free BW (Moulton, 1923; Reid et al., 1968; Reimers et al., 1982; Gerhart et al., 1996a).

Thus, body lean and fat can be estimated from TBW after a correction is made for gut water (above) because lean body mass (LBM) is 73 percent water. Body fat is then estimated as empty body weight minus LBM (Holleman et al., 1982). This approach has been used for deer (Parker et al., 1993a,b; Worden and Pekins, 1995; Parker et al., 1999; Stephenson et al., 2002), reindeer/caribou (Cameron and Luick, 1972; Chan-McLeod et al., 1994; Gotaas and Tyler, 1995), and llamas (Rübsamen and Engelhardt, 1975), but modified for application to muskoxen (Peltier and Barboza, 2003; Peltier et al., 2003).

WATER USE: MATCHING WATER INTAKE, WATER LOSS, AND WATER BALANCE

Water Intake

Meeting requirements for water by providing sufficient water to exceed voluntary consumption is a useful management tool (NRC, 1981), but determining water requirement (WR) is a complex process involving the solution of a water balance equation where water intake (WI) must meet water loss (WL):

$$WI = WL$$

However, it is the voluntary consumption of water by drinking or eating snow and ice, termed free water intake (FWI), that is often identified as the water intake variable that needs to be satisfied to meet WR of the animal. The FWI is a component of the WI equation:

$$WI = FWI + PW + MW + RW + (IW)$$

where PW is preformed water in or on food, MW is metabolic water produced by chemical oxidation of metabolized food nutrients, and RW is water released from tissue physiological pools plus ICF-water released on breakdown of protein (muscle). Although usually ignored, IW is a measure of inspired water, but at least one study (King and Finch,

1982) has found an estimate of IW is necessary to balance the water balance equation. In free-ranging animals, measurement of FWI often cannot be made and estimates of WR must be made from determinations of water turnover using isotope dilution kinetics. Isotopes of water, either TOH or DOH, have been used to estimates water turnover rate (alternatively termed water flux and water transfer rate or WTR) (Richmond et al., 1962; Preston, 1969; Macfarlane and Howard, 1972; Holleman et al., 1982; Nagy and Peterson 1988). The measured WTR gives an excellent estimate of the sum of water input sources (Cameron et al., 1976; King and Finch, 1982), provided the animal is in water balance, i.e. in steady state, and correction is made for the overestimation of the total water pool size using TOH (Sheng and Huggins, 1979). However, studies using multiple isotopes (TOH, DOH, and ^{18}O) for the determination of DEE have revealed several sources of error, especially in growing, finishing, and lactating animals that have conditions typical of animals in non-steady state. These errors include overestimation of the water pool, sequestration of isotope in newly formed tissue, losses in feces, and isotope discrimination, all of which can be corrected for (Nagy and Costa, 1980; Fancy et al., 1986; Midwood et al., 1993; Haggarty et al., 1998; Gotaas et al., 2000a,b). Therefore WTR is a direct measure of WI and WL, provided the animal is in water balance, termed steady state in isotope studies (Macfarlane and Howard, 1972; Cameron et al., 1976; King and Finch, 1982).

Thus:

$$WTR = WI = WL$$

Water Loss

Water is lost from the body by evaporation during breathing, by sweating (cutaneous), through drooling or licking (EWL), in urine (UWL), and in feces (FWL).

Thus, in the WL equation:

$$WL = EWL + UWL + FWL + TWL\ (+\ MWL)$$

where EWL includes respiratory + sweating + licking/drooling (often termed insensible water loss), TWL is water loss to physiological pools expansion, plus tissue water gain during accretion of lean body mass and concepta, and MWL is water loss in milk.

Assuming an animal achieves steady state by the intake of free water, then:

$$FWI = WL - (PW + MW + RW)$$

This, too, is a difficult equation to solve. However, substituting WTR (water transfer rate) for WL gives,

$$FWI = WTR - (PW + MW + RW)$$

The equation is solvable, because WTR can be estimated from BW, and PW and MW can be estimated from dry matter intake (DMI), the water content of the feed, and metabolizability of the diet. Any change in BW or body condition can give an estimate of RW. When the BW trend is positive, RW is replaced by TWL.

Where water requirements are expressed as total water intake (TWI) (NRC, 1985),

$$TWI = FWI + PW$$

Because measures of FWI and TWI underestimate WI and WL, water use determined as WTR has been used extensively in situations where FWI cannot be measured.

Sensible water loss is a function of ambient temperature (T_a) and solar radiation. Adaptations that minimize loss include nasal heat exchangers in species adapted to hot (Schmidt-Nielsen, 1964) and cold (Blix et al., 1983a,b) environments that are responsible for a major reduction in EWL. When WI is reduced in domestic and wild ruminants, a major reduction in EWL occurs (Wallace et al., 1972; Seif et al., 1973; Maloiy, 1973). A reduction in WI also is associated with a reduction in UWL and FWL (Maloiy and Taylor, 1971). The reduction in UWL depends on the capacity to concentrate urine (Macfarlane, 1964; Schoen, 1969; NRC, 2003), while that for FWL depends on the capacity to withdraw water from the gut (Hecker et al., 1964; Little et al., 1976) to produce dry feces (Maloiy, 1973; Ostrowski et al., 2003). Thus, hot desert-adapted species can concentrate urine to over 2,000 mOsm/L. Whereas most ruminants concentrate urine to ~ 500 mOsm/L, the reindeer/caribou produces dilute urine (< 100 mOsm/L; Macfarlane, 1964; Cameron et al., 1982). When water restriction occurs at high (32°C: Maloiy and Taylor, 1971; Maloiy 1973; Seif et al., 1973) or low T_a (–14 or –20 °C: Cameron et al., 1982), UWL may be reduced by about 50 percent, exceeding that loss at normal T_a. Under conditions of low protein intake, FWL can be reduced to less than UWL (Cameron et al., 1982). Water content of feces increases with nitrogen content and with content of other osmotically active molecules. But, like urine, the loss of water in feces shows adaptation, in that at any particular nitrogen concentration, hot desert-adapted species can produce feces with water content < 50 percent WW (Maloiy, 1973; Ostrowski et al., 2003). Other species produce feces of 55–60 percent WW when consuming a very low-protein diet, but when consuming higher nitrogen diets water content of feces is > 65 percent WW (Staaland et al., 1984, 1986). At water contents of < 70 percent WW, feces produced are in the form of pellets. As the osmotic load increases water content exceeds 70 percent WW and feces produced are in the form of paste-like tubes to "cowpats." Production of cowpats by cervids is common in spring in association with the intake of plants high in N, P, and K^+; sometimes it is also associated with high levels of internal parasites. The ability to reduce water content of feces is related to active transport of Na^+ and passive absorption of Cl^-, which provides the osmotic gradient for water absorption in the colon (Skadhauge et al., 1980). Water content normally enters the spiral colon at 80–85 percent WW, and decreases linearly to 70 percent at the distal colon and 55–65 percent WW at the rectum (Skadhauge et al., 1980; Staaland et. al., 1984, 1986; Stevens, 1988).

Most insensible water loss is by respiratory evaporation; however, cutaneous loss increases with exercise in some species and control seems to be mediated through both body core temperature and skin temperature (Finch et al., 1982; Parker and Robbins, 1985a,b). Cutaneous loss increases with sweat gland activity, through epitrichial glands associated with hair follicles and, at low rates, by passive diffusion through the skin (Parker and Robbins, 1985a,b). Highest rates of cutaneous water loss occur in relation to solar radiation, the rate of increase escalating with both body weight and air temperature from two- to eight-fold between 15 and 30–35°C (Parker and Robbins, 1985a,b). Measurements obtained outdoors can be over 5 times higher than the same T_a indoors (Maloiy and Hopcraft, 1971), suggesting that a WR measured indoors will be a conservative estimate. Respiratory heat loss involves both nonevaporative and evaporative processes. Nonevaporative heat loss caused by a higher expired than inspired air temperature is an important avenue of loss at low temperatures. To this heat loss must be added the evaporative respiratory loss that involves water loss. At high T_a, the respiratory component of EWL is the major route of evaporative heat loss, and it increases exponentially with T_a (Blaxter et al., 1959a,b; Parker and Robbins, 1985a). The nasal countercurrent system recovers up to 80 percent of potential respiratory water loss, as well as minimizing heat loss (Withers et al., 1979; Blix and Johnsen, 1983). In order to allow such regulation to occur under a heat load or in the cold, central regulation and vascular control over blood flow to both the nasal mucosa and the brain are necessary (Johnsen et al., 1985a,b; 1987).

WATER USE AND WATER SOURCES

Water Use Relative to Body Weight

When dealing with different species and animals of different BW, a first approximation to estimating water use can be obtained from the well-documented relations between WTR and BW. For fed, adult eutherian mammals, usually held within their TNR and maintaining BW, the relation of WTR (mL/d) with BW (g) is given by the equation

$$\text{WTR} = a\text{BW}^b$$

where a = 0.159–0.326, and slope b = 0.79–0.99 (Richmond et al., 1962; Nagy and Peterson, 1998). For eutherian mammals (99 species and 562 observations), a = 0.159 and b = 0.946 (Nagy and Peterson, 1998). For eutherian mammals in the field (28 species, 28 observations), the intercept "a" is higher (0.326) than for penned animals, but the exponent "b" is less (0.818) (Nagy and Peterson, 1998). However, a comparison of expected values for the field and pens indicates a possible overestimation by the equation for penned animals, possibly due to the large number of observations (562) relative to the species (28). Within species, the range in WTR was often six-fold or higher. Observations were not stratified for season, productivity, or sex (Nagy and Peterson, 1998). Thus, the preferred equation relating WTR (mL/day) to BW (g) for pen-fed eutherian mammals, using species means, is:

$$\text{WTR} = 0.159 \times \text{BW}^{0.946}$$

The equation for field animals is:

$$\text{WTR} = 0.708 \times \text{BW}^{0.795}$$

The latter equation gave better estimates of WTR of deer (Lautier et al., 1988) and reindeer in some studies (Cameron and Luick, 1972; Cameron et al., 1976), but the opposite was noted for reindeer and caribou in another (Fancy et al., 1986). Ostrowski et al. (2002) note that the above equations predict a higher WTR than observed in desert species, and they produced a relation for 10 desert-dwelling species that approximates:

$$\text{WTR} = 0.127 \times \text{BW}^{0.926}$$

where WTR is in mL/d and BW is in g.

Water Use Relative to Dry Matter Intake

When water is freely available, total water intake (TWI = FWI + PW, L/d) correlates with DMI (kg/d) (Forbes, 1968; NRC, 1985) for diets of moderate nitrogen content:

$$\text{TWI} = 3.86 \times \text{DMI} - 0.99$$

The usefulness of this relation is limited to when DMI is either known or can be estimated (see Chapter 3). In other studies, WTR was determined in relation to DMI. The difference WTR – TWI is MW in pen-fed animals, but evaporative losses associated with free ranging must be added to field estimates. Thus, at maintenance the range in TWI/DMI and WTR/DMI (L/kg) overlap across species. Some published values are approximately 1.4–3 in sheep (Forbes, 1968; Wallace et al., 1972), 2–3 in goats (Morand-Fehr and Sauvant, 1978; Giger-Reverdin and Giha, 1991), 2.9 in white-tailed deer (Lautier et al., 1988), 2.1–2.9 in mule deer (Knox et al., 1969), 2.0–3.6 in reindeer/caribou (Cameron et al., 1982; White et al., 1984b; Larsen and Blix, 1985; Fancy et al., 1986), and 2–3 in NWC (Van Saun, 2006). However, Silanikove (1989) considers that the WTR/DMI ratio in goats is highly variable and yields only a first approximation of WR. Factors such as nitrogen, oxalate, and mineral content of feeds can each increase output of water in urine, resulting in an increase in FWI independent of DMI (Wilson, 1966a,b). Wallace et al. (1972) report that the TWI/DMI in sheep (1.37 mL/g) represents one component (FWL + UWL) of WR, the other being attributable to metabolizable energy intake (MEI) (617 mL/kcal), which affects EWL.

Water Use Relative to Energy Intake

Under standardized conditions, it is theorized that water use should relate to energy metabolism (Macfarlane and Howard, 1972) rather than DMI. Therefore, an appropriate relation would be between FWI, or WTR, with digestible energy intake (DEI) or MEI, or with DEE, the latter being determined with doubly labeled water (Nagy, 1989; Haggarty, 1991). In agreement, water requirements for goats relate to daily energy intake at 1 mol water/5 mol oxygen (Silanikove 1989), 1 mL/kcal of MEI in NWC (Fowler, 1998), and 0.62 mL/kcal MEI for one factor, combined with 1.37 mL/kg DMI in sheep (Wallace et al., 1972). The generalized requirement, 1 mL/kcal MEI, is identical to that recommended for nonruminant species and primates (NRC, 1989, 2003). Whether the reported water/energy ratios are the same for body growth, gestation, and lactation is not clear.

Evidence that WTR depends on energy intake or metabolic rate should be that "b" in the interspecies allometry should be the same as for metabolic rate, namely b = 0.75. The exponent "b" (range 0.79–0.90) apparently exceeds the expected 0.75 for energy metabolism (see Chapter 4). Given the variable effect that body fat has on BW, it is not surprising that "b" is variable among studies. It has been suggested that the more appropriate allometry would be to relate WTR to TBW, and the expression would be $aTBW(L)^b$ (Macfarlane and Howard, 1972). Despite this limitation, estimates of "b" are not statistically greater than 0.75 (Nagy and Peterson, 1988). Thus estimates frequently are expressed as kg $BW^{0.75}$. For example, French recommendations for goats give a daily maintenance WR as 146 g[mL]/ kg $BW^{0.75}$ (Morand-Fehr and Sauvant, 1978; NRC, 1981), although a lower value 107 mL/kg $BW^{0.75}$ is recommended by McGregor (2003), and for NWC the maintenance requirement is 122 g[mL]/kg $BW^{0.75}$ (Van Saun, 2006). The strongest direct support for a linkage between water and energy metabolism is for an interspecies data set (9 species, BW range 0.05–28.6 kg) in which WTR and DEI were estimated on the same individuals fed at approximately maintenance and held within the TNR (Silanikove, 1989). The correlation of WTR and DEI was very high ($r^2 = 0.996$, n = 16, $P < 0.001$). Among breeds of goats the correlation of WTR with DEI is equally high ($r^2 = 0.99$, n = 32) (Silanikove, 1989). For Bedouin and Swiss Saanen goats offered two feed types and restricted versus ad libitum feed intake, the slope WTR/DEI (L/Mcal) was 0.91 ± 0.06, not statistically different from a slope of 1.0, and with no differences between desert and temperate breeds. For lactating goats once water loss in milk was subtracted from the estimate of water intake, there was no difference from nonlactating goats. Therefore, there is sufficient evidence to recommend making an estimation of WR based on WTR (mL/kg BW × d^{-1}) and DEI (kcal/kg BW × d^{-1}) in goats using the equation (Silanikove, 1989):

$$WTR = 0.911 \times DEI - 5.38$$

The slope 0.911 mL/kcal DEI should be the same for MEI, provided ME content/kcal DE is constant (0.82, Chapter 3). The TWI/DEI ratio for sheep is 0.524 mL/kcal using a factorial approach (Wallace et al., 1972), and both estimates are lower than WTR/DEI or WTR/MEI for goats (1.2–1.3 mL/kcal) and for NWC (1.0 mL/kcal MEI; Fowler, 1998; NRC, 1989, 2003). Evidence that water use and requirement is linked to DEI and MEI above maintenance has not been adequately evaluated for growing animals. Also, the WTR/DEI ratio would not be applicable when diets result in UWL that is not associated with DEI. Diets containing high protein, oxalates, and salt loads increase UWL. For animals detoxifying secondary compounds in browse-based diets, an increase in UWL may occur in excess predicted from the WTR/DEI ratio. An additional requirement for water could exist for animals in the field if energy costs of activity are not compensated for by DEI, such as in moving between water and feeding sites (Squires and Wilson, 1971; McGregor, 2003) and seasonal migration. Therefore, water requirements may be higher than those based on DEI alone.

Effects of Season and Cold

Water in the R-R can act as a thermal buffer to intake of frozen food and cold water in domestic and cervid species and serves to protect the fermentation capacity (Butcher, 1970; Cameron et al., 1975; White, 1975; Brod et al., 1982). In sheep, ingestion of water lowers rumen temperature and requires a recovery time of 1–1.7 hours depending on initial R-R temperature, which could affect rumen microbial function (Brod et al., 1982). At T_a below the lower critical temperature (T_{lc}), mechanisms that conserve water are important because of the added cost of raising the temperature of free water and preformed water in feed from ambient to deep body temperature (White, 1979). However, at higher T_a (8°C), the energy cost of warming feed and water to body temperature is negligible (Blaxter et al., 1959a,b). Although low water temperature does not affect nitrogen balance or DM, protein, or fiber digestibility (Church, 1971), Nicol and Young (1981) argue that heating consumed water at this T_a could increase ME requirement in lean sheep and cattle. Whatever the heat and water conservation mechanism involved, water turnover in winter is approximately one-fourth that in summer in nonproductive wild ruminants, such as female reindeer (Cameron and Luick, 1972; Cameron et al., 1982; Larsen and Blix, 1985; Fancy et al., 1986). The WTR of reindeer in winter is a function of the requirement to meet fecal, urine, and respiratory water losses. In this species, dilute urine is produced. Thus, both urine and fecal water losses reflect requirements to excrete osmotically active nitrogenous and mineral components of the diet (Cameron et al., 1982).

In north temperate species, it is difficult to separate the effects of cold per se from seasonal acclimatization. The seasonal decrease in resting metabolism is associated with a decrease in metabolizable energy required for maintenance (ME_m), voluntary DMI (Tyler et al., 1999), and WTR in winter (Cameron and Luick, 1972; Larsen and Blix, 1985; White and Fancy, 1986). The seasonal decrease in WTR is > 4-fold, whereas it approximates 2.5-fold for DMI. This suggests an uncoupling of the WTR/DMI relation on a seasonal basis, and/or an increase in EWL for thermoregulation in summer. Whereas seasonal changes in WTR can be as highly correlated with mean daily T_a as with DMI (Larsen and Blix, 1985), WTR also is influenced by seasonal diet quality (Cameron and Luick, 1972). Seasonal changes in WTR of cervids occur even when basal metabolic rate (BMR) does not change seasonally, indicating that WTR reflects the additional energy metabolism of free existence and not simply to BMR. When growth and lactation are included, seasonal differences in WTR of the free-ranging animals approaches six-fold from winter minima to summer maxima (Nagy and Peterson, 1988; Parker et al., 1993b).

Effects of Heat and Water Deprivation

Exposure to high temperatures affects water use in two ways: DMI may decline, but requirements for evaporative and cutaneous cooling increase. Winchester and Morris (1956) showed that TWI/DMI increased exponentially with ambient temperature for both *Bos taurus* and *B. indicus*. Forbes et al. (1968), using pen-fed sheep, found that the ratio of TWI/DMI increased with mean weekly T_a (°C):

$$TWI/DMI = 0.18 \times T_a + 1.25$$

This equation has been adopted for sheep fed at maintenance to account for the effect of T_a on WR (NRC, 1985). These approaches to setting WR do not take into account the extra water requirements associated with water loss by direct exposure to solar radiation (King et al., 1975; King, 1982). For the free-ranging animal, evaporative cooling through respiration and cutaneous loss through sweat glands and drooling or licking onto body surfaces are vital mechanisms for thermoregulation when $T_a > T_{lc}$. Although these cooling mechanisms can increase WR, desert species also show adaptations that minimize water losses behaviorally and through physiological responses involving EWL, UWL, and FWL, and in some species, access to drinking water may not be required (Lynch et al., 1972) when preformed water in feed is adequate at > 70–76 percent WW (King, 1982; Williams et al., 2001; Ostrowski et al., 2002). Other adaptations include the ability to take on a short-term heat load that can be dissipated at night (Finch and Robertshaw, 1979; Finch and King, 1982; Ostrowski et al., 2003), and temporal storage of water for use when water is not available (e.g., black Bedouin goat: Shkolnik et al., 1980). For desert goats, sheep, and cattle, water use, measured as WTR, is approximately twice as high in the wet summer than in the dry summer and winter (Aggrey, 1982; El Hadi and Hassan, 1982; Kamal, 1982; King, 1982; Ranjhan et al., 1982). During the dry period some species, including the Bedouin goat, increase digestive efficiency even as feed quality declines (Brosh et al., 1986) and as resting and field metabolic rate decreases (Finch and King, 1982; Williams et al., 2001).

Species and Breed Effects

In general, those species and breeds that have evolved or been selected for conditions of seasonal water shortage exhibit low water use compared with temperate species and breeds (Macfarlane, 1964; Taylor, 1968a; Macfarlane and Howard, 1970; Maloiy and Taylor, 1971; Macfarlane and Howard, 1972; Shkolnik et al., 1972, 1980; King, 1982; Cameron et al., 1982; Lautier et al., 1988; Ostrowski et al., 2002; McGregor, 2003). Adaptations involve both behavioral and physiological responses that maximize WI and minimize WL. Silanikove (1989) showed that apparent lower WTR by desert species reflected their lower energy requirements. For a wide range in BW, the water use by small ruminants and nonruminant herbivores is relatively constant at 1 mol water/5 mol oxygen. Likewise, differences between races, breeds, or types of sheep and goats show variation in water use. Among breeds of sheep and goats, meat types (e.g., Boer goats: Casey and Van Niekerk, 1988) have a higher water use than wool/Angora types (McGregor, 1986), while under comparable conditions water use by goats of either type is higher than sheep under dry conditions in Australia, Sudan, and East and South Africa (Maloiy and Taylor, 1971; El Hadi and Hassan, 1982; King, 1982; McGregor, 2003), although the opposite has been shown for goats and sheep in India (Ranjhan et al., 1982). Too few deer species have been examined under equivalent nutritional conditions to determine differences in water use. Taylor (1968a) ranked East African bovids for their minimum WR, and an extension of this work shows the minimum WR of the oryx is clearly lower than the Grant's gazelle, which is equivalent to the haired sheep (Maloiy and Taylor, 1971). Based on interspecies allometry, Nagy and Peterson (1988) showed that in winter and under dry conditions, WTR of some deer species are further below the interspecies line (expressed as a percent of interspecies WTR with mule deer 58 and reindeer 17–34) than a number of ruminants considered to have enhanced water economy (bighorn sheep 85; hartebeest 61; wildebeest 64; Thompson's gazelle 90) and are similar to the oryx (35) and the camel (49), both of which are considered to have low minimum WR. Likewise NWC show seasonally low WTR relative to the interspecies line (guanaco 39; llama 29).

The Water Economy Index

Under conditions where DMI, DEI, and MEI are known, it is possible to estimate the component of WTR attributable to FWI above that required for energy metabolism (intake and expenditure). This approach is based on laboratory and ecological field studies that show that daily WTR (mL)/DEE (kcal), termed water economy index (WEI), is a constant independent of BW (Nagy and Peterson, 1988). The WEI for free-living wild animals ranges from 0.42–1.04 mL/kcal for herbivores and the theoretical WEI for a fasting animal is 0.04 mL/kcal (Nagy and Peterson, 1988). Values of WEI in excess of 1.04 mL/kcal indicate an additional intake of water that is required to meet nonenergy-associated costs such as thermoregulatory cooling, excretion of water ingested with feed with excessive preformed water, or a requirement to excrete an osmotic load (nitrogen or solute). A WEI of < 0.71 mL/kcal indicates minimal or no intake of free water, all requirements being met by PW and MW. Nagy and Peterson (1988) report WEI for mule deer at 0.194 and 0.201 mL/kJ (0.81, 0.84 mL/kcal). These values indicate no extra requirement for water independent of DEE. However, WEI calculations that can be made for both penned and free-ranging ruminants exceed 1.04 mL/kcal, suggesting an added WR. For pen-fed reindeer, WEI estimates are lower during winter (1.15 mL/kcal; Gotaas et al., 2000a) than in pen-fed reindeer and sheep in summer (respectively, 1.66 mL/kcal; Gotaas et al., 2000a, and 2.23 mL/kcal; Midwood et al., 1994). For deer at pasture, WEI is high at 1.33 mL/kg for young male reindeer in winter (Gotaas et al., 2000b) vs. 1.98 mL/kcal for nonlactating red deer hinds in summer (Haggarty et al., 1998).

Gestation

Water use during gestation increases 126 percent from the first to fifth month (Head, 1953; ARC, 1980), and 30–136 percent from the third to fifth month in sheep (Head, 1953; Forbes, 1968; ARC, 1980). At 3 months' gestation, TWI is 106 percent greater than nonpregnant ewes, but increases to 138 percent by the fifth month (Forbes, 1968), or a 30 percent increase in the final 2 months (Forbes, 1968). For twin-bearing ewes, the increase in TWI compared with nonpregnant ewes at 3 months (125–150 percent) increased to an even greater extent at 5 months (212–220 percent) (Head, 1953; Forbes, 1968; ARC, 1980); this represents a 46–70 percent increase in the final 2 months. Thus at term, TWI/DMI is 4.3–5.2 L/kg in ewes bearing single lambs, and 7–8 L/kg in twin-bearing ewes, which is almost 2 times that at maintenance (2–3 L/kg) for single and 3.5 times for twins. For sheep with a single fetus in the final trimester, WR is approximately 215–290 mL/kg $BW^{0.75}$, which is very high compared with that for goats of 140 mL/kg $BW^{0.75}$. The latter estimate is 31 percent higher than the comparative WR of maintenance (Giger-Reverdin and Gihad, 1991; McGregor, 2003). There are few comparisons of WTR of pregnant versus nonpregnant animals (Nagy and Peterson, 1988). Field estimates of WTR by nonpregnant reindeer in one year with those pregnant the next (Cameron and Luick, 1972: 186 vs. 236 mL/kg $BW^{0.75}$) suggest a 26 percent increase, considerably less than the experimental findings for sheep but closer to that for goats. Net water flow to the conceptus cannot account for observed increases in TWI of sheep. In ewes 5 months pregnant, net water flow to the conceptus at 80–83 mL/d (Faichney et al., 2004) accounts for an insignificant portion of the increase in WR of pregnancy. Increasing energy demands of pregnancy plus increased urinary excretion are considered to drive the higher TWI of pregnancy (Forbes, 1968). This interpretation is supported by observations that water restriction of pregnant ewes results in reduced DMI, and possibly to ketosis in ewes carrying twin fetuses (Forbes, 1968). Thus it should be possible to estimate WR from increases in DMI, DEI, MEI, or energy expenditure associated with pregnancy as detailed in Chapters 3 and 4 in this publication. More studies are needed to account for the differences for sheep and goats, and also for those animals that are free ranging.

Lactation

The WR for lactation have been expressed as a total requirement, 3.5 kg(L)/kg(L) milk synthesized, as in the dairy goat (Bergmann, 1932), but the factorial approach, adding MWL to WR at maintenance, is also recommended (goats: Morand-Fehr and Sauvant, 1978). The factorial estimation of WR allows for variability in WI associated with energy intake, milk production, and possible increases in EWL. For example, WTR during lactation increases by the amount of milk water produced above maintenance water use, which includes that metabolic water associated with milk synthesis (Silanikove, 1989). For animals in the field, EWL must be added (Macfarlane and Howard, 1972). Thus, WTR increases by 30–150 percent in lactating vs. nonlactating female sheep, goats, and cervids (Forbes, 1968; Brown and Lynch, 1972; Cameron and Luick, 1972; Macfarlane and Howard, 1972; Maltz and Shkolnik, 1980; Wright, 1982; McGregor, 2003). Greater increases in water use are associated with females nursing twins and triplets, because milk yield can double for twins over singles (Sadleir, 1980; Dove, 1988). Under ad libitum feeding, maternal DMI intake increases proportionally to milk production (Sadleir, 1982), and, as a consequence, TWI/DMI in lactating ewes is greater than in nonlactating ewes (Forbes, 1968). However, trends in WTR and DMI are displaced relative to each other, because peak DMI occurs after peak milk production, and also peak WTR.

Although daily peak milk production in ruminants scales at 50–65 mL/kg $BW^{0.75}$ for single offspring (Oftedal, 1984, 1985), it can be up to three times higher in milk-type sheep and goats and in the Bedouin goat (145–152 mL/kg $BW^{0.75}$: Maltz and Shkolnik, 1980; Shkolnik et al., 1980). Water secreted in milk is highly controlled by lactose content, because lactose and Na^+ and K^+ are the primary osmoregulators in milk (Jenness and Sloan, 1970; Martin, 1984). Thus, no simple relation predicts MWL, because it varies between species (Jenness and Sloan, 1970; Martin, 1984) and between types of animals and stage within the lactation cycle (Laben, 1963; Luick et al., 1974). The added water intake that is required to meet MWL, variably determined as 1.43 kg(L)/kg(L) milk (Morand-Fehr and Sauvant, 1978) or 1.0 L water/L MWL (Silanikove, 1989), is that associated with maintenance and milk synthesis (146 mL/kg $BW^{0.75}$: Morand-Fehr and Sauvant, 1978). The combination gives an estimated 200–220 mL/kg $BW^{0.75}$ for female sheep and goats producing milk at 50–60 mL/kg $BW^{0.75}$, and 272 mL/kg $BW^{0.75}$ for a female Bedouin goat producing milk at 145 mL/kg $BW^{0.75}$. Water use by penned goats in mid-lactation is 165 mL/kg $BW^{0.75}$ (McGregor, 2003), which is in good agreement with the factorial estimate.

At pasture, daily WTR of sheep (289–627 mL/kg $BW^{0.75}$: Brown and Lynch, 1972; Russel et al., 1982; Dove, 1988), reindeer (562 mL/kg $BW^{0.75}$; Cameron and Luick, 1972), and Bedouin goats under high T_a (453 mL/kg $BW^{0.75}$: Maltz and Shkolnik, 1980) exceed the WR estimated by the factorial process possibly due to using a low estimate for maintenance. Although not accurately determined, maintenance WR appears higher in summer than winter in animals in the field (Nagy and Peterson, 1988). Daily field WTR in winter (reindeer 186–231 mL/kg $BW^{0.75}$: Cameron and Luick, 1975; Gotaas et al., 2000a,b) is 50–60 percent of that in summer (red deer 359 mL/kg $BW^{0.75}$: Haggarty et al., 1998). If a daily maintenance WR for animals that are lactating in the field of 359 mL/kg $BW^{0.75}$ is assumed, the predicted daily WR for a milk production of 55 mL/kg $BW^{0.75}$ is 412–433 mL/kg $BW^{0.75}$, which is in good agreement with field estimates of WTR. Thus, the factorial approach approximates that for pen-fed lactating animals, but underestimates WR of animals under field and hot conditions by up to 50 percent unless an appropriate field maintenance WR is assumed.

Growth

Water intake in milk satisfies the WR of offspring for the first 2–3 weeks of age (Dove, 1988). However, the contribution made by milk water intake to WTR of the offspring (M, percent) is best described by an exponential decline with age (Dove, 1988):

$$M = 129.5e^{(-0.0225 \times t)}$$

where t is time after birth in days. Because growth rates of nursing offspring correlate with milk intake (Yates et al., 1971; Dove and Freer, 1979; White and Luick, 1984; Dove, 1988; Landete-Castillejos et al., 2001), WTR of offspring also correlate with their growth rates, yielding estimates of 77–129 g BW gain/L WTR (Yates et al., 1971; Dove and Freer, 1979; Dove and Axelsen, 1979; White et al., 1984b), which converts to a WR for growth of 8–13 mL/g BW gain. To this growth requirement must be added a daily maintenance WR of the offspring of 120–140 mL/kg $BW^{0.75}$ (White and Luick, 1984; White et al., 1984b), or 195 mL/kg $BW^{0.75}$. This factorial approach predicts a WR of 255–316 mL/kg $BW^{0.75}$ for offspring average daily gain (ADG) of 100–400 g/d. In nursing offspring, WTR is 232–376 mL/kg $BW^{0.75}$ in sheep, reindeer, and caribou (McEwan and Whitehead, 1971; Dove and Freer, 1979; Dove, 1988; Parker et al., 1990), but can be as high as 450 mL/kg $BW^{0.75}$ in nursing muskox with BW gain of 418–575 g/d (White et al., 1984b). Thus it appears that WR of the nursing offspring can be estimated reasonably from maintenance plus the expected growth rate.

For weaned animals, water use is 32–37 g(DM) gain/L WTR (125–144 g BW gain)/L WTR: Yates et al., 1971; Dove and Axelsen, 1979), which converts to a WR for growth of 7–8 mL/g BW gain. Assuming daily maintenance water use of weaned animals in pens is 143 mL/kg $BW^{0.75}$ (range 137–164 in black-tailed deer: Parker et al., 1993a; 146 mL/kg $BW^{0.75}$ in reindeer/caribou: White et al., 1984b), the predicted WR for BW gain of 200–400 g/d is 244–348 mL/kg $BW^{0.75}$. This range in WR compares favorably with daily WTR of 232 mL/kg $BW^{0.75}$ during growth in pen-fed black-tailed deer (Parker et al., 1993b), 180–582 mL/kg $BW^{0.75}$ in free-ranging, weaned black-tailed deer (Parker et al., 1993b), and 259–484 mL/kg $BW^{0.75}$ for mature animals making BW gain (reindeer: Cameron et al., 1972; sheep: Macfarlane and Howard, 1972; Russel et al., 1982; caribou: White et al., 1984a). The range in WTR of cervids in the field exceeds the predicted WR for growing animals. Although this could be due to a conservative estimate of maintenance WR, a more likely explanation is that the highest daily WTR coincide with availability of high moisture forage (Parker et al., 1993b). Therefore, daily WTR in excess of 350 mL/kg $BW^{0.75}$ may reflect water use in excess of the WR in growing animals utilizing feed of high water content.

WATER QUALITY

Detailed assessments of the effect of water quality on animal requirements and productivity have been published by Church (1971), NRC (1974, 1981), ARC (1980), McGregor (2003), and Van Saun (2006). Contaminants of water for small ruminants, other than high concentrations of mineral salts, include excess microbial loads, toxins such as heavy metals and polychlorinated biphenyls, and debris such as plastic bags. Additionally, contamination of water from agricultural practices or industry (e.g., pesticides, herbicides, and hydrogen cyanide) can result in altered WI and, consequently, DMI. Because almost all contaminants are deleterious to animals, they should be avoided. However, minerals such as calcium, phosphorus, magnesium, and sulfur that are dissolved in drinking water also can affect water intake. Usually an increase in concentration is associated with a decrease in WI that can also result in a decrease in DMI. On the other hand, excessive intake of salts such as NaCl, either in the drinking water or feed, can result in an increase in WI as the animal attempts to eliminate excess Na^+ (Wilson, 1966a). Provided DMI does not decrease and the animal does not display other harmful effects, the animal is said to tolerate the salt load (Peirce, 1959). Thus, total dissolved solid concentrations of 2,000–4,900 ppm may result in temporary water refusal, and young animals will generally show a greater decrease in WI because of increasing total solids than will adults. Abrupt increases in total solid concentrations, as opposed to slower changes, will have a more drastic effect on water consumption. Based on data from Herrick (1971), Church (1971) has compiled a list of limiting levels of solids and salts in drinking water above which productivity will be limited. As a summary, sheep, and by inference goats, cervids, and NWC, may tolerate up to 1.7 percent total dissolved solids, 0.7 percent chlorides, 0.1 percent sulfates, and 1.3 percent sodium chloride (Peirce, 1959). Animals at pasture and in the wild obtain drinking water from a variety of sources that contain variable amounts of mineral and organic substances. Based on concentration ratios of Ca-Mg/CO_3, Ca-Mg/SO_4-Cl, Na-K/CO_3-HCO_3, and Na-K/SO_4-Cl, natural streams in the United States have been classified into these four categories (Ca-Mg/CO_3, Ca-Mg/SO_4-Cl, Na-K/CO_3-HCO_3, and Na-K/SO_4-Cl) for determination of likely consequences for animals of hardness, pH, and mineral balance. In addition, the absolute concentrations of the chemicals in ponds, lakes, and artesian waters can be used to assess the quality of the water supply for animals (Church, 1971). Recommended limits on concentration of potentially toxic minerals (arsenic, cadmium, chromium, cobalt, copper, fluoride, lead, mercury, nickel, nitrate-N, nitrite-N, vanadium, and zinc) in drinking water have been made in a separate NRC publication (NRC, 1974). In many instances these minerals may support animal production when in trace amounts (e.g., copper, cobalt, fluoride, and zinc). Likewise, whereas high concentrations of sulfates may not be tolerated, or may be toxic producing thiamin deficiency and polioencephalomalacia (Chapter 8), low concentrations can support synthesis of amino acids in ruminants (Chapter 7). Depending on the concentrations of major minerals in the water supply, drinking water can supply an appreciable contribution to the full daily requirements, especially of sodium, calcium, magnesium, and potassium (NRC, 1974; Chapter 7). At pasture, where water intake increases to meet requirements to excrete a salt load, providing sufficient water, especially in the summer or dry season, can be a problem. Watering points must be distributed to minimize overgrazing of adjacent pastures (Wilson, 1966a; Squires and Wilson, 1971). Since grazing animals can drink up to five times daily under hot dry conditions, location of watering sites relative to pasture is important to maintaining productivity (Wilson, 1966b). Care in provisioning with water becomes a challenge under drought conditions when water resources become concentrated in minerals and contaminants as water evaporates (McGregor, 2003). In contrast, under cool temperate conditions, water need not be provided because the PW of pasture plants plus dew and other factors can meet requirements (Lynch et al., 1972). Under very wet conditions, intake of fresh pasture has been linked to thiamin deficiency and polioencephalomalacia (Chapter 8).

WATER REQUIREMENTS

Approaches and Methods

In previous recommendations on WR for goats and sheep, values used were based on water use, expressed as FWI or TWI, by animals in relation to DMI at maintenance plus increased allowances for gestation, lactation, and average weekly T_a (ARC, 1980; NRC, 1981, 1985, 2000; McGregor, 2003). This factorial approach also can be used to estimate WR of nursing and weaned offspring; however, estimates of WR have been neither evaluated nor validated in growing animals. For animals in the field, the increased WL of free existence is an added component of WR, but it is difficult to quantify. Therefore, rather than determining a factorial estimate of WR, more confidence can be placed on measures of WTR as estimates of WR for growing animals and for those at pasture or free ranging. The WTR of these animals is assumed to reflect water use that is required to optimize the efficient use of ME for maintenance and production for the given environmental conditions. Other than a study with grazing sheep (Brown and Lynch, 1972; Lynch et al., 1972), few studies have attempted to serially reduce TWI to determine minimal requirements as proposed by Taylor (1968a) and Maloiy and Taylor (1971) when evaluating relative water use and WRs of African ungulates. For African goats and fat-tailed (haired) sheep, daily TWI was reduced from a voluntary 800 mL/kg BW to approximately 400 mL/kg BW as an estimate of minimal WR (Maloiy and Taylor, 1971), but DMI also was reduced. Thus, when WI is restricted, productivity can be affected, and although estimating minimal WR in this way is a valid means for evaluating relative water dependency of breeds and species, its efficacy as a determinant of WR for maintenance and production is questioned. A number of studies confirm that under hot conditions, DMI, BW, and milk production in sheep (Macfarlane et al., 1961; Brown and Lynch, 1972;

Lynch et al., 1972; Bohra and Gosh, 1977; Laden et al., 1987), goats (Maltz and Shkolnik, 1980; Brosh et al., 1986), and white-tailed deer (Lautier et al., 1988) is reduced. In contrast, when sheep and deer are not heat stressed, a limited water restriction does not necessarily result in a decrease in DMI (Singh et al., 1976; Purohit et al., 1976) because behavioral compensation is possible, for example by nighttime grazing, particularly when use of PW, dew, and guttation water on pasture enhances WI (Taylor, 1968b; Brown and Lynch, 1972; Lynch et al., 1972).

Prediction of WR based on FWI—i.e., the minimum amount of drinking water that should be made available to the animal—has many limitations because of the extreme variation in the PW content of feed resources. For example, PW in feed ranges from near zero in cereal grains to 50 percent WW in leafy monocotyledons and dicotyledons, to as high as 70 percent in winter-spring temperate pastures, and 80 percent in fruits and berries. In addition, FWI includes water obtained from dew, guttation (Brown and Lynch, 1972), and snow and ice (Luick and White, 1977). For north temperate species, provision of fresh snow is essential to satisfy preference for snow over water in winter (Luick and White, 1977). Therefore most recommendations of WR are expressed as WTR or as TWI (ARC, 1980; NRC, 1985), where TWI = FWI + PW.

Water Requirements and Water Availability

To overcome limitations in calculating WR by the factorial approach or based on WTR, it has been recommended that water is made freely available. In many instances, making water freely available is a requirement for husbanding confined animals and those at pasture (Church, 1971). Because animals have a wide array of drinking habits, providing water at all times rather than for a limited daily duration also is recommended (Church, 1971). Providing shade in summer and windbreaks in winter, in conjunction with clean water or snow, allows individuals to reach water equilibrium using behavioral responses to balance nutritional and environmental drivers such as PW content of feed, feed quality, feed distribution, feed contaminants, T_a, solar radiation, wind, rain, sleet, or snow. At pasture, denying productive animals, such as lactating sheep, access to water, even when nonproductive types appear to thrive without access to free water, can result in poor health and death of mother and offspring (Lynch et al., 1972).

Factorial Estimation of Water Requirements

Although the factorial approach to estimating WR is based on the sum of WR for maintenance plus the WR for production (gestation, lactation, growth), Wallace et al. (1972), working with penned sheep, recommended determination of WR for maintenance based on two parts: (1) the liquid WI (g/d) that balances UWL + FWL, which was a product of DMI (g/d) (WI = 1.37 × DMI); plus (2) WI (g/d) that balances EWL, which was driven by MEI (Mcal/d) (WI = 617 × MEI). This factorial approach combines two separate components that drive water loss, but it does not account for requirements to excrete excesses of osmotically active components that increase UWL, nor the effects of T_a. Therefore recommendations for determining WR for maintenance are usually based on measures or estimates of TWI at maintenance energy balance, or WTR of free-ranging animals at constant BW. When only BW is known, daily TWI approximates 107–146 mL (g)/kg $BW^{0.75}$. Where DMI is known, the equation for sheep, TWI = 3.86 × DMI – 0.99 (Forbes, 1978), is recommended. For other species, including NWC, published relations on TWI range from 2.0–3.6 L/kg DMI. On a metabolic rate basis, WR approximates 1 mL(g)/kcal energy expenditure (NRC, 1989, 2003) or 1.2–1.3 mL(g) TWI/kcal DEI. However, a better-documented recommendation is between daily WTR and DEI (WTR (mL/kg BW) = –5.4 + 0.911 × DEI (kcal/kg BW: Silanikove, 1989). To determine TWI from WTR, an estimate of MW plus that associated with free existence activity is needed because allometric equations were developed mainly on free-ranging animals. An estimate of MW can be made directly from the composition of digested energy (proportion of carbohydrate, protein, and fat), assuming all is oxidized at maintenance. Metabolic water usually contributes 5–10 percent of TWI.

For pregnancy no factorial approach has been made to separate maternal WR from conceptus growth. Thus, WR for gestation has been reported as TWI or WTR relative to animals at maintenance or to nonpregnant controls. Daily WR is two times maintenance in sheep (215–290 mL/kg $BW^{0.75}$), 31 percent higher in goats (140 mL/kg $BW^{0.75}$), and 26 percent higher than daily field maintenance in reindeer (236 mL/kg $BW^{0.75}$). At term, TWI/DMI estimates for sheep bearing a single fetus is 4.3–5.2 L/kg, and for sheep bearing twin fetuses is 7–8 L/kg.

The WR for lactation can be estimated as the sum of daily maintenance (146 mL/kg $BW^{0.75}$) plus expected water output in milk (peak 50–150 mL/kg $BW^{0.75}$) that declines exponentially following peak MWL. For animals in the field, daily maintenance WTR during summer when animals are lactating approximates 359 mL/kg $BW^{0.75}$ to which must be added MWL. From mid- to late-lactation, maternal BW gains in some species require the additional WR for ADG.

For the preweaned animal, daily maintenance WR approximates 195 mL/kg $BW^{0.75}$ plus WR for growth of 8 mL/g BW ADG. For the weaned animal, daily maintenance WR in pens and free ranging approximates 140 and 236 mL/kg $BW^{0.75}$, respectively, plus a growth requirement of 7.5 mL/g BW ADG. There are too few estimates of WR of the bottle-fed and weaned offspring to verify these equations. In the case of cervids, estimates are even fewer, and many are deduced from field studies that involve added WR of free existence.

TABLE 9-1 Comparison of Estimates of Daily Water Requirements of Goats[a]

Reference	Expression	Unit or Equation	Daily WR (L)	Daily DMI (kg)
Maintenance (TWI)				
Morand-Fehr and Savant, 1978	g/kg $BW^{0.75}$	146	2.75	
Giger-Reverdin and Gihad, 1991	g/kg $BW^{0.75}$	107	2.01	
Giger-Reverdin and Gihad, 1991	L/kg DMI	3	3.36	1.12
Forbes, 1968	DMI (kg)	3.86 × DMI – 0.99	3.33	1.12
Silanikove, 1989	DEI (kcal/kg(BW))	0.911 × DEI – 5.38	1.56	1.12
Literature mean			2.24	
Allometry (WTR)				
Nagy and Peterson, 1988	BW(g), WTR (mL)	0.159 × g $BW^{0.946}$	4.43	
Nagy and Peterson, 1988	BW(g), WTR (mL)	0.708 × g $BW^{0.795}$	3.85	
WEI (mL/kcal)				
Nagy and Peterson, 1988	WTR/DEE		(0.42–1.04)	
Silanikove, 1989	WTR/DEE		0.83	
Mean	WTR/MEI	2,240/(2.04 × 1.12)	0.98	

[a]Assumed BW is 50 kg. Daily DMI is from Sahlu et al., 2004. DEI is based on energy content of 2.0 kcal/kg. DEE is taken as MEI for a pen-fed goat at maintenance.

A Comparison of Estimates of Water Requirements at Maintenance

The most reproducible situation allowing a comparison of estimates of daily WR is the adult animal fed at maintenance. Table 9-1 shows a comparison of recommendations for estimating the WR of a 50 kg meat or indigenous goat at maintenance. To make the comparison, a daily DMI of 1.12 kg was assumed (Sahlu et al., 2004), with a digestible energy content of 2.0 kcal/kg and a daily DEI of 45.1 kcal/kg BW. The mean WR was 2.54 L/d, with a range of 1.56 L/d based on DEI (Silanikove equation for goats), to 3.36 L/d based on a recommendation of 3 L/kg DMI. If WTR is estimated from the allometric equation, the minimal estimate is 3.85 L/d, and is higher than WR due to added contributions of free existence. Using a DEE estimate of 1,873 kcal (100 kcal/kg $BW^{0.75}$), the WEI (Nagy and Peterson, 1988) of 0.83–1.36 mL/kcal suggests a minimum water use for thermoregulation because the upper value of the range where WTR/DEE is balanced is 1.04 mL/kcal.

REFERENCES

Adamczewski, J. Z., C. C. Gates, R. J. Hudson, and M. A. Price. 1987. Seasonal changes in body composition of mature female caribou and calves (*Rangifer tarandus groenlandicus*) on an Arctic island with limited winter resources. Can. J. Zool. 65:1149–1157.

Aggrey, E. K. 1982. Seasonal changes in water content and turnover in cattle, sheep and goats grazing under humid tropical conditions in Ghana. Pp. 133–142 in Use of Tritiated Water in Studies of Production and Adaptation in Ruminants. Vienna: International Atomic Energy Agency.

Andrew, S. M., R. A. Erdman, and D. R. Waldo. 1995. Prediction of body-composition of dairy-cows at 3 physiological stages from deuterium-oxide and urea dilution. J. Dairy Sci. 78:1083–1095.

ARC (Agricultural Research Council). 1980. The Nutrient Requirements of Farm Livestock. Technical Review. Farnham Royal, UK: Commonwealth Agricultural Research Bureau.

Argyle, J. L., and R. L. Baldwin, 1988. Modeling of rumen water kinetics and effects of rumen pH changes. J. Dairy Sci. 71:1178–1188.

Bartle, S. J., O. A. Turgeon, R. L. Preston, and D. R. Brink. 1988. Procedural and mathematical considerations in urea dilution estimation of body composition in lambs. J. Anim. Sci. 66:1920–1927.

Bergmann, H. 1932. Der Wasserbedarf der Ziegen (Water requirements of goats). Der Ziegenzuechter 19:146.

Blaxter, K. L., N. McC. Graham, F. W. Wainman, and D. G. Armstrong. 1959a. Environmental temperature, energy metabolism and heat regulation in sheep. II. The partition of heat losses in closely clipped sheep. J. Agric. Sci. 52:25–40.

Blaxter, K. L., N. McC. Graham, and F. W. Wainman. 1959b. Environmental temperature, energy metabolism and heat regulation in sheep. III. The metabolism and thermal exchanges of sheep with fleeces. J. Agric. Sci. 52:41–49.

Blix, A. S., and H. K. Johnsen. 1983. Aspects of nasal heat exchange in resting reindeer. J. Physiol. 340:443–454.

Blix, A. S., H. K. Johnsen, and J. B. Mercer. 1983a. On nasal heat exchange and the structural basis for its regulation in reindeer. J. Physiol. 343: 108P–109P.

Blix, A. S., H. K. Johnsen, and J. B. Mercer. 1983b. Central control of thermal balance in Norwegian reindeer. J. Physiol. 343:109P–110P.

Bohra, H. C., and P. K. Gosh. 1977. Effect of restricted water intake during summer on the digestibility of cell-wall constituents, nitrogen metabolism and water excretion in Marwari sheep. J. Agric. Sci. 89:605–608.

Brod, D. L., K. K. Bolsen, and B. E. Brent. 1982. Effect of water temperature on rumen temperature, digestion and rumen fermentation in sheep. J. Anim. Sci. 54:179–182.

Brosh, A., A. Shkolnik, and I. Choshniak. 1986. Metabolic effects of infrequent drinking and low-quality feed on Bedouin goats. Ecology 67: 1086–1090.

Brown, G. D., and J. J. Lynch. 1972. Some aspects of the water balance of sheep at pasture when deprived of drinking water. Aust. J. Agric. Res. 23:669–684.

Butcher, J. E. 1970. Is snow adequate and economical as water source for sheep? Nat. Wool Grower 60:28–29.

Cameron, R. D., and J. R. Luick. 1972. Seasonal changes in total body water, extracellular fluid, and blood volume in grazing reindeer. Can. J. Zool. 50:107–116.

Cameron, R. D., R. G. White, and J. R. Luick. 1975. The accumulation of water in reindeer during winter. Biol. Pap. Univ. Alaska Spec. Rep. 1: 374–378.

Cameron, R. D., R. G. White, and J. R. Luick. 1976. Accuracy of the tritium water dilution method for determining water flux in reindeer (Rangifer tarandus). Can. J. Zool. 54:857–862.

Cameron, R. D., J .R. Luick, and R. G. White. 1982. Water turnover in reindeer: Some environmental implications. Pp. 189–194 in Use of Tritiated Water in Studies of Production and Adaptation in Ruminants. Vienna: International Atomic Energy Agency.

Casey, N. H., and W. A. Van Niekerk, 1988. The Boer goats. I. Origin, adaptability, performance testing, reproduction and milk production. Small Ruminant Res. 1:291–302.

Chan-McLeod, A. C. A., R. G. White, and D. F. Holleman. 1994. Effects of protein and energy intake, body condition, and season on nutrient partitioning and milk production in caribou and reindeer. Can. J. Zool. 72:938–947.

Choshniak, I., and A. Shkolnik, A. 1977. Rapid rehydration in the Black Bedouin goats: Red blood cells fragility and role of the rumen. Comp. Biochem. Phys. 56A:581–583.

Church, D. C. 1971. Chapter 2–Water. Pp. 4–24 in Digestive Physiology and Nutrition of Ruminants, vol. 2, 2nd ed., D. C. Church, ed. Portland, OR: O & B Books Inc., Oxford Press.

Clauss, M., R. Frey, B. Kiefer, M. Lechner-Doll, W. Loehlein, C. Polster, G. E. Rossner, and W. J. Streich. 2003. The maximum attainable body size of herbivorous mammals: Morphophysiological constraints on foregut, and adaptations of hindgut fermenters. Oecologia 136:14–27.

Degen, A. A. 1977a. Fat tailed Awassi and German Mutton Merino sheep under semi arid conditions. 1. Total body water, its distribution and water turnover. J. Agric. Sci., Cambridge 88:693–698.

Degen, A. A. 1977b. Fat tailed Awassi and German Mutton Merino sheep under semi arid conditions. 2. Total body water and water turnover during pregnancy and lactation. J. Agric. Sci., Cambridge 88:699–704.

DelGiudice, G. D., L. D. Mech, and U. S. Seal. 1990. Effects of winter undernutrition on body composition and physiological profiles of white-tailed deer. J. Wildl. Manage. 54:430–436.

Donnelly, J. R., and M. Freer. 1974. Prediction of body composition in live sheep. Aust. J. Agric. Res. 25:825–834.

Dove, H. 1988. Estimation of the intake of milk by lambs, from the turnover of deuterium- or tritium-labelled water. Br. J. Nutr. 60:375–387.

Dove, H., and A. Axelsen. 1979. Estimation of milk consumption in beef calves using a tritiated water dilution technique. Aust. J. Exp. Agric. Anim. Husb.19:666–672.

Dove, H., and M. Freer. 1979. The accuracy of tritiated water turnover rate as an estimate of milk intake in lambs. Aust. J. Agric. Res. 30:725–739.

El Hadi, H. M., and Y. M. Hassan. 1982. Seasonal changes in water metabolism of Sudan desert sheep and goats. Pp. 103–115 in Use of Tritiated Water in Studies of Production and Adaptation in Ruminants. Vienna: International Atomic Energy Agency.

Engelhardt, W. V., K. E. Ali, and E. Wipper. 1979. Absorption and secretion in the tubiform forestomach (compartment 3) of the llama. J. Comp. Physiol. 132:337–341.

English, P. B. 1966. A study of water and electrolyte metabolism in sheep. II. The volumes of distribution of antipyrene, thiosulphate and T1824 (Evans Blue) and values for certain extracellular constituents. Res. Vet. Sci. 7:258–275.

Faichney, G. J., and R. C. Boston. 1985. Movement of water within the body of sheep fed at maintenance under thermoneutral conditions. Aust. J. Biol. Sci. 38:85–94.

Faichney, G. C., A. A. Fawcett, and R. C. Boston. 2004. Water exchange between the pregnant ewe, the foetus and its amniotic and allantoic fluids. J. Comp. Physiol. 174B:503–510.

Fancy, S. G., J. M. Blanchard, D. F. Holleman, K. J. Kokjer, and R. G. White. 1986. Validation of doubly labeled water method using a ruminant. Am. J. Physiol. 251:R143–R149.

Finch, V. A., and J. M. King. 1982. Energy-conserving mechanisms as adaptation to undernutrition and water deprivation in the African zebu. Pp. 167–178 in Use of Tritiated Water in Studies of Production and Adaptation in Ruminants. Vienna: International Atomic Energy Agency.

Finch, V. A., and D. Robertshaw. 1979. Thermoregulation in the eland and hartebeest during hydration and dehydration. Am. J. Physiol. 237:R192–R196.

Finch, V. A., I. L. Bennett, and C. R. Holmes. 1982. Sweating response in cattle and its relation to rectal temperature, tolerance of sun and metabolic rate. J. Agric. Sci. 99:479–487.

Foot, J. Z., and J. F. D. Greenhalgh. 1970a. A note on the relation between weights of alimentary tract contents, body fat and the uterus in Blackface ewes. Anim. Prod. 12:669–671.

Foot, J. Z., and J. F. D. Greenhalgh. 1970b. The use of deuterium oxide space to determine the amount of body fat in pregnant Blackface ewes. Br. J. Nutr. 24:815–825.

Forbes, J. M. 1968. The water intake of ewes. Br. J. Nutr. 22:33–43.

Fowler, M. E. 1998. Feeding and nutrition. Pp. 12–48 in Medicine and Surgery of South American Camelids: Llamas, Alpacas, Vicuna, Guanaco, 2nd ed. Ames: Iowa State University Press.

Gad, S. M., and R. L. Preston. 1990. In vivo prediction of extracellular and intracellular water in cattle and sheep using thiocyanate and urea. J. Anim. Sci. 68:3649–3653.

Gerhart, K. L., R. G. White, R. D. Cameron, and D. E. Russell. 1996a. Body composition and nutrient reserves of arctic caribou. Can. J. Zool. 74:136–146.

Gerhart, K. L., R. G. White, R. D. Cameron, and D. E. Russell. 1996b. Estimating fat content of caribou from body condition scores. J. Wildl. Manage. 60:713–718.

Giger-Reverdin, S., and Gihad, E. A. 1991. Water metabolism and intake in goats. Pp. 37–45 (Chapter 4) in Goat Nutrition, P. Morand-Fehr, ed. Wageningen, Netherlands: Pudoc.

Gotaas, G., and N. J. C. Tyler. 1995. Faeces is a reliable source of body water for measuring tritium in reindeer in summer and in winter. Rangifer 15:63–70.

Gotaas, G., E. Milne, P. Haggarty, and N. J. C. Tyler. 2000a. Energy expenditure of free-living reindeer estimated by the doubly labelled water method. Rangifer 20:211–219.

Gotaas, G., E. Milne, P. Haggarty, and N. J. C. Tyler. 2000b. Loss of deuterium in faecal solids and by sequestration in reindeer: Effect on doubly labelled water studies. Rangifer 20:31–41.

Graham, N. McC. 1968. The metabolic rate of Merino rams bred for high or low wool production. Aust. J. Agric. Res. 19:821–824.

Haggarty, P. 1991. Potential of the doubly labelled water method for estimating heat production in farm animals. J. Agric. Sci. 117:141–148.

Haggarty, P., J. J. Robinson, J. Ashton, E. Milne, C. L. Adam, C. E. Kyle, S. L. Christie, and A. J. Midwood. 1998. Estimation of energy expenditure in free-living red deer (*Cervus elaphus*) with the doubly-labelled water method. Br. J. Nutr. 80:263–272.

Head, M. J. 1953. The effect of pregnancy and lactation in the ewe on the digestibility of the ration with a note on the partition of nitrogen in the foetus at full term. J. Agric. Sci. 43:214–217.

Hecker, J. F., O. E. Budtz-Olsen, and M. Ostwald. 1964. The rumen as a water store in sheep. Aust. J. Agric. Res. 15:961–968.

Herrick, J. B. 1971. Water quality for livestock and poultry. Feedstuffs 43:28.

Hobson, P. N., S. O. Mann, and R. Summers. 1976. Rumen microorganisms in red deer, hill sheep and reindeer in the Scottish Highlands. P. Roy. Soc. Edinb. B, 75:171–180.

Holleman, D. F., R. G. White, and J. R. Luick. 1982. The application of isotopic water methods for measuring total body water, body composition and body water turnover. Pp. 9–32 in Use of Tritiated Water in Studies of Production and Adaptation in Ruminants. Vienna: International Atomic Energy Agency.

Jagusch, K. T., B. W. Norton, and D. M. Walker. 1970. Body composition studies with the milk-fed lamb. 2. The effect of the age of the lamb and the protein content of the diet on the chemical composition of the body and its organs. J. Agric. Sci. 75:279–285.

Jenness, R., and R. E. Sloan. 1970. The composition of milk of various species: A review. Dairy Sci. Abstr. 32:599–612.

Johnsen, H. K., A. S. Blix, L. Jorgensen, and J. B. Mercer. 1985a. Vascular basis for regulation of nasal heat exchange in reindeer. Am. J. Physiol. 249:R617–R623.

Johnsen, H. K., A. Rognmo, K. J. Nilssen, and A. S. Blix. 1985b. Seasonal changes in the relative importance of different avenues of heat loss in resting and running reindeer. Acta Physiol. Scand. 123:73–79.

Johnsen, H. K., A. S. Blix, J. B. Mercer, and K. D. Bolz. 1987. Selective cooling of the brain in reindeer. Am. J. Physiol. 253:R848–R853.

Kamal, T. H. 1982. Tritiated-water heat-tolerance index to predict the growth rate in calves in hot deserts. Pp. 155–165 in Use of Tritiated Water in Studies of Production and Adaptation in Ruminants. Vienna: International Atomic Energy Agency.

Kay, R. N. B., W. V. Engelhardt, and R. G. White. 1980. The digestive physiology of wild ruminants. Pp. 743–761 in Digestive Physiology and Metabolism in Ruminants, Y. Ruckebusch and P. Thivend, eds. Lancaster, UK: MTP Press Ltd.

Kay, R. N. B., G. A. M. Sharman, W. J. Hamilton, E. D. Goodall, K. Pennie, and A. G. P. Coutts. 1981. Carcass characteristics of young red deer farmed on hill pasture. J. Agric. Sci., Cambridge 96:79–87.

King, J. M. 1982. Field studies of game and livestock under African ranching conditions. Pp. 179–188 in Use of Tritiated Water in Studies of Production and Adaptation in Ruminants. Vienna: International Atomic Energy Agency.

King, J. M., and V. A. Finch. 1982. Value and limitations of using tritiated water for predicting body composition and water intake in the African zebu. Pp. 57–67 in Use of Tritiated Water in Studies of Production and Adaptation in Ruminants. Vienna: International Atomic Energy Agency.

King, J. M., G. P. Kingaby, J. G. Colvin, and B. R. Heath. 1975. Seasonal variation in water turnover by oryx and eland on the Galana Game Ranch Research Project. E. Afr. Wildl. J. 13:287–296.

Kleiber, M. 1975. The Fire of Life: An Introduction to Animal Energetics. Huntington, NY: R. E. Krieger.

Knox, K. L., J. G. Nagy, and R. D. Brown. 1969. Water turnover in mule deer. J. Wildl. Manage. 33:389–393.

Laben, R. C. 1963. Factors responsible for variation in milk composition. J. Dairy Sci. 46:1–8.

Laden, S., L. Nehmadi, and R. Yagil. 1987. Dehydration tolerance in Awassi fat-tailed sheep. Can. J. Zool. 65:363–367.

Landete-Castillejos, T., A. Garcia, and L. Gallego. 2001. Calf growth in captive Iberian red deer (*Cervus elaphus hispanicus*): Effects of birth date and hind milk production and composition. J. Anim. Sci. 79: 1085–1092.

Larsen, T. S., and A. S. Blix. 1985. Seasonal changes in total body water; Body composition and water turnover in reindeer. Rangifer 5:2–9.

Lautier, J. K., T. V. Dailey, and R. D. Brown. 1988. Effect of water restriction on feed intake of white-tailed deer. J. Wildl. Manage. 52:602–606.

Lifson, N., and R. McClintock. 1966. Theory of use of the turnover rates of body water for measuring energy and material balance. J. Theor. Biol. 12:46–74.

Little, W., B. F. Sansom, R. Manston, and W. M. Allen. 1976. Effects of restricting the water intake of dairy cows upon their milk yield, body weight and blood composition. Anim. Prod. 22:329–339.

Longhurst, W. M., N. F. Baker, G. E. Connolly, and R. A. Fisk. 1970. Total body water and water turnover in sheep and deer. Am. J. Vet. Res. 31:673–677.

Luick, J. R., and R. G. White. 1977. Preferences of reindeer for various physical and chemical forms of water. Res. Coord. Meeting on Res. Prog. on Water Requirements of Tropical Herbivores. Joint FAO/IAEA sponsorship, Khartoum, Sudan, 7–10 September.

Luick, J. R., R. G. White, A. M. Gau, and R. Jenness. 1974. Compositional changes in the milk secreted by grazing reindeer. I. Gross composition and ash. J. Dairy Sci. 57:1325–1333.

Lynch, J. J., G. D. Brown, P. F. May, and J. B. Donnelly. 1972. The effect of withholding drinking water on wool growth and lamb production of grazing Merino sheep in a temperate climate. Aust. J. Agric. Res. 23:659–668.

Macfarlane, W. V. 1964. Terrestrial animals in dry heat: Ungulates. Pp. 509–531 in Handbook of Physiology: Section 4, Adaptation to the Environment, D. B. Dill, ed. Washington, DC: American Physiological Society.

Macfarlane, W. V., and B. Howard. 1966. Water content and turnover of identical twin *Bos indicus* and *B. taurus* in Kenya. J. Agric. Sci., Cambridge 66:297–302.

Macfarlane, W.V., and B. Howard. 1970. Water in the physiological ecology of ruminants. Pp 362–374 in The Physiology of Digestion and Metabolism in the Ruminant. A.T. Phillipson, ed. Aberdeen: Oriel Press.

Macfarlane, W.V., and B. Howard. 1972. Comparative water and energy economy of wild and domestic animals. Symp. Zool. Soc. London 31:261–296.

Macfarlane, W. V., R. J. Morris, and B. Howard. 1956. Water economy of tropical merino sheep. Nature 178:304–305.

Macfarlane, W. V., R. J. Morris, B. Howard, J. McDonald, and O. E. Budtz-Olsen. 1961. Water and electrolyte changes in tropical Merino sheep exposed to dehydration during summer. Aust. J. Agric. Res. 12:889–912.

Maloiy, G. M. O. 1973. The water metabolism of a small East African antelope: the dik-dik. Proc. R. Soc. Lond. B. 184:167–178.

Maloiy, G. M. O., and D. Hopcraft. 1971. Thermoregulation and water relations of two East African antelopes: The hartebeest and impala. Comp. Biochem. Physiol. 38A:525–534.

Maloiy, G. M. O., and C. R. Taylor. 1971. Water requirements of African goats and haired-sheep. J. Agric. Sci. 77:203–208.

Maltz, E., and A. Shkolnik. 1980. Milk production in the desert: Lactation and water economy in the black Bedouin goat. Physiol. Zool. 53: 12–18.

Martin, R. D. 1984. Scaling effects and adaptive strategiesin mammalian lactation. Symp. Zool. Soc. London. 51:87–117.

McEwan, E. H., and P. E. Whitehead. 1971. Measurement of the milk intake of reindeer and caribou calves using tritiated water. Can. J. Zool. 49:443–447.

McGregor, B. A. 1986. Water intake of grazing Angora wether goats and Merino wethers. Aust. J. Exp. Agric. 26:639–642.

McGregor, B. A. 2003. Nutrition of goats during drought. RIRDC Publication No. 03/016. Barton, ACT, Australia.

Midwood, A. J., P. Haggarty, and B. A. McGaw. 1993. The doubly labeled water method—errors due to deuterium-exchange and sequestration in ruminants. Am. J. Physiol. 264:R561–R567 Part 2.

Midwood, A. J., P. Haggarty, B. A. McGaw, G. S. Mollison, E. Milne, and G. J. Duncan. 1994. Validation in sheep of the doubly labeled water method for estimating CO_2 production. Am. J. Physiol. 266: R169–R179.

Moen, A. N. 1973. Wildlife ecology: An analytical approach. San Francisco: W. H. Freeman.

Morand-Fehr, P., and D. Sauvant. 1978. Nutrition and optimum performance of dairy goats. Livest. Prod. Sci. 5:203–213.

Morris, R. J. H., B. Howard, and W. V. Macfarlane. 1962. Interaction of nutrition and air temperature with water metabolism of Merino wethers shorn in winter. Aust. J. Agric. Res. 13:320–334.

Moulton, C. R. 1923. Age and chemical development in mammals. J. Biol. Chem. 57:79–87.

Nagy, J. G., and W. L. Regelin. 1975. Comparison of digestive organ size of three deer species. J. Wildl. Manage. 39:621–624.

Nagy, K. A. 1989. Doubly-labeled water studies of vertebrate physiological ecology. Pp. 268–287 in Stable Isotopes in Ecological Research, P. W. Rundel, J. R. Ehleringer, and K. A. Nagy, eds. New York: Springer-Verlag.

Nagy, K. A., and D. P. Costa. 1980. Water flux in animals: Analysis of potential errors in the tritiated water method. Am. J. Physiol. 238:R454–R465.

Nagy, K. A., and C. C. Peterson. 1988. Scaling of water flux rate in animals. Univ. Calif. Pub. Zool. 120:1–172.

Nicol, A. M., and B. A. Young. 1981. The heat of warming feed. Proc. NZ. Soc. Anim. Prod. 41:152–162.

NRC (National Research Council). 1974. Nutrients and Toxic Substances in Water for Livestock and Poultry. Washington, DC: National Academy Press.

NRC. 1981. Effect of Environment on Nutrient Requirements of Domestic Animals. Washington, DC: National Academy Press.

NRC. 1985. Nutrient Requirements of Sheep. Washington, DC: National Academy Press.

NRC. 1989. Nutrient Requirements of Dairy Cattle, 6th rev ed. Washington, DC: National Academy Press.

NRC. 2000. Nutrient Requirements of Beef Cattle. Update 2000. Washington, DC: National Academy Press.

NRC. 2001. Nutrient Requirements of Dairy Cattle, 7th rev ed. Washington, DC: National Academy Press.

NRC. 2003. Nutrient Requirements of Nonhuman Primates, 2nd rev ed. Washington, DC: The National Academies Press.

Odwongo, W. O., H. R. Conrad, A. E. Staubus, and J. H. Harrison. 1985. Measurement of water kinetics with deuterium oxide in lactating dairy cows. J. Dairy Sci. 68:1155–1164.

Oftedal, O. T. 1984. Milk composition, milk yield and energy output at peak lactation: A comparative review. Symp. Zool. Soc. London. 51: 33–85.

Oftedal, O. T. 1985. Pregnancy and lactation. Pp. 215–238 in Bioenergetics of Wild Herbivores, R. J. Hudson and R. G. White, eds. Boca Raton, FL: CRC Press.

Ostrowski, S., J. B. Williams, E. Bedin, and K. Ismail. 2002. Water influx and food consumption of free-living oryxes (*Oryx leucoryx*) in the Arabian desert in summer. J. Mammal. 83:665–673.

Ostrowski, S., J. B. Williams, and K. Ismael. 2003. Heterothermy and the water economy of free-living Arabian oryx (*Oryx leucoryx*). J. Exp. Biol. 206:1471–1478.

Ouellet, J. P., D. C. Heard, S. Boutin, and R. Mulders. 1997. A comparison of body condition and reproduction of caribou on two predator-free Arctic islands. Can. J. Zool. 75:11–17.

Pace, N., and E. N. Rathbun. 1945. Studies on body composition. 3. The body water and chemically combined nitrogen content in relation to fat content. J. Biol. Chem.158:685–691.

Panaretto, B. A. 1963. Body composition in vivo—the composition of living ruminants and its relation to the tritiated water spaces. Aust. J. Agric. Res.14:944–952.

Panaretto, B. A. 1968. Body composition in vivo. 9. The relation of body composition to the tritiated water spaces of ewes and wethers fasted for short periods. Aust. J. Agric. Res.19:267–272.

Panaretto, B. A., and A. R. Till. 1963. Body composition in vivo. 2. The composition of mature goats and its relationship to the antipyrine, tritiated water, and N-acetyl-4-aminoantipyrine spaces. Aust. J. Agric. Res. 14:926–943.

Parker, K. L., and C. T. Robbins. 1985a. Thermoregulation in mule deer and elk. Can. J. Zool. 62:1409–1422.

Parker, K. L., and C. T. Robbins. 1985b. Thermoregulation in ungulates. Pp. 161–182 in Bioenergetics of Wild Herbivores, R. J. Hudson and R. G. White, eds. Boca Raton, FL: CRC Press.

Parker, K. L., R. G. White, M. P. Gillingham, and D. F. Holleman. 1990. Comparison of energy metabolism in relation to daily activity and milk consumption by caribou and muskox neonates. Can. J. Zool. 68: 106–114.

Parker, K. L., G. D. Delgiudice, and M. P. Gillingham. 1993a. Do urinary urea nitrogen and cortisol ratios of creatinine reflect body-fat reserves in black-tailed deer. Can. J. Zool. 71:1841–1848.

Parker, K. L., M. P. Gillingham, T. A. Hanley, and C. T. Robbins. 1993b. Seasonal patterns in body-mass, body-composition, and water transfer rates of free-ranging and captive black-tailed deer (*Odocoileus-hemionus-sitkensis*) in Alaska. Can. J. Zool. 71:1397–1404.

Parker, K. L., M. P. Gillingham, T. A. Hanley, and C. T. Robbins. 1999. Energy and protein balance of free-ranging black-tailed deer in a natural forest environment. Wildl. Mono. 143:5–48.

Peirce, A. W. 1959. Studies on salt tolerance of sheep. II The tolerance of sheep to mixtures of sodium chloride and magnesium chloride in the drinking water. Aust. J. Agric. Res. 10:725–735.

Peltier, T. C., and P. S. Barboza. 2003. Growth in an arctic grazer: Effects of sex and diet nitrogen on yearling muskoxen. J. Mammal. 84:915–925.

Peltier, T. C., P. S. Barboza, and J. E. Blake. 2003. Seasonal hyperphagia does not reduce digestive efficiency in an Arctic grazer. Physiol. Biochem. Zool. 76:471–483.

Preston, R. L. 1969. Influence of diethylstilbestrol on body water space in ruminants. Proc. Soc. Exp. Biol. Med. 132:401–404.

Purohit, G. R., P. K. Ghosh, and G. C. Taneja. 1972. Water metabolism in desert sheep. Effects of various degrees of water restriction on the distribution of body water in Marwari sheep. Aust. J. Agric. Res. 23: 685–691.

Ranjhan, S. K., A. P. Kalanidhi, T. K. Gosh, U. B. Singh, and K. K. Saxena. 1982. Body composition and water metabolism in tropical ruminants using tritiated water. Pp. 117–132 in Use of Tritiated Water in Studies of Production and Adaptation in Ruminants. Vienna: International Atomic Energy Agency.

Reid, J. T., A. Bensadoun, L. S. Bull, J. G. Burton, P. A. Gleeson, I. K. Han, Y. D. Joo, D. E. Johnson, W. R. McManus, O. L. Paladines, J. W. Strond, H. F. Tyrrell, B. D. H. Van Niekerk, and G. W. Wellington. 1968. Some peculiarities in body composition of animals. Pp. 19–44 in Body Composition in Animals and Man, J. T. Reid, ed. Washington, DC: Natl. Acad. Sci.

Reimers, E., T. Ringberg, and R. Sørumgärd. 1982. Body composition of Svalbard reindeer. Can. J. Zool. 60:1812–1821.

Richmond, C. R., W. H. Langham, and T. T. Trujillo. 1962. Comparative metabolism of tritiated water by mammals. Cell. Comp. Physiol. 59: 45–53.

Ringberg, T. M., R. G. White, D. F. Holleman, and J. R. Luick. 1981. Body growth and carcass composition of lean reindeer (*Rangifer tarandus tarandus* L.) from birth to sexual maturity. Can. J. Zool. 59:1040–1044.

Robbins, C. T. 1993. Wildlife Feeding and Nutrition, 2nd ed. San Diego, CA: Academic Press.

Robbins, C. T., A. N. Moen, and J. T. Reid. 1974. Body composition of white-tailed deer. J. Anim. Sci. 38:871–876.

Robinson, J. R. 1957. Functions of water in the body. Proc. Nutr. Soc. 16:108–112.

Rosenmann, M., and P. Morrison. 1963. Physiological response to heat and dehydration in the guanaco. Physiol. Zool. 36:45–51.

Rübsamen, K., and W. V. Engelhardt. 1975. Water metabolism in the llama. Comp. Biochem. Physiol. 52A:595–598.

Russel, A. J. F., J. M. Doney, and R. G. Gunn. 1969. Subjective assessment of body fat in live sheep. J. Agric. Sci. 72:451–454.

Russel, A. J. F., J. Z. Foot, and D. M. McFarlane, 1982. Use of tritiated water for estimating body composition in grazing ewes. Pp. 45–56 in Use of Tritiated Water in Studies of Production and Adaptation in Ruminants. Vienna: International Atomic Energy Agency.

Sadleir, R. M. F. S. 1980. Milk yield of black-tailed deer. J. Wildl. Manage. 44:472–478.

Sadleir, R. M. F. S. 1982. Energy consumption and subsequent partitioning in lactating black-tailed deer. Can. J. Zool. 60:382–386.

Sahlu, T., A. L. Goetsch, J. Luo, I. V. Nsahlai, J. E. Moore, M. L. Galyean, F. N. Owens, C. L. Ferrell, and Z. B. Johnson. 2004. Nutrient requirements of goats: Developed equations, other considerations and future research to improve them. Small Ruminant Res. 53:191–219.

Schmidt-Nielsen, K. 1964. Desert animals: Physiological problems of heat and water. Oxford: Clarendon Press.

Schoen, A. 1969. Water conservation and the structure of the kidneys of tropical bovids. J. Physiol. 204:143P–144P.

Searle, T. W. 1970a. Body composition in lambs and young sheep and its prediction in vivo from tritiated water space and body weight. J. Agric. Sci. 74:357–362.

Searle, T. W. 1970b. Prediction of body composition of sheep from tritiated water space and body weight tests of published equations. J. Agric. Sci. 75:497–500.

Searle, T. W., and M. Hilmi. 1977. In vivo prediction with tritiated water of chemical and dissectible components of the dressed carcass of sheep growing at different rates. Aust. J. Agric. Res. 28:963–970.

Seif S. M., H. D. Johnson, and L. Hahn. 1973. Environmental heat and partial water restriction effects on body fluid spaces, water loss, body temperature, and metabolism of holstein cows. J. Dairy Sci. 56(5):581–586.

Sheng, H. P., and R. A. Huggins. 1979. A review of body composition studies with emphasis on total body water and fat. Am. J. Clin. Nutr. 32:630–647.

Shkolnik, A., A. Borut, and J. Choshniak. 1972. Water economy of the Bedouin goat. Symp. Zool. Soc. London. 31:229–242.

Shkolnik, A., A. Borut, I. Choshniak, and E. Maltz. 1975. The black Bedouin goat—a desert ruminant that "stores" water. FASEB J. 34:472.

Shkolnik, A., E. Maltz, and I. Choshniak. 1980. The role of the ruminant's digestive tract as a water reservoir. Pp. 731–742 in Digestive Physiology and Metabolism in Ruminants, Y. Ruckebusch and P. Thivend, eds. Lancaster, UK: MTP

Silanikove, N. 1989. Interrelationships between water, food and digestible energy intake in desert and temperate goats. Appetite 12:163–170.

Singh, N. P., T. More, and K. L. Sahni. 1976. Effect of water deprivation on feed intake, nutrient digestibility and nitrogen retention in sheep. J. Agric. Sci. 86:431–433.

Skadhauge, E., E. Clements, and G. M. O. Maloiy. 1980. The effects of dehydration on electrolyte concentrations and water content along the large intestine of a small ruminant: the Dik-dik antelope. J. Comp. Physiol. 135B:165–173.

Squires, V. R., and A. D. Wilson, 1971. Distance between food and water supply and its effect on drinking frequency, and food and water intake of Merino and Border Leicester sheep. Aust. J. Agric. Res. 22:283–290.

Staaland, H., K. Hove, and R.G. White. 1986. Mineral absorption in relation to nutritional ecology of reindeer. Rangifer Spec. Iss. No.1:279–287.

Staaland, H., D. F. Holleman, J. R. Luick, and R. G. White. 1982. Exchangeable sodium pool size and turnover in relation to diet in reindeer. Can. J. Zool. 60:603–610.

Staaland, H., E. Jacobsen, and R. G. White. 1984. The effect of mineral supplements on nutrient concentrations and pool sizes in the alimentary tract of reindeer fed lichens or concentrates during the winter. Can. J. Zool. 62:1232–1241.

Stephenson, T. R., V. C. Bleich, B. M. Pierce, and G. P. Mulcahy. 2002. Validation of mule deer body composition using in vivo and post-mortem indices of nutritional condition. Wildl. Soc. B. 30:557–564.

Stevens, C. E. 1988. Comparative Physiology of the Vertebrate Digestive System. Cambridge, UK: Cambridge University Press.

Taylor, C. R. 1968a. The minimum water requirements of some East African bovids. Symp. Zool. Soc. Lond. 21:195–206.

Taylor, C. R. 1968b. Hygroscopic food: A source of water for desert antelopes? Nature, Lond. 219:181–182.

Torbit, S. C., L. H. Carpenter, D. M. Swift, and A. W. Alldredge. 1985. Differential loss of fat and protein by mule deer during winter. J. Wildl. Manage. 49:80–85.

Tyler, N. J. C., P. Fauchald, O. Johansen, and H. R. Christiansen. 1999. Seasonal inappetance and weight loss in female reindeer in winter. Ecol. Bull. 47:105–106.

Van Saun, R. J. 2006. Nutrient requirements of South American camelids: A factorial approach. Small Ruminant Res. 61:165–186.

Wallace, J. D., D. N. Hyder, and K. L. Knox. Water metabolism in sheep fed forage rations differing in digestibility. 1972. Am. J. Vet. Res. 33:921–927.

White, R. G. 1975. Some aspects of nutritional adaptations of arctic herbivorous mammals. Pp. 239–268 in Physiological Adaptation to the Environment, F. J. Vernberg, ed. New York: Educ. Publ.

White, R. G. 1979. Nutrient acquisition and utilization in arctic herbivores. Pp. 13–50 in Comparative Mechanisms of Cold Adaptation in the Arctic, L. S. Underwood, L. L. Tieszen, A. B. Callahan, and G. E. Folk, eds. New York: Academic Press.

White, R. G., and S. G. Fancy. 1986. Nutrition and energetics of indigenous northern ungulates. In Grazing Research at Northern Latitudes, O. Gudmundsson, ed. NATO ASI Series A: Life Sciences Vol. 108:259–269. New York: Plenum Press.

White, R. G., and J. R. Luick. 1984. Plasticity and constraints in the lactational strategy of reindeer and caribou. Pp. 215–232 in Physiological Strategies in Lactation, M. Peaker, R. G. Vernon, and C. H. Knight, eds. Symp. Zool. Soc. Lond. No. 51: Academic Press.

White, R. G., E. Jacobsen, and H. Staaland. 1984a. Secretion and absorption of nutrients in the alimentary tract of reindeer fed lichens or concentrates during the winter. Can. J. Zool. 62:2364–2376.

White, R. G., K. Frisby, B. Sammons, D. F. Holleman and M. Jourdan. 1984b. Seasonal changes in water metabolism of captive muskoxen. Biol. Papers of the Univ. of Alaska, Spec. Report No. 4:205–206.

Widdowson, E. M., and J. W. T. Dickerson. 1960. The effect of growth and function on the chemical composition of soft tissues. Biochem. J. 77: 30–43.

Williams, J. B., S. Ostowski, E. Bedin, and K. Ishmail. 2001. Seasonal variation in energy expenditure, water flux and food consumption of Arabian oryx *Oryx leucoryx*. J. Exp. Biol. 204:2301–2311.

Wilson A. D. 1966a. The intake and excretion of sodium by sheep fed on species of *Atriplex* (saltbush) and *Kochia* (bluebush). Aust. J. Agric. Res. 17:155–163.

Wilson, A. D. 1966b. The tolerance of sheep to sodium chloride in food or drinking water. Aust. J. Agric. Sci. 17:503–514.

Winchester, C. F., and M. J. Morris. 1956. Water intake rates of cattle. J. Anim. Sci. 15:722–740.

Withers, P. C., T. M. Casey, and K. K. Casey. 1979. Allometry of respiratory and haematological parameters of Arctic mammals. Comp. Biochem. Physiol 64A:343–350.

Woodford, S. T., M. R. Murphy, and C. L. Davis. 1984. Water dynamics of dairy cattle as affected by initiation of lactation and feed intake. J. Dairy Sci. 67:2336–2343.

Worden, K. A., and P. J. Pekins. 1995. Seasonal change in feed-intake, body-composition, and metabolic-rate of white-tailed deer. Can. J. Zool. 73:452–457.

Wright, D. E. 1982. Use of labelled water in studies on the nutrition and physiology of grazing ruminants in New Zealand. Pp. 91–102 in Use of Tritiated Water in Studies of Production and Adaptation in Ruminants. Vienna: International Atomic Energy Agency.

Yates, N. G., W. V. Macfarlane, and R. Ellis. 1971. The estimation of milk intake and growth of beef calves in the field by using tritiated water. Aust. J. Agric. Res. 22:291–306.

10

Plant Factors Affecting Nutrient Availability

INTRODUCTION

In both natural systems and in livestock production, small ruminants rely upon their ability to utilize plant carbohydrate. This commodity represents not only the most abundant, but also the most renewable source of carbon on earth, and is the major resource that allows ruminants to provide humans with food, fiber, and draught power. Of the carbon fixed by photosynthesis, nearly half is found in the lignocellulose of plant cell walls (Bhat, 2000). Mammals lack the enzymes to degrade the structural carbohydrates of plants (Van Soest, 1994), and the anaerobic fermentation of plant cell wall material is a major role of gut microorganisms. The capacity of herbivorous animals to use these carbohydrates as a feed resource thus depends on this fermentative ability of microorganisms; on the evolution of a digestive tract, which can provide an anaerobic chamber in which fermentation can take place; and on the evolution of the host animal to make use of the end products of fermentation (see Van Soest, 1994, and Chapter 2 of this volume). Ruminant animals have evolved to use plant cell wall carbohydrates in just this manner.

Since ruminants provide much of the meat, milk, animal fiber, and draught power used in the world, there is an obvious economic dimension to their utilization of plant carbohydrate. However, ruminant digestion also plays a crucial and global ecological function in recycling the carbon fixed by photosynthesis into a labile form (principally carbon dioxide), which allows its re-use in the world's carbon flows.

Cellulose and the other polymers of glucose that make up plant cell walls are the most abundant carbohydrates in the world and represent a huge feed resource for organisms, which can utilize them either directly or indirectly. Paradoxically, this also limits the energy content of the diet of grazing or browsing ruminants, unless they are also given high-energy supplements. Since carbohydrate makes up most of the plant and the lipid content of plant material is usually relatively low, the gross energy (GE) of plant material is related closely to the carbohydrate content. This results in a GE of about 4.3 Mcal/kg dry matter (DM). Higher GE levels than this have been observed (R. G. White, personal communication, 2006) found in good-quality browse containing 20–34 g/100 g DM acid-detergent lignin+proanthocyanidin and which had GE contents (by bomb calorimetry) in the range 4.7–5.5 Mcal/kg DM. Nevertheless, energy provision to the animal is usually very much a function of the digestibility of the carbohydrate component and the efficiency with which metabolizable energy (ME) is used (itself a function of digestibility).

THE CHEMICAL NATURE OF PLANT CARBOHYDRATES

The simple sugars in plant tissue are mostly combined by glycosidic linkages into disaccharides, oligosaccharides, and polysaccharides, and with noncarbohydrate moieties. The structure of the individual polymers, and especially the relationships between the polymers in both chemical and physical terms, is extremely complex; for detailed treatment of these aspects, see Van Soest (1982, 1994) and Mertens (2003). The main components of the plant cell wall constituents (CWC) comprise polymers of glucose, galactose, xylose, arabinose, and mannose and a complex of lignin with cellulose. Depending upon the stage of maturity of the plant, and on plant species, the cell wall components can account for 25–80 percent of forage DM.

Cellulose is the major polymer of the cell wall of terrestrial plants and the most abundant carbohydrate in the world. It consists of β1-4 glycosidic bonds, with glucose rings arranged in a trans-configuration. In monocotyledons such as grasses and sedges, the cellulose usually forms a ribbon or chain-like structure, which has been described as "stringy." These species can also include varying amounts of silica deposited in the fiber bundles, which can lower the digestibility of the fiber. As Van Soest (1982) has emphasized, pure cellulose ". . . in nature is a genetic rarity . . ." and all structural celluloses are intimately associated with varying amounts of hemicellulose, lignin, cutin, and minerals. The nutritional availability of such cellulose thus depends largely upon this degree of lignification.

The exact nature of hemicellulose is more difficult to delineate. It is actually a mixture of complex polysaccharides, the composition of which varies. The common factor in the mixture is a series of β1-4 bonds in a xylan core polymer. In the leaf and the stem of grasses and in legumes, hemicellulose consists largely of arabinoxylan with linkages to lignin and glucuronic acid.

The walls of adjacent plant cells appear to be "cemented" by pectin, which consists of long chains of galacturonic acid substituted with araban and possibly galactan side units. The chain is coiled because it is based on α1-4 linkages. In grasses, the contribution of pectin to total CWC is about 1–2 percent, but can be much higher in legumes (Wilson, 1994).

The remaining major component of cell wall is lignin, which is technically not a carbohydrate but a high molecular weight phenylpropanoid polymer. One of the problems associated with the term "lignin" and with its description is that, in part, the composition of an isolated "lignin fraction" depends on the method of preparation. For a more complete description of the chemistry and analysis of "lignin," see Van Soest (1982, 1994), Krause and Pell (2003), and Mertens (2003).

Lignin can constitute 2–24 percent of DM, but the effect of lignin, plus cutin, on herbage digestibility is often out of proportion to its actual content. Potential digestibility of neutral detergent fiber (NDF) is lowered from 90 to 20 percent as lignin content of cell wall increases from 5 to 15 percent (Schwartz and Renecker, 1998), and lignin content of NDF increases from 3 to 45 percent (Robbins, 1992). This is because lignin bonds to cell wall polysaccharides and restricts microbial access during digestion (Wilson, 1994). The bonding between lignin and cellulose as plants mature is essential in conferring strength to the plant, but also results in a major physical constraint for the ruminant in terms of physical resistance to prehension, chewing, rumination, and susceptibility to microbial digestion. Because stem usually contains more cell wall, the effect of increased lignification is exacerbated by a higher stem:leaf ratio in grasses and a higher lignified cortex:outer bark (cambium layer) ratio in mature plants. The CWC of browse plants, and particularly of woody browse, are distinguished from grasses and grass-like species (sedges) by the lignin content of the cell wall (woody browse 22–70 percent, leafy browse 8–48 percent, graminoids 5–13 percent). The high lignin:cellulose ratio (0.6–1.9:1 in browse, < 0.2:1 in grass hay as calculated from Lawler and White, unpub.) is associated with a short-structured or "blocky" fiber that shatters to small cuboids during mastication (Milchunas et al., 1978; Clauss et al., 2003). Time required for particle size reduction by mastication is therefore less than that for a grass of equivalent CWC (Schwartz and Renecker, 1998). Many dicotyledons, shrubs, and forbs have a lower CWC than monotyledons (grasses and sedges) (Robbins, 1992); however, a higher lignin content typical of dicotyledon cell wall results in a lower digestibility (Schwartz and Hobbs, 1985). In addition, both the cambium and the woody fiber of woody browse may contain secondary compounds, which act as a deterrent to herbivory (see Chapter 3 and below).

PLANT SECONDARY METABOLITES AND THEIR EFFECT ON NUTRIENT SUPPLY

A detailed discussion of the effects of plant secondary metabolites (PSM) is beyond the scope of this publication, but their effects on the availability of nutrients require mention. As Iason (2005) discussed, many PSM do not appear to have functions within the primary metabolism of the plant, and in early studies (for citations, see Launchbaugh, 1996), they were considered merely as a mechanism for the plant to dispose of "excess carbon." However, they are now known to have many ecological functions, among them the protection of the plant from attack and consumption by pathogens or herbivores (both vertebrate and invertebrate). The presence of PSM appears to reduce both the incidence and the extent of such "attacks." This concept was first suggested in the late 19th century (see Launchbaugh, 1996) but did not achieve prominence until the work of Fraenkel (1959). While these "anti-herbivory" aspects are undoubtedly a major component of the role of PSM, the wide range of such metabolites in the higher plants suggests that they did not evolve to confer the single evolutionary advantage of the minimization of herbivory (see Iason, 2005).

The incidence and effects of PSM and of plant toxins in the pasture and weed species in grazed pastures have been the subjects of many reviews, and the reader is referred to Launchbaugh (1996), Cheeke (1998), and Waghorn et al. (2002) for a range of viewpoints. Reviews by McArthur et al. (1991) and Iason (2005) provide a more ecological perspective, covering the wider range of plant foods such as grasses, forbs, and browse.

When consumed by herbivores, some PSM function as frank toxins, such as the pyrrolizidine alkaloids or the cyanogenic glycosides, which are found in a range of plants (Table 15.1 in Waghorn et al., 2002). Other toxins are more plant species-specific, such as those associated with toxicoses arising from the consumption of phalaris (Bourke, 1992; Waghorn et al., 2002), kikuyu (Cheeke, 1998), or the brassica forages (Waghorn et al., 2002).

Other PSM reduce the availability of nutrients from the consumed diet, and it is now clear that the same PSM can have either toxic or nutritional effects, depending on the dose. Indeed, some PSM, such as the condensed tannins, exemplify the dictum by Paracelsus that "Sola dosis facit venenum" or "Only the dose makes the poison" (quoted in Launchbaugh, 1996), in that they can have marked negative or positive effects on digestion, depending on their concentration in consumed material. A summary of some of

TABLE 10-1 Summary of Some Observed Positive and Negative Effects of Plant Secondary Metabolites after Consumption by Mammalian Herbivores[a]

Negative Effect	Counter-adaptation	Positive Effect	Reference
Tissue damage (e.g., pyrrolizidine and other alkaloids)	Detoxification system (e.g., conjugation and excretion; mixed-function oxidases)	—	see Iason (2005)
Increased energy expenditure	Detoxification and excretion	—	see Foley et al. (1999)
Oxidative damage (e.g., many phenolics)	Antioxidant system	Antioxidant function (e.g., flavonoids)	see Iason (2005)
Sodium imbalance	—	—	see Foley et al. (1999); Iason (2005)
Diuresis	—	—	Dearing et al. (2001)
Depression of activity of rumen microbial digestion (e.g., condensed tannins)	Tannin-binding salivary proteins (e.g., some cervids)	Reduction in rumen protein degradation ("protein protection"). Anthelminthic effects on nematode larvae. Reduced methane production.	Barry et al. (2002); Waghorn et al. (2002); White and Lawler (2002); Athanasiadou and Kyriazakis (2004)

[a]Adapted from Waghorn et al. (2002), White and Lawler (2002), and Iason (2005).

the positive and negative effects of PSM is given in Table 10-1.

In domesticated livestock, condensed tannins are a typical example of a PSM that can have marked positive or, at higher plant concentrations, negative effects. If concentrations in consumed plant material exceed, for example, about 5 percent DM, then the negative effects on microbial enzymes predominate and the digestibility of herbage is reduced. In turn, this reduces intake. By contrast, at levels of about 2–5 percent of plant DM, the reduction in rumen protein degradability can increase the postruminal supply of protein, without reducing herbage digestibility (for discussion, see Waghorn et al., 2002).

Similarly, it has been suggested that the sometimes substantial energy costs of detoxification of PSM might be at least partially offset by reductions in rumen methane production, though in muskoxen fed woody or leafy browse, White and Lawler (2002) found the compensation was relatively small. When consuming tannins, some mammals secrete salivary proline-rich proteins (PRPs) that bind to the tannins with high affinity. It has been suggested that the salivary PRPs bind to the tannins in the gastrointestinal tract, forming indigestible complexes that are excreted in the feces, thus protecting the animal from the negative effects of tannin ingestion (Hagerman et al., 1992). The quantitative significance of this mechanism in ruminants and its energetic costs have yet to be established (see discussion in Skopec et al., 2004).

More recently, the possible anthelminthic effects of PSM have shown promise (Athanasiadou and Kyriazakis, 2004). Given the costs of nematode control in domesticated ruminants and the problems being encountered with the development of anthelminthic resistance, this is an area worthy of further study.

THE NUTRIENT CONTENT OF FORAGES CONSUMED BY NONDOMESTICATED LIVESTOCK

Some classes of forage, such as the mushrooms, lichens, and mosses, are nonvascular, and therefore have fiber characteristics different from vascular plants. When available, mushrooms become important dietary components of many ruminants' grazing natural systems, and lichens and mosses are consumed seasonally by wild ruminants.

Mushrooms constitute the fruiting body of fungi that are made up of hyphae forming complex tissues and cell walls. Edible mushrooms are high in protein (16–45 percent DM: Courtright, 1959; Skjenneberg and Slagsvold, 1979), but estimates of protein content based on Kjeldahl analysis could be in error due to the effects of compounds such as chitin (Danel and Eaker, 1992). Crude fiber analyses are variable (32–45 percent DM: Courtright, 1959; Skjenneberg and Slagsvold, 1979) and fat levels are low (6–7 percent DM: Diez and Alvarez, 2001). The few estimates on digestibility of mushrooms by ruminants are variable, and the "cellulose" component of the fiber is reported to be indigestible (Skjenneberg and Slagsvold, 1979). Because the fractional absorption of the fallout radionuclide cesium-137 from mushrooms by cervids exceeds 73 percent (Hove et al., 1990), digestion of the fiber component is inferred. A high nutritive value would support the wide use and preference for mushrooms by ruminants, especially the cervids, as well as many other mammals (Carey, 1996).

The lichen body, or thallus, is composed of fungal and algal cells in a symbiotic association that has many growth forms and is harvested by ruminants from trees (arboreal lichens), the ground surface (terrestrial foliose lichens), or rocks (crustaceous lichens). Cell wall of the thallus is usually dominated by the carbohydrate lichenin, with isolichenin and hemicellulose as less important components.

These polysaccharides are dominated by glucose, galactose, and mannose (Solberg, 1970; Svihus and Holand, 2000). However, lichens also contain polyhydric alcohols, oligosaccharides, oils, free amino acids (16 identified), vitamins, and a highly variable array of minerals. A huge array of organic lichen acids (> 100) are secreted into the extracellular fluids (cell contents) and often crystallize on the surface of the fungal hyphae (Hale, 1968; Dahl and Krog, 1970). Many lichen chemicals are toxic to animals and can be bactericidal. Both effects deter herbivores. Of the cervids, only the reindeer/caribou specializes in the use of lichens as a seasonal (winter) food resource, but most other north temperate cervids make use of arboreal lichens whenever available. Neutral detergent analyses of lichens indicate that they can be grouped as low (< 30 percent) or high (> 50 percent) in NDF (White et al., 1975; Svihus and Holand, 2000). A limited number of analyses indicate that those species with < 30 percent NDF were high in soluble crude fiber (CF), highest in lichenin content, highest in initial gas production in vitro, and the highest in vitro dry matter digestibility (DMD). These terrestrial and arboreal species of low NDF are preferred by reindeer/caribou and deer, but other factors, including the content of plant secondary compounds, also influence choice (Svihus and Holand, 2000). Digestibility of lichens in vitro (9–82 percent) and in sacco (20–90 percent) is highly variable (Person et al., 1980), and controlling factors have not been well defined. Nitrogen content is high in only the nitrogen (N)-fixing species, but these species are avoided because of toxicity and are rarely used by ruminants. The most preferred and most used lichen species by ruminants are low in N (< 1.5 percent DM), but most contain < 1.0 percent N (Skjenneberg and Slagsvold, 1979). Those herbivores that selectively feed on lichens digest thallus carbohydrates by microbial fermentation with DM digestibilities often exceeding 80 percent. Dietary adaptation to overcome effects of anti-microbial chemicals in many lichen species is inferred from results with in vitro and in sacco systems (Trudell et al., 1980).

Mosses are generally low in protein (about 10 percent DM), moderate to high in fiber (> 27 percent DM) and low in vitro and in sacco DM digestibility (1–25 percent: Person et al., 1980; Trudell et al., 1980), except for reports of higher digestibility for high Arctic reindeer and caribou (48 percent in vivo: Staaland et al., 1988; 11–35 percent in vitro: Thomas and Kroeger 1980; 11–36 percent in vitro: Orpin and Mathiesen, 1990). The calcium (Ca) and phosphorus (P) contents of mosses are high, and mosses could be taken as a mineral supplement (Batzli, 1975; Batzli et al., 1980; Staaland et al., 1988).

The seasonal phenology of potential forage plants involves the production of buds, inflorescences, seed/fruits, and vegetative storage units (such as tubers and roots) that are potentially important food resources to small ruminants in the wild, and these plant parts are frequently consumed as part of small ruminant diets. Depending on the ecosystem and geographical location, the supply of overwintering buds of woody shrubs and trees, new buds, and unfurling leaves and flowers in spring, as well as fruits and vegetative storage units that become available from mid-summer to autumn and early winter, can be either predictable or highly variable. Just as in grazed pastures, these phenological events represent a series of pulses that are superimposed on a seasonal trend in forage biomass, with a generally declining quality from spring to winter, or wet to dry season (Crampton and Harris, 1969; Kubota et al., 1970; Albon and Langvatn, 1992; Johnstone et al., 1999). Although the seasonal timing of reproduction in most plants is temporally set and is reliable, there are examples, such as mast production, that vary greatly in amount from year to year (McCullough, 1979). Foraging ecology in relation to phenology and seasonal progression in biomass and plant quality is well documented for small ruminants in the wild and under rangeland grazing conditions (Klein, 1970; Moen, 1973; Van der Wal et al., 2000; Mysterud et al., 2001; Owen-Smith, 2002), and can be the basis for migratory movements in ruminants (Fryxell and Sinclair, 1988). Overwintering buds of plants such as poplar and birch represent a reliable and potentially nutritious food resource at 10–12 percent crude protein (CP); however they are usually coated in a waxy cuticle high in chemicals that deter feeding (Reichardt et al., 1990) and in condensed tannins (> 1.5 percent) that potentially lower CP and DM digestibility (Hanley et al., 1992). Hence, they are rarely used by most browser-concentrate selectors (CS) species. By contrast, new spring buds of many shrubs and forage trees are heavily utilized by both CS species and intermediate mixed foragers (IM). Goats, deer, reindeer/caribou, and wapiti strip buds and unfurling young leaves to maximize foraging efficiencies. Buds and leaves low in lignin content (approximately 4 percent for blackberry, red dogwood, gray dogwood, red alder) are higher in NDF (43 vs. 29 percent), lower in acid detergent fiber (ADF) (18 vs. 23 percent), and lower in condensed tannins (0.25 vs. 0.41 percent) than buds and leaves with a higher lignin content (approximately 11 percent for willows, birches, and silky dogwood) (McCullough and Ullrey, 1985; Robbins et al., 1987b; Klein, 1990; Manseau, 1996; Van der Wal, 2000; Jorgenson et al., 2002). Although CP was slightly higher for buds and new leaves high in lignin content (22 vs. 18 percent), the higher condensed tannin content should result in a reduction in CP digestibility (Robbins et al., 1987a; Hanley et al., 1992). Despite the anti-nutrient effects of condensed tannins in leaf buds, these buds are important to the diets of postcalving deer (McCullough and Ullrey, 1985) and wapiti (Hudson et al., 1985), and early lactation in caribou and reindeer (Russell et al., 1993; Griffith et al., 2002). Flowering buds and inflorescences of most forage plants are high in CP (18 percent, range 14–25 percent) and low in lignin (3.3 percent). Mean NDF of inflorescences is approximately 43 percent, ADF 20 percent, and in sacco and in vitro dry matter digestibility (IVDMD) > 70 percent. However, condensed tannins in some inflorescences (e.g., fireweed) lower CP digestibility (from 14 percent CP to 5 percent digestible CP: Hanley et al., 1992) and DMD (from approximately 60 percent to 42 percent digestibility of NDF: Robbins et al., 1987b). Flower buds and early inflorescences of tussock cotton grass are extremely important to milk production and survival of caribou and reindeer calves on the calving grounds in spring (Griffith et al., 2002). During summer an array of flowering plants, including legumes and louseworts, raise the CP content of grass- and sedge-based diets (White et al., 1981). Among the most important influences over animal productivity, through autumn fattening that indirectly affects overwinter survival in deer, is the availability of mast, especially acorns (Moen, 1973; McCullough and Ullrey, 1985). The food value of acorns is related to their very high lipid levels in the "meat" (24 percent DM) that is lowered to 18 percent when the acorn is eaten whole as opposed to eating the "meat" only (McCullough and Ullrey, 1985). Likewise, seed grains of monocotyledons are efficiently stripped from the plant by goats. Although these grains are moderately high in CP (17 percent), digestibility is low (digestible CP 9 percent). However the combination of low structural carbohydrate (CHO) (CF 4 percent) and high nonstructural CHO content results in a high ME (3.08 kcal/g DM). Seedpods of legumes are very high in CP (41 percent) but somewhat lower (21 percent) in digestible CP. When associated with a high CF and low ME content (see NRC, 1981), their potential as a supplement needs careful evaluation. In wet-cool areas of the Arctic and in high alpine wet-meadows, many monocotyledons are viviparous. As judged by the improvement in nutrition of germinating seeds, these viviparous seed heads are likely high in CP, low in NDF, and high in cell solubles. A field evaluation of volatile fatty acid (VFA) production rates in Svalbard reindeer (White and Staaland, 1983) suggested that a diet dominated by viviparous seed heads supported VFA production indicative of a daily DM intake in excess of 100 g/kg$^{0.75}$, which is very high for small ruminants (see Chapter 3).

THE NUTRIENT CONTENT OF PLANT-BASED FEEDS UNDER ZOO CONDITIONS

Diets for herbivores under zoo conditions are frequently based on commercially available, formulated feeds designed to be "nutritionally complete" and for which nutritional compositions are available. Unfortunately, it can be difficult to relate these to diet compositions of herbivores in the wild, for want of data about the latter (Schmidt et al., 2005). Nevertheless, these commercial feeds are often supplemented with plant products such as the fruit and vegetables (produce) consumed by humans. As Schmidt et al. (2005) discussed, this poses two problems in trying to relate the nutrient intake from the total diet to the animals' nutrient requirements:

1. When zoo animals are given produce items, they often consume the entire item, by contrast with humans who may only consume specific parts. The published information on nutrient composition often only relates to these specific parts, but the nutrient composition of the whole and its parts may well differ.

2. While nutritional composition data are available for produce items (e.g., Pennington, 1998; Wildlife Conservation Society, 2001; USDA-ARS, 2004), these are often related to human requirements and not couched in the terms normally used by animal nutritionists in diet formulation. For example, fiber is commonly reported as "dietary fiber," rather than NDF and ADF as would be used with animal feeds. This makes it difficult to use such data in ration formulation.

Much less information is available on the nutrient content of produce items as fed to and consumed by zoo herbivores, especially in relation to structural carbohydrate content. The publication by Schmidt et al. (2005) provides valuable data on the proximate analyses, structural and nonstructural carbohydrate content, and free sugars content of a wide range of fruits and vegetables. A selection of these data is reproduced in the feed composition tables.

RELATING CARBOHYDRATE ANALYSES TO NUTRITIVE VALUE AND ANIMAL RESPONSE

To be useful in establishing feeding standards, information such as the plant content of various CWC must ultimately be expressed in ME terms, or at least in terms of the effect of the content of CWC on digestibility. This in turn means that methods for the analysis of CWC must be both reproducible and nutritionally relevant. As Mertens (2003) has recently discussed, dietary fiber is unique among the constituents of feed because, while chemical techniques are used to measure it, it is defined only in nutritional terms (the digestive and physiological consequences of fiber consumption). "Relevance" in this context means that analytical procedures must describe the feed in quantitative terms that provide nutritional information.

Techniques are available for the analysis of plant structural and nonstructural carbohydrates in terms of their constituent monomers; however, the use of such analyses assumes that they will provide nutritional insight. Unfortunately, this is usually not the case, so that such analyses involve two practical problems for animal feeding. First, the analyses are time-consuming and expensive, because they involve extensive hydrolysis and the use of complex laboratory equipment. Second, even when results are obtained, they can be difficult to relate to animal response or, even more importantly, are difficult to use to predict animal response. As Mertens (2003) puts it, "The nonuniform digestibility of fibrous carbohydrates suggests that knowing their monomeric composition, no matter how accurately, provides little information about their availability to the animal."

In general terms, these difficulties have been recognized for over a century and have generated a series of attempts to

TABLE 10-2 Fractionation of Forage Organic Matter According to the Detergent System (constructed in part from Van Soest, 1994; see also AOAC, 2002, methods 2002.04 and 973.18)

Fraction	Reagent	Component
Neutral detergent solubles (NDS)	Na lauryl sulfate; EDTA, pH 7.0	Lipids, sugars, organic acids, starch, pectin, soluble protein and nonprotein N
Neutral detergent fiber (NDF)		Plant cell wall less pectin
Acid detergent solubles	Cetyl trimethylammmonium bromide in 1N H_2SO4	Hemicellulose, fiber-bound protein
Acid detergent fiber (ADF)		Cellulose, lignin, lignified N

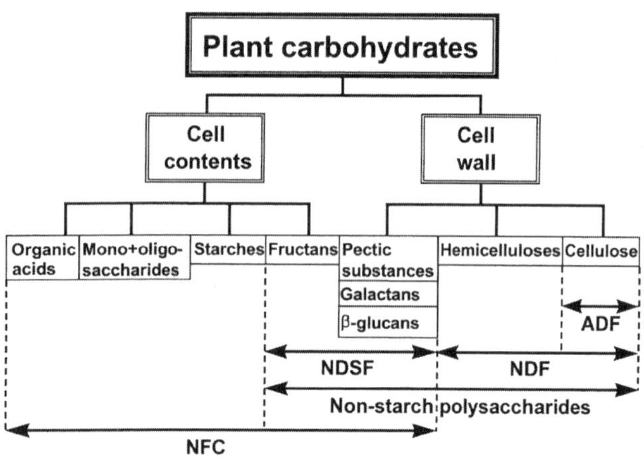

FIGURE 10-1 Relationship between plant carbohydrate fractions and analytical components used to describe them (from Hall, 2003). ADF = acid detergent fiber, NDF = neutral detergent fiber, NDSF = neutral detergent-soluble fiber, NFC = non-NDF carbohydrates.

devise simpler and more rapid chemical assays, usually gravimetric in whole or in part, which could provide a prediction of the nutritive value of a feed for animals, principally by relating the assay to digestibility (see Van Soest, 1994, and Mertens, 2003, for discussion). This can function as a surrogate for ME or provide input data for empirical relationships between ME and digestibility (ARC, 1980; SCA, 1990) or between ME and digestibility and fat content (AFRC, 1993; Freer et al., 1997). The estimation of CF and nitrogen-free extract (NFE) within the proximate system of analysis is an example of these simpler assays. Although initially established to reflect the plant cell wall and "highly digestible carbohydrates," respectively, these fractions are both highly error-prone, as Van Soest (1994) and Mertens (2003) have discussed. The CF component is not well related to any accepted definitions of dietary fiber and is not uniformly available to the animal. This is also true for NFE, with the added disadvantage that this fraction is obtained by subtraction and thus contains the accumulated errors from all other fractions.

Although CF is still used by regulatory agencies to specify feeds in terms of their minimum CF content, its use in research and practical feeding has now been supplanted by the "detergent system" developed by Van Soest and colleagues (see Van Soest, 1994, for general discussion). This approach attempts to fractionate feed material into classes of compound that are completely available to the animal (soluble in detergent), partially available (cellulose and hemicellulose), and unavailable (lignin, cutin, silica). A brief outline of this system is given in Table 10-2, while the relationship with plant carbohydrate fractions is shown in Figure 10-1 (from Hall, 2003).

A major advantage of the detergent system is that because detergents such as cetyl trimethylammonium bromide form strong protein complexes that are soluble above pH 6, plant protein can be removed as a potential source of contamination in preparing a sample that represents plant cell wall material. The ethylenediaminetetraacetic acid (EDTA) in the neutral detergent is included to prevent interference from heavy metal and alkaline earth metal ions. The use of neutral detergent thus provides a fraction that essentially consists of the major cell wall components hemicellulose, cellulose, and lignin. By contrast, extraction with acid detergent (Table 10-2) removes hemicellulose, the content of which can thus be computed as NDF-ADF. Although NDF and ADF extractions are usually conducted separately, there are occasions when ADF is measured sequentially after neutral detergent extraction. This almost always results in a lower ADF content than if the ADF extraction had been conducted separately (Mertens, 2003) because the neutral detergent removes components not well removed by acid detergent (e.g., pectins, tannins, and phenolic complexes).

FACTORS INFLUENCING CARBOHYDRATE CONTENT

The carbohydrate content, and especially the structural carbohydrate content of plants, is influenced by a range of factors, including:

1. Photosynthetic pathway. As a generalization, plants exhibiting the Hatch-Slack (C4) pathway of photosynthesis exhibit higher levels of structural carbohydrate at a given stage of maturity than do plants exhibiting the Calvin (C3) pathway. This is in part due to the higher temperatures in which C4 species frequently grow (Henry et al., 2000) but is primarily related to the unique leaf vascular anatomy of C4 plants (Wilson, 1994).

2. Species of plant, especially legumes vs. grasses. At a given digestibility, legumes contain less cell wall than do grasses, but this is compensated for by the fact that within their cell wall, legumes generally contain a higher ratio of lignin to cellulose. This results in legumes having about twice the lignin content of grasses at the same digestibility (see Van Soest, 1964; Figure 6.5 in Van Soest, 1982). Nevertheless, the structural relationship between lignin/cellulose/hemicellulose in legumes is such that at a given digestibility, sheep will consume about 25 percent more legume than grass (Freer and Jones, 1984). Moreover, the weight gain of young sheep is higher with legumes than with grasses of the same digestibility (Freer and Jones, 1984).

3. Season of the year. The decline with season of the year in the nutritive value of plant material, especially its digestibility, is well documented both for legumes and particularly for grasses (Figure 10-2). This is especially marked beyond flowering and has major repercussions for the management of the herbage resource by livestock producers. The effect can be due to increased cell wall content of forage, both in absolute terms and also as a result of increased stem:leaf ratios. However, data with annual grasses indicate that the amount of cell wall is reasonably constant after flowering (Ballard et al., 1990; for a detailed discussion, see Dove, 1996). In annual ryegrass, for example, it was the neutral detergent solubles (NDS) (1-NDF) content (and especially water-soluble carbohydrate) that declined most dramatically beyond flowering (Ballard et al., 1990; Armstrong et al., 1992). The reduction in digestible DM yield in the sward beyond flowering was almost entirely attributable to the reduction in cell contents, rather than to an increase in CWC.

4. Plant part. As a generalization, grass stems contain more structural carbohydrate than leaves and are thus less digestible (Figure 10-3). This is less the case with legumes, in which petioles and leaves can be of similar digestibility.

5. Environmental effects. Higher environmental temperatures usually result in greater accumulation of structural carbohydrate and also in greater metabolic activity, which reduces the pool size of cell contents and thus soluble carbohydrates (Ford et al., 1979; Henry et al., 2000), resulting in lower DM digestibility. This appears less so with C4 plants (Henry et al., 2000). Perhaps an even greater environmental effect is that of temperature and light on plant phenology, especially the onset of reproductive development. This results in a rapid increase in the stem:leaf ratio in grasses, for example, with concomitant reduction in digestibility. In contrast, for those grass species with distribution to temperate and north temperate regions, and to higher elevations, a cline to higher digestibility and cell contents is noted with latitude and altitude, which has been attributable to lower temperature and to longer daylength for the latitude cline (Van Soest, 1964).

Given the close relationship between the digestibility of plant material and its content of CWC, and the response of

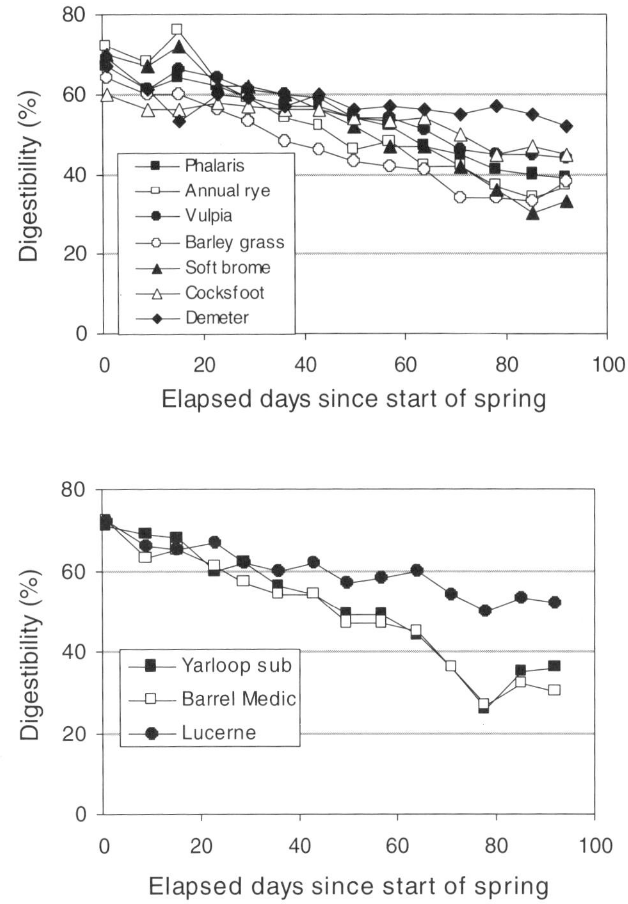

FIGURE 10-2 Typical changes in dry matter digestibility of a range of pasture grasses (upper panel) and legumes (lower panel) as spring progresses (from Radcliffe and Cochrane, 1970). Phalaris = *Phalaris aquatica*; Annual rye = *Lolium rigidum*; Barley grass = *Hordeum leporinum*; Soft brome = *Bromus mollis*; Cocksfoot = Orchard grass = *Dactylis glomerata*; Demeter = *Festuca arundinacea* cv. Demeter; Yarloop sub = *Trifolium subterraneum* cv. Yarloop; Barrel medic = *Medicago truncatula*; Lucerne = Alfalfa = *Medicago sativa*.

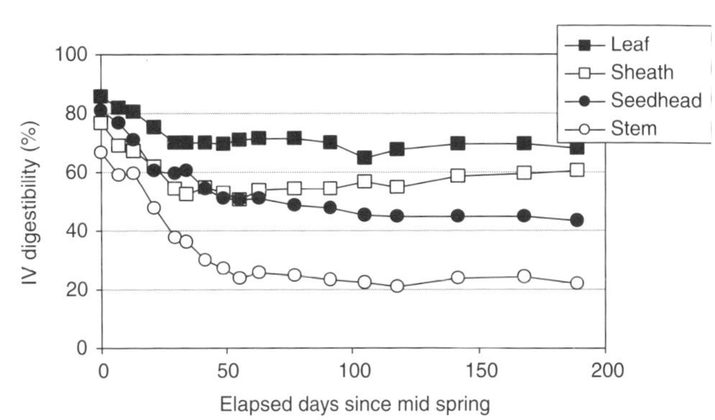

FIGURE 10-3 Changes in the digestibility of different plant parts of annual grass pasture during spring-autumn (from the data of Gatford et al., 1999).

TABLE 10-3 Estimated Digestibility of Neutral Detergent Solubles (NDS) in a Range of Grass Species (adapted from Ballard, 1990 and Dove, 1996)

Grass Species	Digestibility of NDS (%)	Supporting Reference
Dactylis	90	Colburn et al. (1968)
Digitaria	35–61	Minson (1984)
Lolium perenne	72–92	Radojevic et al. (1994)
Lolium rigidum	39–95	Ballard et al. (1990)
Lolium rigidum	40–100	Armstrong et al. (1992)
Panicum	46–67	Minson (1971)
Triticum	83	Moir (1971)

animal performance to digestibility, an emphasis on the structural carbohydrate content of plant material has been both understandable and warranted. However, this emphasis may, inadvertently, have led to an underemphasis on the role of plant cell contents.

The main components of cell contents (Table 10-2, Figure 10-1) include the nonstructural carbohydrates (sugars and storage polysaccharides), protein and nonprotein N, lipids, organic acids, and the vitamins and minerals. While NDF is known to vary in digestibility, it is usually assumed that as a group, the cell contents are 100 percent digestible (Mertens, 2003). The data collated by Van Soest (1982) indicate that the true mean DM digestibility of NDS is 98 percent (see Figure 4-3, Table 4-2) and thus lend support to this assumption. In vitro digestibility of some leafy browses is less than the NDS content suggesting that digestibility of NDS is less that 98 percent (Person et al., 1980). This cannot be attributed to analytical errors, because there is published evidence that at least in some grass species, the digestibility of NDS can be as low as 35–40 percent (Table 10-3). The data in Table 10-3 require cautious interpretation, as Dove (1996) has emphasized, because they are, of necessity, based on in vitro digestibilities. However, they suggest a need for equal caution about the assumption that the NDS fraction is completely digestible.

The levels of storage carbohydrates are usually higher in legumes (Culvenor et al., 1989), in which the storage carbohydrate is usually starch (Jones and Wilson, 1987; Culvenor et al., 1989). Carbohydrate is also stored as starch in C4 grasses (Norton, 1982) but the storage carbohydrates of temperate C3 grasses are fructans of varying degrees of polymerization (Smouter and Simpson, 1989). The temperate grasses contain about 5–40 percent storage carbohydrate in their DM, mainly in stems (Ballard et al., 1990; Armstrong et al., 1992; Ciavarella et al., 2000a,b), with a peak content at about anthesis. The decline observed beyond this point can be associated with seed development and the storage of carbohydrate in perennating organs.

The water-soluble carbohydrate (WSC) content of forage (Yemm and Willis, 1954), which includes the simple sugars, is markedly affected by conditions of growth. High light intensity and increased photosynthetic rate will increase WSC content while shading will decrease it (e.g., Ciavarella et al., 2000a,b). Higher ambient temperatures increase metabolic rate and will result in a decrease in WSC. These effects combine to generate marked diurnal variation in total WSC content and the content of most of its component sugars (Ciavarella et al., 2000b).

There is increasing evidence that WSC also plays an important role in preference for and intake of plant material by herbivores, with downstream consequences for rumen fermentation and animal performance. The role of WSC as a determinant of diet selection has been noted over a wide range of herbage maturities and in both grazing and indoor trials (e.g., Michell, 1973; Orr et al., 1997; Leury et al., 1999; Siever-Kelly et al., 1999; Ciavarella et al, 2000a). Using annual grass pasture treated with glyphosate to reduce the loss of stem WSC during senescence, Siever-Kelly et al. (1999) showed that housed sheep preferred stem from sprayed pasture to leaf material from unsprayed pasture. WSC concentrations in the former fraction were much higher and preference was not related to in vitro digestibility, but was directly related to the WSC content of a plant part. Leury et al. (1999) confirmed that the same patterns of diet selection occurred when sheep grazed sprayed vs. unsprayed pasture.

In green herbage, Fisher et al. (1999) demonstrated that animals preferred hay made from forage in the afternoon, when WSC content was high, to hay made from the same area in the morning, when WSC content was lower. In sheep grazing vegetative phalaris/subterranean clover pasture, Ciavarella et al. (2000a) used a shade treatment to create swards that differed only in their WSC content. When given free choice between the low-WSC pasture and the high-WSC pasture, sheep had an almost threefold preference for the latter.

It appears that the preference for material with higher WSC content is also associated with higher intakes of the material, when compared with low-WSC herbage (Michell, 1973; Jones and Roberts, 1991; Leury et al., 1999). Efficiency of utilization, whether measured indirectly as yield of lamb/unit DOM intake (Davies et al., 1991) or directly by calorimetry (Corbett et al., 1966) is also improved.

An obvious mechanism for an effect of dietary WSC on animal production would be via an effect on the efficiency of microbial protein synthesis, by bringing the rates of volatile fatty acid and ammonia production in the rumen into better synchrony (SCA, 1990). This has been difficult to demonstrate under grazing conditions. However, Dove and Milne (1994) reported higher non-ammonia nitrogen and microbial flows from the rumen in ewes grazing a perennial ryegrass pasture with almost identical digestibility in summer (high WSC) and autumn (low WSC).

These results suggest that the response to soluble carbohydrates, particularly in green herbage, is of practical, economic significance, and there may be a need for a reassessment of their role in the process of diet selection. This in turn would suggest a need to pay more attention, in assays of the nutritive value of animal feeds, to the content of nonstructural carbohydrates, especially WSC. This will further fuel the debate over which of these fractions are nutritionally relevant and warrant analysis, and which methods should be used for their analysis (Hall, 2003).

Although the dominating factor influencing diet selection between typical browser (e.g., deer) vs. grazer (e.g., wapiti/elk) species appears to be plant cell wall thickness (Spalinger et al., 1986), nonstructural carbohydrates play a dominant role in diet selection by grazer species (e.g., elk, mountain sheep). Grazers more strongly select for those grasses and sedges with highest cell content concentration from a wide array of plant species in nature (Hobbs et al., 1983). Determining selection criteria by browser species is further complicated by the complexing effects of tannins on neutral detergent solubles, lowering the availability of proteins and other components of the solubles (Hanley et al., 1992; Robbins, 1992). In some herbivores, salivary PRP are produced and function as a first line of defense against dietary tannins (Austin et al., 1989; Makkar, 2003) by complexing with them in the mouth and then passing intact through the gut (Austin et al., 1989). As pointed out by Makkar, this not only ensures that quantitatively less dietary protein is complexed with the tannins, but also ensures that the excreted tannin complex is relatively rich in nonessential amino acids, rather than essential amino acids (see Makkar, 2003 for further discussion). Sheep and goats do not produce salivary PRP (Villalba et al., 2002; Makkar, 2003), and the observation that goats cope better with dietary tannins may relate to greater saliva production by goats (Domingue et al., 1991; Villalba et al., 2002).

A further approach to alleviating the effects of dietary condensed tannins is supplementation with polyethylene glycol (PEG). Depending on the original dietary tannin concentrations, this has been shown to influence feeding behavior (Landau et al., 2002; Villalba et al., 2002) and have positive effects on feed intake (Pritchard et al., 1992; Villalba et al., 2002) and animal production (Pritchard et al., 1992). Possible approaches to PEG supplementation under practical conditions are discussed by Makkar (2003).The response to PEG seems to depend not only on the relative doses of tannin and PEG but also on the rumen conditions in different herbivores (Frutos et al., 2004).

REFERENCES

AFRC (Agricultural and Food Research Council). 1993. Energy and Protein Requirements of Ruminants. An advisory manual prepared by the AFRC Technical Committee on Responses to Nutrients. Wallingford, UK: CABI Publishing.

Albon, S. D., and R. Langvatn. 1992. Plant phenology and the benefits of migration in a temperate ungulate. Oikos 65:502–513.

AOAC (Association of Official Analytical Chemists). 2002. Official Methods of Analysis of AOAC International, 15th ed., William Horwitz, ed. Arlington, VA: AOAC International.

ARC (Agricultural Research Council). 1980. The Nutrient Requirements of Ruminant Livestock. Technical review by the Agricultural Research Council Working Party. Farnham Royal, UK: Commonwealth Agricultural Bureaux.

Armstrong, R. D., R. J. Simpson, G. R. Pearce, and I. Radojevic. 1992. Digestibility of senescing annual ryegrass following applications of glyphosate. Aust. J. Agric. Res. 43:871–885.

Athanasiadou, S., and I. Kyriazakis. 2004. Plant secondary metabolites: Antiparasitic effects and their role in ruminant production systems. Proc. Nutr. Soc. 63:631–639.

Austin, P. J., A. Suchar, C. T. Robbins, and A. E. Hagerman. 1989. Tannin-binding proteins in saliva of deer and their absence in saliva of sheep and cattle. J. Chem. Ecol. 15:1335–1347.

Ballard, R. A., R. J. Simpson, and G. R. Pearce. 1990. Losses of the digestible components of annual ryegrass (*Lolium rigidum* Gaudin) during senescence. Aust. J. Agric. Res. 41:719–731.

Barry, T. N., S. O. Hoskin, and P. R. Wilson. 2002. Novel forages for growth and health in farmed deer. New Zealand Vet. J. 50:244–251.

Batzli, G. O. 1975. The role of small mammals in arctic ecosystems. Pp. 243–268 in Small Mammals: Their Productivity and Population Dynamics, F. B. Golley, K. Petrusewicz, and L. Ryszkowski, eds. Cambridge, UK: Cambridge University Press.

Batzli, G. O., R. G. White, S. F. MacLean, Jr., F. A. Pitelka, and B. D. Collier. 1980. The herbivore-based trophic system. Pp. 335–410 in An Arctic Ecosystem: The Coastal Tundra at Barrow, Alaska, J. Brown, P. C. Miller, L. L. Tieszen, and F. L. Bunnell, eds. Stroudsburg, PA: Dowden, Hutchinson and Ross.

Bhat, M. K. 2000. Cellulases and related enzymes in biotechnology. Biotechnol. Adv. 18:355–383.

Bourke, C. A. 1992. Toxins in pasture plants—phalaris toxicity. Anim. Prod. Aust. 19:399–401.

Carey, A. B. 1996. Interactions of Northwest forest canopies and arboreal mammals. Northwest Sci. Spec. Iss. 70:72–78.

Cheeke, P. R. 1998. Natural Toxicants in Feeds, Forages and Poisonous Plants. Danville, IL: Interstate Publishers.

Ciavarella, T. A., H. Dove, B. J. Leury, and R. J. Simpson. 2000a. Diet selection by sheep grazing *Phalaris aquatica* L. pastures of differing water-soluble carbohydrate content. Aust. J. Agric. Res. 51:757–764.

Ciavarella, T. A., R. J. Simpson, H. Dove, B. J. Leury, and I. M. Sims. 2000b. Diurnal changes in the concentration of water-soluble carbohydrates in *Phalaris aquatica* L. pasture, and the effect of short-term shading. Aust. J. Agric. Res. 51:749–756.

Clauss, M., M. Lechner-Doll, and W. J. Streich. 2003. Ruminant diversification as an adaptation to the physicomechanical characteristics of forage. A reevaluation of an old debate and a new hypothesis. Oikos 102:253–262.

Colburn, M. W., J. L. Evans, and C. H. Ranage. 1968. Apparent and true digestibility of forage nutrients by ruminant animals. J. Dairy Sci. 51: 1450–1457.

Corbett, J. L., J. P. Langlands, I. McDonald, and J. D. Pullar. 1966. Comparison by direct energy calorimetry of the net energy values of an early and late season growth of herbage. Anim. Prod. 8:13–27.

Courtright, A. M. 1959. Range management and the genus Rangifer: A review of selected literature. M.Sci. thesis, University of Alaska. 172 pp.

Crampton, E. W., and L. E. Harris. 1969. Applied Animal Nutrition, 2nd ed. San Francisco: W. H. Freeman.

Culvenor, R. A., I. A. Davidson, and R. J. Simpson. 1989. Regrowth of swards of subterranean clover after defoliation. 1. Growth, non-structural carbohydrate and nitrogen content. Ann. Bot. 64:545–556.

Dahl, E., and H. Krog. 1970. Macrolichens of Denmark, Finland, Norway and Sweden. Universitetsforlaget. Oslo, Bergen, Tromsø.

Danel, E., and D. Eaker. 1992. Amino acid and total protein content of the mushroom Cantharellus cibarius (Freis). J. Sci. Food Agric. 60:333–337.

Davies, D. A., M. Fothergill, and D. Jones. 1991. Assessment of contrasting perennial ryegrass, with and without white clover, under continuous sheep stocking in the uplands. 3. Herbage production, quality and intake. Grass Forage Sci. 46:39–49.

Dearing, M. D., A. M. Magnione, and W. H. Karasov. 2001. Plant secondary compounds as diuretics: An overlooked consequence. Am. Zool. 41:890–901.

Diez, V. A., and A. Alvarez. 2001. Compositional and nutritional studies on two wild edible mushrooms from northwest Spain. Food Chem. 75: 417–422.

Domingue, B. M. F., D. W. Dellow, and T. N. Barry. 1991. The efficiency of chewing during eating and ruminating in goats and sheep. Br. J. Nutr. 65:355–363.

Dove, H. 1996. The ruminant, the rumen and the pasture resource: nutrient interactions in the grazing animal. Pp. 219–246 in The Ecology and Management of Grazing Systems, J. Hodgson and A. W. Illius, eds. Wallingford, UK: CABI Publishing.

Dove, H., and J. A. Milne. 1994. Digesta flow and rumen microbial protein production in ewes grazing perennial ryegrass. Aust. J. Agric. Res. 45:1229–1245.

Fisher, D. S., H. F. Mayland, and J. C. Burns. 1999. Variation in ruminants' preference for tall fescue hays cut either at sundown or at sunup. J. Anim. Sci. 77:762–768.

Foley, W. J., G. R. Iason, and C. McArthur. 1999. The role of plant secondary metabolites in the nutritional ecology of mammalian herbivores: How far have we come in 25 years? Pp. 130–209 in Nutritional Ecology of Herbivores, H. J. G. Jung and G. C. Fahey, eds. Savoy, IL: American Society of Animal Science.

Ford, C. W., I. M. Morrison, and J. R. Wilson. 1979. Temperature effects on lignin, hemicellulose and cellulose in tropical and temperate grasses. Aust. J. Agric. Res. 30:621–633.

Fraenkel, G. S. 1959. The raison d'etre of secondary plant substances. Science 129:1466–1470.

Fryxell, J. M., and A. R. E. Sinclair. 1988. Causes and consequences of migration by large herbivores. Trends Ecol. Evol. 3:237–241.

Freer, M., and D. B. Jones. 1984. Feeding value of subterranean clover, lucerne, phalaris and wimmera ryegrass for lambs. Aust. J. Exp. Agric. Anim. Husb. 24:156–164.

Freer, M., A. D. Moore, and J.R. Donnelly. 1997. GRAZPLAN: Decision support systems for Australian grazing enterprises. II. The animal biology model for feed intake, production and reproduction and the GrazFeed DSS. Agric. Systems. 54:77–126.

Frutos, P., G. Hervás, F. J. Giráldez, and R. Mantecón. 2004. An *in vitro* study on the ability of polyethylene glycol to inhibit the effect of quebracho tannins and tannic acid on rumen fermentation in sheep, goats, cows and deer. Aust. J. Agric. Res. 55:1125–1132.

Gatford, K. L., R. J. Simpson, C. Siever-Kelly, B. J. Leury, H. Dove, and T. A. Ciavarella. 1999. Spray-topping annual grass pasture with glyphosate to delay loss of feeding value during summer. I. Effects on pasture yield and nutritive value. Aust. J. Agric. Res. 50:453–464.

Griffith, B., D. C. Douglas, N. E. Walsh, D. D. Young, T. R. McCabe, D. E. Russell, R. G. White, R. D. Cameron, and K. R. Whitten. 2002. The porcupine caribou herd. Pp. 8–37 in Arctic Refuge Coastal Plain Terrestrial Wildlife Research Summaries. D. C. Douglas, P. E. Reynolds, and E. B. Rhode, eds. U.S. Geological Survey, Biological Resources Division, Biological Science Report USGS/BRD/BSR-2002-0001.

Hagerman, A. E., C. T. Robbins, Y. Weerasuriya, T. C. Wilson, and C. McArthur. 1992. Tannin chemistry in relation to digestion. J. Range Manage. 45:57–62.

Hale, M. E. 1968. Lichen Handbook, 3rd reprint. Washington, DC: Smithsonian Institution Press.

Hall, M. B. 2003. Challenges with nonfiber carbohydrate methods. J. Anim. Sci. 81:3226–3232.

Hanley, T. A., C. T. Robbins, A. E. Hagerman, and C. McArthur. 1992. Predicting digestible protein and digestible dry matter in tannin-containing forages consumed by ruminants. Ecology 73:537–541.

Henry, D. A., R. J. Simpson, and R. H. Macmillan. 2000. Seasonal changes and the effect of temperature and leaf moisture content on intrinsic shear strength of leaves of pasture grasses. Aust. J. Agric. Res. 51: 823–831.

Hobbs, N. T., D. L. Baker, and R. B. Gill 1983. Comparative nutritional ecology of montane ungulates during winter. J. Wildl. Manage. 47: 1–16.

Hove, K., O. Pedersen, T. H. Garmo, H. S. Hansen, and H. Staaland. 1990. Fungi: A major source of radiocesium contamination of grazing ruminants in Norway. Health Phys. 59:189–192.

Hudson, R. J., W. G. Watkins, and R. W. Pauls. 1985. Bioenergetics of wapiti in western Canada. Pp. 447–452 in Biology of Deer Production, P. Fennessy and K. R. Drew, eds. Wellington: Royal Society of New Zealand.

Iason, G. 2005. The role of plant secondary metabolites in mammalian herbivory: Ecological perspectives. Proc. Nutr. Soc. 64:123–131.

Johnstone, J., D. E. Russell, and G. Griffith. 1999. Variations in plant forage quality in the range of the Porcupine caribou herd. Rangifer 22:83–91.

Jones, D. I. H., and J. R. Wilson. 1987. Nutritive quality of forage. Pp. 65–89 in The Nutrition of Herbivores, J. B. Hacker and J. H. Ternouth, eds. Sydney: Academic Press.

Jones, E. L., and J. E. Roberts. 1991. A note on the relationship between palatability and water-soluble carbohydrates content in perennial ryegrass. Irish. J. Agric. Res. 30:163–167.

Jorgenson, J. C., M. S. Udevitz, and N. A. Felix. 2002. Forage quantity and quality. Pp. 46–50 in Arctic Refuge Coastal Plain Terrestrial Wildlife Research Summaries, D. C. Douglas, P. E. Reynolds, and E. B. Rhode, eds. U.S. Geological Survey, Biological Resources Division, Biological Science Report USGS/BRD/BSR-2002-0001.

Klein, D. R. 1970. Tundra ranges north of the boreal forest. J. Range Manage. 23:8–14.

Klein, D. R. 1990. Variation in quality of caribou and reindeer forage plants associated with season, plant part, and phenology. Rangifer Spec. Iss. No. 3:123–130.

Krause, D. O., and A. N. Pell. 2003. Plant cell wall degradation in the rumen: Ecology, constraints to digestion and modelling. Pp. 129–150 in Matching Herbivore Nutrition to Ecosystems Biodiversity, L.'t Mannetje, L. Rámirez-Avilés, C. Sandoval-Castro, and J. C. Ku-Vera, eds. Mérida, Mexico: Universidad Autónoma de Yucatán.

Kubota, J., S. Rieger, and V. A. Lazar. 1970. Mineral composition of herbage browsed by moose in Alaska. J. Wildl. Manage. 34:565–569.

Landau, S. Y., A. Perevolotsky, D. Kbabya, N. Silanikove, R. Nitzan, H. Baram, and F. D. Provenza. 2002. Polyethylene glycol affects goats' feeding behavior in a tannin-rich environment. J. Range Manage. 55:598–603.

Launchbaugh, K. L. 1996. Biochemical aspects of grazing behaviour. Pp. 159–184 in The Ecology and Management of Grazing Systems, J. Hodgson and A. W. Illius, eds. Wallingford, UK: CABI Publishing.

Leury, B. J., C. Siever-Kelly, H. Dove, K. L. Gatford, and R. J. Simpson. 1999. Spray-topping annual grass pasture with glyphosate to delay loss of feeding value during summer. IV. Herbage intake, digestibility, diet selection and animal production in grazing sheep. Aust. J. Agric. Res. 50:487–495.

Makkar, H. P. S. 2003. Effects and fate of tannins in ruminant animals, adaptation to tannins, and strategies to overcome detrimental effects of feeding tannin-rich feeds. Small Ruminant Res. 49:241–256.

Manseau, M. 1996. Relation Réciproque entre les Caribous et la Végétation des Aires d'Estivage: Le Cas du Troupeau de Caribous de la Rivière George. PhD thesis, Université Laval, Quebec, Canada. 167 pp. (p. 90).

McArthur, C., A. E. Hagerman, and C. T. Robbins. 1991. Physiological strategies of mammalian herbivores against plant defences. Pp. 103–114 in Plant Defenses against Mammalian Herbivory, R. T. Palo and C. T. Robbins, eds. Boca Raton, FL: CRC Press.

McCullough, D. 1979. The George River Deer Herd: Population Ecology of a K-Selected Species. Caldwell, NJ: Blackburn Press.

McCullough, D. R., and D. E. Ullrey. 1985. Chemical composition and gross energy of deer forage plants on the George Reserve. Michigan Agricultural Experiment Station Research Report 465.

Mertens, D. R. 2003. Challenges in measuring insoluble dietary fiber. J. Anim. Sci. 81:3233–3249.

Michell, P. J. 1973. Relationships between the neutral detergent fibre, acid detergent fibre and water soluble carbohydrate contents of pasture species and their digestibility and voluntary intake by sheep. Aust. J. Exp. Agric. Anim. Husb. 13:165–170.

Milchunas D. G., M. I. Dyer, O. C. Wallmo, and D. E. Johnson. 1978. In-vivo/in-vitro relationships of Colorado mule deer forages. Spec. Rept. No 43. Colorado Div. Wildl., Ft. Collins, CO.

Minson, D. J. 1971. Influence of lignin and silicon on a summative system assessing the organic matter digestibility of *Panicum*. Aust. J. Agric. Res. 22:589–598.

Minson, D. J. 1984. Digestibility and voluntary intake by sheep of five *Digitaria* species. Aust. J. Exp. Agric. Anim. Husb. 24:494–500.

Moen, A. N. 1973. Wildlife Ecology, an Analytical Approach. San Francisco: W. H. Freeman.

Moir, K. W. 1971. The *in vivo* and *in vitro* digestible fractions in forage. J. Sci. Food Agric. 22:338–341.

Mysterud, A., R. Langvatn, N. G. Yoccoz, and N. C. Stenseth. 2001. Plant phenology, migration and geographical variation in body weight of a large herbivore: the effect of variable topography. J. Anim. Ecol. 70: 915–923.

Norton, B. W. 1982. Differences between species in forage quality. Pp. 88–110 in The Nutrition of Herbivores, J. B. Hacker and J. H. Ternouth, eds. Sydney: Academic Press.

NRC (National Research Council). 1981. Nutrient Requirements of Goats: Angora, Dairy, and Meat Goats in Temperate and Tropical Countries. Washington, DC: National Academy Press.

Orpin C. G., and S. D. Mathiesen. 1990. Microbiology of digestion in the Svalbard reindeer (Rangifer tarandus platyrhyncus). Rangifer Spec. Iss. No. 3:187–199.

Orr, R. J., P. D. Penning, A. Harvey, and R. A. Champion. 1997. Diurnal patterns of intake rate by sheep grazing monocultures of ryegrass or white clover. Appl. Anim. Behav. Sci. 52:65–77.

Owen-Smith, R. N. 2002. Adaptive Herbivore Ecology. Cambridge, UK: Cambridge University Press.

Pennington, J. A. T. 1998. Bowes and Church's food values of portions commonly used, 17th rev. ed. Philadelphia: J. B. Lipincott Williams and Wilkins.

Person, S. J., R. E. Pegau, R. G. White, and J. R. Luick. 1980. In vitro and nylon bag digestibilities of reindeer and caribou forages. J. Wildl. Manage. 44:613–622.

Pritchard, D. A., P. R. Martin, and P. K. O'Rourke. 1992. The role of condensed tannins in the nutritional value of mulga (*Acacia aneura*) for sheep. Aust. J. Agric. Res. 43:1739–1746.

Radcliffe, J. C., and M. J. Cochrane. 1970. Digestibility and crude protein changes in ten maturing pasture species. Proc. Aust. Soc. Anim. Prod. 8:531–536.

Radojevic, I., R. J. Simpson, J. A. St. John, and M. O. Humphreys. 1994. Chemical composition and *in vitro* digestibility of lines of *Lolium perenne* selected for high concentrations of water-soluble carbohydrate. Aust. J. Agric. Res. 45:901–912.

Reichardt, P. B., J. P. Bryant, B. R. Mattes, T. P. Clausen, F. S. Chapin, and M. Meyer. 1990. Winter chemical defense of Alaskan balsam poplar against snowshoe hares. J. Chem. Ecol. 16:1941–1959.

Robbins, C. T. 1992. Wildlife Feeding and Nutrition, 2nd ed. San Diego, CA: Academic Press.

Robbins, C. T., T. A. Hanley, A. E. Hagerman, O. Hjeljord, D. L. Baker, C. C. Schwartz, and W. W. Mautz. 1987a. Role of tannins in defending plants against ruminants: Reduction in protein availability. Ecology 68:98–107.

Robbins, C. T., S. Mole, A. E. Hageman, and T. A. Hanley. 1987b. Role of tannins in defending plants against ruminants: Reduction in dry matter digestion? Ecology 68:1606-1615.

Russell, D. E., A. M Martel, and W. A. C. Nixon. 1993. Range ecology of the porcupine caribou herd in Canada. Rangifer Spec. Iss. No. 8.

SCA (Standing Committee on Agriculture). 1990. Feeding Standards for Australian Livestock: Ruminants. Standing Committee on Agriculture, Ruminants Subcommittee. Melbourne, Australia: CSIRO.

Schmidt, D. A., M. S. Kerley, J. H. Porter, and J. L. Dempsey. 2005. Structural and nonstructural carbohydrate, fat and protein composition of commercially available, whole produce. Zoo Biol. 0:1–15.

Schwartz, C. C., and T. N. Hobbs 1985. Forage and range evaluation. Pp. 25–51 in Bioenergetics of Wild Herbivores, R. J. Hudson and R. G. White, eds. Boca Raton, FL: CRC Press.

Schwartz C. C., and L. A. Renecker 1998. Nutrition and energetics. Pp. 441–478 in Ecology and Management of the North American Moose, A. W. Franzmann and C. C. Schwartz, eds. Washington, DC: Smithsonian Institution Press.

Siever-Kelly, C., B. J. Leury, K. L. Gatford, R. J. Simpson, and H. Dove. 1999. Spray-topping annual grass pasture with glyphosate to delay loss of feeding value during summer. II. Herbage intake, digestibility and diet selection in penned sheep. Aust. J. Agric. Res. 50:465–474.

Skjenneberg S., and L. Slagsvold. 1979. Reindeer Husbandry and Its Ecological Principles. English translation of Norwegian (T. T. Deer). Reindriften og dens Naturgrunnlag, Universitetsforlaget, Oslo, 1968, C. M. Anderson and J. R. Luick, eds. U.S. Dept. Interior Bureau of Indian Affairs, Juneau, AK.

Skopec, M. M., A. E. Hagerman, and W. H. Karasov. 2004. Do salivary praline-rich proteins counteract dietary hydrolysable tannin in laboratory rats? J. Chem. Ecol. 30:1679–1692.

Smouter, H., and R. J. Simpson. 1989. Occurrence of fructans in the Gramineae (Poaceae). New Phytol. 111:359–368.

Solberg, Y. T. 1970. Studies on the chemistry of lichens. IX. Quantitative determination of monosaccharides and amino acids in hydrolysates of several Norwegian lichen species. Lichenologist 4:283–288.

Spalinger, D. E., C. T. Robbins, and T. A. Hanley. 1986. The assessment of handling time in ruminants: The effect of plant chemical and physical structure on the rate of breakdown of plant particles in the rumen of mule deer and elk. Can. J. Zool. 64:312–321.

Staaland, H., N. A. Øritsland, and R. G. White. 1988. Digestion of energy and nutrients in Svalbard reindeer. Rangifer 8:2–10.

Svihus, B., and Ø. Holand. 2000. Lichen polysaccharides and their relation to reindeer/caribou nutrition. J. Range Manage. 53:642–648.

Thomas, D. C., and P. Kroeger. 1980. In vitro digestibilities of plants in rumen fluids of Peary caribou. Arctic 33:757–767.

Trudell, J., R. G. White, E. Jacobsen, H. Staaland, E. Ekern, and K. Kildemo. 1980. Comparison of some factors affecting the in vitro digestibility estimate of reindeer forages. Pp. 262–273 in Proc. 2nd Int. Reindeer and Caribou Symp., E. Reimers, E. Gaare, and S. Skjenneberg, eds. Trondheim, Norway: Directoratet for vilt og ferskvannsfisk.

USDA-ARS (U.S. Department of Agriculture, Agricultural Research Service). 2004. USDA National Nutrient Database for Standard Reference, Release 17. Nutrient Data Laboratory. Available: http://www.nal.usda.gov/fnic/foodcomp/Data/SR17/sr17.html. Accessed June 1, 2005.

Van der Wal, R., N. Madan, S. van Lieshout, C. Dormann, R. Langvatn, and S. D. Albon. 2000. Trading forage quality for quantity? Plant phenology and patch choice by Svalbard reindeer. Oecologia 123:108–115.

Van Soest, P. J. 1964. Symposium on nutrition and forage and pastures: New chemical procedures for evaluating forages. J. Anim. Sci. 23:838–845.

Van Soest, P. J. 1982. Nutritional Ecology of the Ruminant: Ruminant Metabolism, Nutritional Strategies, the Cellulolytic Fermentation and the Chemistry of Forages and Plant Fibers. Corvallis, OR: O & B Books.

Van Soest, P. J. 1994. The Nutritional Ecology of the Ruminant, 2nd ed. Ithaca, NY: Cornell University Press.

Villalba, J. J., F. D. Provenza, and R. E. Banner. 2002. Influence of macronutrients and polyethylene glycol on intake of a quebracho tannin diet by sheep and goats. J. Anim. Sci. 80:3154–3164.

Waghorn, G. C., N. R. Adams, and D. R. Woodfield. 2002. Deleterious substances in grazed pastures. Pp. 333–356 in Sheep Nutrition, M. Freer and H. Dove, eds. Wallingford, UK: CABI/CSIRO Publishing.

White, R. G., and Lawler, J. P. 2002. Can methane suppression during digestion of woody and leafy browse compensate for energy costs of detoxification of plant secondary compounds? A test with muskoxen fed willows and birch. Comp. Biochem. Physiol. 133A:849–859.

White, R. G., and Staaland, H. 1983. Ruminal volatile fatty acid production as an indicator of forage quality in Svalbard reindeer. Acta Zool. Fenn. 175:61–63.

White, R. G., B. R. Thomson, T. Skogland, S. J. Person, D. E. Russell, D. F. Holleman, and J. R. Luick. 1975. Ecology of caribou at Prudhoe Bay, Alaska. Pp. 151–201 in Ecological Investigations of the Tundra Biome in the Prudhoe Bay Region, Alaska, J. Brown, ed. Biol. Papers, Univ. Alaska, Spec. Report No. 2.

White, R. G., F. L. Bunnell, E. Gaare, T. Skogland, and B. Hubert. 1981. Ungulates on Arctic ranges. Pp. 397-483 in Tundra Ecosystems: A Comparative Analysis. IBP Vol. 25, L. C. Bliss, O. W. Heal, and J. J. Moore, eds. Cambridge, UK: Cambridge University Press.

Wildlife Conservation Society. 2001. Zootrition, version 2.0. Bronx, NY.

Wilson, J. R. 1994. Cell wall characteristics in relation to forage digestion by ruminants. J. Agric. Sci., Cambridge 122:173–182.

Yemm, E. W., and A. J. Willis. 1954. The estimation of carbohydrates in plant extracts by anthrone. Biochem. J. 57:508–514.

11

Nutrient Sources and Feeding Practices

IMPORTANCE AND CLASSIFICATION OF SOURCES OF NUTRIENTS

Previous chapters addressed the nutrients energy, protein, minerals, vitamins, and water required in diets of small ruminants. These nutrients are derived from feeds (diet) that are consumed and subjected to the digestive processes of the gastrointestinal tracts of the various animal species. Diets may be obtained directly by grazing or browsing growing or senesced plants still in place or may be provided in a trough in a planned manner to animals in confinement or dry-lot. Intensively managed pastures or mixed pastures through rotational grazing may maximize forage quality and provide complete diet. A third common practice is a combination of the first two in which animals are allowed to graze freely and are provided a supplement containing nutrients that may be inadequate in the feeds otherwise consumed. Whether the diet is adequate for providing the required nutrients depends on which ingredients are chosen and consumed by the animal during grazing and in what amounts and/or which complete diets or supplements are fed. The Feed Composition Tables 15-11, 15-12, and 15-13 provide estimates of the nutrient contents of most common feeds. Some nutrient concentrations were not estimated because of the lack of data. Actual levels of nutrients in feeds vary and can be estimated more accurately by sampling and analysis. All nutrient contents are listed considering that other nutrients are available in the diet in adequate amounts. Water is a special case. Although a portion is derived from other dietary components, most water is consumed as liquid from existing sources in the landscape or a trough and will not be considered further in this discussion of feeds (although water is covered more thoroughly in Chapter 9).

The availabilities of the organic nutrients (protein and energy-releasing compounds) from grazed or formulated feedstuff sources are determined largely by the chemical makeup of the cell walls that regulate accessibility of the nutrients to digestive processes and secondary plant chemicals that impose various levels of chemical interference. These governing processes are discussed in detail in Chapter 10.

Estimates of the nutrient contents of feedstuffs are presented in three tables:

Feed Composition Table 15-11: Common Feedstuffs for Small Ruminants

- A) Green and senesced forages either grazed or harvested and fed fresh
- B) Silages
- C) Other roughages including harvested and cured forages
- D) High-protein sources
- E) High-energy sources

Feed Composition Table 15-12: Browse and Other Novel Sources

Feed Composition Table 15-13: Mineral Sources

Feed Composition Table 15-11: Common Feedstuffs for Small Ruminants

Green and Senesced Forages Either Grazed or Harvested and Fed Fresh

Forages vary in nutrient density depending largely on fiber and protein contents determined by species differences, stage of growth, and cultural practices (Chapter 10). Forages that are low in fiber and high in protein, such as ryegrass in the early vegetative stage of growth, provide the required nutrients for animals in high levels of productivity. Conversely, forages in advance stages of growth (e.g., wheat straw and mature or senesced range grasses) often are high in fiber and low in available nutrients. They are suited only for animals in lower stages of production and may require concurrent feeding of supplements.

Green forages may be grazed or stall-fed in a zero grazing system. Small ruminants can consume large amounts of forages by grazing; however, intake may be higher at the trough with cut-and-carry feeding systems (Morand-Fehr, 1981). On heterogeneous resources (browse and graze), small ruminants, particularly goats, are more selective and choose a diet of higher quality than that offered in trough (Van et al., 2004). The relationship between the nutritive value of forages and voluntary intake and its importance is presented in detail in Chapter 3. Also described is the positive relationship between forage quality (and voluntary intake) and the opportunity of the small ruminant to be selective for diet ingredients whether grazing/browsing or in confinement. Therefore, increasing refusal allowance by providing greater amounts (de Simiane, 1978) and types of forage may increase diet quality and voluntary intake.

Silages

Common silages are partially fermented grain crops, grass, and legume forages and should be produced free of molds. Whereas the feeding of silage to small ruminants is not rare, the technology for its use in cattle feeding systems is more highly developed. Grass silage has been successfully used in goat diet when compared to hay (Trodahl et al., 1981). However, many high-moisture residues from food industries, such as apple pomace, cull apples, potatoes, beet pulp, and cannery refuse, can also be preserved as silage and fed to small ruminants. Other crops in the tropics, such as banana residue (stems and leaves) mixed with sugar cane or molasses, can produce satisfactory silage (Pieltain et al., 1998). Cassava leaves, though high in cell wall contents, can produce a good low-energy silage (Ly, 2003).

Other Roughages Including Harvested and Cured Forages

Dry forages include hays, pelleted forages, and some byproducts such as straws and hulls. Hays are partially dried forages with less than 15 percent allowable moisture. Hay harvested in an early stage of growth may have lower dry matter (DM) content and a lower yield per unit of land area, but will be higher in protein and digestibility compared with hay harvested in later stages (Fick and Mueller, 1989). Properly cured hays with minimum shattering (loss of leaves), leaching (rain damage and loss of soluble nutrients), and bleaching (excessive exposure to sunlight) will maintain nutritive value for prolonged periods. Roughages are often fed to add a bulk factor (Perry et al., 1999) to the diet thereby reducing digestive disturbances. Dry forages (or other roughages) added to high-concentrate diets can increase rumen buffering capacity, optimize rumen fermentation, and improve milk fat synthesis (Allen, 1997). However, higher plant cell wall and neutral detergent fiber (NDF) content of forages can reduce intake and digestibility (see Chapter 10). Straws, most hulls, and stovers are of lower quality (digestibility) (Torrent et al., 1994) but not necessarily of low value in mixed feed because of the associated effects on the animal's use of the complete diet. Cottonseed hulls have higher palatability and feeding value than peanut hulls and oat hulls. All are generally low-quality roughages that contribute mostly to the bulk factor of the ration (Perry et al., 1999). Soybean hulls are an exception; in combination with hay, they are excellent forages for small ruminants (Martin and Hibberd, 1990).

High-Protein Sources

Feeds containing crude protein at levels greater than 20 percent of DM are considered high-protein sources because they exceed the minimum protein concentrations required by small ruminants. High-protein alfalfa hay, meal, or cubes are desirable protein sources, but other plant high-protein concentrates such as the oil seed byproduct meals (e.g., cottonseed, peanut, and soybean) may be more economical sources, especially for mixed rations. Animal protein concentrates such as blood meal, fish meal, feather meal, bone meal, or meat and bone meal have high amounts of undegradable intake protein (UIP), but some may not be approved for feeding animals that provide products used in human food. Concentrates containing high UIP proportions vary in their amino acid balance and, thus, supply amino acids for digestion in the lower gastrointestinal tract that differ in value. Corn gluten meal is high in UIP and has a poor balance of amino acids, whereas fish meal and heat-treated soybean meal provide a good and beneficial balance (Santos et al., 1998). Soybean meal is a high-quality protein with high degradable intake protein (DIP). Readers are advised to refer to Chapters 2 and 5 for detailed discussions on the importance of protein solubility and site of digestion.

Urea provides nonprotein nitrogen (source of ammonia to the rumen microorganisms) that is efficiently used by microorganisms of the rumen during fermentation and protein synthesis but should be used with caution (Chapter 13). Urea does not provide energy in the diet; therefore, it should be included only with adequate readily digestible carbohydrates. Its use with low-energy feeds, such as low-quality forages, is not recommended unless adequate time for adaptation and other sources of readily available energy are provided. Also, it should not be included in the diets of young ruminants when the rumen is not fully functional. Ammonia toxicity can occur when a large amount of urea is introduced in the diet or the ration containing urea is improperly mixed (Chapter 13).

There are numerous varieties of commercial protein supplements available, such as byproduct meals (most common in ration formulation), cubes or pellets, liquid supplements, and blended and cooked containerized products. Protein is the most expensive part of the diet; therefore, cost comparison, presence of other dietary components, palatability, feeding facilities, labor cost/convenience, and uniformity of intake must be considered. Many factors that can influence supplement consumption by individual animals are discussed by Bowman and Sowell (1997). These factors include amount provided, supplement formulation, form, and delivery methods. Also included are animal-related factors, including exposure time, previous experiences, and social interactions and forage factors such as quality and availability.

High-Energy Sources

Energy feeds are quantitatively the most important feeds in practical livestock rations. Concentrates that are high in energy usually contain less than 20 percent protein and 18 percent fiber. They include, but are not limited to, all cereal grains, some root crops, flour-mill byproducts, bakery byproducts, and other food manufacturing byproducts such as beet pulp and citrus pulp. Vegetable oil or animal fats are also used to increase energy density of the diet.

Cereal grains such as barley, corn, wheat, oats, and sorghum contain large amounts of readily digestible carbohydrates (Rowe and Pethick, 1994), but also contain certain nonstarch polysaccharides, fiber, and protein (Van Barneveld, 1999). High-energy feeds yield absorbable energy-yielding compounds such as volatile fatty acids (VFA) and increase the flow of protein to the lower gastrointestinal tract by increasing both rumen fermentation rate and microbial protein synthesis (Hirstov et al., 2005). However, high levels of grain feeding can reduce the rate of fermentation of plant cell wall constituents (CWC), as discussed in Chapter 10. The net result of feeding grain to animals, which are also receiving roughage, will depend on the relative qualities and intakes of both the grain and roughage and on the nutritive requirements and expected productivity of the animals.

There is little difference in the net values of corn, sorghum, barley, and wheat as energy concentrates for small ruminants, and cost usually is the determining factor. Rapid fermentation of the starch in grains can cause acute and recurring acidosis (Chapter 13) if not increased in the diet in increments over time (Mackie et al., 2002). Wheat has the highest starch content followed by corn, sorghum, barley, and oats (Nocek and Tamminga, 1991). Ground wheat fed at 33 percent of diet DM had no negative effect on animals (Faldet et al., 1989); however, it should be fed with caution if included in the grain mixture at greater amount. Oats, on the other hand, are less likely to produce acidotic conditions. Gelaye et al. (1997) reported that pearl millet grain could be substituted successfully for corn in complete diets for lactating dairy goats but not for immature (growing) animals. Although the metabolizable energy of pearl millet is only 92 percent that of corn for mature goats and the crude protein may be less efficiently utilized, the energy intake and nitrogen balance were similar for both grains because of the increased intake of pearl millet (Terrill et al., 1998).

Some unprocessed seeds containing elevated lipids such as cottonseed and soybeans can be used as energy concentrates. Whole cottonseed (WCS), perhaps the most common, contains high levels of both crude protein (CP) (20–24 percent) and energy (3.4 Mcal ME [metabolizable energy]/kg) and requires no processing, which makes it a very desirable byproduct feed (Poore and Rogers, 1995). Most of the energy in WCS is from fat. Whole cottonseed also contains gossypol, a polyphenolic yellow pigment that can reduce male reproduction function (Randel et al., 1992) if consumed at high levels. Adding WCS (0, 8, 14, and 24 percent of diet) to medium- or low-quality forage diets for growing male goats had detrimental effects on animal production (Luginbuhl et al., 2000). However, feeding WCS at 15 percent of the diet improved DM digestibility and increased rate of passage (Solaiman et al., 2002) and had no adverse effect on growth or sperm quality in growing male goats (McCrary, 1998).

Brewer's grains and distillers grains are also good energy feed. Distillers grains include distillers dried grains, distillers dried grains with solubles, condensed distillers solubles, and wet distillers grains. These co-products of the distiller industry are good sources of energy and protein; however, drying may produce changes that reduce their nutritional quality (Weiss et al., 1989; Van Soest, 1989). Wet distillers grains (Firkins et al., 1985) and thin stillage (Rust et al., 1990) have been used as good sources of energy and protein for cattle.

Roots and tubers such as dried sweet potatoes and sweet potato meals are high in digestible starch and carotene and can substitute for corn in the diet (Aregheore, 2004). Although cassava is a tropical root crop, significant amounts of dehydrated cassava meal are used in animal feeds in the United States and Europe. It is a high-energy feed and can replace most of the grain portion of the diet (Dunga et al., 2005). However, fresh cassava may contain cyanogenic glucosides, linamarin, and lotaustralin that convert to hydrocyanic acid and produce prussic acid in the rumen and must be heat processed before use. Prussic acid inhibits oxygen transport at the cellular level and causes the animal to suffocate (Stoltenow and Lardy, 1998).

Lipid supplements are used commonly as ingredients in concentrate feeds to increase the caloric value (energy concentration), to serve as a carrier of fat-soluble ingredients (including vitamins A and E, and essential fatty acids), to facilitate the digestion of these fat-soluble ingredients, and to improve the physical nature of the mixed ration (Palmquist, 1987). Dietary lipids may be protected to alter the profile of fatty acids in meat or milk fat to be more desirable for the food industry (Keeney, 1970). Although the process of biohydrogenation in the rumen (Reiser, 1951) greatly alters the fatty acids available to the animal for metabolism, long-chain fatty acid composition of the dietary ingredients may influence the energetic value of the diet (NRC, 2001). As noted in Chapter 6, fatty acid composition of the diet is particularly important when attempting to alter the fatty acid profile of food products derived from small ruminants. Long-chain fatty acid composition of selected feedstuffs is listed in Table 11-1.

Lipid content and fatty acid profile varies considerably among feedstuffs. Small differences may be noted between the total fatty acids in Table 11-1 and the ether extract (EE) values shown in Table 15-11. These differences are not surprising because variability exists among sample of ingredients, and fatty acids are only a portion of total lipids.

TABLE 11-1 Long-Chain Fatty Acids in Some Feedstuffs Fed to Small Ruminants[a]

Feedstuff	Total Fatty Acids g/100 g DM	Fatty Acid Profile (g/100 g of fatty acid)						
		16:0	16:1	18:0	18:1	18:2	18:3	Other
Cereal Grains								
Barley	1.6	29.1	0.8	2.8	18.4	37.9	2.9	8.1
Corn, high oil	7.9	12.7	0.6	2.5	30.8	47.9	1.0	4.5
Corn, yellow	4.0	13.0	0.5	2.0	26.4	52.5	1.7	3.9
Oats	3.2	22.1	1.0	1.3	38.1	34.9	2.1	0.5
Sorghum grain (milo)	2.3	20.0	5.2	1.0	31.6	40.2	2.0	—
Wheat	1.0	20.0	0.7	1.3	17.5	55.8	4.5	0.2
Roughages								
Alfalfa hay	1.5	35.8	—	3.3	3.4	15.5	21.5	20.7
Alfalfa meal, dehy	1.4	28.5	2.4	3.8	6.5	18.4	39.0	1.4
Alfalfa pellets, dehy	1.1	27.0	1.9	4.9	6.2	20.5	25.7	13.8
Alfalfa silage	1.9	22.0	2.1	3.4	3.5	19.5	27.1	22.4
Barley silage	0.7	21.7	—	3.3	18.5	28.1	6.4	22.0
Bromegrass hay	1.2	28.0	—	3.8	7.5	18.7	22.8	18.0
Citrus pulp	2.7	32.0	3.9	1.8	23.8	36.7	1.8	—
Cocksfoot		11.2	6.4	2.6	—	76.5	—	3.3
Corn silage	2.7	16.4	1.7	2.4	19.8	49.0	2.8	7.9
Foxtail millet hay	2.2	22.0	—	3.0	11.6	25.0	20.2	17.9
Orchardgrass	1.8	16.5	—	1.5	0.8	8.9	27.9	42.6
Ryegrass, perennial		11.9	1.7	1.0	2.2	14.6	68.2	0.4
Ryegrass pellets, dehy	1.9	14.0	1.8	1.3	1.9	10.5	64.1	6.4
Ryegrass pasture, perennials		14.2	—	4.2	2.2	11.2	47.5	20.7
Ryegrass silage, perennial	1.8	20.2	0.2	2.0	2.7	15.0	46.4	13.5
Red clover	1.2	23.0	—	3.7	5.7	13.5	46.2	2.2
Red clover silage	2.2	24.0	0.1	3.0	2.1	18.0	43.9	8.9
Sugarbeet tops		25.2	2.1	5.7	19.1	19.8	18.3	9.8
Tyfon		22.6	2.0	5.6	8.7	12.5	32.7	15.9
Turnip tops		26.9	1.3	6.4	7.8	10.4	35.5	11.7
White clover		6.5	2.5	0.5	6.6	18.5	60.7	4.7
White clover silage	2.4	22.4	0.2	2.7	3.0	18.6	44.8	8.3
Oilseeds								
Canola (rapeseed)	38.0	4.0	0.3	1.6	57.1	23.9	9.6	3.5
Cottonseed	18.6	25.3	—	2.8	17.1	53.2	0.1	1.4
Safflower seed, high-oleate	34.0	7.0	—	0.1	75.6	11.3	0.5	5.5
Safflower seed, high-linoleate	36.5	7.7	—	2.6	10.3	73.8	0.4	5.2
Soybeans	19.6	10.9	0.2	4.0	22.8	50.9	6.8	4.4
Sunflower seed, high-oleate	43.5	0.1	—	4.4	87.3	2.1	0.1	6.0
Sunflower seed, high-linoleate	37.5	6.2	—	3.0	17.8	70.7	0.2	2.1
Fat supplements	90.0[b]							
				Animal Fats and Animal-Vegetable Fat Blends				
Animal-vegetable fat blend		23.8	1.6	16.8	31.7	14.9	1.7	9.5
Grease, choice white		23.4	4.3	13.3	43.4	10.9	1.3	3.4
Lard		24.4	6.5	10.6	38.4	19.3	—	0.8
Poultry fat		22.1	7.2	6.5	43.0	18.5	1.0	1.7
Tallow		27.2	4.1	18.8	40.6	2.6	0.5	6.2
Yellow grease		22.1	3.5	11.5	43.7	14.6	1.0	3.6
					Fish Oils[c]			
Herring		11.7	9.6	0.8	12.0	1.1	0.8	56.8
Menhaden		19.2	13.5	4.7	14.9	2.5	1.7	43.5
Salmon		19.0	2.0	6.0	24.0	3.0	13.0	33.0
Squid		18.3	5.3	2.8	13.0	1.7	1.4	42.5
Tuna		22.5	3.0	6.1	14.3	1.5	0.4	52.2
					Vegetable Oils			
Canola (rapeseed)		4.6	0.5	1.8	60.9	19.0	7.1	6.1
Corn		10.7	—	1.9	25.6	57.7	0.9	3.2

TABLE 11-1 continued

Feedstuff	Total Fatty Acids g/100 g DM	Fatty Acid Profile (g/100 g of fatty acid) 16:0	16:1	18:0	18:1	18:2	18:3	Other
Coconut[d]		12.3	—	3.4	8.5	1.2	—	74.6
Cottonseed		22.7	0.7	2.5	16.5	54.9	0.2	2.5
Linseed		5.5	—	3.9	19.9	14.1	55.3	1.3
Olive		12.0	1.0	2.3	72.5	8.5	1.3	2.4
Palm		43.0	0.2	3.7	42.8	5.6	0.2	4.5
Peanut		10.9	0.1	2.7	48.2	32.6	—	5.5
Safflower, high-linoleate		7.1	0.2	2.6	12.6	74.6	0.5	2.4
Sesame		8.9	0.2	4.8	39.3	41.3	0.3	5.2
Soybean		10.9	0.2	4.0	21.5	53.5	7.3	2.6
Sunflower		5.4	0.2	3.5	45.3	39.8	0.2	5.6
				Granular and Rumen-Protected Fats				
Linoleate, calcium salts		4.8	—	2.4	53.1	29.3	—	10.4
Linoleamide	84.7	2.5	—	0.9	28.9	61.8	5.3	0.6
Palm oil fatty acids, calcium salts	84.0	44.3	1.1	4.1	35.1	7.9	0.3	7.2
Tallow fatty acids, hydrolyzed		39.7	0.7	42.7	10.9	1.0	—	2.6
Tallow, partially hydrogenated[e]		25.6	0.5	44.9	22.9	0.5	0.2	5.4

[a]Averaged from the scientific literature. The proportion of a fatty acid was not listed if its value was less than 0.1 percent. Values reported in Table 11-1 are representative only.
[b]Triacylglycerol (90 percent fatty acid) was assumed to be the major lipid class of fats and oils (Palmquist and Jenkins, 2003).
[c]Other fatty acids consist predominantly of polyunsaturated fatty acids greater than 18 carbons in length (e.g., 20:4, 20:5, and 22:6).
[d]Other fatty acids consist predominantly of medium-chain fatty acids (8:0, 10:0, 12:0, and 14:0).
[e]Composition of partially hydrogenated tallow is reported as an average; however, composition varies considerably among products due to varying degrees of hydrogenation.

Acylglycerols constitute the major lipid class of most cereals, oilseeds, and fat supplements. For forage plants, the cuticular fraction is composed of 28- to 40-carbon fatty acids, hydroxyl and epoxy fatty acids, alcohols, and hydrocarbons that are unlikely to be digested and utilized by the animal (Palmquist, 1988). Fatty acids of nutritional significance comprise only about one-half of the total lipid content of forages. These long-chain fatty acids exist largely as glycolipids and phospholipids in the chloroplasts, which decrease as the plant matures (Hawke, 1973). Harvesting and processing (in forms of hays and silages) also alter the long-chain fatty acid profile of forage lipids (Dewhurst et al., 2003). Slow oxidation and polymerization of unsaturated fatty acids form resins and reduce ether-soluble substances and carotenoids in harvested plants (Couchman, 1959). However, the extent of this alteration depends on the degree of unsaturated fatty acids in the plant oil.

Feed Composition Table 15-12: Browse and Other Novel Sources

Habitats and diets of small ruminants are characterized by variation and variety. Free-ranging sheep, goats, and deer prefer foliage from trees and shrubs (browse) and herbaceous dicots over grasses (McMahan, 1964; Ramircz, 1999). Feed resources appropriate for one species may be inadequate for another, although the species may be very similar in appearance and form (Evers, 1997). Diets selected by the different species of New World camelids (NWC) are not the same and differ from those selected by small ruminant domestic and nondomestic species (Chapter 3). Although classifying a feedstuff as typical or novel is sometimes arbitrary, Table 15-12 contains estimates of nutrient contents of feeds that commonly are not listed in tables used to evaluate and formulate diets of cattle. Small ruminants, considered as a worldwide population, depend heavily on these feedstuffs.

Foliage classified as browse may be rich in nutrients (Devendra, 1979; Huston et al., 1981; Fagan and Solaiman, 1993) but often contains secondary plant chemicals such as tannins, terpenes/terpeniods, or other compounds (Chapter 3) that restrict the availabilities of the nutrients or otherwise harm the animal (Hegarty et al., 1964; Short et al., 1992). In some instances, nutritional values indicated by laboratory analyses are higher than is realized in animal performance (Solaiman et al., 2006). Under other circumstances, browse offers the best opportunity for animals to satisfy their requirements and provides a collateral benefit in reducing parasite infestations (Min and Hart, 2003; Solaiman et al., 2006). Available browse can serve as a supplement in pastures in declining forage quality and help sustain grazing animal performance (Papachristou et al., 1999). Supplementation with conventional feeds (e.g., barley) can reduce secondary compound overload (Ben Salem et al., 2003) and improve the value of pastures that are predominantly browse.

Other novel sources of nutrients include seeds, fruits, byproducts, and fresh or discarded produce that can be consumed on site of production or harvested and delivered to the animals. High moisture contents of many of these feeds preclude long-term storage or transporting long distances. Nutrient concentrations for these sources listed in Table 15-12 are incomplete because of lack of data, but most entries are described for DM, CP, and total digestible nutrients (TDN), which are good indicators of nutritive value.

Feed Composition Table 15-13: Mineral Sources

Small ruminants require several mineral elements in their diets for normal metabolic activities and as components of various products (e.g., calcium [Ca] in milk, sulfur [S] in wool, Ca and phosphorus [P] in antlers). Those required in small amounts (micro elements or trace minerals) are infrequently of concern, but those required in relatively higher concentrations (macro elements or major minerals) receive primary consideration. Requirements for Ca and P, two of the most deficient of the macro elements, are given in Tables 15-1, 15-2, 15-4, 15-5, 15-6, 15-9, and 15-10 for sheep, goats, cervids, and NWC. Detailed discussions and specific requirements for all necessary minerals are topics of Chapter 7.

Sources of minerals include the major dietary components (e.g., forages, hays, and grains), which vary in their mineral content (Adams, 1975; Kertz, 1998), and supplementary mineral concentrates fed selectively to provide specific minerals to balance the total diet. Table 15-13 lists the sources of minerals in concentrate form and is arranged to show the available choices from individual minerals of interest. Mineral supplements can be as simple as common salt (NaCl) or as complex mixtures of several macro and trace elements along with vitamins provided free choice in loose or block forms or mixed with the total ration. Commercial mineral blocks ordinarily contain salt alone, salt and sulfur, or salt plus a formulated balance of trace minerals. Some sources listed in Table 15-13 contain more than one of the required minerals (e.g., dicalcium phosphate) and are listed under more than one mineral, whereas others (e.g., calcium carbonate) are listed for only one mineral. An important consideration is availability of the minerals from the different sources, a topic addressed in Chapter 7.

FEED PROCESSING AND MANUFACTURING

Forages

Processing of forages to change physical structure and, sometimes, chemical content involves considerations of feeding value, feeding convenience, and economic return. Fahey et al. (1993) and Berger et al. (1994) reviewed processing methods of forages for ruminants in the early 1990s. The most common processing methods addressed in these reviews are highlighted below, with special consideration given for small ruminants.

Chopping, grinding, and pelleting are common methods for changing the physical characteristics of forages. Chopping or coarse grinding of forage has little or no impact on intake or digestibility but does increase the ease of handling. Fine grinding, however, can alter feed intake and/or digestion (Goetsch et al., 1997). The decrease in particle size with fine grinding increases both the exposed surface area and the rate at which microbes attach, thereby increasing rate of digestion of potentially digestible cell walls (Fadel, 1984). Grinding does not necessarily increase the extent of digestion. With ad libitum intake and relative smaller particle size of ingesta, both rate of digesta flow through the gastrointestinal tract and intake increase, typically resulting in decreased extent of digestion (Fahey et al., 1993). Grinding coarsely chopped forages decreased salivary flow, pH, and chewing activity, and depressed milk fat (Shaver et al., 1986; Grant et al., 1990). However, a minimum of 3 mm particle size was needed for optimum chewing and buffering (Allen, 1997). Finely ground alfalfa hay had lower retention time and resulted in lower fiber digestion (Rodrique and Allen, 1960). Further, finely ground forages are often pelleted to avoid dustiness and for further improvements in ease of handling. Pelleting also increases intake and digesta flow thereby possibly decreasing extent of digestion. For both processes, fine grinding and pelleting, increases in feed intake (Van Soest, 1994b) are relatively greater than declines in digestibility for an overall rise in ME intake.

Treatment of forages with hydrolytic chemicals (alkali), including sodium hydroxide, ammonia, and urea (via ammoniation), improves rate and extent of ruminal digestion (Haddad et al., 1994). This occurs primarily by partial hemicellulose solubilization, including that of linkages with noncore lignin. Other changes impacting nutritive value are increases in particle fragility and partial solubilization of silica, disruptions of intermolecular hydrogen bonding in cellulose, and decreases in time for fiber hydration and the rate and extensiveness of microbial attachment and colonization (Jackson, 1977; Berger et al., 1979; Males, 1987). Effects of alkali treatment are greater with monocots than with dicots because of differences between the two forage types in chemical linkages involving lignin. Generally, effects of sodium hydroxide have been greater than those achieved by ammoniation. An attribute of the addition of ammonia or urea, especially with low-quality forages, is an increase in nitrogen (CP) concentration (Schneider and Flachowsky, 1990).

As with fine grinding and pelleting, treatment with alkali can increase feed intake for an increased rate of particle passage from the rumen to a degree that extent of digestion is unchanged, but ME intake is increased (Animut et al., 2002; Abebe et al., 2004). Maximal improvements in ME intake will occur only with adequate ruminally available nitrogenous compounds and animals with high production potential.

There are other treatments of forages and diets but none that are receiving widespread usage. One possible exception for the future is exogenous fibrolytic enzymes. Beauchemin et al. (2003) proposed that enzyme application to feedstuffs or diets before feeding results in binding with the substrate that impacts resistance to proteolysis and retention time in the rumen. Added enzymes may also cause structural changes in feed that enhance later digestion by ruminal microbes. Future research is necessary to better understand how exogenous enzymes work, proper methods of application, and production scenarios with greatest positive responses to specific products.

Concentrates

Concentrate feedstuffs can be ground and pelletized to decrease dustiness and selectivity, although fine grinding and pelleting has less effect on rate of digestion compared with forages. Because of more thorough mastication by small ruminants, grinding of corn generally is less advantageous than with cattle. Advantages of physical processing become greater for grains with slower rates of ruminal starch digestion, such as sorghum grain (Rowe et al., 1999). Performance benefits from more extensive processing of sorghum grain, such as steam flaking for starch gelatinization, may depend primarily on animal production potential. Benefits may also be coupled with protein sources that are degraded rapidly in the rumen (Matras et al., 1991). Using processing methods to increase fermentation rate of feed grains also increases the management risk of creating acute lactic acidosis during the initial feeding stage or after feeding mistakes (e.g., inadvertent failure to keep feed available at all times, as described in Chapter 13).

In some instances it is desirable to increase ruminal outflow of intact dietary protein. A common method of feed processing to achieve this is heat treatment. Heat denatures protein, which decreases solubility in the rumen and slows the rate at which protein is degraded (Van Soest, 1994a). Heat also causes formation of indigestible Maillard complexes (nonenzymatic browning reaction products), the rate and extent of which depend on temperature, length of processing, and presence of reducing sugars. This reaction involves the condensation of sugar residues with amino acids followed by polymerization. Through this process, proteins are rendered indigestible, particularly those amino acids with free nucleophilic group such as amine or sulfur in lysine, cystine, methionine, or phenolic group in tyrosine (Van Soest, 1994a). Other compounds, such as unsaturated oils and phenols, are also produced. The rate of the complete sequence of these reactions is slow until the temperature reaches 60–65°C (Van Soest, 1965). At lower temperatures, the extent of Maillard reaction product formation is small relative to the decrease in protein solubility and associated change in rate and extent of ruminal degradation.

Manufactured Feeds

Manufactured feeds are blends of ingredients that are formulated to supply all (full feed) or defined portions (supplement) of the requirements of targeted animals. Some blended mixes are intended to supply only a portion of the diet to be added to another portion (e.g., concentrate mix and hay, respectively) at feeding. Other blends may contain quantitatively minor ingredients (pre-mixes) that can be best prepared separately, then mixed with the larger portions.

The ingredients used in manufactured feeds and their proportions may differ, even under the same label, as determined by the similarities in the nutrients and physical characteristics provided among the ingredients and their relative costs. Most manufactured feeds will be blends of ingredients described in Tables 15-11 and 15-13. However, other byproduct feeds may be especially common in feeds for small ruminants around the world. Ben Salem and Nefzaoui (2003) reviewed the potential use of feed blocks from agroindustrial byproducts as alternative sources of supplement for grazing small ruminants. Other unusual byproducts include green tea waste (Kondo et al., 2004), dehydrated citrus pulp (Bueno et al., 2002), mustard cake (Anil Kumar et al., 2002), coffee pulp (Abate and Pfeffer, 1986), olive leaves (Yanez Ruiz et al., 2004), cowpea husks (Adeloye, 1995), and poultry waste (Qureshi, 1988; Bartlett, 1989). These are only examples of investigations in the use of byproduct feeds. Readers are advised to search the available scientific literature in determining the merits and disadvantages (e.g., variability in composition or potential carriers of micotoxins) of an ingredient to be used in a specific circumstance.

Various feed additives are included in diets, usually in pre-mixes, for health purposes and to stimulate animal performance (e.g., growth rate). These additives are usually classified as drugs and are regulated in the United States by the Food and Drug Administration (FDA). They include antibiotics, arsenicals, coccidiostats, nitrofurans, sulfas, hormone-like growth stimulants, and other special purpose additives (Chapter 12). Other additives intended for special purposes, such as polyethylene glycol (PEG) for binding tannins in browse (Gilboa et al., 2000), are under investigation.

Manufactured feeds are prepared as loose mixes, pellets, blocks, tubs (cooked and hardened simi-liquid blends), and liquids. Small ruminants have the ability to select for and against specific dietary ingredients because of the smaller size of their mouths and mouthparts, as well as the nimbleness of their lips and tongues. Also, individuals within a group vary considerably in their practice of food selection. Some small ruminants (concentrate selectors) may be highly selective for concentrate parts of a plant (shoots, fruits, nuts) and are highly intolerant of high fibrous forages (Hofmann, 1973); however, others (grass eaters) may be completely the opposite (Hofmann, 1988). Hence, the composition of total mixed diets or rations in loose form can differ markedly from that actually consumed by individuals. Each form carries advantages and disadvantages, especially when considering convenience as a value (Bowman and Sowell, 1997; Taylor et al., 2002a,b; Ben Salem and Nefzaoui, 2003; Ben Salem et al., 2003).

ASSOCIATIVE EFFECTS OF FEEDING

Associative effects between feedstuffs are very important considerations when balancing rations and determining proper supplements. Some feedstuffs may either impair or enhance utilization of others when fed together. The "supplement response," discussed in Chapter 3, describes the multiple responses possible when a feed containing high levels of one or more nutrients is fed to grazing animals. Forage consumption can increase (complementary effect), decrease (substitutive effect), or remain unchanged (additive effect), depending on the nutrient composition of the forage and the chemical composition of the supplement. Similar effects can be observed for the extent of digestion. Positive associative effects on intake and digestibility are common when animals consuming low-quality forages are fed a relatively low level of supplement containing adequate amounts of one or more nutrients that are deficient (e.g., P and/or DIP) (Bodine et al., 2000). Negative associative effects on intake and digestibility (although possibly an economically sound practice) occur when the supplement is fed at relatively high levels (requirements are met), or when the supplement contains liberal amounts of soluble carbohydrates or lipids that substantially change the rumen environment and the microbial population (Bodine et al., 2000, 2001). Although high amounts of soluble carbohydrates decrease fiber digestibility and intake, small amounts can increase fiber digestion by increasing rumen microbial activity.

Other associative effects of feeding are possible as well. The efficiency of energy utilization for protein synthesis is enhanced by feeds providing extra UIP, thereby increasing the amounts of absorbed amino acids (Chapters 4 and 5). A mineral supplement that provides too much Ca will result in a decrease in the absorption of several of the trace element cations that are supplied in other ingredients (Chapter 7). A supplement of vitamin D can alleviate a marginal Ca deficiency by facilitating the absorption of Ca from the small intestine (Chapter 8).

Therefore, an animal's diet has the net nutritional value of the combined interacting ingredients. The withdrawal of one ingredient may change the net value of the diet more or less than the value of that one ingredient. The nutrient contents of the ingredients described in Tables 15-11, 15-12, and 15-13 are estimated considering all other nutrients to be supplied are in appropriate balance.

FEEDING SYSTEMS

Feeding systems are strategies for supplying the required nutrients to animals from available nutrient sources. Sheep, goats, NWC, and a range of cervids occupy many environmental settings throughout the climatic zones of the earth. Likewise, many successful feeding systems have developed that are characteristic of local conditions and opportunities. Figure 11-1 depicts the generalized pattern of weight change for sheep for the annual production cycle (ASIA, 2002). Recognizable changes in weight during pregnancy, lactation, and recovery are typical in ewes receiving nutrients in the amounts specified in the Requirements Tables 15-1 and 15-2. Similar patterns of typical weight change apply to species of small ruminants. Feeding systems provide nutrients at changing levels mirroring more or less the levels required. That is, higher than average nutrients must be supplied during late pregnancy and early lactation to support adequate weight gain (growth of fetus and reproductive tissues) and allow only minimal weight loss (during milk synthesis), respectively. Lower than average nutrient supplies are needed after weaning and while recovering slowly to breeding condition. Thus, relatively low-quality feed or pasture may be acceptable for ewes after weaning but inadequate for ewes during late pregnancy.

Where the aim is to optimize profit, attempting to perfectly match nutrient supply and demand for individual animals may not be appropriate (Freer, 2002; Dove, 2004). In most grazing systems with domestic ruminants, profit accrues from animal production/area (total flock) rather than production/head. This almost always involves compromise and compensatory nutrition. Animals often will be below their requirements at some stage through the year in order to save costs or take advantage of other periods. Animals may be allowed to gain weight on a spring flush of plant growth and then utilize body energy reserves and lose weight over dry summers. It may be more profitable to accept the nutritional stress that results if ewes give birth well before the spring flush of pasture growth in order to ensure that lambs are weaned onto good-quality pasture. Livestock grazing systems that attempt to match nutrient supply and demand so that nutrient requirements of individual animals are always met are likely to be unprofitable.

The Livestock and Environmental Toolbox (LEAD, 1999) classified livestock management systems as grassland-based, mixed farming, and landless systems. Further, LEAD (1999) describes the agroecological regions as temperate and tropi-

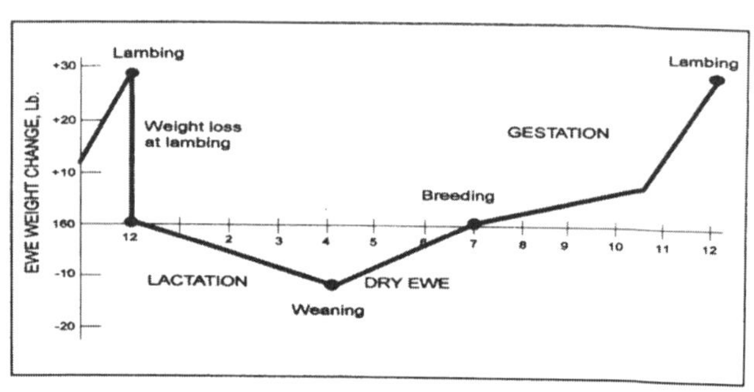

FIGURE 11-1 Annual weight change for single-bearing ewe. Reprinted, with permission, from the American Sheep Industry Association (2006). Sheep Production Handbook, Copyright 2003, All rights reserved.

cal highland, humid/subhumid tropics and subtropics, and arid/semi-arid tropics and subtropics. Forage growth patterns in temperate and tropical highlands are temperature-controlled. The temperate zone is characterized by distinct seasons and limited growth periods. Grasses growing during the warm season (C_4) and those growing during the cool season (C_3) coexist on the same land, but either can be favored by management practices to dominate the vegetation of an area for a special purpose. In tropical highlands (e.g., high mountain ranges of central South America), mean daily temperatures range from 5 to 20° C and the growing season often approaches 365 days depending on rainfall patterns. The tropics are warm areas with distinct rainy and dry seasons. Areas in the humid tropics often receive enough rainfall during the dry season to sustain some plant growth, whereas the dry season in the arid tropics can last up to 11 months. Forage quality is a limiting characteristic in the humid tropics and during the dry season in the arid zone. Grassland-based systems are common throughout all agroecological regions, whereas mixed farming systems are most commonly located in the temperate and subtropical regions where climatic conditions are favorable for alternative agricultural enterprises. Landless systems (e.g., livestock feedlots and confinement dairies) are found in all regions.

Examples of Feeding Systems

Feeding systems in the tropics include both grazing (grassland-based) and mixed systems. The grazing system involves natural or introduced pastures and forages grown under perennial cultivars. The main constraint for livestock production in the humid tropics is forage quality, a production challenge that must be addressed (Chapters 3 and 10). During the rainy season, forage dry matter accumulates and matures with the concomitant reduction in quality. The mixed system involves grazing and use of agricultural byproducts. Major opportunities for small ruminants in the tropics are in the use of forage/feed combinations including potentially available and high-yielding crops such as cassava (Hillocks et al., 2002), sugarcane (Sansoucy et al., 1988), foliage trees (Leng, 1997), grasses, and legumes, while maintaining soil fertility and the environment.

The subtropical and temperate zones are highly suited to small ruminants. Many systems, especially in New Zealand and Australia, are grassland-based and intensively managed using fertilization and variable stocking rates to manipulate forage quality and harvest efficiency. Nutrient content and forage quality changes as plants progress through vegetative, reproductive, and mature stages of growth (Minson, 1990) and as environmental factors change (Buxton and Fales, 1994). Grass-legume mix pastures may provide a more consistent production pattern than grasses alone and partially replace the need for nitrogen fertilization (Wen et al., 2002). Supplementation is used to increase production in grazing animals. Supplementation of low-quality forages with protein and/or nonprotein nitrogen increases forage intake (Huston, 1994; Paterson et al., 1994), but supplementation with energy supplements has a minimal or negative impact on forage intake (Huston, 1994; Poppi and McLennen, 1995; Matejovsky and Sanson, 1995; see also Chapter 3). Other systems combine the use of forage and byproducts to meet requirements. Solaiman et al. (2006) proposed a year-round foraging system for goats that included annual Marshall ryegrass (cool season grass) for winter grazing (December–April); peas or soybean greens (legume) for late spring and early summer (May–June); mimosa browse, sorghum, or bermudagrass (warm season grasses) for summer (July–October); and hay/concentrates to be used sparingly when needed.

Rangelands in the arid/semiarid regions support different vegetation types, including shrublands, chaparral, grasslands, steppes, woodlands, temporarily treeless areas in forests, as well as areas with dry, sandy, rocky, saline, or wet soils, or steep topography that preclude the growing of commercial farm and timber crops (Heady and Child, 1994). Rangeland occupies over 50 percent of Earth's land surface (World Resources Institute, 2003). Satisfying animal nutritional requirements on rangelands is challenging because of low and uncertain precipitation (erratic plant growth), variable nutrient content of a complex native forage base, and the expanse and variable topography of pastures (Launchbaugh and Hunt, 2000). The vegetation supplies the nutritional base for optimal production during the spring and summer months (or rainy seasons) provided forage availability is adequate. However, free-ranging ruminants may be unable to meet their nutritional requirements during periods created by erratic environmental conditions, especially during the dryer and more inclement seasons (DelCurto et al., 2000). The nutritive value (both nutrient content and nutrient availability) of rangeland vegetation typically decreases with advancing stages of phenological development. Thus, supplemental nutrients are usually (but not always) essential for small ruminant animals maintained on rangelands dominated by dormant and decedent vegetation. Recommendations for specific supplements are difficult because of the uncertainty of diet quality, a product of the erratic nature of rangeland environments. The successful feed manager must have a keen eye to assess range condition, nutrient needs, and body condition of the animals to determine the quantity and type of supplement needed to optimize production (Thomas and Kott, 1996).

An example of a landless system is the lamb feedlot that most frequently relies on concentrate/grain diets to finish lambs for market (ASIA, 2002). Lamb-feeding operations may be highly specialized and focus solely on the production of market lambs that are attained at some stage of postweaning growth and taken to market weight for sale as finished lambs. Most specialized lamb feeders purchase lambs to feed rather than manage the flocks that produce the lambs. However, in the farm flock areas, many of the ewe flock operations are also lamb-feeding operations and finish the lambs produced in that flock to market weight. These lamb-feeding operations may therefore be part of any of the production systems discussed above. High grain/concentrate diets that support rapid rates of gain are typically used. In some cases, high-quality pasture may be used for part or all of the lamb-feeding period.

Some sheep flocks are managed successfully in confinement or partial confinement systems (ASIA, 2002). These systems are equally successful for sheep and goats and are attractive when land values preclude or limit their use for agricultural production and when predation is severe under grazing systems. The nutritional management of confinement sheep flocks will depend on availability and cost of harvested forages and concentrate feeds. Diets will be formulated to meet the changing nutritional demands throughout the production stages.

Intensive and extensive systems for cervids managers of wildlife species, including those cervids specified in this publication, address nutritional requirements of individuals and populations held under five general systems: (1) individually penned animals held in zoos; (2) those retained in small groups on improved pastures for high-end productivity such as venison, milk production, or the antler and oriental byproducts market, usually termed deer farming (Haigh and Hudson, 1993; Evers, 1997); (3) unconfined animals on large acreage of native rangelands for recreational hunting, termed game ranching (Hudson et al., 1989; Renecker and Hudson, 1991); (4) communal grazing and quasi-nomadic herding of semi-domesticated reindeer for production of meat, byproducts, and antlers (Skjenneberg and Slagsvold, 1979; Zhigunov, 1986; Helle et al., 1990); and (5) wild populations managed for recreational and subsistence hunting, wildlife viewing, and natural components of ecosystems in parks, forests, preserves, and wilderness areas, where no exploitation necessarily occurs.

Although constituting diets for year-round feeding of cervids is the basic means of feeding animals in zoos, animals in most systems obtain most of their nutritional needs from grazing. Provision of supplements on a seasonal basis for various classes of animals provides nutrient intake in addition to that achieved through range management techniques. Those cervid species capable of adaptation to pastures, the intermediate, mixed foragers and grazers, are currently used for deer farming (Haigh and Hudson, 1993; Evers, 1997). In North America, the white-tailed deer, a more browser-adapted species, is farmed only to a limited extent because it does not adapt well to utilizing warm-season perennial grasses (Evers, 1997). Thus, in North America, deer farming is based mainly on exotic species and wapiti. Formulation of diets and supplements (Baker and Hobbs, 1985; Baker et al., 1998), combined with pasture or range management, has the objective of meeting maintenance requirements in winter for north temperate deer and during the dry season in the tropics. In zoos, frequent reproduction by individuals must be restricted to control numbers, and feeding at maintenance is required to maintain healthy animals by preventing individuals from becoming overly fat (Ratcliffe, 1966). For a number of species, e.g. white-tailed deer, wapiti, red deer, and reindeer/caribou, diet formulation is well established (Ullrey et al., 1971; Skjenneberg and Slagsvold, 1979; Bøe and Jacobsen, 1981; Haigh and Hudson, 1993; Baker et al., 1998), and little or no supplementation with native forage is necessary to maintain healthy individuals held in pens. For browser specialists, formulated diets require some supplementation with fresh browse such as willows in summer and a woody browse source in winter. Grazer specialists, such as wapiti, need diets based on monocotyledons (hay) combined with additions of legumes, such as alfalfa or clover, during spring and summer. For intermediate-mixed foragers and browsers, any hay supplement must be restricted to high quality, and with intake limited to avoid rumen impaction. The same considerations need to be met when feeding individuals and groups, especially when cut-and-carry feeding systems are in use, or when single-species pastures constitute the basic grazing system. Management of pastures and rangelands to meet seasonal requirements for high-quality feed (digestibility and protein) in spring to meet lactation demands and compensatory growth will minimize supplementation with protein. In native rangeland systems, individual animals are expected to meet their requirements by selective feeding and avoiding negative effects of plant toxins and secondary compounds (Provenza et al., 1990; Du Toit et al., 1991), provided there is relative topographical relief and a sufficiently low population density that a diverse seasonal phenology can be expressed (Albon and Langvatn, 1992; Van der Wal et al., 2000; Mysterud et al., 2001). However, in many pastoral and unimproved native rangeland systems, maximizing the use of available feed resources by increased stocking rates and a reduction in pasture size becomes an economic necessity. The resulting reduction in range species richness, combined with a narrow seasonal phenology, usually necessitates provision of supplements on a seasonal basis (Baker et al., 1998; Kumpula et al., 2002). Use of targeted mineral and nutrient-supplement blocks may be required to meet seasonal demands, such as salt in spring and urea-molasses in winter for communal grazing of reindeer. In natural systems the use of seasonal supplementation sometimes becomes necessary to maintain individual species abundance as a management objective. But supplemental feeding usually has major implications for other components of the ecosystem, including a decrease in biodiversity of the range and its consumers. Therefore, supplemental feeding needs to be carefully targeted in game ranching and communal–nomadic herding systems, and it is difficult to justify if natural regulation (i.e., free of human manipulation) is, or becomes, management policy of natural ecosystems. An example is supplemental feeding of elk (wapiti) in Yellowstone National Park and the Greater Yellowstone Ecosystem

(NRC, 2002). Modifying animal movements and numbers (stocking rate) to achieve management goals for animal population size and sustainable yield are the tools used by wildlife managers. Assessing range carrying capacity in relation to seasonal and annual animal requirements is both complex and an evolving process in theoretical and adaptive management. Estimating local, regional, and seasonal availability of metabolic energy, metabolic protein, and minerals in the food resource in relation to dietary preferences and requirements of the various species and cohorts of the ecosystem is a major research task, which makes heavy demands on the ARC (1980) and NRC (1981, 1985) publications (Russell et al., 1992; Moen et al., 1998; Parker et al., 1999; NRC, 2002). Achieving the goals is difficult given the number of environmental factors that can influence feed and supplement intake. Therefore, monitoring of some, if not all, animals to provide timely adjustments to the designed range-supplementary feeding protocol is necessary.

Live weight and body condition estimates are probably the most basic monitoring parameters. However, understanding whether the pasture/range and/or supplement are meeting goals requires additional, and often sophisticated and costly, determinations. Determination of the driving forces on animal populations due to density-dependent effects (DelGiudice et al., 1991, 2001; Taper and Gogan, 2002), food resource use and diet selection (Hanley, 1997; Parker et al., 1999; Mysterud et al., 2001), and competition for food resources (Barboza and Bowyer, 2001; Owen-Smith, 2002) all involve a strong nutritional ecology component that is sometimes overlooked because of difficulties in matching habitat supply with nutritional demands. New technologies based on landscape measures of range quality and productivity determined remotely from satellite images are finding new applications based on nutritional ecology, for example in studies involving impacts of industrial development on tundra rangelands and caribou (Griffith et al., 2002; NRC, 2002; Cameron et al., 2005), and implications of habitat and animal responses to climate change (Post et al., 1997; Weladji et al., 2002). A thorough understanding of habitat, and therefore nutritional effects, is needed because small differences in plant quality and biomass can affect body growth substantially (White, 1983).

Simulation modeling is frequently used to help understand the system and to analyze the many nutritional interactions involved. Those models simulating individual animal performance are based on the energy, protein, and mineral requirements as recommended in previous ARC (1980) and NRC (1981, 1985) publications (Swift, 1983; Hudson and White, 1985; Hobbs, 1989; Moen and DelGiudice, 1997; Moen and Pastor, 1998). In conjunction with the metabolizable energy and protein systems for determining nutrient requirements, some highly pragmatic solutions are required to reduce the number of variables that exist.

Supplement Feeding and Protein Metabolism in Cervids

The first priority for ruminants is to satisfy the rumen requirement for readily fermentable energy in support of microbial growth through the incorporation of urea-N, or a DIP supplement such as soybean meal, in order to maximize digestion of fiber. The second priority is to determine if the basic system provides nutrients that can escape rumen fermentation and be used efficiently in postruminal digestion. If the system does not provide the necessary rumen escape nutrients (protein, starch, lipid), then locally available supplements are needed. In this way the products of ruminal and postruminal digestion are balanced with maintenance or productive requirements of the animal. Rumen escape supplements include protein sources such as nutcakes, legumes, and legume trees with 2–4 percent condensed tannins, browse, and fish meal, which can ensure a steady supply of DIP (in order to estimate UIP, as discussed in Chapter 3). The contribution of high-protein native legumes and browse plants to DIP and UIP of cervids under free-ranging conditions has not been well addressed. The DIP-UIP status of native plant species has not been determined using assessment approaches such as rumen cannulated animals and the in situ technique. Rumen escape lipids provided by mast production have major implications for production in years of plentiful mast. Natural provision of bypass starch is not commonly reported, but could be present in native grains, and is available by supplementary feeding of cereal grains that are not readily fermented (Waldo, 1973), such as cracked maize or rice shavings. Cereal grain-based supplements have been used extensively with cervids, although a preferred supplement for wapiti is hay. Caution should be exercised when providing cereal grain as the single feed base under confined feeding, because animals fed whole-grain barley ad libitum deposit excess fat, which leads to adverse affects on fetal development and can be associated with dystocia and stillborns (Blanchard and Hauer, 1986). The approach to meeting husbandry requirements by identifying the main biomass forage, ensuring the supply of readily fermentable energy and protein for the rumen and providing bypass nutrients, has been advocated for developing countries in the humid and dry topics (Preston and Leng, 1987). Although the technology appears different to the metabolizable energy and protein systems as presented in NRC publications, the fundamental basis for satisfying rumen function and provisioning bypass nutrients is a component for understanding diet selection by cervids (Hanley, 1982; Provenza, 1995). Preston and Leng (1987) justify the balance of rumen and postrumen balance as a mechanism to meet the animal's nutrient supply that satisfies glucose requirements for maintenance, growth, and milk production (Weekes, 1986), as well as providing a balance of nitrogen and protein that is ruminally degradable and nondegradable. Thus, provision of fermentable carbohydrate (CHO) that results in a higher proportion of propionate relative to acetate is recommended, as is a recommendation for starch that can escape rumen fermentation (Waldo, 1973) and can directly provide glucose (Stangassinger and Giesecke, 1986) when the gluconeogenic precursor supply cannot meet glucose requirements. At least for cervids that display a wide food choice, understanding the extent that the rumen balance–rumen escape hypothesis could operate under natural selection is a research priority. Although the potential productive and health benefits of ingesting plant species and parts that contain phenolics, particularly condensed tannins, is now well recognized for domestic species (Barry and McNabb, 1999; Waghorn and McNabb, 2003; Min et al., 2003), the likely effects in cervids could be different (Min et al., 1997) due to production of high proline-containing salivary proteins (Hagerman and Robbins, 1993) that may reduce tannin toxicity and minimize effects on cell wall digestion (Robbins et al., 1987a,b, 1991). While positive effects of UIP appear substantial, an overall decrease in digestion of protein measured in vivo is attributable to condensed tannins (Hanley et al., 1992). Iason (2005) recommends more research on subclinical effects of plant secondary metabolites as there is little doubt that toxic effects can direct food choice to plant species and parts low in secondary metabolites that also may be low in nutrients (Foley et al., 1999).

REFERENCES

Abate, A., and E. Pfeffer. 1986. Changes in nutrient intake and performance by goats fed coffee pulp-based diets followed by a commercial concentrate. Anim. Feed Sci. and Tech. 14:1–10.

Abebe, G., R. C. Merkel, G. Animut, T. Sahlu, and A. L. 2004. Effects of ammoniation of wheat straw and supplementation with soybean meal or broiler litter on feed intake and digestion in yearling Spanish wether goats. Small Ruminant Res. 51:37–46.

Adams, R. S. 1975. Variability in mineral and trace element content of dairy feeds. J. Dairy Sci. 58:1538–1548.

Adeloye, A. A. A. 1995. The value of cowpea husk to the goat. Biore. Technol. 52:281–282.

Albon, S.D., and R. Langvatn. 1992. Plant phenology and the benefits of migration in a temperate ungulate. Oikos 65:502–513.

Allen, M. S. 1997. Relationship between fermentation acid production in the rumen and the requirement for physically effective fiber. J. Dairy Sci. 80:1447–1462.

Anil Kumar, G. K., V. S. Panwar, K. R. Yadavand, and S. Sihag. 2002. Mustard cake as a source of dietary protein for growing lambs. Small Ruminant Res. 44:47–51.

Animut, G., R. C. Merkel, G. Abebe, T. Sahlu, and A. L. Goetsch. 2002. Effects of level of broiler litter in diets containing wheat straw on performance of Alpine doelings. Small Ruminant Res. 44:125–134.

ARC (Agricultural Research Council). 1980. The Nutrient Requirements of Ruminant Livestock. Slough, UK: Commonwealth Agricultural Bureaux.

Aregheore, E. M. 2004. Nutritive value of sweet potato (*Ipomea batatas* (L) Lam) forage as goat feed: Voluntary intake, growth and digestibility of mixed rations of sweet potato and batiki grass (*Ischaemum aristatum* var. *indicum*). Small Ruminant Res. 51:235–241.

ASIA (American Sheep Industry Association). 2002. Nutrition. Pp. 701–747 in Sheep Production Handbook. Fort Collins, CO: ADS/Nightwing Publishing.

Baker, D. L., and N. T. Hobbs. 1985. Emergency feeding of mule deer during winter: tests of a supplemental ration. J. Wildl. Manage. 49:934–942.

Baker, D. L., G. W. Stout, and M. W. Miller. 1998. A diet supplement for captive wild ruminants. J. Zoo Wildl. Med. 29:150–156.

Barboza, P. S., and R. T. Bowyer. 2001. Seasonality of sexual segregation in dimorphic deer: Extending the gastrocentric model. Alces 37: 275–292.

Barry, T. N., and W. C. McNabb. 1999. The implications of condensed tannins on the nutritive value of temperate forages fed to ruminants. Br. J. Nutr. 81:263–272.

Bartlett, J. 1989. Passage kinetics and digestion of different broiler litter diets in Nubian dry does. M.S. thesis, Tuskegee University, Tuskegee, AL.

Beauchemin, K. A., D. Colombatto, D. P. Morgavi, and W. Z. Yang. 2003. Use of exogenous fibrolytic enzymes to improve feed utilization by ruminants. J. Anim. Sci. 81(E. Suppl. 2):E37–E47.

Ben Salem, H., and A. Nefzaoui. 2003. Feed blocks as alternative supplements for sheep and goats. Small Ruminant Res. 49:275–288.

Ben Salem, H., I. Ben Salem, A. Nefzaoui, and M. S. Ben Said. 2003. Effect of PEG andolive cake feed blocks supply on feed intake, digestion, and health of goats given kermes oak (*Quercus coccifera* L.) foliage. Anim. Feed Sci. Tech. 110:45–59.

Berger, L., T. Klopfenstein, and R. Britton. 1979. Effect of sodium hydroxide on efficiency of rumen digestion. J. Anim. Sci. 49:1317–1323.

Berger, L. L., G. C. Fahey, Jr., L. D. Bourquin, and E. C. Titgemeyer. 1994. Modification of forage quality after harvest. Pp. 922–966 in Forage Quality, Evaluation, and Utilization, G. C. Fahey, Jr., ed. Madison, WI: Amer. Soc. of Agron, Inc., Crop Sci. Soc. of America, Inc., Soil Sci. Soc. of America, Inc.

Blanchard J. M., and W. E. Hauer. 1986. Reproductive performance of reindeer fed all-grain rations. Rangifer Spec. Iss. No. 1:39–41.

Bodine, T. N., H. T. Purvis, 2nd, C. J. Ackerman, and C. L. Goad. 2000. Effects of supplementing prairie hay with corn and soybean meal on intake, digestion, and ruminal measurements by beef steers. J. Anim. Sci. 78:3144–3154.

Bodine, T. N., H. T. Purvis, 2nd, and D. L. Lalman. 2001. Effects of supplement type on animal performance, forage intake, digestion, and ruminal measurements of growing beef cattle. J. Anim. Sci. 79:1041–1051.

Bøe, U. B., and E. Jacobsen 1981. Trials with different feeds to reindeer. Rangifer 1:39–43.

Bowman, J. G. P., and B. F. Sowell. 1997. Delivery method and supplement consumption by grazing ruminants: A review. J. Anim. Sci. 75:543–550.

Bueno, M. S., E. Ferrari, Jr., D. Bianchini, F. F. Leinz, and C. F. C. Rodrigues. 2002. Effect of replacing corn with dehydrated citrus pulp in diets of growing kids. Small Ruminant Res. 46:179–185.

Buxton, D. R., and S. L. Fales. 1994. Plant environment and quality. Pp. 155–199 in Forage Quality, Evaluation and Utilization, G. C. Fahey, Jr., ed. Madison, WI: Amer. Soc. of Agron, Inc., Crop Sci. Soc. of America, Inc., Soil Sci. Soc. of America, Inc.

Cameron, R. D., W. T. Smith, R. G. White, and B. Griffith. 2005. Central Arctic caribou and petroleum development: Distributional, nutritional, and reproductive implications. Arctic 58:1–9.

Couchman, J. F. 1959. Storage of hay. I. Effect of temperature on the "soluble" nitrogen, sugar and fat contents. J. Sci. Food Agric. 10:513–519.

de Simiane, M. 1978. Pp. 124–189 in Advances in Goat Feeding, P. Morand-Fehr et al., eds. Paris: INRA.

DelCurto, T., B. W. Hess, J. E. Huston, and K. C. Olson. 2000. Optimum supplementation strategies for beef cattle consuming low-quality roughages in the western United States. Proc. Am. Soc. Anim. Sci., 1999. Available: http://www.asas.org/jas/symposia/proceedings/0922.pdf [accessed March 15, 2005].

DelGiudice, G. D., F. J. Singer, and U. S. Seal. 1991. Physiological assessment of winter nutritional deprivation of elk in Yellowstone National Park. J. Wildl. Manage. 55:653–664.

DelGiudice, G. D., R. A. Moen, F. J. Sinfer, and M. R. Riggs. 2001. Winter nutritional restriction and simulated body condition of Yellowstone elk and bison before and after the fires of 1988. Wildl. Monog. 147:1–62.

Devendra, C. 1979. Malaysian Feedstuffs. Serdang, Selangor, Malaysia: Malaysian Agricultural Research & Development Institute (MARDI).

Dewhurst, R. J., N. D. Scollan, M. R. F. Lee, H. J. Ougham, and M. O. Humphreys. 2003. Forage breeding and management to increase the beneficial fatty acid content of ruminant products. Proc. Nutr. Soc. 62:329–336.

Dove, H. 2004. Sheep: Nutrition management. Pp. 800–802 in Encyclopedia of Animal Science, A. W. Bell and W. G. Pond, eds. New York: Marcel Dekker.

Du Toit, J. T., F. D. Provenza, and A. Nastis. 1991. Condition taste aversion: How sick must a ruminant get before it learns about toxicity in foods? Appl. Anim. Behav. Sci. 30:35–46.

Dunga, N. T., N. T. Mui, and I. Ledin. 2005. Effect of replacing a commercial concentrate with cassava hay (Manihot esculenta Crantz) on the performance of growing goats. Anim. Feed Sci. Tech. 119:271–281.

Evers, G. W. 1997. Introduction to deer farming. Pp. 1–3 in Non-native Deer Farming Symposium. Res. Center Tech. Rep. No. 97–1, Texas Agric. Expt. Stn., College Station, TX.

Fadel, J. G. 1984. Development of mathematical techniques to model ruminant fiberdigestion systems. Ph.D. dissertation, Cornell University, Ithaca, NY.

Fagan, G. L., and S. G. Solaiman. 1993. Nutritional analysis of forest vegetation in 1991 and 1992 browsing season. Goat Forestry Seminar, Tuskegee University, January 1993, Tuskegee, AL.

Fahey, G. C., L. D. Bourquin, E. C. Titgemeyer, and D. G. Atwell. 1993. Postharvest treatment of fibrous feedstuffs to improve their nutritive value. Pp. 715–766 in Forage Cell Wall Structure and Digestibility, H. G. Jung, D. R. Buxton, R. D. Hatfield, and J. Ralph, eds. Madison, WI: Amer. Soc. of Agron, Inc., Crop Sci. Soc. of America, Inc., Soil Sci. Soc. of America, Inc.

Faldet, M. A., T. Nalsen, L. J. Bush, and G. D. Adams. 1989. Utilization of wheat in complete rations for lactating cows. J. Dairy Sci. 72: 1243–1251.

Fick, G. W., and S. C. Mueller. 1989. Alfalfa quality, maturity, and mean stage of development. Cornell Univ. Agron. Dept., Info. Bull. 217.

Firkins, J. L., L. L. Berger, and G. C. Fahey, Jr. 1985. Evaluation of wet and dry distillers grains and wet and dry corn gluten feeds for ruminants. J. Anim. Sci. 60:847–860.

Foley, W. J., G. R. Iason, and C. McArthur. 1999. The role of plant secondary metabolites in the nutritional ecology of mammalian herbivores: How far have we come in 25 years? Pp. 130–209 in Nutritional Ecology of Herbivores, H. J. G. Jung and G. C. Fahey, eds. Savoy, IL: American Society of Animal Science.

Freer, M. 2002. The nutritional management of grazing sheep. Pp. 357–376 in Sheep Nutrition, M. Freer and H. Dove, eds. Wallingford, UK and Melbourne, Australia: CABI Publishing/CSIRO Publishing.

Gelaye, S., T. Terril, E. A. Amoah, S. Miller, R. N. Gates, and W. W. Hanna. 1997. Nutritional value of pearl millet for lactating and growing goats. J. Anim. Sci. 75:1409–1414.

Gilboa, N., A. Perevolotsky, S. Landau, Z. Nitsan, and N. Silanikove. 2000. Increasing productivity in goats grazing mediterranean woodland and scrubland by supplementation of polyethylene glycol. Small Ruminant Res. 38(2):183–190.

Goetsch, A. L., A. R. Patil, D. L., Galloway, B. Kouakou, Z. S. Wang, K. K. Park, and J. E. Rossi. 1997. Net flux of nutrients across splanchnic tissues in wethers consuming ad libitum different grass sources and physical forms. Br. J. Nutr. 77:769–781.

Grant, R. J., V. F. Colenbrander, and D. R. Mertens. 1990. Milk fat depression in dairy cows: Role of particle size of alfalfa hay. J. Dairy Sci. 73: 1823–1833.

Griffith, B., D. C. Douglas, N. E. Walsh, D. D. Young, T. R. McCabe, D. E. Russell, R. G. White, R. D. Cameron, and K. R. Whitten. 2002. The porcupine caribou herd. Pp. 8–37 in Arctic Refuge Coastal Plain Terrestrial Wildlife Research Summaries, D. C. Douglas, P. E. Reynolds, and E. B. Rhode, eds. U.S. Geological Survey, Biological Resources Division, Biological Science Report USGS/BRD/BSR-2002-0001.

Haddad, S. G., R. J. Grant, and T. J. Klopfenstein. 1994. Digestibility of alkali-treated wheat straw measured in vitro or in vivo using Holstein heifers. J. Anim. Sci. 72:3258–3265.

Hagerman, A. E., and C. T. Robbins. 1993. Specificity of tannin-binding salivary proteins relative to diet selection by mammals. Can. J. Zool. 71:628–633.

Haigh, J. C., and R. J. Hudson. 1993. Farming Wapiti and Red Deer. St. Louis, MO: Mosby.

Hanley, T. A. 1982. The nutritional basis for food selection by ungulates. J. Range Manage. 35:146–151.

Hanley, T. A. 1997. A nutritional view of understanding and complexity in the problem of diet selection by deer (Cervidae). Oikos 79:209–218.

Hanley, T. A., C. T. Robbins, A. E. Hagerman, and C. McArthur. 1992. Predicting digestible protein and digestible dry matter in tannin-containing forages consumed by ruminants. Ecology 73:537–541.

Hawke, J. C. 1973. Lipids. Pp. 213–231 in Chemistry and Biochemistry of Herbage, vol. 1. G. W. Butler and R. W. Bailey, eds. New York: Academic Press.

Heady, H. F., and R. D. Child. 1994. P. 1 in Rangeland Ecology and Management. Boulder, CO: Westview Press.

Hegarty, M. P., P. G. Schinckel, and R. D. Court. 1964. Reaction of sheep to the consumption of *Leucaena glauca* Benth. and to its toxic principle mimosine. Aust. J. Agric. Res. 15:153–167.

Helle, T., S.-S. Kilpelä, and P. Aikio. 1990. Lichen ranges, animal densities and production in Finnish reindeer management. Rangifer Spec. Iss. No. 3:115–121.

Hillocks, R. J., J. M. Thresh, and A. Bellotti, eds. 2002. Cassava: Biology, Production and Utilization. Wallingford, UK: CABI Publishing.

Hirstov, A. N., J. K. Ropp, K. L. Grandeen, S. Abedi, R. P. Etter, A. Melgar, and A. E. Foley. 2005. Effect of carbohydrate source on ammonia utilization in lactating dairy cows. J. Anim. Sci. 83:408–421.

Hobbs, N. T. 1989. Linking energy balance to survival in mule deer: Development and test of a simulation model. Wildl. Monog. 101:1–39.

Hofmann, R. R. 1973. P. 354 in The Ruminant Stomach: Stomach Structure and Feeding Habits of East African Game Ruminants. Nairobi, Kenya: East Afr. Lit. Bureau.

Hofmann, R. R. 1988. Anatomy of gastrointestinal tract. P. 14 in The Ruminant Animal, D. C. Church, ed. Englewood Cliffs, NJ: Prentice Hall.

Hudson, R. J., and R. G. White. 1985. Computer simulation of energy budgets. Pp. 261–290 in Bioenergetics of Wild Herbivores, R. J. Hudson and R. G. White, eds. Boca Raton, FL: CRC Press.

Hudson, R. J., K. R. Drew, and L. M. Baskin, eds. 1989. Wildlife Production Systems. Economic Utilization of Wild Ungulates. Cambridge, UK: Cambridge University Press.

Huston, E. 1994. Effects of supplemental feeding on intake by kid, yearling, and adult Angora goats on rangeland. J. Anim. Sci. 72:768–773.

Huston, J. E., B. S. Rector, L. B. Merrill, and B. S. Engdahl. 1981. Nutritional value of range plants in the Edwards Plateau region of Texas. Texas Agric. Expt. Stn., College Station, TX, Bulletin B 1357.

Iason, G. 2005. The role of plant secondary metabolites in mammalian herbivory: Ecological perspectives. Proc. Nutr. Soc. 64:123–131.

Jackson, M. G. 1977. Review article: The alkali treatment of straws. Anim. Feed Sci. Technol. 2:105–130.

Keeney, M. 1970. Lipid metabolism in the rumen. Pp. 489–503 in Physiology of Digestion and Metabolism in Ruminants, A. T. Phillipson, ed. Newcastle upon Tyne, UK: Oriel Press.

Kertz, A. 1998. Variability in delivery of nutrients to lactating dairy cows. J. Dairy Sci. 81:3075–3084.

Kondo, M., K. Kita, and H. Yokota. 2004. Feeding value to goats of whole-crop oat ensiled with green tea waste. Anim. Feed Sci. Tech. 113:71–81.

Kumpula, J., A. Colpaert, and M. Nieminen. 2002. Productivity factors of the Finnish semi-domestic reindeer (*Rangifer t. tarandus*) stock during the 1990s. Rangifer 22:3–12.

Launchbaugh, K. L., and C. W. Hunt. 2000. New approaches for enhancing grazing productivity: Meeting the challenges of variable environments. Proc. Am. Soc. Anim. Sci., 1999. Available: http://www.asas.org/symposia/0646.pdf [accessed March 15, 2005].

LEAD (Livestock, Environment and Development) Initiative. 1999. Livestock and Environment Toolbox. Food and Agriculture Organization of the United Nations. Available: http://www.fao.org/lead/ [accessed March 31, 2005].

Leng, R. A. 1997. Tree foliage in ruminant nutrition. FAO Animal Production and Health Paper 139, Rome. Pp.100.

Luginbuhl, J. M., M. H. Poore, and A. P. Conrad. 2000. Effect of level of whole cottonseed on intake, digestibility, and performance of growing male goats fed hay-based diets. J. Anim. Sci. 78:1677–1683.

Ly, J. 2003. The effect of methionine on digestion indices and N balance of young Mong Cai pigs fed high levels of ensiled cassava leaves. Livestock Research for Rural Development 15(1). Available: http://www.cipav.org.co/lrrd/lrrd15/1/ly151.htm [accessed June 22, 2005].

Mackie, R. I., C. S. McSweeney, and A. V. Klieve. 2002. Microbial Ecology of the Ovine Rumen. Pp. 71–94 in Sheep Nutrition, M. Freer and H. Dove, eds. Wallingford, UK: CABI Publishing.

Males, J. R. 1987. Optimizing the utilization of cereal crop residues for beef cattle. J. Anim. Sci. 65:1124–1130.

Martin, S. K., and C. A. Hibberd. 1990. Intake and digestibility of low quality native grass hay by beef cows supplemented with graded levels of soybean hulls. J. Anim. Sci. 68:4319–4325.

Matejovsky, K. M, and D. W. Sanson. 1995. Intake and digestion of low-, medium-, and high-quality grass hays by lambs receiving increasing levels of corn supplementation. J. Anim. Sci. 73:2156–2163.

Matras, J., S. J. Bartle, and R. L. Preston. 1991. Nitrogen utilization in growing lambs: Effects of grain (starch) and protein sources with various rates of ruminal degradation. J. Anim. Sci. 69:339–347.

McCrary, Q. 1998. Effect of feeding whole cotton seed on reproductive performance in goats, M.S. thesis, Tuskegee University, Tuskegee, AL.

McMahan, C. A. 1964. Comparative food habits of deer and three classes of livestock. J. Wildl. Manage. 28:798–808.

Min, B. R., and S. P. Hart. 2003. Tannins for suppression of internal parasites. J. Anim. Sci. 81:102–109.

Min, B. R., T. N. Barry, P. R. Wilson, and P. D. Kemp. 1997. The effects of grazing chicory and Birdsfoot trefoil on venison and velvet production by young red and hybrid deer. NZ J. Agric. Res. 40:337–349.

Min, B. R., T. N. Barry, G. T. Attwood, and W. C. McNabb. 2003. The effect of condensed tannins on the nutrition and health on ruminants fed fresh temperate forages: A review. Anim. Feed Sci. Technol. 106: 1–4.

Minson, D. J. 1990. Forage in Ruminant Nutrition. San Diego, CA: Academic Press.

Moen, R., and G. D. DelGiudice. 1997. Simulating nitrogen metabolism and urinary urea nitrogen: Creatinine ratios in ruminants. J. Wildl. Manage. 61:881–894.

Moen, R., and J. Pastor. 1998. Simulating antler growth and energy, nitrogen, calcium and phosphorus metabolism in caribou. Rangifer Spec. Iss. No. 10:85–97.

Moen, R., Y. Cohen, and J. Pastor. 1998. Linking moose population and plant growth models with a moose energetics model. Ecosystems 1: 52–63.

Morand-Fehr, P. 1981. Growth. Pp. 253–283 in Goat Production, C. Gall, ed. New York: Academic Press.

Mysterud, A., R. Langvatn, N. G. Yoccoz, and N. C. Stenseth. 2001. Plant phenology, migration and geographical variation in body weight of a large herbivore: The effect of a variable topography. J. Anim. Ecol. 70:915–923.

Nocek, J. E., and S. Tamminga. 1991. Site of digestion of starch in the gastrointestinal tract of dairy cows and its effect on milk production. J. Dairy Sci. 74:3598–3629.

NRC (National Research Council). 1981. Nutrient Requirements of Goats: Angora, Dairy, and Meat Goats in Temperate and Tropical Countries. Washington, DC: National Academy Press.

NRC. 1985. Nutrient Requirements of Sheep, 6th rev. ed. Washington, DC: National Academy Press.

NRC. 2001. Nutrient Requirements of Dairy Cattle, 7th rev. ed. Washington, DC: National Academy Press.

NRC. 2002. Ecological Dynamics on Yellowstone's Northern Range. Washington, DC: National Academy Press.

Owen-Smith, R. N. 2002. Adaptive Herbivore Ecology. Cambridge, UK: Cambridge University Press. 374 pp.

Palmquist, D. L. 1987. Feed ingredients and management to maximize use of fat in dairy rations. P. 106 in Proc. California Anim. Nutr. Conf., Fresno.

Palmquist, D. L. 1988. The feeding value of fats. Pp. 293–311 in Feed Science, E. R. Orskov, ed. Amsterdam: Elsevier.

Palmquist, D. L., and T. C. Jenkins. 2003. Challenges with fats and fatty acid methods. J. Anim. Sci. 81:3250–3254.

Papachristou, T. G., P. D. Platis, V. P. Papanastasis, and C. N. Tsiouvaras. 1999. Use of deciduous woody species as a diet supplement for goats grazing Mediterranean shrublands during the dry season. Anim. Feed Sci. and Technol. 80:267–279.

Parker, K. L., M. P. Gillingham, T. A. Hanley, and C. T. Robbins. 1999. Energy and protein balance of free-ranging black-tailed deer in a natural forest environment. Wildl. Monog. 143:1–48.

Paterson, J. A., R. L. Belyea, J. P. Bowman, M. S. Kerley, and J. E. Williams. 1994. The impact of forage quality and supplementation regimen on ruminant animal intake and performance. Pp. 59–114 in Forage Quality, Evaluation and Utilization, G. C. Fahey, Jr., ed. Madison, WI: Amer. Soc. of Agron, Inc., Crop Sci. Soc. of America, Inc., Soil Sci. Soc. of America, Inc.

Perry, T.W., A. E. Cullison, and R. S. Lowrey. 1999. Feeds and Feeding, 5th ed. Upper Saddle River, NJ: Prentice Hall.

Pieltain, M. C., J. I. R. Castanon, M. R. Ventura, and M. P. Flores. 1998. Nutritive value of banana (*Musa acuminata* L.) fruits for ruminants. Anim. Feed Sci. and Technol. 73:187–191.

Poore, M. H., and G. Rogers. 1995. Feeding whole cottonseed and other cotton by-products to beef cattle. Vet. Med. 90:1077–1087.

Poppi, D. P., and S. R. McLennan. 1995. Protein and energy utilization by ruminants at pasture. J. Anim. Sci. 73:278–290.

Post, E., N. C. Stenseth, R. Langvatn, and J. M. Fromentin. 1997. Global climate change and phenotypic variation among red deer cohorts. Proc. Royal Soc. London. Series B 264:1317–1324.

Preston, T. R., and R. A. Leng. 1987. Matching ruminant production systems with available resources in the tropics and sub-tropics. Armidale, Australia: Penambul Books.

Provenza, F. D. 1995. Postingestive feedback as an elementary determinant of food preference and intake in ruminants. J. Range Manage. 48:2–17.

Provenza, F. D., E. A. Burritt, T. P. Clausen, J. P. Bryant, P. B. Reichardt, and R. A. Distel. 1990. Conditioned flavor aversion: A mechanism for goats to avoid condensed tannins in blackbrush. Am. Nat. 136:810–828.

Qureshi, A. 1988. Intake, digestibility and passage kinetics of different broiler litter rations in goats, M.S. thesis, Tuskegee University, Tuskegee, AL.

Ramirez, R. G. 1999. Feed resources and feeding techniques of small ruminants under extensive management conditions. Small Ruminant Res. 34:215–230.

Randel R. D., C. C. Chase Jr., and S. J. Wyse. 1992. Effects of gossypol and cottonseed products on reproduction of mammals. J. Anim. Sci. 70: 1628–1638.

Ratcliffe, H. L. 1966. Diets of zoological gardens: Aids to conservation and disease control. Int. Zoo Yearb. 6:4–23.

Reiser, R. 1951. Hydrogenation of polyunsaturated fatty acids by the ruminants. Fed. Proc. 10:236.

Renecker, L. A., and R. J. Hudson, eds. 1991. Wildlife Production: Conservation and Sustainable Development. Fairbanks: Agricultural and Forestry Experiment Station, University of Alaska, Fairbanks.

Robbins, C. T., S. Mole, A. E. Hagerman, and T. A. Hanley. 1987a. Role of tannins in defending plants against ruminants: Reduction in dry matter digestion? Ecology 68:1606–1615.

Robbins, C. T., T. A. Hanley, A. E. Hagerman, O. Hjeljord, D. L. Baker, C. C. Schwartz, and W. W. Mautz. 1987b. Role of tannins in defending plants against ruminants: Reduction in protein availability. Ecology 69:98–107.

Robbins, C. T., A. E. Hagerman, P. J. Austin, C. McArthur, and T. A. Hanley. 1991. Variation in mammalian physiological responses to a condensed tannin and its ecological implications. J. Mammal. 72:480–486.

Rodrique, C. B., and N. N. Allen. 1960. The effect of fine grinding of hay on ration digestibility, rate of passage, and fat content of milk. Can. J. Anim. Sci. 40:23–29.

Rowe, J. B., and D. W. Pethick. 1994. Starch digestion in ruminants—problems, solutions and opportunities. Proc. Nutr. Soc. Aust. 18:40–52.

Rowe, J. B., M. Choct, and D. W. Pethick. 1999. Processing cereal grains for animal feeding. Aust. J. Agric. Res. 50:721–736.

Russell, J. B., J. D. O'Conner, D. G. Fox, P. J. Van Soest, and C. J. Snoffen. 1992. A net carbohydrate and protein system for evaluating cattle diets: I. Ruminal fermentation. J. Anim. Sci. 70:3551–3561.

Rust, S. R., J. R. Newbold, and K. W. Metz. 1990. Evaluation of condensed distillers' solubles as an energy source for finishing cattle. J. Anim. Sci. 68:186–192.

Sansoucy, R., G. Aarts, and T. R. Preston. 1988. Sugarcane as feed. FAO Animal Production and Health Paper 72, Rome. 319 pp.

Santos, F. A. P., J. E. P. Santos, C. B. Theurer, and J. T. Huber. 1998. Effects of rumen + – undegradable protein on dairy cow performance: A 12-year literature review. J. Dairy Sci. 81:3182–3213.

Schneider, M., and G. Flachowsky. 1990. Studies on ammonia treatment of wheat straw: Effects of level of ammonia, moisture content, treatment time and temperature on straw composition and degradation in the rumen of sheep. Anim. Feed Sci. Technol. 29:251–264.

Shaver, R. D., A. J. Nytes, L. D. Satter, and N. A. Jergensen. 1986. Influence of amount of feed intake and forage physical form on digestion and milk production in lactating dairy cows. J. Dairy Sci. 69: 1545–1559.

Short, R. E., L. F. James, K. E. Panter, R. B. Staigmiller, R. A. Bellows, J. Maclcolm, and S. P. Ford. 1992. Effects of feeding ponderosa pine needles during pregnancy: Comparative studies with bison, cattle, goats and sheep. J. Anim. Sci. 70:3498–3504.

Skjenneberg, S., and L. Slagsvold. 1979. Reindeer Husbandry and Its Ecological Principles. English translation of Norwegian (T. T. Deer). Reindriften og dens Naturgrunnlag, Universitetsforlaget, Oslo, 1968. C. M. Anderson and J. R. Luick, eds. U.S. Dept. Interior Bureau of Indian Affairs, Juneau, Alaska. pp. 395.

Solaiman, S. G., Y. P. Smoot, and F. N. Owens. 2002. Impact of EasiFlo cottonseed on feed intake, apparent digestibility, and rate of passage by goats fed a diet containing 45 percent hay. J. Anim. Sci. 80:805–811.

Solaiman, S. G., D. Bransby, C. Kerth, B. Blagburn, and R. Noble. 2006. A sustainable year-round forage system for goat production in the Southern U.S. Annual Report, Project # LS02-141, Southern SARE.

Stangassinger, M., and D. Giesecke. 1986. Splanchnic metabolism of glucose and related energy substrates. Pp. 347–366 in Control of Digestion and Metabolism in Ruminants, L. P. Milligan, W. L. Grovum, and A. Dobson, eds. Englewood Cliffs, NJ: Prentice Hall.

Stoltenow C., and G. Lardy. 1998. Prussic acid poisoning. North Dakota State University, V-1150. Available: http://www.ext.nodak.edu/extpubs/ansci/livestoc/v1150w.htm [accessed March 8, 2006].

Swift, D. M. 1983. A simulation model of energy and nitrogen balance for free-ranging ruminants. J. Wildl. Manage. 47:620–645.

Taper, M. L., and P. J. P. Gogan. 2002. The Northern Yellowstone elk: Density dependence and climate conditions. J. Wildl. Manage. 66: 106–122.

Taylor, N., P. G. Hatfield, B. F. Sowell, J. G. P. Bowman, J. S. Drouillard, and D. V. Dhuyvetter. 2002a. Pellet and block supplements for grazing ewes. Anim. Feed Sci. and Technol. 96:193–201.

Taylor, N., P. G. Hatfield, B. F. Sowell, and G. S. Lewis. 2002b. Influence of supplement form on ewe performance and reproduction. Sheep Goat Res. J. 17:52–54.

Terrill, T. H., S. Gelaye, E. A. Amoah, S. Miller, B. Kouakou, R. N. Gates, and W. W. Hanna. 1998. Protein and energy value of pearl millet grain for mature goats. J. Anim. Sci. 76:1964–1969.

Thomas, V. M., and R. W. Kott. 1996. Winter range supplementation of sheep: A historical perspective of ewe winter range supplementation. In Proc. 3rd Grazing Livestock Nutrition Conference. Proc. West. Sec. Amer., M. B. Judkins and F. T. McCollum III, eds. Soc. Anim. Sci. 47(Suppl. 1):19–29.

Torrent, J., D. E. Johnson, and M. A. Kujawa. 1994. Co-product fiber digestibility kineticsand in vivo assessment. J. Anim. Sci. 72:790–795.

Trodahl, S., T. Skjevdal, and T. A. Steine. 1981. Goats in cold and temperate climates. Pp. 489–513 in Goat Production, C. Gall E., ed. New York: Academic Press.

Ullrey, D. E., H. E. Johnson, W. G. Youatt, F. D. Fay, B. L. Schoepke, and W. T. Magee. 1971. A basal diet for deer nutrition research. J. Wildl. Manage. 35:57–62.

Van, D. T. T., N. T. Mui, and I. Ledin. 2004. Tropical foliages: Effect of presentation method and species on intake by goats. Anim. Feed Sci. Technol. 118:1–17.

Van Barneveld, S. L. 1999. Chemical and physical characteristics of grain related to variability in energy and amino acid availability in ruminants: A review. Aust. J. Agric. Res. 50:651–666.

Van der Wal, R., N. Madan, S. van Lieshout, C. Dorman, R. Langvatn, and S. D. Albon. 2000. Trading forage quality for quantity? Plant phenology and patch choice by Svalbard reindeer. Oecologia 123:108–115.

Van Soest, P. J. 1965. Use of detergent in analysis of fibrous feeds. III. Study on effects of heating and drying on yield of fiber and lignin in forages. J. Assoc. Off. Anal. Chem. 48:785–790.

Van Soest, P. J. 1989. On the digestibility of bound N in distillers grains: A reanalysis. Proc. Cornell Nutrition Conf. 39:127–131.

Van Soest, P. J. 1994a. Carbohydrates. Pp. 156–176 in Nutritional Ecology of the Ruminant, 2nd ed. Ithaca, NY: Cornell University Press.

Van Soest, P. J. 1994b. Forage preservation. Pp. 229 in Nutritional Ecology of the Ruminant, 2nd ed. Ithaca, NY: Cornell University Press.

Waghorn, G. C., and W. C. McNabb. 2003. Consequences of plant compounds for productivity and health of ruminants. Proc. Nutr. Soc. 62:383–392.

Waldo, D. R. 1973. Extent and partition of cereal grain starch digestion in ruminants. J. Anim. Sci. 37:1062–1074.

Weekes, T. E. C. 1986. Carbohydrate metabolism. Pp.187–209 in Digestive Physiology and Nutrition of Ruminants, vol. 2, Nutrition, D. C. Church, ed. Corvallis, OR: O & B Books.

Weladji, R. B., D. R. Klein, Ø. Holand, and A. Mysterud. 2002. Comparative response of Rangifer tarandus and other northern ungulates to climatic variability. Rangifer 22:33–50.

Weiss, W. P., D. O. Erickson, G. M. Erickson, and G. R. Fisher. 1989. Barley distillers grains as a protein supplement for dairy cows. J. Dairy Sci. 72:980–987.

Wen, L., R. L. Kallenbach, J. E. Williams, C. A. Roberts, P. R. Beuselinck, R. L. McGraw and H. R. Benedict. 2002. Performance of steers grazing rhizomatous and nonrhizomatous birdsfoot trefoil in pure stands and in tall fescue mixtures. J. Anim. Sci. 80:1970–1976.

White, R. G. 1983. Foraging patterns and their multiplier effects on productivity of northern ungulates. Oikos 40:377–384.

World Resources Institute. 2003. Available: http://earthtrends.wri.org/pdf library/data tables/for2_2003.pdf [accessed March 31, 2005]

Yanez Ruiz, D. R., A. I. Martin Garcia, A. Moumen, and E. Molina Alciade. 2004. Ruminal fermentation and degradation pattern, protozoa population and urinary purine derivatives excretion in goats and wethers fed diets based on olive leaves. J. Anim. Sci. 82:3006–3014.

Zhigunov, G. I., ed. 1986. Reindeer Husbandry. (Translated from Russian). Jerusalem: Israel Program for Scientific Translations.

12

Environmental Impact

BENEFITS OF SMALL RUMINANT USE IN FORAGING SYSTEMS AND RANGE RESTORATION

When rangeland grazing/foraging is left unbalanced, particularly by maintaining single species (cow or horse) herds, overgrazing will occur and result in desertification and/or noxious weed or woody plant overgrowth. Sustaining rangeland agriculture requires the ability to balance plant growth and plant harvesting. Multispecies grazing in a controlled fashion can effectively alter the amounts of poorly usable plant material to a more harvestable biomass (Heitschmidt et al., 2004). The debarking, defoliation habits of goats can alter the viability of many species of woody brush. Including goats in a forage harvesting system with sheep, cattle, and/or horses is a low-cost, yet environmentally friendly method of increasing income and improving range sustainability (Villalba et al., 2002). Sheep will reportedly consume diets of 15 percent forbs and 31 percent browse, whereas goats prefer diets high in browse (70 percent) and forbs (10 percent) (Hart, 2001).

Goats co-grazing with cattle and/or horses will consume plant species not utilized by these other species (Taylor, 1985). Goats are very useful in the control of woody plants, weeds, and brush that can depress range productivity, such as leafy spurge, Sericea lespedeza, post oak, black jack, black locust, shinnery oak, thistle, sumac, poison ivy, multiflora rose, eastern red cedar, iron weed, sumac, sweet briar, green briar, brambles, and honeysuckle (Walker et al., 1994; Allan and Holst, 1996; Escobar et al., 1998; Luginbuhl et al., 1999, 2000; Hart, 2001). This is an added benefit to the primary purpose of range management to produce meat and fiber. Co-grazing traditional cattle-used rangeland with small ruminants will help reduce the added production costs of either chemical or mechanical control of weeds and will allow for an increase in biomass of harvested livestock (Hart, 2001).

Many woody plants not readily eaten by cattle or horses have extensive root systems allowing them to become well established and to sequester soil nutrients. In addition, goats can aid in the reestablishment of grassy species in some overgrazed and eroded range conditions by consuming and, thus, recycling nutrients held in the weeds (Hart, 2001). Goats grazing undesirable weeds and brush have been shown to increase available soil nitrogen, phosphorus, and potassium, aiding in reestablishment of grasses (Escobar et al., 1998). This is a valuable tool in helping to minimize erosion, while maximizing grassland restoration. When goats or sheep are allowed to graze rangeland with restoration in mind, supplemental feeding can be valuable in the promotion of more uniform grazing, particularly in underused areas (Bailey, 2004). The "moving" of the flock or herd, as previously stated, can help to redistribute some nutrients (e.g., phosphates).

Co-grazing of small ruminants, horses, and cattle will reduce parasitism of any one animal species and apparently reduce animal losses to poisonous plants (Taylor and Ralphs, 1992; Hart, 2001; Hoste et al., 2001). Both sheep and goats will consume and control tannin-rich vegetation, even in areas and/or during times of reduced water availability (Villalba et al., 2002). An added benefit of tannin-rich ingestion, as previously discussed, is the potential reduction in internal parasites, reduced incidence of bloat, and possible improvement of other health conditions (Hart, 2001; Waghorn and McNabb, 2003).

Sheep and goats reduce the spread of weeds and woody plant species via seed (Fay, 1991; Mayo, 2000) and have been used successfully to reduce brush overgrowth for the improvement of wildlife habitats (Hart, 2001). In summary, small ruminant species are well suited for range restoration and increase the production of livestock biomass in both range and woodland production systems, particularly when integrated into multispecies grazing systems.

CONCERNS

The effects of animals on the environment in which they live depend on the intensity of grazing-browsing, species and/or number of animals, type of land (e.g., feedlot, pasture, range, woodland, or other type), amount of usable forage, and other husbandry practices connected with livestock production (e.g., administration of some endectocides or sheep dipping). Overgrazing, improper grazing management, and many practices linked to intensive production agriculture can result in loss of desirable forages, soil erosion, sequestration of soil nutrients in less desirable plants, and accumulation of potentially toxic chemicals and/or animal use medicines used in animals' care. Although desirable in weed control, goats' ability to debark plants can be an undesirable trait when they browse on and kill desirable trees. Overgrazing of all small ruminants that result in loss of valuable browse and grass species should be avoided. Sound forage and livestock management will enhance ground cover with crops suitable for grazing, resist weed or woody plant overgrowth, enhance soil fertility and soil water retention, and minimize the introduction of toxic substances to soils, ground water, and air. Emphasis should be placed on production systems that are both sustainable and environmentally safe.

Livestock waste disposal and the potential contamination of air and groundwater is a major concern in animal production. Although some work has been conducted on the gas production associated with small ruminants (Misi and Forster, 2001), much more work is needed in this area. There may be a conflict between modern or "improved" agricultural practices where more animal waste products are produced in smaller, confined areas and the reduction of greenhouse gases (Moore et al., 2001). Sheep, goats, cervids, and camelids will all contribute to the production of these gases. Yang et al. (2003) reported a reduction in two greenhouse gases, methane and nitrous oxide, produced by livestock waste management in Taiwan from 1990 to 2000. Goat production is a major contributor to livestock waste because it ranks second to swine production in Taiwan. Much work is required in order to determine the exact contribution of small ruminants, and how best to reduce associated emissions worldwide.

Disposal of livestock waste is a growing concern. Improper waste disposal is environmentally damaging. Moral et al. (2005) reported that goat manure had lower concentrations of organic carbon than horse, pig, or rabbit manure and had significantly higher concentrations of biodegradable organic compounds than pig or rabbit manure. Improper manure disposal has devastating zoonotic consequences. Livestock waste produced by animals consuming predominately forages appears to be less likely than waste from grain-fed animals to contain pathogenic E. coli or salmonella (Hutchinson et al., 2005). Thus, low-input, range-managed, small-ruminant production may reduce the potential for transmission of pathogens from manure handling and reduce the amount of nonbiodegradable livestock waste produced, as compared to some other species. Furthermore, keeping small ruminants on range will allow more dispersal of manure, reduce the need for manure handling, reduce parasitism associated with heavy stocking rates of small ruminants, and dilute any pesticides and antibiotics over greater areas of land (Hooda et al., 2000). Siddiqui (2004) showed that composted goat feces have value in reducing soilborne nematode growth and improving tomato growth. Composted goat feces were superior to similarly handled horse manure in promoting tomato plant health. However, where handling and disposal of small ruminant manure is required, procedures such as composting, spreading onto large areas, and minimizing water shed contamination may be required. Management practices that rely heavily on high stocking rates, high-grain diets (e.g., feedlots or dairy), and confinement systems will require greater future scrutiny in order to diminish effects on animal and human health.

Soil and water contamination of phosphates, nitrates, and other chemicals from livestock production is a growing environmental concern. Although the contribution of these chemicals by sheep, goats, cervids, and camelids is minor as compared to other North American livestock entities such as poultry, swine, and cattle, it is nonetheless significant. Placing animals on larger range areas vs. small intensely managed areas reduces the potential contamination of water sources via simple dilution. Constantly moving and grazing sheep on different areas of pastures, woodlands, or rangelands seems to be useful for the redistribution of phosphates accumulated in contaminated wetland to other areas or range (Haynes and Williams, 1993). Sheep grazing around North American streams reportedly had no measurable impact on nitrates and phosphates in the stream water (Darling and Coltharp, 1973). The ratio of chloride/bromide, which is useful in the identification and quantification of groundwater contamination, is reportedly lower in leachate from goat waste than in that of domestic wastewater, and is within the range of oil field brine (Hudak, 2003). Some agricultural practices tend to increase nitrate-N concentrations in underlying groundwater. However, sheep ranch areas seem to result in lower nitrate-N groundwater concentration than most agronomic-horticultural production practices (McLay et al., 2001). Much research is needed in this area to better quantify the extent of sheep, goat, cervid, and camelid contribution to this growing concern.

Chemicals and medications used in livestock production may have some environmental implications. Examples are some of the compounds used to control external and internal parasite control, which have garnered much of the concern with respect to potential environmental damage (Virtue and Clayton, 1997; Hooda et al., 2000). Compounds used in livestock care find their way into the environment by accidental spills, runoff or washoff, urinary and/or fecal excretion, and improper chemical container disposal and/or use. Methods for diminishing contamination from these products have been described (Virtue and Clayton, 1997; Hooda et al., 2000). Although just one of many such compounds, the avermectin class of endectocides is an example of commonly used chemicals that have beneficial effects for animal production but can result in unwanted altering of the environment. These chemicals have toxic effects on some terrestrial and aquatic organisms (Bloom and Matheson, 1993). After their use, avermectins reach the environment via excretion in feces and through other previously described avenues. They can result in a population reduction of many beneficial insects, including the dung beetle (Fincher, 1992; Holter et al., 1994; Floate and Gill, 1998; Wardhaugh et al., 2001). As tannin intake can help reduce internal parasitism, one potential benefit in using goats and sheep in the control of tannin-rich forages in range conditions is the decreased need for some endectocides. Allowing sheep and goats to browse in range conditions will diminish the need for many pharmaceuticals that are required for intensive farming, thus, further reducing potential contamination (Boxal et al., 2003).

The spread of disease between domestic small ruminants and wildlife populations is a concern and needs to be prevented when ever co-grazing occurs (Meagher et al., 1992; Pugh et al., 1995; Ward et al., 1997; Li et al., 1999, 2003a,b; Rudolph et al., 2003; Kreeger et al., 2004). Many diseases, including malignant catarrhal fever, pasteurellosis, infectious keratoconjunctivitis, and brucellosis, are transmissible from domestic livestock to wildlife populations (Meagher et al., 1992; Ward et al., 1997; Li et al., 2003a,b; Kreeger et al., 2004). Attempts should be made to introduce only healthy animals into range areas where they are to co-graze with wild ruminant species. Whenever possible, animals should be quarantined and appropriate diagnostic tests utilized in order to identify any infection in the domestic animals prior to introduction into the range where they will co-graze with susceptible wildlife populations. Whenever co-grazing, domestic creatures are also capable of becoming infected by some diseases from wildlife such as parelaphostrongylosis.

REFERENCES

Allan, C. J., and P. J. Holst. 1996. The ecological role of the goat in maintaining pasture and range. Pp. 427–435 in Proc. VI Intl. Conf. on Goats, Beijing, China.

Bailey, D. W. 2004. Management strategies for optimal grazing distribution and use of arid rangelands. J. Anim. Sci. 82(E Suppl.):E147–E153.

Bloom, R. A., and J. C. Matheson. 1993. Environmental assessment of avermectins by the US Food and Drug Administration. Vet. Parasitol. 48:281–294.

Boxall, A. B., L. A. Fogg, P. Kay, P. A. Blackwell, E. J. Pemberton, and A. Crawford. 2003. Prioritization of veterinary medicine in the UK environment. Toxicol. Lett. 142:207–218.

Darling, L. A., and G. B. Coltharp. 1973. Effects of livestock grazing on the water quality of mountain streams. Water-Animal Relations Proc. USDA-ARS, Kimberly, ID.

Escobar, E. N., F. Pinkerton, and T. S. McKinney. 1998. Use of goats as a vegetation management tool. Mimeo Report of E. (Kika) de la Garza Institute for Goat Research, Langston University, Langston OK.

Fay, P. K. 1991. Controlling leafy spurge with grazing animals. Pp. 193–199 in Noxious Range Weeds, L. F. James, J. O. Evans, M. H. Ralphs, and R. D. Child, eds. Boulder, CO: Westfield Press.

Fincher, G. T. 1992. Injectable ivermectin for cattle: Effects on some dung-inhabiting insects. Environ. Entomol. 21:871–876.

Floate, K. D., and B. D. Gill. 1998. Seasonal activity of dung beetles (Coleoptera:Scarabaeidae) associated with cattle dung in southern Alberta and their geographic distribution in Canada. Can. Entomol. 130: 131–151.

Hart, S. P. 2001. Recent perspectives in using goats for vegetation management in the USA. J. Dairy Sci. 84(E Suppl.):E170–E176.

Haynes, R. J., and P. H. Williams. 1993. An overview of pasture response, nutrient turnover and nutrient accumulation on the grazed, long-term superphosphate trial at Winchmore, New Zealand. Pp. 1430–1433 in Proc. XVII Int. Grassland Congress.

Heitschmidt, R. K., L. T. Vermeire, and E. E. Gring. 2004. Is rangeland agriculture sustainable? J. Anim. Sci. 82 (E Suppl.):138–146.

Holter, P., L. Strong, R. Wall, K. Wardhaugh, and R. Herd. 1994. Effects of ivermectin on pastureland ecology. Vet. Rec. 135:211–212.

Hooda, P. S., A. C. Edwards, H. A. Anderson, and A. Miller. 2000. A review of water quality concerns in livestock farming areas. Sci. Total Environ. 250:143–167.

Hoste, H., H. Leveque, and P. Dorchies. 2001. Comparison of nematode infections of the gastrointestinal tract in Angora and dairy goats in a rangeland environment: Relations with the feeding behavior. Vet. Parasitol. 101:127–135.

Hudak, P. F. 2003. Chloride/bromide ratios in leachate derived from farm-animal waste. Environ. Pollut. 121:23–25.

Hutchinson, M. L., L. D. Walters, S. M. Avery, F. Munro, and A. Moore. 2005. Analyses of livestock production, waste storage, and pathogen levels and prevalences in farm manures. Appl. Environ. Microbiol. 71: 1231–1236.

Kreeger, T. J., W. E. Cook, W. H. Edwards, and T. Cornish. 2004. Brucellosis in captive Rocky Mountain bighorn sheep (Ovis canadensis) caused by Brucella abortus biovar 4. J. Wildl. Dis. 40:311–315.

Li, H., W. C. Westover, and T. B. Crawford. 1999. Sheep-associated malignant catarrhal fever in a petting zoo. J. Zoo Wildl. Med. 30:408–412.

Li, H., K. Gailbreadth, L. C. Bender, K. West, J. Keller, and T. B. Crawford. 2003a. Evidence of three new members of malignant catarrhal fever virus group in muskox (Ovibos moschatus), Nubian ibex (Capra nubiana), and gemsbok (Oryx gazella). J. Wildl. Dis. 39:875–880.

Li, H., A. Wunschmann, J. Keller, D. G. Hall, and T. B. Crawford. 2003b. Caprine herpesvirus-2-associated malignant catarrhal fever in white-tailed deer (Odocoileus virginianus). J. Vet. Diagn. Invest. 15:46–49.

Luginbuhl, J-M., T. M. Harvey, J. T. Green, Jr., M. H. Poore, J. P. Mueller. 1999. Use of goats as biological agents for renovation of pastures in Appalachian regions of the United States. Agroforestry Systems 44:241–252.

Luginbuhl, J-M., J. T. Green, Jr., M. H. Moore, A. P. Conrad. 2000. Use of goats to manage vegetation in cattle pastures in Appalachian region of North Carolina. Sheep Goat Res. J. 16:124–135.

Mayo, J. M. 2000. The effects of goats grazing on sericea lespedeza. Pp. 14–15 in Symp. Proc. Lespedeza and the Future of Invasive species, Kansas State Univ. Dept. of Agron., Manhattan, KS.

McLay, C. D., R. Dragten, G. Sparling, and N. Selvarajah. 2001. Predicting groundwater nitrate concentrations in a region of mixed agricultural land use: A comparison of three approaches. Environ. Pollut. 115:191–204.

Meagher, M., W. J. Quinn, and L. Stackhouse. 1992. Chlamydial-caused infectious keratoconjunctivitis in bighorn sheep of Yellowstone National Park. J. Wildl. Dis. 28:171–176.

Misi, S. N., and C. F. Forster. 2001. Batch co-digestion of multi-component agro-wastes. Bioresource Technol. 80:19–28.

Moore, J. L., S. M. Howden, G. M. McKeon, J. O. Carter, and J. C. Scanlan. 2001. The dynamics of grazed woodlands in Southwest Queensland, Australia and their effect on greenhouse gas emissions. Environ. Int. 27:147–153.

Moral, R., J. Moreno-Casellas, M. D. Perez-Murcia, A. Perez-Espinosa, B. Rufette, and C. Paredes. 2005. Characterization of the organic matter pool in manure. Bioresource Technol. 96:153–158.

Pugh, D. G., B. L. Blagburn, K. Causey, and D. F. Wolfe. 1995. Clinical parelaphostrongylosis in llamas. Comp. Cont. Ed. Pract. Vet. 17:600–607.

Rudolph, K. M., D. L. Hunter, W. J. Foreyt, E. F. Cassirer, R. B. Rimler, and A. C. Ward. 2003. Sharing of Pasteurella ssp. between free-ranging bighorn sheep and feral goats. J. Wildl. Dis. 39:897–903.

Siddiqui, Z. A. 2004. Effects of plant growth promoting bacteria and composed organic fertilizers on the reproduction of *Meloidogyne incognita* and tomato growth. Bioresource Technol. 95:223–227.

Taylor, C. A. 1985. Multispecies grazing research overview (Texas). Pp 39–45 in Proc. C Multispecies Grazing, F. H. Baker and R. K. Jones, eds. Morrilton, AR: Winrock International Institute for Agricultural Development.

Taylor, C. A., and M. H. Ralphs. 1992. Reducing livestock losses from poisonous plants through grazing management. J. Range Manage. 45:9–12.

Villalba, J. J., F. D. Provenza, and R. E. Banner. 2002. Influence of macronutrients and polyethylene glycol on intake of a quebracho tannin diet by sheep and goats. J. Anim. Sci. 80:3154–3164.

Virtue, W. A., and J. W. Clayton. 1997. Sheep dip chemicals and water pollution. Sci. Total Environ. 195:207–217.

Waghorn, G. C., and W. C. McNabb. 2003. Consequences of plant phenolic compounds for productivity and health of ruminants. Proc. Nutr. Soc. 62:383–392.

Walker, J. W., S. L. Kronberg, A. L. Rowaily, and N. E. West. 1994. Comparison of sheep and goat preferences for leafy spurge. J. Range Manage. 47:429–434.

Ward, A. C., D. L. Hunter, M. D. Jaworski, P. J. Benolkin, M. P. Dobel, J. B. Jeffress, and G. A. Tanner. 1997. Pasteurella spp. in sympatric bighorn and domestic sheep. J. Wildl. Dis. 33:544–557.

Wardhaugh, K. G., P. Holter, and B. Longstaff. 2001. The development and survival of three species of coprophagous insect after feeding on the faeces of sheep treated with controlled-release formulations of ivermectin or albendazole. Aust. Vet. J. 79:125–132.

Yang, S. S., C. M. Liu, and Y. L. Liu. 2003. Estimation of methane and nitrous oxide emission from animal production sector in Taiwan during 1990–2000. Chemosphere 52:1381–1388.

13

Nutritional and Metabolic Diseases, Ailments, and Modifiers

INTRODUCTION

This chapter is a short review of the common diseases that have a major nutritional/metabolic component, or have direct applications to nutritional or feeding practices. The diseases are listed alphabetically, except for parasites, which are discussed last. Parasites appear later in this text as they are not a true nutritional or metabolic disorder, but are the most significant and important disease affecting small ruminant production in the world; they both affect nutrition and have elements of their management in proper feeding. This review should not serve as a substitute for a more complete veterinary–health care text, and a medical text should be consulted to treat these conditions.

BLOAT

Bloat is distention of a portion of the forestomachs (i.e., rumen, compartment 1 resulting from the accumulation of free gas or froth (Chennells, 1981; Van Metre et al., 2000; Navarre and Pugh, 2002). Frothy bloat is associated with the ingestion of either leguminous forages or lush pastures (usually winter annuals or cereal grains), and it also may occur with high-grain diets (Navarre and Pugh, 2002). At a low pH of the rumen fluid (or compartment 1 [C1] in camelids) encountered with ingestion of finely ground diets, mucoprotein released from protozoa stabilizes any accumulated foam, resulting in distention. With legume-associated frothy bloat, plant chloroplasts and their components are released into the rumen, trapping gas bubbles. Regardless of the cause of frothy bloat, the small bubbles fill much of the rumen (or C1), preventing clearance and resulting in a depressed eructation. Free gas bloat also occurs with grain diets, particularly when the animals are not adapted to the diet. Physical obstructions of the esophagus (e.g., choke or swollen mediastinal lymph nodes) can interfere with eructation and result in bloat. In addition, endotoxemia, hypocalcemia, pain, peritonitis, and some pharmaceutical agents (e.g., xylazine) can all interfere with rumen eructation (Chennells, 1981; Van Metre et al., 2000; Navarre and Pugh, 2002). Enlargement of the left paralumbar fossa is the most consistent clinical sign, but may be very subtle in nonshorn sheep, fiber-producing goats, or unshorn camelids. Other clinical signs include colic, anxiety, rumen or C1 hypo- or hyper-motility, respiratory distress, and, if left untreated, death (Van Metre et al., 2000; Navarre and Pugh, 2002).

Regardless of the etiology, bloat is a medical emergency, and therapy should be immediate. Where possible, an orogastric tube should be passed through the esophagus and into the rumen. If bloat is not relieved by orogastric intubation, the animal should be checked for frothy bloat. Frothy bloat can be treated by infusing poloxalene (44 mg/kg), dioctyl sodium sulfosuccinate (28 ml), peanut oil (20 to 50 mg/kg), vegetable oil (100 to 200 ml), and/or hand soap (10 ml) into the rumen via the nasogastric tube. In cases where frothy bloat occurs secondary to the excessive ingestion of carbohydrates, mineral oil (100 ml) should also be administered through a nasogastric tube (Navarre and Pugh, 2002). If the animal is in severe respiratory distress, a trocar or large needle can be inserted into the rumen or C1 through the paralumbar fossa. This, however, may result in peritonitis and other abnormalities, and should be performed only with caution.

The prevention of frothy bloat may be aided by limiting access to offending feedstuffs, providing supplemental feed and poloxalene in mineral supplements, and adding ionophores to the ration (Van Metre et al., 2000; Navarre and Pugh, 2002). Animals should be introduced to the bloat-producing feed (green lush forages, finely ground feeds) or pasture (legumes) slowly, over 2 to 3 weeks. Legumes containing sufficient quantities of condensed tannins (≥ 5 g/kg DM) may reduce or prevent bloat (Li et al., 1996; Min et al., 2003). Feeding dry, stemmy hay prior to grazing the legume pasture, grazing mixed grass-legume pastures, or grazing legumes with high leaf tannin concentrations (e.g., arrowleaf clover or kudzu) will all help reduce the incidence of bloat (Chennells, 1981; Van Metre et al., 2000; Navarre and Pugh, 2002).

ENTEROTOXEMIA

Enterotoxemia (overeating disease, pulpy kidney disease) results in sudden death in sheep, goats, elk, and camelids due to a toxin produced in the intestine by the bacteria *Clostridium perfringens* type D. It is more common in small ruminants that are fed, housed, and maintained as livestock, but is relatively rare in wild species. This disease is associated with the feeding of energy-rich diets, usually in very young sucklings and growing animals (NRC, 1981, 1985; Belknap and Pugh, 2002). With excess consumption of carbohydrate from grains or immature succulent forage, the causative bacteria rapidly multiply, producing toxin resulting in increased intestinal permeability. The toxin's pathogenicity is enhanced by gut stasis or parasite damage (NRC, 1981, 1985; Belknap and Pugh, 2002). Symptoms include diarrhea, depression, incoordination, coma, or acute death. Pregnant females should be vaccinated against *C. perfringens* type D 1 to 2 months prior to parturition. This prepartum vaccination will help to maximize colostral antibodies to the disease-producing toxin. Lambs, kids, and crias should be vaccinated twice, preferably pre- and post-weaning. Young born from vaccinated dams should be immunized at 1 to 2 weeks of life, then boostered in 3 to 4 weeks. Young animals born from vaccinated dams should be vaccinated at 1 to 3 months of life, then boostered 3 to 4 weeks later. Other preventative measures include reducing the consumption of fermentable dietary carbohydrate (< 20 percent of a creep feed formulation), avoiding overeating by feeding small frequent meals, and treating young susceptible animals with antiserum (NRC, 1981, 1985; Belknap and Pugh, 2002). Creep feed should be composed of ground forage and a protein source (e.g., soybean meal), and have < 15 to 25 percent fermentable carbohydrates (e.g., corn, oats, and wheat midds). Enterotoxemia type D is most commonly associated with heavy concentrate feeding or an abrupt change in the diet, usually to a better feed. It usually affects weaned lambs that are consuming at least 0.35 kg of grain per day. In contrast, enterotoxemia type C most often affects nursing lambs within the first few weeks of life, causing a bloody diarrhea.

GLUCOSINOLATE TOXICITY

Plants of the *Brassicaceae (Cruciferae)* and related families contain glucosinolate compounds that, upon mastication, ingestion, and hydrolysis in the rumen, form toxins (e.g., epithionitriles, isothiocyanates, and nitriles) capable of interfering with the uptake of iodine by the thyroid gland. This may result in an inhibition in a normal thyroxine formation and secretion (Bell, 1984; Cox-Ganser et al., 1994). Glucosinolate-containing plants include *Amoracia lapathifolia, Brassica campestris, B. napus, B. nigra, B. oleracea, Limnanthes alba, Nasturtium officinalis, Raphanus sativus,* and *Thiaspi arvense,* among others. Ruminants may tolerate 10 percent of their diet in the form of glucosinolate-containing plants without signs of thyroid deficiencies. Symptoms of excessive intake are depressed milk production, growth, and reproduction; goiters; decreased immunity; and chronic illness. The best mode of therapy is to reduce intake, remove offending plants from the diet, and/or supplement with iodine in the diet (Bell, 1984; Cox-Ganser et al., 1994).

HYDROGEN CYANIDE TOXICITY

Acute depression in the blood's ability to transport oxygen may result from the ingestion of plants where damage (wilt, frost, drought) has resulted in the accumulation of hydrogen cyanide (HCN, also called hydrocyanic acid or prussic acid). HCN consumption from contaminated forages alters cytochrome oxidase enzyme activity and blocks cellular respiration. Blood in the affected animals is bright red due to the inability of hemoglobin to release bound oxygen. Although many species of plants may contain potentially toxic concentrations of HCN, cassava, cherry tree, corn, Johnson grass, Sudan grass, and sorghum are some of the most commonly associated plants (Galey, 1996). The symptoms of HCN toxicosis include apparent anxiety, staggering, difficult breathing, dilated pupils, salivation, muscle tremors, bright red blood, and convulsions. Treatment of this condition should be instituted swiftly, to include the intravenous administration of sodium nitrate followed by methylene blue, or singularly sodium thiosulfate (Belknap, 2002).

HYPOCALCEMIA

Hypocalcemia is occasionally encountered in all classes of small ruminants and camelids (NRC, 1981; Smith, 1989; Rankins et al., 2002), but most commonly affects females in late gestation through early lactation. When sudden demand for ionized calcium occurs, the body requires one or more days to accrue the enzyme systems needed for mobilization of calcium from bone storage, and enhanced calcium absorption from the bowel. High dietary intake of calcium, phosphorus, or other cations (e.g., potassium, sodium) results in a decreased production of parathyroid hormone, resulting in decreased production of 1,25 dihydroxycholecalciferol. With inadequate production of 1,25 dihydroxycholecalciferol, there is a lowered absorption and mobilization of calcium from the intestines and bones (Rankins et al., 2002). Stressful events (e.g., hauling, predator attack, or lack of feed) also contribute to the pathophysiology of this condition. Clinical symptoms/signs are a result of low concentrations of ionizable blood calcium during early lactation in heavily lactating animals or late gestation in animals with high calcium demand (i.e., calcification of fetal bones). Multiple fetuses (sheep and goats), hypophosphatemia, and/or hypomagnesemia or hypermagnesemia may complicate and exacerbate this condition (NRC, 1981; Rankins et al., 2002). Symptoms include ataxia, constipation, depressed rumen motility, tremors, tetany, bloat, progressing to recumbency, and/or death (NRC, 1981; Smith, 1989; Rankins et al., 2002). In clinical cases, treatment should be initiated immediately in the form of intravenous administration of calcium salts. Dietary modifications used for the prevention of milk fever in cattle, such as reducing or eliminating diets rich in cations or calcium (e.g., legumes) and phosphorus (e.g., corn and oats) in the late dry period, may be of value in dairy sheep and goats. Immediately after parturition, the calcium levels in the diet should be increased to meet requirements (Rankins et al., 2002). Hauling, shearing, re-sorting groups of animals, predator attacks, predator control, or other forms of stress should be minimized in sheep, goats, and camelids during the final 3 weeks of gestation.

NITRATE-NITRITE TOXICITY

Nitrate toxicity may occur in all ruminant or ruminant-like animals due to the anaerobic conversion of nitrate to nitrite in the forestomach. Nitrite is approximately 10 times more toxic than nitrate in its binding of "heme" iron and subsequent conversion of hemoglobin into methemoglobin. This process results in decreased blood oxygen transport to tissues. When blood methemoglobin concentrations exceed 30 percent, affected blood will have a brown appearance. Certain plants (e.g., alfalfa, beets, corn, sorghum, and Johnson grass) are capable of accumulating greater quantities of nitrates. Nitrate accumulation in plants is enhanced by alteration in plant growth or husbandry practices, such as recent fertilization, moist or acidic soils, rapid growth, freeze damage, or drought. Symptoms include difficulty breathing, exercise intolerance, trembling, weakness, and sudden death. Diagnosis is confirmed by assessing the nitrite levels of the blood, urine, or aqueous humor of the anterior chamber of the eye (Burrows, 1984; Belknap, 2002). Therapy should be instituted immediately and include intravenous methylene blue. Nitrate-nitrite toxicity may be prevented by ensuring that total feed nitrate concentrations are ≤ 0.6 percent (Osweiler et al., 1985; Belknap, 2002).

POLIOENCEPHALOMALACIA

Polioencephalomalacia is a form of cerebrocortical necrosis, secondary to thiamin deficiency, and most commonly is diagnosed in growing ruminants fed high-concentrate diets (Smith, 1979; NRC, 1985; Smith, 1989; Pugh, 1993). Nutritional factors associated with this disease include sudden changes in diet, feeds rich in molasses (horse feed), moldy hay, rumen acidosis, and the dietary stress of weaning and secondary to heat stress (Pugh, 1993). Ruminal bacteria normally produce sufficient thiamin (vitamin B_1) to meet the animal's requirements; however, lowered pH associated with the feeding of high concentrated diets predisposes to this condition. Reduction of the rumen pH can reduce the amount of thiamin-producing bacteria, increase bacterial thiaminase activity in the rumen, and increase the activity of bacteria-produced thiamin antimetabolite (Smith, 1979; NRC, 1985; Rammell and Hill, 1986; Pugh, 1993). Overdosage of certain drugs (e.g., amprolium) may also predispose to this condition (Loew and Dunlop, 1972; Pugh, 1993). Glucose derived through the pentose phosphate pathway requires thiamin diphosphate as a coenzyme for a critical enzyme, transketolase. When thiamin deficiency exists, glucose production via this pathway is compromised. In the case of neurological tissue, glucose deficiency cellular osmotic gradients cannot be maintained and brain swelling occurs, producing polioencephalomalacia (Pugh, 1993; Rankins et al., 2002). Excessive dietary intake of sulfur resulting from mixing errors, high-sulfur water sources, feed intake limiters (e.g., calcium sulfate), and urinary acidifiers (e.g., ammonium sulfate) may cause clinical symptoms and necropsy lesions consistent with polioencephalomalacia (Bulgin et al., 1996). High concentrations of sulfates that are reduced in the rumen to sulfides appear to interfere with energy production in the brain by inhibiting cytochrome oxidase, which participates in the electron transport chain to eventually produce adenosine triphosphate (ATP). Dietary concentrations of sulfur ≥ 0.43 percent have been reported to be associated with clinical cases of polioencephalomalacia in sheep (Gooneratne et al., 1989; Low et al., 1996). Regardless of the pathogenesis, symptoms of polioencephalomalacia include anorexia, blindness, convulsions, depression, diarrhea, head pressing, incoordination, opisthotonos, recumbence, coma, and death (Loew and Dunlop, 1972; Pierson and Jensen, 1975; Smith, 1979; Rammell and Hill, 1986; Pugh, 1993; Bulgin et al., 1996). The initial treatment for polioencephalomalacia should be intravenous and/or intramuscular injection of thiamin (10 mg/kg IV-IM). Prevention should include the avoidance of sudden dietary changes to energy-dense feedstuffs, including some long-stem roughage, allowing free access to a good quality trace mineral salt, and monitoring animals fed diets or water sources rich in sulfate (Rankins et al., 2002).

PREGNANCY TOXEMIA

Pregnancy toxemia (ketosis, hepatic lipidosis) is encountered most commonly during late-term gestation of sheep or goats, and possibly other small ruminant species carrying multiple fetuses, exacerbated by an inability to consume adequate energy to match metabolic demands (NRC, 1981, 1985; Anderson et al., 1994; Tornquist et al., 1999). Environmental conditions that increase energy requirements or decrease energy intake predispose the pregnant female to this condition. Obese or extremely thin sheep and goats may be more prone to developing the condition. Llamas and alpacas of all ages appear to be susceptible to hepatic lipidosis with stressful episodes and inadequate feed intake the initiating cause (Anderson et al., 1994; Tornquist et al., 2001). Other chapters in this publication address adequate energy intake in ewes carrying one or more fetuses. Some animals may not be capable of consuming enough feedstuffs to meet the demands required for late gestation. Environmental stresses or chronic illnesses that result in weight loss, depressed appetite, and a negative energy balance all lead to alterations in the insulin-glucagon ratio. Fatty acids and glycerol are mobilized from body fat and used for energy production. If energy supply does not keep pace with demands, the liver may become overwhelmed with free fatty acids, and release toxic levels of ketones (Marteniuk and Herdt, 1988; Navarre and Pugh, 2002).

The symptoms of pregnancy toxemia are depression, incoordination, circling, teeth grinding, recumbency, tremors, and stargazing. The diagnosis is confirmed by detecting an increase in urine and blood ketone concentrations. Treatment should include oral propylene glycol, sodium propionate, or intravenous glucose solutions, and be initiated immediately. Strategies aimed at prevention include meeting energy, protein, mineral, and vitamin requirements; decreasing stress in late gestation (e.g., parasite control, predator control); dietary supplementation of niacin and/or ionophores; and shearing of pregnant sheep in late gestation (Austin and Young, 1977; Navarre and Pugh, 2002). Providing adequate bunk space, identifying those animals carrying twins or triplets (e.g., transabdominal ultrasonography) and feeding them accordingly, maintaining proper body condition throughout gestation, isolation of affected or high-risk animals in order to monitor feed intake, and decreasing the incidence of chronic disease all may help prevent this condition (Tornquist et al., 1999; Navarre and Pugh, 2002).

RICKETS

Rickets is a metabolic bone disease of young animals resulting from the failure of proper cartilage mineralization and may be caused by vitamin D, phosphorus, and/or calcium deficiency (Reilly et al., 2002). Rickets is more commonly encountered in young rapidly growing animals with limited sunlight exposure (e.g., heavily wooled or fall born) and deficient blood concentrations of vitamin D (Bonniwell et al., 1988; Van Saun et al., 1996; Smith and Van Saun, 2001; Van Saun, 2004). Lambs, kids, and crias living in northern latitudes in winter and animals that are housed indoors and/or consume diets low in phosphorus or calcium are prone to this condition (Bonniwell et al., 1988; Smith and Van Saun, 2001; Parker et al., 2002). Chronic parasitism, ingestion of some poisonous plants (i.e., oxalate-containing plants), chronic lead, or fluoride-aluminum toxicity can all produce or add to the pathogenesis of rickets (Reilly et al., 2002). Symptoms of rickets include a stiff gait, shifting leg lameness, enlarged joints and bones, humped back stance, recumbency, swelling at the costochondral junctions, deformed and possibly bowed limbs, and mottled teeth with delayed eruption. Prevention of this condition includes allowing access to sunlight, adjusting the diet to maintain adequate intake of all nutrients with emphasis on phosphorus and calcium, maintaining a proper calcium-phosphorus ratio of 1-2:1, and removal of any potentially toxic substances or plants from the diet. Where latitude or season result in inadequate sunlight exposure in growing animals, adding vitamin D3 to the diet or via injection may be of benefit in prevention of rickets (Judson and Feakes, 1999).

RUMEN ACIDOSIS

Rumen or compartment 1 (C1 in the camelid) acidosis results from the rapid fermentation of carbohydrates when ingested in excessive amounts (Nour et al., 1977; Braun et al., 1992; Cebra et al., 1996; Van Metre et al., 2000; Navarre and Pugh, 2002). The feeding of finely ground cereal grains (corn, barley, oats, wheat) is the major contributor. Finely ground feedstuffs with small particle size are more rapidly fermented in the forestomachs, resulting in decreased rumen pH. "Grain overload" can also be caused by the ingestion of breads, candy, fruits, beets, potatoes, and other sources of readily fermentable carbohydrate, particularly in those animals that have been fed a forage-based ration and are suddenly allowed access to these highly fermentable feedstuffs (Nour et al., 1977; Braun et al., 1992; Cebra et al., 1996; Van Metre et al., 2000; Navarre and Pugh, 2002).

During the fermentation process in the forestomachs, lactic acid producing bacterial species (e.g., *Lactobacillus* sp.) proliferate, resulting in a lowering of the rumen pH. As the pH drops, many rumen protozoa and lactate using bacteria begin to die, resulting in acid accumulation, fluid influx into the forestomachs, increased osmotic pressure, dehydration, and possibly hypovolemic shock. As the liver's ability to process is overwhelmed, lactate concentrations in the blood increase and may result in systemic lactic acidosis (Van Metre et al., 2000; Navarre and Pugh, 2002). The lactic acid accumulation and associated osmotic changes are toxic to the rumen epithelium, and damage may result in bacterial and toxin leakage into the portal and systemic circulation. Sequelae to rumen acidosis include liver abscesses, fungal rumenitis, bloat, polioencephalomalacia, and/or chronic diarrhea (Braun et al., 1992; Van Metre et al., 2000).

Clinical signs first appear 12 to 36 hours after feed engorgement, and include anorexia, depression, diarrhea, colic, bloat, seizures, weakness, recumbency, shock, and death (Nour et al., 1977; Van Metre et al., 2000; Navarre and Pugh, 2002). Diagnosis is based on clinical signs and the rumen fluid with a pH below 5.5, milky gray rumen fluid and particles of the inciting feed visible, and reduced or absent number of protozoa, and the presence of large gram-positive rods (*Lactobacillus* sp.) visualized with a Gram's stain.

Orally administered magnesium hydroxide and magnesium oxide (1 g/kg) can neutralize the acidic pH and may be sufficient in mild cases. If, however, much of the feed is still present in the rumen, these two alkalinizing agents will only work temporarily (Van Metre et al., 2000; Navarre and Pugh, 2002). Appropriate antibiotics given orally can kill rumen microflora and inhibit continued fermentation (Nour et al., 1977; Van Metre et al., 2000; Navarre and Pugh, 2002). After the rumen pH is corrected, transfaunation of the rumen microflora is beneficial in order to reestablish normal rumen function. Thiamin supplementation and systemic antimicrobials may be indicated until rumen function returns. Forage feeding and water should be limited until rumen contractions return (Van Metre et al., 2000; Navarre and Pugh, 2002).

Dietary change from high fiber to high fermentable carbohydrates should occur slowly and preferably over a 2- to 3-week period. When group feeding concentrate, adequate feeding space should be maintained in order to minimize excessive intake, and allowing for management practices that restrict meal size. Buffering agents can be added to the diet of animals being fed high-grain rations (e.g., club lambs, feedlot lambs, and dairy goats). Feeding buffers may improve milk production, increase feed intake, and increase rate of gain. Sodium bicarbonate is probably the most commonly used buffer; it can be offered free choice or included in the diet as 1 percent of dry matter (DM) intake. Calcium carbonate or magnesium oxide (0.5–0.8 percent of DM intake) may also be useful if fed as buffering agents (Navarre and Pugh, 2002).

STRESS ABORTION IN ANGORAS

The goat is dependent on the corpus luteum for pregnancy maintenance; therefore, prevention of its normal production of progesterone may predispose to abortion (NRC, 1981; Mobini et al., 2002). A habitual abortion syndrome has been described in Angora goats and appears to be associated with hypoadrenocorticism (Van Rensburg, 1971; Van Tonder, 1975; Wentzel et al., 1976; Ruffin et al., 2002). Some Angoras cannot adequately respond to stress during gestation, apparently due to small adrenal glands with less than optimal plasma cortisol secretion in times of need (Wentzel et al., 1976). Stressful situations (e.g., decreased feed availability or weather changes), coupled with the does' inability to respond by increasing cortisol output and maternal hypoglycemia, result in hypertrophy of fetal adrenal glands and excessive fetal cortisol output. The parturition cascade is initiated due to increasing blood cortisol concentrations resulting in delivery of premature, stillborn, or aborted fetuses (Wentzel et al., 1976; Ruffin et al., 2002). Most abortions occur between 90 and 110 days of gestation. Aborted fetuses are typically dysmature and anemic and have adrenocortical hyperplasia (Wentzel et al., 1976). Preventative measures include identifying animals with this trait and removing them from the breeding flock, feeding to meet nutritional requirements, and minimizing stressful times and husbandry practices (particularly with respect to energy).

ULCERATIVE POSTHITIS (PIZZLE ROT)

Rams, bucks, and wethers are all susceptible to bacterial posthitis-balanoposthitis (Shelton and Livingston, 1975; NRC, 1981; Belknap and Pugh, 2002). This is the most common bacterial infection of the prepuce in small ruminants and is referred to as ulcerative posthitis, pizzle rot, or sheath rot (NRC, 1981). This condition is caused by an interaction between excess protein intake and the bacteria *Corynebacterium renale* (NRC, 1981). Diets containing significant quantities of legumes or other sources of protein will result in alkaline urine and excess urinary urea. In the presence of the urease enzyme-producing *C. renale*, excess urinary urea is converted to ammonia, which may damage mucosal surfaces of the prepuce. This condition is more common during wet springs when animals are grazing lush legume or legume-grass pastures (Shelton and Livingston, 1975; NRC, 1981; Belknap and Pugh, 2002). Symptoms include straining during urination, swelling of the prepuce, necrosis and ulceration of the preputial mucosa, abdominal discomfort, and stiff-stilted gait. The urine of affected animals may be thick or semi-solid, and very malodorous (Belknap and Pugh, 2002). Preventative measures include shearing the preputial wool or mohair; allowing a free-choice access to fresh, clean water; and maintaining adequate, yet not excessive, protein intake. Where dietary changes are difficult due to management constraints, such as animals being fed to a high degree of "finish" and blood donor animals, the feeding of urine acidifiers (e.g., ammonium chloride) and/or antimicrobial agents (e.g., chlortetracycline) may aid in prevention (NRC, 1981; Belknap and Pugh, 2002).

UREA (AMMONIA) TOXICITY

Urea (ammonia) toxicity is seen in animals newly introduced to diets containing nonprotein nitrogen (e.g., urea or ammoniated feeds) as the predominant protein source (NRC, 1981; Divers, 1999; Rankins et al., 2002). When urea or other sources of nonprotein nitrogen (NPN) are fed with inadequate available fermentable carbohydrates or when an elevated rumen pH exists (usually due to the intake of poor quality forages), there is an enhanced function of the rumen's bacterial-produced urease enzyme, and the bacterial protein production ability of the rumen is overwhelmed. This will result in excessive ruminal production of ammonia, systemic alkalosis, and encephalopathy. Symptoms of urea toxicity include trembling, facial twitching, incoordination, bloating, dyspneia, hyperesthesia, blindness, recumbency, and possibly death (NRC, 1981; Divers, 1999; Rankins et al., 2002).

In cases of this disease, infusing cold, weak acetic acid solution via nasogastric tube into the rumen improves the blood acid-base status and slows bacterial production of ammonia. Oral charcoal may also be helpful in decreasing ammonia absorption (Divers, 1999; Rankins et al., 2002). If nonprotein nitrogen sources are to be fed in order to enhance bacterial protein production of the rumen, then they should be: (1) introduced very slowly over a 2- to 3-week period, (2) calculated to supply less than one-third of the total crude protein of the diet, (3) calculated to supply less than one-half of the crude protein in the concentrate portion of the diet, and (4) fed along with a readily fermentable source of carbohydrates (NRC, 1981; Rankins et al., 2002).

UROLITHIASIS

Urolithiasis is occasionally encountered in intact or castrated male goats, sheep, or camelids. This condition is much more common in males than females, probably due to the longer, smaller urethra, and the sigmoid flexure in the male (NRC, 1981; Kock and Fowler, 1982; NRC, 1985; Smith, 1989). Early castration may result in a decreased urethral diameter, with resultant increase in incidence. The composition of urinary calculi (urolith) varies according to geographic location, but is commonly composed of calcium salts, magnesium, and phosphatic complexes (Belknap and Pugh, 2002). Phosphatic calculi are formed in response to diets rich in concentrates (e.g., cereal grains), low in roughages, low dietary calcium:phosphorus ratios (diets rich in cereal grains), high magnesium diets, and alkaline urine (NRC, 1981, 1985; Smith, 1989; Belknap and Pugh, 2002). Animals with diets rich in cations (e.g., legumes and grass hays) or animals with urinary infections are both prone to have alkaline urine (NRC, 1981, 1985). Silicate calculi are occasionally identified in small ruminants fed plants grown in sandy soil or water containing high levels of silica. Oxalate calculi are associated with the ingestion of excessive quantities of oxalate-containing plants, and are more commonly encountered in browsing conditions (Belknap and Pugh, 2002). Uroliths can be formed in any part of the tract by obstructing of urine flow and resulting in the symptoms of straining to urinate, difficult urination, urinary dripping, abdominal pain, crystal formation on preputial hairs, blood in the urine, and possibly death. If the urinary bladder or urethra ruptures, urine may be released into the abdomen or the subcutaneous areas of the ventral abdomen. This condition is commonly referred to as "water belly" (NRC, 1981; Kock and Fowler, 1982; NRC, 1985; Smith, 1989; Belknap and Pugh, 2002).

There are many methods useful in prevention of urolithiasis. Increasing the calcium to phosphorus ratio (e.g., 2:1) by the addition of a calcium-containing mineral (e.g., calcium carbonate) and/or the reduction of oil seed meals, cereal grains, and the addition of sodium chloride up to 4 percent of the diet may result in increased water intake with resultant urinary dilution (NRC, 1985; Belknap and Pugh, 2002). Molasses and legumes are both rich sources of potassium and should be avoided in the diet of animals either predisposed or affected by this condition. Other strategies useful in minimizing urolithiasis are reduction of dietary phosphorus, reducing the urinary excretion of phosphorus, and increasing water intake. From an applied standpoint, reducing the urinary output of phosphorus and increasing the fecal output of phosphorus can be accomplished by reducing dietary cereal grains, avoiding the feeding of pelleted feeds, and enhancing the intake of forages. Increasing fiber intake and decreasing pelleted feeds is a dietary strategy that may increase rumen "mat" formation and rumination, thus increasing the fecal output and decreasing urinary output of phosphorus. In the case of stones containing oxalate, silica, or calcium carbonate, avoiding these substances in the diet (oxalate-containing plants, silica soils, and excessive legume intake) will help reduce the incidence (Belknap and Pugh, 2002).

Dietary supplements that acidify the urine and/or reduce urinary tract infection may be useful in stone prevention (NRC, 1981, 1985; Belknap and Pugh, 2002). Ammonium chloride and ammonia sulfate (0.5 percent of diet or 100–200 mg/kg BW) may be useful in acidifying the urine, while oral tetracycline may help control bacterial urinary tract infection, thus reducing urinary alkalinity (NRC, 1981; Belknap and Pugh, 2002).

PARASITES

Pasture-range, the most important component of a complete nutritional program for small ruminants, is also the source of internal parasites, which, paradoxically, pose the most serious limits to productivity. Internal nematode parasites are the most common disease processes in many temperate, subtropical, and tropical areas of the world. Sheep, goats, many species of deer, and camelids share most of the same species of internal cestodes, nematodes, and trematodes. The control of these parasites is as varied as animal usage, land types, husbandry practices, and feeding protocols. Specific control programs are not discussed in this text. The genetic potential of animals will never be met regardless of the nutritional program utilized, unless sound, sustainable internal parasite control programs are instituted, and are based on excellent husbandry-grazing systems applicable for specific species of animals and individual locales (Pugh et al., 1998; Pugh and Navarre, 2001). Small ruminants fed diets that meet nutritional requirements for optimal growth and production are more prone to resist parasite infection and more likely to make a quicker recovery after the infection is controlled (Wallace et al., 1996; Coop et al., 1997).

As noted in Chapter 4 on Energy, subclinical parasitism can influence nutrient requirements, although impacts have not been well characterized regarding site of infestation (e.g., abomasums vs. small intestine for internal parasites) and level (e.g., linear, threshold, quadratic, and/or cubic change). Likewise, type of infection could have impact, with parasites eliciting primarily blood loss (e.g., ticks) or ingesting nutrients from the gut lumen (e.g., tapeworms) presumably affecting protein turnover and loss relatively more than ones principally causing gastrointestinal tract tissue damage. The effect on metabolizable protein (MP) requirement appears to be related to the greater use of amino acids (AA) to mount the immune response, to repair and replace gastrointestinal tract tissues (i.e., leakage of plasma protein, sloughing of epithelial cells, secreted mucoproteins), and to support higher rates of liver export protein synthesis (Liu et al., 2003). In sheep, gastrointestinal parasite infection increases nitrogen flow into the gastrointestinal tract and reduces the efficiency of dietary nutrient use for production (Sykes, 2000). Thus, subclinical internal parasitism has relatively greater impact on MP than on metabolizable energy (ME) requirements with influences on the optimum or required dietary MP:ME ratio (Liu et al., 2003). Liu et al. (2003) estimated that the immunity-associated response to an infection of sheep with the small intestinal parasite *Trichostrongylus colubriformis* increases MP requirements for maintenance by 0.69-fold for ewes in late pregnancy and by 2.5-fold for ewes in early lactation. In addition to the increased competition for MP with internal parasitism, there are effects on the profile of AA (e.g., lower sulfur-AA) available to nonvisceral tissues, with likely impact on the efficiencies of MP utilization.

Numerous studies now support the view that providing supplemental MP to sheep and goats with subclinical infections of gastrointestinal parasites improves their resilience and resistance to parasites (Kyriazakis et al., 1996; Coop and Kyriazakis, 1999; Torres-Acosta et al., 2004). And, for the most part, the response to supplementation is greater when the protein source is protected (i.e., rumen undegradable) such as with fish meal (Donaldson et al., 1998). However, less degradable protein sources (SBM), along with supplemental carbohydrates (sorghum), appear to improve postnematode infection resilience in browsing goats (Torres-Acosta et al., 2004). Economic analysis of supplementation with protein and carbohydrates (SBM and sorghum) on browse-fed kids suggested an economic return by supplementation, but less of a return than when compared to the use of anthelmintics (Torres-Acosta et al., 2004). Best cost-benefit returns were observed with a combination of supplemental feeding and the use of anthelmintics. Interestingly, supplemental feeding of molasses-urea blocks may have some effect on reduction of gastrointestinal parasites in lambs (Anindo et al., 1998).

Feed selection is also influenced during parasitism, presumably as part of a coordinated effort to counter the effects of infestation and to mount an effective immune response. Parasitized sheep and goats, given the choice, will select for a higher nutrient content diet, particularly one higher (206 vs. 86 g crude protein (CP)/kg) in protein (Aumont et al., 1984; Kyriazakis et al., 1994, 1996). It is expected that the requirement for sulfur-AA will be greater when small ruminants have gastrointestinal parasitism (Coop et al., 1997).

Feeding forages with condensed tannins may help reduce or allow better tolerance of gastrointestinal parasites by grazing ruminants by interfering with the parasite life cycle (Niezen et al., 1995; Min and Hart, 2003; Min et al., 2003), inhibiting nutrient availability for parasite larval growth directly by causing larval death (Athanasiadou et al., 2001) and stimulating the immune system (Min and Hart, 2003; Min et al., 2003). Future research into this area may help identify more naturally occurring compounds that enhance parasite control (Stepek et al., 2005).

Widespread anthelmintic resistance by gastrointestinal parasites in small ruminant species has been documented (Barton et al., 1985; Mwamachi et al., 1995; Maingi et al., 1996; Terrill et al., 2001; Mortensen et al., 2003). As anthelmintic efficacy continues to be reduced, new and more innovative strategies will be required in order to control gastrointestinal parasites. Some of these control measures include nutritional supplementation to meet dietary requirements for all major nutrients; grazing strategies that reduce stocking rate, optimize pasture rotation systems, and employ multispecies grazing; the selection of animals with natural resistance; and the use of naturally occurring plant compounds that reduce parasitism (Hart, 2001; Hoste et al., 2001; Waghorn and McNabb, 2003; Stepek et al., 2005)

METABOLIC MODIFIERS

Metabolic modifiers are classified as agents that affect metabolism to improve nutrient utilization and product synthesis. Included in this class of compounds are antibiotics and ionophores, which improve digestion through influences on the gut microbiota, and anabolic steroids, somatotropin, and β-adrenergic agonists. The latter only affect postabsorptive nutrient use through regulation of muscle protein metabolism (i.e., protein synthesis and/or degradation). It is recommended that prior to considering the feeding or administration of any metabolic modifier or feed additive, the U.S. Food and Drug Administration website (http://dil.vetmed.vt.edu/NADA/) be consulted for current information on approved and banned substances and recommended effective withdrawal measures for those that have been approved. Information on those approved for use in Canada can be found on the Veterinary Drugs Directorate of Canada website (http://www.hc-sc.gc.ca/vetdrugs-medsvet/).

The effects of metabolic modifiers such as anabolic implants, somatotropin (ST), and β-adrenergic agonists on protein (amino acid) and energy utilization occur primarily postabsorptive. Metabolic modifiers promote increased tissue gain by shifting the partition nutrients away from catabolic pathways and towards greater protein deposition. In common with administration of ST, growth hormone releasing factor (GRF), β-agonists, and anabolic steroids is that they all improve rates of skeletal muscle growth. However, these agents differ in their effects on protein, lipid, and carbohydrate metabolism. They further differ in whether organ and bone growth are also increased along with the enhanced muscle growth. Given the different modes of action and partition of nutrient use, it would be expected that the requirements for dietary nutrients and the nutrient influences on the efficacy of the metabolic modifier will differ. Few data are available on lambs and meat goats, however, that have addressed the adequacy of nutrient intake with respect to responses to metabolic modifiers, although considerable information exists about beef and dairy cattle. A further factor that will influence the magnitude of effect of growth modifiers on growth and carcass composition changes is sex. Where lambs of similar genetic background and fed the same diet are compared, carcass protein accretion rates in ram lambs are ~ 30 percent greater than for ewes and wethers, whereas lipid accretion rates are proportionally less in rams (Beermann et al., 1990).

Somatotropin and Release Factor

Somatotropin is a naturally occurring protein hormone produced in the pituitary gland of all farm animal species. This hormone is the major regulator of animal growth and especially of milk production. To date, there is yet to be commercial production of recombinant forms of caprine and ovine ST, although recombinant forms of these are available commercially for research use.

Since the last NRC reports for sheep (NRC, 1985) and goats (NRC, 1981), many new and emerging roles of ST in coordination of growth, fetal development, and lactating have emerged, with new technologies and on-farm applications soon to appear. In concert with estradiol, ST promotes morphogenesis of terminal end buds in the mammary fat pads to increase the amount of parenchymal tissues (McFadden et al., 1990). In gestating ewes (Stelwagen et al., 1993) and goats (Knight et al., 1994) administered bST, mammary growth was stimulated, and this was accompanied by increased milk yields during the subsequent lactation. Furthermore, sustained-release bovine ST (bST) given to ewes at breeding resulted in larger lambs at birth and heavier singleton lambs at 30, 60 and 75 d of age compared to singleton lambs from control (untreated) ewes (Costine et al., 2005). In overnourished adolescent sheep, which produce small and unthrifty lambs, ST administration increases utero-placental growth leading to increased fetal size and survivability after lambing (Wallace et al., 2004b).

The responses in milk yield and quality by lactating ewes and goats administered ST are generally similar to those reported for ST-treated dairy cows. The effects of ST administration have also been shown to enhance mammary growth and extend lactation persistency in goats (Knight et al., 1990) and in sheep (Stelwagen et al., 1993). Enhancement of milk production by administration of ST has been observed in various breeds of lactating goats (Alpine, Saanen) where increases in milk yield of 5–30 percent are reported (Mepham et al., 1984; Nielsen, 1988; Knight et al., 1990; Knight, 1992; Disenhaus et al., 1995; Gallo et al., 1997; Chadio et al., 2000).

Growing lambs administered either recombinant bST or ovine ST (oST) increased daily live weight gain from 10–35 percent (bST: Johnsson et al., 1985; Pell and Bates, 1987; McLaughlin et al., 1991; oST: Beermann et al., 1990; McLaughlin et al., 1993) and increased feed conversion efficiency by 14–20 percent. Administration of bST, but not oST, to wool breeds of sheep has been shown to increase wool growth either during (Johnsson et al., 1985, 1987) or after discontinuing (Wheatley et al., 1966; Reklewska, 1974; Wynn et al., 1988) bST treatment, although reduced wool growth (diameter) has also been reported during bST treatment (Wynn et al., 1988). Angora does and wether goats given bST also showed increased daily gain but with no effect on mohair growth (Davis et al., 1999a,b; Puchala et al., 2001).

In ewes and goats, there tends to be a delayed increase in dry matter intake (DMI) after bST administration. In growing or finishing lambs administered ST, Zainur et al., (bST: 1989) and McLaughlin et al. (bST: 1991; oST: 1993) failed to observe effects on DMI. The magnitude of the effect and the responsiveness to ST is largely determined by level of protein intake and the extent that the metabolizable protein component meets the amino acid requirements for optimal growth and milk production potential. Thus, both the source (fish meal > soybean meal) and quantity of dietary protein intake have been shown to improve responses to ST and GRF by growing lambs (Beermann et al., 1991; MacRae et al., 1991), but these effects appear to be additive (i.e., independent) for body weight gain, feed conversion, and hindleg muscle weights.

β-Adrenergic Agonists

To date, none of the β-adrenergic agonist compounds have been given governmental approval for feeding to small ruminants raised for meat or milk production in the United States or in any other country. Of the β-agonists, clenbuterol has been directly linked with incidences of toxicity in humans that have consumed liver from medicated animals (Mitchell and Dunnavan, 1998). Nonetheless, the entire class of β-agonist compounds are being treated similarly by regulatory agencies until substantive information to the contrary can be provided by pharmaceutical companies. To date, ractopamine has not been approved for use in sheep or goats, and such use is illegal.

Included in this category are the synthetic compounds clenbuterol, cimaterol, ractopamine, salbutamol, and L-644,969, all of which affect various aspects of metabolism leading to increased lean deposition and reduced fat accretion. The predominant target for β-adrenergic agonists is skeletal muscle via specific binding to β_1- or β_2-adrenergic receptors in muscle. These compounds promote an initial increase in muscle protein gain by either stimulation of protein synthetic mechanisms (Claeys et al., 1989; Smith et al., 1989) or by inhibition of muscle proteolytic pathways

(Bohorov et al., 1987; Wang and Beermann, 1988), both mechanisms variously shown to be temporally influenced at some time after β-adrenergic administration. Unlike ST, the anabolic effects of β-agonists are transient as target tissues eventually become desensitized by 14 to 21 d after initial feeding. General effects in sheep include a 15 percent increase in gain and feed efficiency and a 25 percent increase in muscle gain compared to a 25 percent reduction in body fat, albeit these effects all tend to be transient. In most studies, β-agonists have not been found to alter feed intake consistently (Mersmann, 1995, 1998).

Steroidal Growth Promoters

These growth promoters are given as implants (pellets) that contain specified dosages of one or usually more hormones. They are inserted in the fleshy part of the ear using a special implant gun; the implants do not enter the human food chain as ears are discarded at slaughter. The hormones are gradually released over a period of 50–60 days to ensure a relatively constant and slightly elevated level in the blood. At present, none of the growth promoters listed below have been approved for use in sheep and goats in Canada, and only Zeranol (Ralgro®) is approved for sheep (but not goats) in the United States.

Estradiol-17β is a naturally occurring female sex hormone that is typically included as estradiol benzoate as a minor component in combination with another hormone. Progesterone is another naturally occurring female sex hormone often given as the major component of a dual combination implant. Testosterone is the primary naturally occurring male sex hormone, often administered as the propionate form as the major component of a dual combination implant. Trenbolone acetate is a synthetic hormone that mimics the action of testosterone.

Zeranol (Ralgro®) is a synthetic hormone that mimics the action of estradiol and is often given as the sole component of implants. Studies indicate that Zeranol reduces the percentage of fat while increasing the proportion of lean tissue in carcasses of lambs (Sinnett-Smith et al., 1983). Hutcheson et al. (1992) and Nold et al. (1992) demonstrated that zeranol improves daily gain and feed efficiency of lambs.

Prenatal androgenization is a technique to manipulate growth rate and carcass composition of female animals by altering the prenatal sexual differentiation. Normal ewe lambs have lower daily gain and feed efficiency, and they produce carcasses with greater proportions of fat, compared to their male (intact or castrates) counterparts (Ferrell et al., 1979). The higher carcass fat content of ewe lambs reduces the value of their carcasses and increases the cost of meat production. Prenatal androgenization of ewe lambs is shown to increase daily gain and feed efficiency (Klindt et al., 1987) and decrease carcass fat content (DeHaan et al., 1987; Jenkins et al., 1988) compared to control ewe lambs.

Ionophores

Ionophores may be used in small ruminant production to increase feed efficiency, improve growth rates on high roughage diets, increase utilization of dietary nitrogen, decrease bloat, decrease acidosis, and aid in the control of coccicidosis (Richardson et al., 1976; Orskov et al., 1979; Chalupa et al., 1984; Foreyt, 1990; Raun, 1990; McGuffey et al., 2001; Tedeschi et al., 2003). Ionophores appear to alter the movement of certain ions across biologic membranes, which, in the rumen, results in an alteration of microflora. These microflora changes result in increased production of propionate, improved nitrogen utilization, increased digestibility of dry matter, and decreased acetate and methane production. Of the ionophores (laidlomycin, lasalocid, monensin, narasin, salinomycin), lasalocid is approved for use in sheep, while monensin is approved for use in goats. Ionophores have a beneficial effect in altering the deamination and decarboxylation reactions that occur in the rumen in degradation of tryptophan. These reactions result in the formation of the toxic chemical 3-methylindole. The inhibition by monensin and the formation of ruminal 3-methylindole concentrations reduce the incidence of the toxin produced pulmonary edema and emphysema (Carlson and Breeze, 1984). The feeding of monensin to lactating goats may effect endogenous growth hormone concentrations, in addition to improved productivity (Brown and Hogue, 1987). Lasalocid may be more palatable than monensin to both sheep and goats (Huston et al., 1990). Whenever ionophores are included in the ration of both sheep and goats, care should be taken to minimize mixing errors, feed at appropriate dietary concentrations, and follow all governmental feed guidelines, as ionophores can be toxic to sheep, goats, camelids, and other small ruminant species (Anderson et al., 1984; Mathieson et al., 1990; Dalvi and Sawant, 1990; Miller et al., 1990; Jones, 2001)

REFERENCES

Anderson, D. E., P. D. Constable, K. E. Yvorchuk, N. V. Anderson, G. St-Jean, and L. Rock. 1994. Hyperlipidemia and ketonuria in an alpaca and a llama. J. Vet. Int. Med. 8:207–211.

Anderson, T. D., W. G. Van Alstine, M. D. Ficken, D. W. Miskimins, T. L. Carson, and G. D. Osweiler. 1984. Acute monensin toxicosis in sheep: Light and electron microscopic changes. Am. J. Vet. Res. 45:1142.

Anindo, F., S. Toe, E. Tembely, A. Mukasa-Mugerwa, S. Lahlou-Kassi, and S. Sovani. 1998. Effect of molasses-urea-block (MUB) on dry matter intake, growth, reproductive performance and control of gastrointestinal nematode infection of grazing Menz ram lambs. Small Ruminant Res. 27:63–71.

Athanasiadou, S., I. Kyriazakis, F. Jackson, and R. L. Coop. 2001. Direct anthelmintic effects of condensed tannins towards different gastrointestinal nematodes of sheep: *In vitro* and *in vivo* studies. Vet. Parasitol. 99:205–219.

Aumont, G., P. Yvox, and A. Esnault. 1984. Experimental coccidiosis in goats. 1. Experimental model: Effects of parasitism on the feeding behaviour and the growth of animals; intestinal lesions. Ann. Recherche. Vet. 15:467–473.

Austin, A. R., and N. E. Young. 1977. The effect of shearing pregnant ewes on lamb birth weights. Vet. Rec. 100:527–529.

Barton, N. J., B. L. Trainor, J. S. Urie, J. W. Atkins, M. F. S. Pyman, and I. R. Wolstencroft. 1985. Anthelmintic resistance in nematode parasites of goats. Aust. Vet. J. 62:224–227.

Beermann, D. H., D. E. Hogue, V. K. Fishell, S. Aronica, H. W. Dickson, and B. R. Schricker. 1990. Exogenous human growth hormone releasing factor and ovine somatotropoin improve growth performance and composition of gain in lambs. J. Anim. Sci. 68:4122–4133.

Beermann, D. H., T. F. Robinson, T. M. Byrem, D. E. Hogue, A. W. Bell, and C. L. McLaughlin. 1991. Abomasal casein infusion and exogenous somatotropin enhance nitrogen utilization by growing lambs. J. Nutr. 121:2020–2028.

Bell, J. M. 1984. Nutrients and toxicants in rapeseed meal: A review. J. Anim. Sci. 58:996–1010.

Belknap, E. B. 2002. Diseases of the urinary system. Pp. 257–272 in Sheep and Goat Medicine, D. G. Pugh, ed. Philadelphia: W. B. Saunders.

Belknap, E. B., and D. G. Pugh. 2002. Diseases of the urinary system. Pp. 125–126 in Sheep and Goat Medicine, D. G. Pugh, ed. Philadelphia: W. B. Saunders.

Bohorov, O., P. J. Buttery, J. I. R. D. Corrcia, and J. B. Soar. 1987. The effect of the β_2-adrenergic agonist clenbuterol or implantation with oestradiol plus trenbolone acetate on protein metabolism in wether lambs. Br. J. Nutr. 57:99–107.

Bonniwell, M. A., B. S. Smith, J. A. Spence, H. Wright, and D. A. Ferguson. 1988. Rickets associated with vitamin D deficiency in young sheep. Vet. Rec. 122:386–388.

Braun, U., T. Rihs, and U. Schefer. 1992. Ruminal lactic acidosis in sheep and goats. Vet. Rec. 130(16):343–349.

Brown, D. L., and D. E. Hogue. 1987. Effects of feeding monensin to lactating goats: Acetyl coenzyme A carboxylase, hormone-sensitive lipase, plasma glucose, and circulating hormones. J. Dairy Sci. 70:823–830.

Bulgin, M. S., S. D. Lincoln, and G. Mather. 1996. Elemental sulfur toxicosis in a flock of sheep. J. Am. Vet. Med. Assoc. 208:1063–1065.

Burrows, G. E. 1984. Methylene blue: Effect and disposition in sheep. J. Vet. Pharmocol. Therap. 7:225–231.

Carlson, J. R., and R. G. Breeze. 1984. Ruminal metabolism of plant toxins with emphasis in indolic compounds. J. Anim. Sci. 58:1040–1049.

Cebra, C. K., M. L. Cebra, F. B. Garry, and E. B. Belknap. 1996. Forestomach acidosis in six New World camelids. J. Amer. Vet. Med. Assoc. 208:901–904.

Chadio, S. E., G. Servas, K. Kiriakou, C. Goulas, and J. Menegatos. 2000. Effects of recombinant bovine somatotropin administration to lactating goats. Small Ruminant Res. 35:263–269.

Chalupa, W. H., B. Rickabaugh, D. S. Kronfeld, and D. Sklan. 1984. Rumen fermentation in vitro as influenced by long chain fatty acids. J. Dairy Sci. 67:1439–1444.

Chennells, D. 1981. Bloat in kids. Goat Vet. Soc. J. 2:16–17.

Claeys, M. C., D. R. Mulvaney, F. D. McCarthy, M. T. Gore, D. N. Marple, and J. L. Sartin. 1989. Skeletal muscle protein synthesis and growth hormone secretion in young lambs treated with clenbuterol. J. Anim. Sci. 67:2245–2254.

Coop, R. L., and I. Kyriazakis. 1999. Parasite infection. Vet Parasitol. 84: 187–204.

Coop, R. L., I. Kyriazakis, J. F. Huntley, E. Jackson, and F. Jackson. 1997. The influence of protein and amino acid on the resilience of sheep to intestinal parasitism. Pp. 196–198 in Proc. 4th Int. Congress for Sheep Veterinarians, Armidale, N.S.W., Australia.

Costine, B. A., E. K. Inskeep, and M. E. Wilson. 2005. Growth hormone at breeding modifies conceptus development and postnatal growth in sheep. J. Anim. Sci. 83:810–815.

Cox-Ganser, J. M., G. A. Jung, R. T. Pushkin, and R. L. Reid. 1994. Evaluation of Brassicas in grazing systems for sheep: II. Blood composition and nutrient status. J. Anim. Sci. 72:1832–1845.

Dalvi, R, R., and S. G. Sawant. 1990. Studies on monensin toxicity in goats. Zentralbl Veterinarmed A 37:352–355.

Davis, J. J., T. Sahlu, R. Puchala, M. J. Herselman, J. M. Fernandez, J. P. McCann, and S. W. Coleman. 1999a. The effect of bovine somatotropin treatment on production of lactating Angora does with kids. J. Anim Sci. 77:17–24.

Davis, J. J., T. Sahlu, R. Puchala, M. J. Herselman, S. P. Hart, E. N. Escobar, S. W. Coleman, J. P. McCann, and A. L. Goetsch. 1999b. Effects of bovine somatotropin and ruminally undegraded protein on feed intake, live weight gain, and mohair production by yearling Angora wethers. J. Anim. Sci. 77:1029–1036.

DeHaan, K. C., L. L. Berger, D. J. Kesler, F. K. McKeith, D. L. Thomas, and T. G. Nash. 1987. Effect of prenatal androgenization on lamb performance, carcass composition and reproductive function. J. Anim. Sci. 65:1465–1470.

Disenhaus, C., H. Jammes, J. Hervieu, F. Ternois, and D. Sauvant. 1995. Effects of recombinant bovine somatotropin on goat milk yield, composition and plasma metabolites. Small Ruminant Res. 15:139–148.

Divers, T. J. 1999. Diseases of the nervous system. In Current Veterinary Therapy 4, Food Animal Practice, J. L. Howard and R. A. Smith, eds. Philadelphia: W. B. Saunders.

Donaldson, J. D., M. F. J. van Houtert, and A. R. Sykes. 1998. The effect of nutrition on the periparturient parasite status of mature sheep. Anim. Sci. 67:523–533.

Ferrell, C. L., J. D. Crouse, R. A. Field, and J. L. Chant. 1979. Effects of sex, diet and stage of growth upon energy utilization by lambs. J. Anim. Sci. 49:790–801.

Foreyt, W. J. 1990. Coccidiosis and cryptosporidiosis in sheep and goats. Vet. Clin. North Am. Food Anim. Pract. 6:655–670.

Galey, F. D. 1996. Disorders caused by toxicants. Pp. 1874–1919 in Large Animal Internal Medicine, B. P. Smith, ed. St Louis, MO: Mosby.

Gallo, L., L. Bailoni, S. Schiavon, P. Carnier, M. Ramanzin, I. Andrighetto, and G. Bittante. 1997. Effect of slow-release somatotropin on the pattern of milk yield between and within injection intervals. J. Dairy Sci. 80:46–51.

Gooneratne, S. R., A. A. Olkowski, and D. A. Christensen. 1989. Sulfur-induced polioencephalomalacia in sheep: Some biochemical changes. Can. J. Vet. Res. 53:462–467.

Hart, S. P. 2001. Recent perspective in using goats for vegetation management in the USA. J. Dairy Sci. 84 (E Suppl.):E170–E176.

Hoste, H., H. Leveque, and P. Dorchies. 2001. Comparison of nematode infections of the gastrointestinal tract in Angora and dairy goats in a rangeland environment: Relations with the feeding behavior. Vet. Parisitol. 101:127–135.

Huston, J. E., B. S. Engdahl, and M. C. Calhoun. 1990. Effects of supplemental feed with or without ionophores on lambs and Angora goats on rangeland. J. Anim. Sci. 68:3980–3986.

Hutcheson, J. P., L. W. Greene, G. E. Carstens, and F. M. Byers. 1992. Effects of zeranol and two dietary levels of calcium and phosphorus on performance, carcass and bone characteristics, and calcium status in growing lambs. J. Anim. Sci. 70:1346–1351.

Jenkins, T. G., J. J. Ford, and J. Klindt. 1988. Postweaning growth, feed efficiency and chemical composition of sheep as affected by prenatal and postnatal testosterone. J. Anim. Sci. 66:1179–1185.

Johnsson, I. D., I. C. Hart, and B. W. Butler-Hogg. 1985. The effects of exogenous bovine growth hormone and bromocriptine on growth, body development, fleece weight and plasma concentrations of growth hormone, insulin and prolactin in female lambs. Anim. Prod. 41:207–217.

Johnsson, I. D., D. J. Hathorn, R. M. Wilde, T. T. Treacher, and B.W. Butler-Hogg. 1987. The effects of dose and method of administration of biosynthetic bovine somatotropin on live-weight gain, carcass composition and wool growth in young lambs. Br. Soc. Anim. Prod. 44: 405–414.

Jones, A. 2001. Monensin toxicosis in 2 sheep flocks. Can. Vet. J. 42:135.

Judson, G. J., and A. Feakes. 1999. Vitamin D doses for alpacas (*Lama pacos*). Austr. Vet. J. 77:310–315.

Klindt, J., T. G. Jenkins, and J. J. Ford. 1987. Prenatal androgen exposure and growth and secretion of growth hormone and prolactin in ewes postweaning. Proc. Soc. Exp. Biol. Med. 185:201–205.

Knight, C. H. 1992. Milk yield responses to sequential treatments with recombinant bovine somatotrophin and frequent milking in lactating goats. J. Dairy Res. 59:115–122.

Knight, C. H., P. A. Fowler, and C. J. Wilde. 1990. Galactopoietic and mammogenic effects of long-term treatment with bovine growth hormone and thrice daily milking in goats. J. Endocrinol. 127:129–138.

Knight, C. H., J. R. Brown, and K. Sejrsen. 1994. A comparison of growth hormone-induced mammogenesis in pregnant and lactating goats. Endocrinol. Metab. 1 (Suppl B) 52.

Kock, M. D., and M. E. Fowler. 1982. Urolithiasis in a three month old llama. J. Am. Vet. Med. Assoc. 81:1410.

Kyriazakis, I., J. D. Oldham, R. L. Coop, and F. Jackson. 1994. The effect of subclinical intestinal nematode infection on the diet selection of growing sheep. Brit. J. Nutr. 72:665–677.

Kyriazakis, I., D. H. Anderson, J. D. Oldham, R. L. Coop, and F. Jackson. 1996. Long-term subclinical infection with Trichostrongylus colubriformis: Effects on food intake, diet selection and performance of growing lambs. Vet. Parasitol. 61:297–313.

Li, Y. G., G. Tanner, and P. Lankin. 1996. The DMCA-Hel protocol and the threshold proanthocyanidin content for bloat safety in forage legumes. J. Sci. Food Agric. 70:89–101.

Liu, S. M., D. G. Master, and N. R. Adams. 2003. Potential impact of nematode parasitism on nutrient partitioning for wool production, growth and reproduction in sheep. Austr. J. Exp. Agric. 43:1409–1417.

Loew, F. M., and R. H. Dunlop. 1972. Induction of thiamine inadequacy and polioencephalomalacia in adult sheep with amprolium. Am. J. Vet. Res. 33:2195–2205.

Low, J. C., P. R. Scott, F. Howie, M. Lewis, J. Fitzsimons, and A. Spence. 1996. Sulfur-induced polioencephalomalacia in lambs. Vet. Rec. 138:327–329.

MacRae, J. C., L. A. Bruce, F. D. Hovell, I. C. Hart, J. Inkster, A. Walker, and T. Atkinson. 1991. Influence of protein nutrition on the response of growing lambs to exogenous bovine growth hormone. J. Endocrinol. 130:53–61.

Maingi, N., M. Bjorn, S. M. Thamsborg, H. O. Bogh, and P. Nansen. 1996. A survey of anthelmintic resistance in nematode parasites of goats in Denmark. Vet. Parasit. 66:53–66.

Marteniuk, J. V., and T. H. Herdt. 1988. Pregnancy toxemia and ketosis of ewes and does. Vet. Clin. North Am.: Food Anim. Pract. 4:307.

Mathieson, A. O., B. D. Hosie, and G. L. Caldow. 1990. Monesin and ovine toxoplasmosis. Vet. Rec. 126:20.

McFadden, T. B., T. E. Daniel, and R. M. Akers. 1990. Effects of plane of nutrition, growth hormone and unsaturated fat on growth hormone, insulin and prolactin receptors in prepubertal lambs. J. Anim. Sci. 68:3180–3189.

McGuffey, R. K., L. F. Richardson, and J. I. D. Wilkinson. 2001. Ionophores for dairy cattle: Current status and future outlook. J. Dairy Sci. 84(E Suppl.):E194–E203.

McLaughlin, C. L., G. J. Rogan, F. C. Buonomo, W. J. Cole, G. F. Hartnell, S. Hudson, T. R. Kasser, M. A. Miller, and C. A. Baile. 1991. Finishing lamb performance responses to bovine and porcine somatotropins administered by Alzet pumps. J. Anim. Sci. 69:4039–4048.

McLaughlin, C. L., H. B. Hedrick, J. J. Veenhuizen, R. F. Finn, R. L. Hintz, G. F. Hartnell, T. R. Kasser, and C. A. Baile. 1993. Comparison of performance, clinical chemistry, and carcass characteristics of finishing lambs treated with recombinant ovine or bovine somatotropins. J. Anim. Sci. 71:1453–1463.

Mepham, T. B., S. E. Lawrence, A. R. Peters, and I. C. Hart. 1984. Effects of exogenous growth hormone on mammary function in lactating goats. Horm. Metab. Res. 16:248–253.

Mersmann, H. G. 1995. Species variation in mechanisms for modulation of growth by beta-adrenergic receptors. J. Nutr. 125(6 Suppl): 1777S–1782S.

Mersmann, H. G. 1998. Overview of the effects of beta-adrenergic receptor agonists on animal growth including mechanisms of action. J. Anim. Sci. 76:160–172.

Miller, R. E., W. J. Boever, R. E. Junge, L. P. Thornburg, and M. F. Raisbeck. 1990. Acute monensin toxicosis in Stone sheep (Ovis dalli stonei), bles-bok (Damaliscus dorcus phillipsi), and a Bactrian camel (Camelus bactrianus). J. Amer. Vet. Med. Assoc. 196:131–134.

Min, B. R., and S. P. Hart. 2003. Tannins for suppression of internal parasites. J. Anim. Sci. 81(E Suppl. 2):E102–E109.

Min, B. R., T. N. Barry, G. T. Atwood, and W. C. McNabb. 2003. The effect of condensed tannins on the nutrition and health of ruminants fed fresh temperate forages: A review. Anim. Feed Sci. and Technol. 106:3–19.

Mitchell, G. A., and G. Dunnavan. 1998. Illegal use of β-adrenergic agonists in the United States. J. Anim. Sci. 76:208–211.

Mobini, S., A. M. Heath, and D. G. Pugh. 2002. Theriogenology of sheep and goats. Pp. 185–186 in Sheep and Goat Medicine, D.G. Pugh, ed. Philadelphia: W. B. Saunders.

Mortensen, L. L., L. H. Williamson, T. H. Terrill, R. A. Kircher, M. Larsen, and R. M, Kaplan. 2003. Evaluation of prevalence and clinical implications of anthelmintic resistance in gastrointestinal nematodes in goats. J. Am. Vet. Med. Assoc. 223:495–500.

Mwamachi, D. M., J. O. Audho, W. Thorpe, and R. L. Baker. 1995. Evidence for multiple anthelmintic resistance in sheep and goats reared under the same management in Coastal Kenya. Vet. Parasitol. 60: 303–313.

Navarre, C. B., and D. G. Pugh. 2002. Diseases of the gastrointestinal system. Pp. 74–99 in Sheep and Goat Medicine, D. G. Pugh, ed. Philadelphia: W. B. Saunders.

Nielsen, M. O. 1988. Effect of recombinantly derived bovine somatotropin on mammary gland synthetic capacity in lactating goats. J. Anim. Physiol. 59A:263–272.

Niezen, J. H., T. S. Waghorn, W. A. Charleston, and G. C. Waghorn. 1995. Growth and gastrointestinal parasitism in lamb grazing one of seven herbages and dosed with larvae for six weeks. J. Agric. Sci. 125: 281–289.

Nold, R. A., J. A. Unruh, C. W. Spaeth, and J. E. Minton. 1992. Effects of zeranol implants in ram and wether lambs on performance traits, carcass characteristics, and subprimal cut yields and distribution. J. Anim. Sci. 70:1699–1701.

Nour, M. S. M., M. T. Abusamara, and B. E. D. Hago. 1977. Experimentally induced lactic acidosis in Nubian goats: Clinical, biochemical, and pathological investigators. Small Ruminant Res. 31(1):7.

NRC (National Research Council). 1981. Nutritional Requirements of Goats: Angora, Dairy, and Meat Goats in Temperate and Tropical Countries. Washington, DC: National Academy Press.

NRC. 1985. Nutrient Requirements of Sheep. Washington, DC: National Academy Press.

Orskov, E. R., D. A. Grubb, J. S. Smith, A. J. F. Webster, and W. Corrigall. 1979. Efficiency of utilization of volatile fatty acids for maintenance and energy retention by sheep. Br. J. Nutr. 41:541–552.

Osweiler, G. D., T. L. Carson, W. B. Buck, and G. A. Van Gelder. 1985. Clinical and Diagnostic Veterinary Toxicity, 3rd ed. Dubuque, IA: Kendall Hunt.

Parker, J. E., K. I. Timm, B. B. Smith, R. J. Van Saun, K. M. Winters, P. Sukon, and C. M. Snow. 2002. Seasonal interaction of vitamin D and bone density in the llama. Am. J. Vet. Res. 63:948–953.

Pell, J. M., and P. C. Bates. 1987. Collagen and non-collagen protein turnover in skeletal muscle of growth hormone-treated lambs. J. Endocrinol. 115:R1–R4.

Pierson, R. E., and R. Jensen. 1975. Polioencephalomalacia in feedlot lambs. J. Am. Vet. Med. Ass. 166:257–259.

Puchala, R., I. Prieto, V. Banskalieva, A. L. Goetsch, M. Lachica, and T. Sahlu. 2001. Effects of bovine somatotropin and thyroid hormone status on hormone levels, body weight gain, and mohair fiber growth of Angora goats. J. Anim. Sci. 79:2913–2919.

Pugh, D. G. 1993. Polioencephalomalacia in a llama herd. Eq. Pract. 15:24–26.

Pugh, D. G., and C. B. Navarre. 2001. Internal parasite control strategies. Vet. Clin. North Am. (Update Small Ruminant Med.) 17:231–244.

Pugh, D. G., C. D. Hilton, and S. M. Mobini. 1998. Contol programs for gastrointestinal nematodes in sheep and goats. Comp. Cont. Ed. Pract. Vet. 20:5112–5123.

Rammell, C. G., and J. H. Hill. 1986. A review of thiamine deficiency and its diagnosis, especially in ruminants. New Zealand Vet. J. 34:202–204.

Rankins, D. C., D. C. Ruffin, and D. G. Pugh. 2002. Feeding and Nutrition. Pp. 19–60 in Sheep and Goat Medicine, D. G. Pugh, ed. Philadelphia: W. B. Saunders.

Raun, A. P. 1990. Rumensin "then and now." Pp. A1–A20 in Rumensin in the 1990s. Denver: Elanco Animal Health.

Reilly, L. K., A. N. Baird, and D. G. Pugh. 2002. Diseases of the Musculoskeletal System. Pp. 248–249 in Sheep and Goat Medicine, D. G. Pugh, ed. Philadelphia: W. B. Saunders.

Reklewska, B. 1974. A note on the effect of bovine somatotrophic hormone on wool production in growing lambs. Anim. Prod. 19:253–255.

Richardson, L. F., A. P. Raun, E. L. Potter, C. O. Cooley, and R. P. Rathmacher. 1976. Effect of monensin on rumen fermentation in vitro and in vivo. J. Anim. Sci. 43:657–664.

Ruffin, D. C., V. Christman, and D. G. Pugh. 2002. Diseases of the Endocrine System. Pp. 187–196 in Sheep and Goat Medicine, D. G. Pugh, ed. Philadelphia: W. B. Saunders.

Shelton, M., and C. W. Livingston. 1975. Posthitis in Angora wethers. J. Am. Vet. Med. Assoc. 167:154–155.

Sinnett-Smith, P. A., N. W. Dumelow, and P. J. Buttery. 1983. Effects of trenbolone acetate and zeranol on protein metabolism in male castrate and female lambs. Br. J. Nutr. 50:225–234.

Smith, B. B., and R. J. Van Saun. 2001. Seasonal changes in serum calcium, phosphorus and vitamin D concentration in llamas and alpacas. Am. J. Vet. Res. 62:1187–1193.

Smith, J. A. 1989. Noninfectious Diseases, Metabolic Diseases, Toxicities, and Neoplastic Diseases of South American Camelids. Vet. Clin. North Am.: Food Anim. Pract. 5:101–143.

Smith, M. C. 1979. Polioencephalomalacia in goats. J. Am. Vet. Med. Assoc. 174:1328–1332.

Smith, S. B., D. K. Garcia, and D. B. Anderson. 1989. Elevation of a specific mRNA in longissimus muscle of steers fed ractopamine. J. Anim. Sci. 67:3495–3502.

Stelwagen, K., D. G. Grieve, J. S. Walton, J. L. Ball, and B. W. McBride. 1993. Effect of prepartum bovine somatotropin in primigravid ewes on mammogenesis, milk production and hormone concentrations, J. Dairy Sci. 76:992–1001.

Stepek, G., D. J. Buttle, I. R. Duce, A. Lowe, and J. M. Behnke. 2005. Assessment of the anthelmintic effect of natural plant cysteine proteinases against the gastrointestinal nematode, Heligmosomoides polygyrus, in vitro. Parisitol. 130:203–211.

Sykes, A. R. 2000. Environmental effects on animal production: The nutritional demands of nematode parasite exposure in sheep. Asian-Australas J. Anim. Sci. 13(Suppl):343–350.

Tedeschi, L. O., D. G. Fox, and T. P. Tylutki. 2003. Potential environmental benefits of ionophores in ruminant diets. J. Environ. Qual. 32:1591–1602.

Terrill, T. H., R. M. Kaplan, M. Larsen, O. M. Samples, J. E. Miller, and S. Gelayes. 2001. Anthelmintic resistance on goat farms in Georgia: Efficacy of anthelmintics against gastrointestinal nematodes in two selected goat herds. Vet. Parasitol. 97:261–268.

Tornquist, S. J., R. J. Van Saun, B. B. Smith, and C. K. Cebra. 1999. Histologically confirmed hepatic lipidosis in llamas and alpacas: 31 cases (1991–1997). J. Am. Vet. Med. Assoc. 214:1368–1372.

Tornquist, S. J., C. K. Cebra, R. J. Van Saun, B. B. Smith, and J. S. Matoon. 2001. Metabolic changes and induction of hepatic lipidosis in llamas. Am. J. Vet. Res. 62:1081–1087.

Torres-Acosta, J. F. J., D. E. Jacobs, A. Aguilar-Caballero, C. Sandoval-Castro, M. May-Martinez, and L. A. Cob-Galera. 2004. The effect of supplementary feeding on the resilience and resistance of browsing criollo kids against natural gastrointestinal nematode infections during the rainy season in tropical Mexico. Vet. Parasitol. 124:217–238.

Van Metre, D. C., J. W. Tyler, and S. M. Stehman. 2000. Diagnosis of enteric disease in small ruminants. Vet. Clin. North Am.: Food Anim. Pract. 16:87–115.

Van Rensburg, S. J. 1971. Reproductive physiology and endocrinology of normal and habitually aborting Angora does. Onderstepoort J. Vet. Res. 38:1–62.

Van Saun, R. J. 2004. Vitamin D-responsive rickets in neonatal lambs. Can. Vet. J. 45:841–844.

Van Saun, R. J., B. B. Smith, and B. J. Waltrous. 1996. Evaluation of Vitamin D status of llamas and alpacas with hypophosphatemic rickets. J. Am. Vet. Med. Assoc. 209:1128–1133.

Van Tonder, E. M. 1975. Notes on some disease problems in Angora goats in South Africa. Vet. Med. Rev. 1-2:109–138.

Waghorn, G. C., and W. C. McNabb. 2003. Consequences of plant phenolic compounds for productivity and health of ruminants. Proc. Nutr. Soc. 62:383–392.

Wallace, D. S., K. Bairden, J. L. Duncan, G. Fishwick, M. Gill, and P. H. Holms. 1996. Influence of soybean meal supplementation on the resistance of Scottish black face lambs to *Haemonchosis*. Res. Vet. Sci. 60: 138–143.

Wallace, J. M., R. P. Aitken, J. S. Milne, and W. W. Hay. 2004a. Nutritionally mediated placental growth restriction in the growing adolescent: Consequences for the fetus. Biol. Reprod. 71:1055–1062.

Wallace, J. M., D. A. Bourke, J. S. Milne, and R. P. Aitken. 2004b. Maternal growth hormone treatment from day 35 to day 80 of gestation alters nutrient partitioning in favor of utero-placental growth in the overnourished adolescent sheep. Biol. Reprod.70:1277–1285.

Wang, S. Y., and D. H. Beermann. 1988. Reduced calcium-dependent proteinase activity in cimaterol induced muscle hypertrophy in lambs. J. Anim. Sci. 66:2545–2550.

Wentzel, D., M. M. LeRoux, and L. J. Botha. 1976. Effect of the level of nutrition on blood glucose concentrations and reproductive performance of pregnant Angora goats. Agroanimalia 8:59–61.

Wheatley, I. S., A. L. C. Wallace, and J. M. Bassett. 1966. Metabolic effects of ovine growth hormone in sheep. J. Endocrinol. 35:341–353.

Wynn, P. C., A. L. C. Wallace, A. C. Kirby, and E. F. Annison. 1988. Effects of growth hormone administration on wool growth in Merino sheep. Austr. J. Biol. Sci. 41:177–187.

Zainur, A. S., R. Tassell, R. C. Kellaway, G. H. McDowell, W. R. Dodemaide, and A. Kirby. 1989. Recombinant growth hormone in growing lambs: Effects on growth, body and carcass characteristics, hormones and metabolites. Austr. J. Agric. Res. 40:663–674.

14

Providing Required Nutrients to Small Ruminants

As is stated in Chapter 1, this chapter is intended to be a synopsis of the entire publication in easy to understand language and to provide an aid to using the information for practical purposes. It specifically addresses nutrient requirements for the different species, symptoms that may occur during deficiencies, and means and methods for using available feed resources to feed animals properly. It is written without citations, but does refer the reader to other chapters for greater detail. It is intended as a stand-alone chapter with recommendations for how to access more information as needed.

SHEEP

Sheep are distributed widely throughout the regions of the world. The array of social and climatic circumstances provide for many breeds differing in body characteristics and productivity. Mature body size of breeding females, which can range from less than 40 kg to more than 130 kg, has a major influence on total nutrients required and on adaptation to the various conditions. Reproductive rate, milk production, and wool growth of adults and growth rate of young animals greatly influence requirements of nutrients and the grazing circumstances and/or commercially available feeds that are most suited for supplying the required nutrients.

Determining Nutrient Requirements and Deficiencies of Sheep

Requirements for energy, protein, minerals, and vitamins were determined by reviews of the scientific literature (Chapters 4, 5, 7, and 8, respectively). Requirements were determined by the factorial method and individual entries in recommendations are sums of requirements of the different functions (maintenance, pregnancy, lactation, growth, and fiber growth) as they relate to individual circumstances. Maximum concentrations were determined in cases where toxicities pose a common threat. Tables 15-1 and 15-2 contain the nutrient requirement information according to body size and expectations of productivity as indicated by breeding, reproductive rate (0, 1, 2, or 3 fetuses), milk production (number of nursing lambs or kg milk/d), and rate of gain. Requirements for wool production are included in the maintenance component because they add relatively small amounts to the annual budget of requirements. Requirements for water were considered separately in Chapter 9.

Breeds and genetically selected lines that have greater genetic potential also generally have greater nutrient requirements and suffer the most from limited nutrients. Reduced level of productivity such as slowed growth and lowered milk production is the most commonly seen result of undernutrition. However, some acute consequences of nutrient deficiencies—such as behavioral changes, loss of normal mobility and appearances, specific malfunctions of other normal processes, and death—can occur (Chapter 13).

Critical Periods in Development and Production Cycles in Sheep

Reproduction

Some consequences of undernutrition during breeding and pregnancy are low conception, severe embryo wastage, pregnancy toxemia, and low birth weights (poor lamb survival). Increasing the nutrient intake, especially energy intake, during the breeding season increases ovulation and conception rates. Response to this practice, commonly called "flushing," is confounded with body condition of the breeding ewes. Success is more pronounced in ewes of average body condition (2.5–3.5 on a scale of 1 to 5) and less pronounced in ewes that are overly thin and overly fat. Nutrient requirements of ewes during early pregnancy are only slightly higher than those at maintenance but increase slowly during the first 15 weeks of pregnancy as the embryos grow and exert greater demands on the maternal tissue. Requirements during the final 6 weeks of pregnancy are greatly elevated. Deficiencies that occur early in pregnancy (at implantation of the embryos to the uterine wall or shortly thereafter) result in embryo wastage, thereby reducing the numbers that develop into fetuses. Losses by abortion during the later stage of pregnancy are not as common in sheep as in some other small ruminants (e.g., goats). In sheep, hypoglycemia (low blood sugar) results in **pregnancy toxemia** and is usually fatal to the pregnant ewe. Also known as "twin lamb disease," pregnancy toxemia is caused by the heavy demand for glucose by the lamb fetuses, thereby depriving the ewe of her specific requirements for glucose, especially in nerve (brain) tissue. Twin lambs demand more glucose than a single lamb, thus the name of twin lamb disease. The incidence of pregnancy toxemia can be greatly reduced or eliminated by increasing nutrient intake during the last 6 weeks of pregnancy, especially with feeds (containing soluble sugars and other carbohydrates and protein) that will increase the blood glucose level. Often, ewes that are underfed during late pregnancy escape pregnancy toxemia but give birth to small, underdeveloped lambs that may die at birth or shortly thereafter or may require extraordinary care. Commonly, these undernourished ewes do not produce adequate amounts of milk, thereby exacerbating the circumstance. Good management that includes good general nutrition (including attention to vitamins, minerals, and water) and elevated nutrients at breeding, during late pregnancy, and early in the lactation phase will result in lamb crops equal to or near the potential of the flock. Recommended levels of the most commonly critical vitamins and minerals are listed along with requirements for energy and protein in Tables 15-1 and 15-2.

Lactation

Nutrient requirements in sheep reach the highest levels during the first month of lactation. During this period, high-producing ewes cannot consume enough feed to supply these required nutrients. Several nutrition-related crises may occur at this time. The nutritional demand eases during mid-lactation (about the 7th through 12th week of lactation). Thereafter until weaning, ewes can gain weight during a much reduced demand for nutrients to support a reduced milk yield. **Ketosis**, a metabolic state that is expressed during gestation as pregnancy toxemia, may occur as a result of mobilization of fat to provide the elevated energy requirement. Concurrent with this ketotic state, **hypocalcaemia** may occur. The high demand for calcium in milk requires mobilization from the bone. The parathyroid gland is involved in this mobilization. Sometimes there is a delay in activation of the parathyroid gland after onset of heavy milk synthesis. This general state, commonly called milk fever in cattle, is less common in sheep but can occur as outbreaks involving up to 25 percent of the flock. Greater detail on these complex relationships are given in Chapter 13. Attempts to avoid undernutrition and associated problems during early lactation by feeding high levels of concentrates can cause **lactic acidosis,** which is an intraruminal consequence of an accumulation of products of rapid carbohydrate fermentation. Mobilization of fat and losses in body condition and weight during early lactation are normal occurrences and not of great concern unless they become extreme. Giving early attention to nutritional needs and avoiding sudden changes in diet and movement usually prevents or reduces the common nutritional maladies associated with lactation.

Growth

Growing lambs encounter various acute nutritional strains that result in an array of abnormal conditions. Although some occur during the nursing phase, most are first noticed after lambs have been weaned and transferred to new diets. **Rickets**, although seldom observed during modern times, occasionally occurs. Lambs with this malady have weak and misshapen bones, usually as a result of poor mineralization of the protein matrix of the immature bone. Rickets is no longer an important problem because synthetic vitamin D is a common ingredient in all commercial feeds and premixes. **Lactic acidosis** occurs when concentrates (including high-starch ingredients, such as corn) are increased in the diet. Small incremental increases in acidity (lowering of pH) in the rumen are collateral occurrences with 10 to 20 percent increases in the concentrate portion of the diet. These gradual changes are expected and are not harmful. However, a large and sudden increase in concentrates in the diet results in a rapid decline in ruminal pH, the accumulation of lactic acid, and severe damage to the linings of the gastrointestinal tract. Acute lactic acidosis as a major problem can be avoided by changing the diet gradually. Using five or more rations with incremental increases in concentrates in a stepwise manner will minimize the risk of this problem. **Enterotoxemia** results in the sudden death of rapidly growing lambs. This nutritional disease may occur in nursing lambs receiving large quantities of milk, in feedlot lambs given high-concentrate rations, or in lambs grazing high-quality pastures. A toxin produced by the bacterium *Clostridium perfringens* type D in the lamb's intestinal tract causes death. Proliferation of this organism is encouraged by the presence of high-energy substances in the intestines as is common with lambs having high feed intakes and rapid growth. This disease can be controlled with two or three sequential vaccinations of a toxoid. **Urinary calculi** (water belly) occur as a result of mineral precipitates lodging in the urinary tract usually causing the bladder to rupture and spill urine into the abdominal area. Death from uremic poisoning occurs within days. Urinary calculi occur mainly in male lambs fed diets with a calcium/phosphorous imbalance (low calcium) and/or a low water intake. Attention to the calcium:phosphorous ratio (2 to 1 or greater) and the water supply (fresh, clean, plentiful) will minimize the incidence of this problem. The inclusion of urine acidifiers (e.g., ammonium chloride) in the diet will prevent the formation of calculi in the urinary tract. **Polioencephalomalacia** is a brain disorder that seems more common in lambs fed high-concentrate diets in the feedlot. Although not the single cause, a thiamin deficiency is a complicating factor. Including thiamin in the diet may help prevent the onset of the disorder. Sheep, especially lambs, are more likely than other small ruminants to suffer from **copper toxicity**. Copper is an essential element, but high levels of copper should be avoided, especially when molybdenum is low. Mineral concentrates formulated for other livestock species may not be appropriate for sheep.

Wool Growth

Nutrient requirements for wool growth in wool-producing sheep are included with the maintenance component. At present, evidence does not indicate these small amounts of additional nutrients increase maintenance detectably above those of wool-less or hair sheep. However, several circumstances uniquely affect wool quantity and quality. The potential to grow wool is related to density of wool follicles and is determined during the fetal stage. Underfed pregnant ewes give birth to lambs having a diminished capacity for wool production. Wool growth (fleece weight) is greatly affected by nutrition throughout the annual cycle. High nutrition (especially high protein) results in greater wool growth and slightly coarser fibers. Ewes fed at a medium level produce wool that is both fine (high quality; low-fiber diameter) and strong. During periods of extremely low nutrition, fiber diameter is greatly restricted and may result in fiber weakness (breaks) that makes the fleece worthless. In range sheep, wool breaks often are associated with severe weather storms, traumatic events (e.g., predator chase), and parturition under stressful circumstances that markedly reduce intake for a short period.

GOATS

Goats occupy all continents of the Earth (except for Antarctica) and are of some social and economic value in essentially every nation. Perhaps they are the most widely adapted domestic species. Perceptions of goats vary. Some consider goats a highly destructive influence in creating widespread desertification, while others recognize them as major means of survival of small landholders in developing countries. The global distribution of goats corresponds with an array of genotypes reflecting local environmental conditions and selection pressures. Thus, the goat population consists of many breeds that have emerged to suit the needs of local producers and consumers of the goat products. Breeds differ according to body size and fertility and the ability to produce meat, milk, and fleece. However, a substantial proportion of the world goat population is nondescript in appearance, not belonging to any recognized breed. These goats vary greatly in body size, color pattern, occurrence and shape of horns, size and attachment of udder, occurrence of waddles, and characteristics of fleece. Goats of all genotypes share the common characteristic of peculiarity in selection of diet (Chapter 3). They are aggressive browsers of foliage of trees and shrubs, but opportunistically select high-quality portions of grasses and other herbaceous plants when available. A small mouth and mobile lips and tongue enable the goat to discriminate effectively among available plant species and parts in diet selection.

Determining Nutrient Requirements and Deficiencies of Goats

The requirements of goats for energy, protein, minerals, and vitamins were determined after review of available literature reporting definitive experimental data (Chapters 4, 5, 7, and 8). In instances where quantitative data relating to particular nutrients were not available for goats, estimates were made from data collected using similar species (usually sheep and/or cattle). Major determinants of nutrient requirements include maturity, body size, physiological stage (growth, pregnancy, lactation, etc.), and productivity (growth rate, number of embryos/fetuses, milk production, and fleece growth). Other influences on requirements include age, activity, climate, body composition, and parasitism, and these influences were considered in forming the nutrient requirements tables, usually by applying adjustment factors.

Energy

Requirements for energy include amounts of metabolizable energy (ME) attributed to maintenance (ME_m), growth (ME_g), pregnancy (ME_{preg}), and lactation (ME_l). Maintenance requirements for energy vary with body weight (BW).

The maintenance portion of the energy requirements varies only slightly among animals in the different physiological states except for growing dairy goat kids, which have a maintenance energy requirement approximately 21 percent higher than the average for the remaining types and classes. Requirements for gain are dependent on composition of gain (i.e., proportions of protein, fat, and water) that is related to age and maturity. As animals age, greater portions of the gain are fat, which on a weight basis is energetically more expensive to produce. In the special case of the Angora, body weight gain is comprised of both wet body tissue (tg; nonfiber tissue) and mohair growth (f). Energy requirements for these are expressed as ME_{tg} and ME_f, respectively, and sum to the total requirements for gain.

Energy required for pregnancy is related to birth weight (influenced by mature weights of dam and sire), stage of pregnancy, and litter size according to an inclusive formula described in Chapter 4. For example, a doe carrying either single, twin, or triplet fetuses during late gestation (average =

day 135) would require energy above maintenance for pregnancy according to the expected birth weight(s) of the kid(s).

Energy requirements for lactation vary with the amount and composition of milk produced. During a normal lactation, production peaks a few weeks after parturition then tapers off during the subsequent weeks. Early in lactation, does producing large amounts of milk will be unable to consume adequate energy to support milk synthesis and must mobilize energy from stored body fat and protein. Later in lactation after milk production has declined, the requirement can be met and often weight gain can occur to restore depleted tissue reserves.

Protein

Protein nourishment to the body is actually in the form of the breakdown products of protein, amino acids. Protein is digested to amino acids in the small intestines, where the amino acids are absorbed and become available for synthesis of body protein. Sources of protein to the small intestine include microbial protein that is formed during ruminal fermentation and protein that is consumed and escapes fermentation in the rumen (Chapter 2).

The actual protein requirement of an animal is the sum of the amino acids that must be present in the correct proportions for the metabolic processes that are occurring. This amount is less than the required crude protein (CP; an approximation of total protein) because of its incomplete digestion and the imperfect balance of amino acids produced during protein degradation. The metabolic processes considered during the construction of the requirements table included maintenance, growth, milk synthesis, processes related to pregnancy, and mohair growth (Tables 15-4, 15-5, and 15-6). Metabolizable protein required for maintenance (MP_m) is the amount needed to replace protein tissue that is continuously being broken down and exiting the body and signaled by the appearance of nitrogen-containing compounds in the feces and urine. Therefore, MP_m can be estimated by the sum of protein equivalents excreted in the feces (MFCP, metabolic fecal crude protein related to dry matter intake) and in the urine (EUCP, endogenous urinary crude protein related to body size) plus a factor adjusting for the inefficiency of protein synthesis. Metabolizable protein required for growth in dairy, indigenous, meat, and Angora goats are 29.0, 29.0, 40.4, and 28.1 g/100 g of wet tissue gain, respectively. Milk and mohair synthesis requires 1.45 and 1.65 g, respectively, of MP per g of protein synthesized.

Metabolizable protein required for pregnancy (MP_{preg}) was estimated by a formula (Chapter 5) that included birth weight of kids, day of gestation, and litter size.

Other Nutrients

Requirements for minerals and vitamins are discussed in Chapters 7 and 8, respectively. Values for macro minerals calcium (Ca) and phosphorus (P) and vitamins (A and E) are given along with energy and protein requirements in Tables 15-4, 15-5, and 15-6 for the different weights and classes of goats at the various levels of productivity. Water requirements are discussed in Chapter 9.

Critical Periods in Development and Production Cycles in Goats

The considerable variation that exists within the goat population and among breeds results in recognizable differences in nutrient requirements and symptoms of deficiencies. Chapter 13 contains detailed discussions of nutritional and metabolic diseases that are briefly referred to here.

Reproduction

Ovulation, conception, gestation, and parturition all share in the importance of the reproductive process. The period surrounding the breeding event determines the potential for reproductive rate and is influenced by nutritional status and strategy. **Flushing** is a strategy for increasing ovulation rate in females by feeding high-energy feeds just before and during the breeding period. Goats that are at or below average in body condition (fatness) usually respond well to flushing, whereas goats that are above average in body condition have a high ovulation rate without extraordinary energy intake. Once conception has occurred, good nutrition at a level only slightly above maintenance will prevent **embryo wastage**. During this 2- to 3-month, early-gestation period, diet stability is as important as nutritional level. Large fluctuations in nutrient intake should be avoided, especially soon after conception and toward the end of the third month. The later stage of the mid-trimester of pregnancy is very critical in goats prone to **nutritional abortion**. Angora females, in particular, are likely to abort during 75 to 100 days of pregnancy when nutritional homeostasis is disrupted by inclement weather, predator chase, or management errors causing physical stress. Substantial increases in nutrient levels are required during the last trimester of gestation, especially in litter-bearing females, to prevent **pregnancy toxemia** and provide for normal fetal development. Kids that are too small and weak at parturition are less likely to stand and nurse quickly after birth and less likely to survive, especially if environmental conditions are unfavorable (e.g., cold, wet weather). However, overfeeding that results in fetuses becoming too large and causing difficult births should be avoided.

Lactation

Nutrient requirements in goats are highest during lactation compared with the other periods of the production cycle. High-producing goats are unable to consume adequate amounts of typical diets to supply enough energy and must rely on mobilizing energy from body fat to satisfy their energy requirements. The sudden onset of milk synthesis causes several metabolic disorders that should be addressed in the management plan. **Ketosis** results from the breakdown of body fat in combination with low blood sugar (glucose). Similarly, the high requirement for calcium for milk synthesis requires mobilization of calcium from the bone, a process triggered by the parathyroid gland. When this process is delayed or not functioning at full capacity, **hypocalcemia** develops. Together, ketosis and hypocalcemia result in **milk fever**, a condition characterized by sluggish movement, semi-comatose appearance, and inability to stand. Administering a combination of calcium and glucose intravenously will result in a dramatic recovery from milk fever. Another condition common during early lactation is **lactic acidosis**, which occurs after sudden increases in concentrates in the diet in efforts to meet high requirements. This condition can be aided by the use of buffers or by more gradual increases in the concentrate contents in the diet.

Growth

The developing kid has high levels of requirements for all nutrients. Quantitatively, protein and energy may be considered most important, but minerals and vitamins must be supplied in adequate amounts and in proper balance for satisfactory growth. Although retarded growth is the most common result of underfeeding, several undesirable conditions often appear during the development period that are related to nutrition level and/or nutrient balance. **Lactic acidosis** develops when the concentrate level is increased in the diet. Small increases over time in the level of starchy feeds allow the animal to adapt with only minimal signs of acidosis. Sudden, large changes result in severe acidosis that may cause chronic illness and wasting because of permanent damage to the gastrointestinal tract or lead to death. **Enterotoxemia** results in sudden death, usually in the most rapidly growing animals. This condition results when soluble carbohydrates (from starchy feeds or lush pasture) bypass rumen fermentation and appear in the small intestine where they provide a substrate for the development of the *Clostridium* toxin. This condition can be reduced or eliminated by vaccination of the pregnant female or a few weeks before the onset of heavy carbohydrate feeding. **Urinary calculi** (urolithiasis or kidney stone formation) is a common condition that develops in young, growing animals as a result of mineral imbalance. Grains and oilseed meals (such as soybean or cottonseed meal) are common ingredients in growing rations but contain high levels of phosphorus and low levels of calcium compared with requirements. This imbalance (low Ca:P ratio) favors the formation of insoluble mineral crystals in the kidney that lodge in the ureter or urethra causing extreme pain and possibly rupture of the urinary tract and death. This is of greater risk in male kids. Proper balance of calcium to phosphorus in the diet (> 2:1) greatly decreases the likelihood of urinary calculi. Also, feeding an agent (i.e., ammonium chloride) to acidify the urine is a very effective preventative strategy. Several conditions can occur as a result of vitamin deficiencies. Among the most dramatic is **polioencephalomalacia** that occurs with a thiamin deficiency. This condition can be treated/prevented by administering thiamin in the diet or by injection.

Mohair Growth

This discussion relates only to the Angora, although fiber is produced on all goats. The mohair produced by the Angora has a greater diameter than wool from fine-wool sheep breeds or the primary fiber (down) on cashmere-producing goats. However, mohair is smaller in diameter than the wool from long-wool breeds of sheep and the coarse secondary fibers of goats. It is a specialty product used in exclusive lines of clothing and upholstery because of its softness, durability, and luster in revealing bright colors. The quality of mohair is defined mainly by fiber diameter, which is related to both genetics and nutrition. Increased protein intake stimulates both growth rate and fiber diameter of mohair. Requirements reported in Table 15-6 were derived considering both level of production and quality of the product.

CERVIDS

Cervids belong to a subgroup among thousands of wildlife species. Even within the family *Cervidae*, many sizes and forms of species occupy habitats around the world and are not addressed in this publication. The species in this subgroup are considered because of their anatomical, behavioral, locational, and/or socioeconomic similarities with other small ruminant and ruminant-like animals. The species included are white-tailed deer (*Odocoileus virginianus*), red deer/elk/wapiti (*Cervus elaphus*), and reindeer/caribou (*Rangifer tarandus*). Whereas the red deer shares the same genus and species with the elk/wapiti of North America, they are divided for discussion purposes because of differences in behavior, body size, and physiological traits that have developed over time. No guidelines are offered for extrapolating the estimated nutrient requirements to similar wildlife species, although in some cases when alternative information might not be available, this might be appropriate if body size and level of productivity are considered. However, the reference to "cervids" in this publication is intended to refer only to those species listed.

The nutritional requirements information in this publication pertains to cervids under five circumstances: (1) fully confined individuals or groups in low productivity; (2) animals under full confinement in pens or small pastures with expectations for higher productivity; (3) unconfined resident populations on large acreages under single or multi-ownership for commercial recreational purposes; (4) nomadic herds providing meat and other products for dependent human populations along migratory routes; and (5) large and extensive wild populations under minimal direct management and available for recreational viewing and hunting or as natural inhabitants in national and state parks and wilderness areas not intended for exploitation (see Chapter 11).

Total confinement with little expectations for productivity characterizes zoo conditions. Zoo animals being held for viewing require maintenance feeding with only occasional elevated needs for reproduction and nursing of offspring. Although conventional feedstuffs can be used in formulating diets for this purpose, certain surplus produce and similar excellent nutrient sources listed in Table 15-12 are attractive for use in zoos. These products are nutritious but difficult to manage in other circumstances. They are easy to meter out to individuals or small groups of animals (e.g., number of heads of lettuce or medium-sized turnips, cups of peas), are often very economical, and add to the joy of the observers.

Full confinement in pens or small pastures where a high level of productivity is expected (deer farming) resembles conventional livestock management. This management system as it exists in the United States usually applies to exotic deer species (e.g., fallow deer or sika deer) and wapiti. Farming of red deer is a large commercial enterprise in New Zealand. Similarly, reindeer commonly are farmed in other regions. As with livestock species, these confined animals are managed for high levels of production of meat and other products considering optimal growth rate, reproductive rate, and other factors. Therefore, developing complete rations for animals in total confinement and supplements for those grazing pasture forages are appropriate uses of the information presented in the requirements tables and tables of nutrient composition of feedstuffs.

Nutritional management of unrestrained populations of cervids (circumstances 3, 4, and 5 listed above) is more complex, involving alternative land uses related to forage type and availability, human desires and intentions, and climatic events, along with physiological needs of the animals. In each circumstance, the forage type, availability, and distribution over time, along with water availability and quality, set the baseline for the population. In many instances, the human element prefers that this balance not be interrupted. The population fluctuates up and down, sometimes catastrophically, as climate and other forces change the habitat. Others favor a policy that protects only against catastrophic events such as severe drought, fire, or dieoff following a buildup in population to an unsustainable level. In all of these circumstances, knowledge of the nutrient contents of the vegetation and feedstuffs as presented in Tables 15-11 and 15-12 can be used in estimating the nutrients provided by the habitat and what could be used to supply the balance of the required nutrients.

If the decision is made to manage the diet of unconstrained cervids, several strategies can be employed to change and supplement the habitat. Various control measures—such as mechanical, chemical, biological, hydrological (irrigation or drainage), and thermal (prescribed fire)—can be used to favorably modify the species composition of the vegetation. Food plots can be installed that provide desirable forage during crucial periods. Animal population control, including the reduction of both the species of interest and competing species, will lower the grazing/browsing pressure and improve the diet of remaining individual animals. Supplemental feeds can be provided to supply limiting nutrients, thereby increasing the utilization of the existing dietary ingredients and improving the animals' nutritional status. Also, complete feeds or feeds intended to supply large portions of the diet can be provided in order to reduce the animals' dependency on the natural resource (i.e., range, forest, or wetland vegetation). This latest strategy might be employed for wapiti herds trapped by severe winter storms, various species stranded on barren land caused by wildfires or extended droughts, or other situations. However, full-feeding animals on concentrated areas for extended periods can decimate the natural vegetation of those areas, and the practice should be used sparingly and with caution.

Management systems for white-tailed deer in resident herds for commercial recreational purposes (circumstance 3) often employ feeding strategies to increase the number and attractiveness of individuals in the herd and to increase hunter success. Installing high fences around large areas to control ingress and egress is now a common practice. This allows the manager to impose practices such as supplemental feeding on the resident herd without the concern of losing any benefit to neighboring enterprises. Supplemental feeding is a controversial issue because of concern about destroying the wild nature of white-tailed deer and the associated hunting challenge, as well as the danger of creating herds that overpopulate and destroy healthy ecosystems. Baiting is a common practice by hunters to lure animals into range using very palatable feed (e.g., corn grain) released from a spin cast feeder at timed intervals. Nutrient requirements and animal health are secondary considerations under most circumstances where feeding is practiced only leading up to and during the hunting season. Feeding higher protein supplements (20–45 percent) during late fall and winter (times of low availability of quality forage) and during late spring and summer (late gestation and early lactation) is generally more appropriate management to improve the nutritional status of white-tailed deer herds.

The body of information on cervid nutrition has increased substantially during recent decades. However, the nature of wildlife and the difficulties those wildlife populations present in collecting definitive data under natural conditions continue to challenge wildlife scientists and, in some instances, limit detailed recommendations. The nutrient requirements being presented represent the latest and most accurate estimates. Future editions will further update and refine these requirements based on the scientific findings that accumulate.

NEW WORLD CAMELIDS

New World camelids (NWC) include species from the *Lama* and *Vicugna* genera and are related to, but distinguished from, the one- and two-hump camels (*Camelus* spp.) in Asia. This discussion will address specifically the llama (*Lama glama*) and alpaca (*Vicugna pacos*), but generally applies to all NWC. Though not true ruminants in all anatomical features (Chapter 2), NWC are nutritionally similar to ruminants and are referred to in this publication and elsewhere as "ruminant-like," being indistinguishable in many aspects of gastrointestinal tract physiology. Terms such as regurgitation and cud-chewing, microbial populations, fermentation and products thereof, microbial protein synthesis, passage rate, retention time, hydrolytic digestion, and absorption in the lower tract refer equally well to NWC as to ruminants, although compartmental sizes and rates of various processes and transfers may differ slightly.

Daily energy and protein requirements presented in Table 15-10 were estimated according to the equations and factors developed in Chapters 4 and 5, respectively, and presented below:

	ME	CP
Maintenance	73 kcal/kg $BW^{0.75}$	3.5 g/kg $BW^{0.75}$
Activity:		
Pens, stalls, small lots	0	
Typical rangeland	$0.25 \times ME_m$	
Semiarid rangeland	$0.50 \times ME_m$	
Arid rangeland	$0.75 \times ME_m$	
Growth	7.25 kcal/g ADG	0.284 g/g ADG
Pregnancy:		
8 months	$65.3 \times TBW_{kg}{}^{a} - 33.5$ kcal	0.95 g/kg $BW^{0.75}$
9 months	$131.7 \times TBW_{kg} - 39.7$ kcal	1.94 g/kg $BW^{0.75}$
10 months	$203.5 \times TBW_{kg} + 86.1$ kcal	3.23 g/kg $BW^{0.75}$
Lactation	946 kcal/kg milk	60.6 g/kg milk
Fiber production	30 kcal/g fleece	4.3 g/g fleece

[a]Total birth weight

The requirements for minerals and vitamins presented in Table 15-10 were derived mostly from sheep, goat, and cattle data. These estimates, along with those for energy and protein, should be considered with a degree of uncertainty until more definitive data are accumulated from studies involving the camelid species under various conditions. However, it is believed that these values are reasonably accurate for most circumstances.

Somewhat greater uncertainty accompanies the quality values of feeds and forages determined for other species and applied to camelids. Camelids consume less feed on a body weight basis than do ruminants, hold it in the gastrointestinal tract longer, and digest it more completely. Moreover, camelids seem to be very efficient in nitrogen recycling (Chapter 2), which may increase the value of low-protein feeds and forages for these species. Therefore, feeds and especially lower quality forages listed in Tables 15-11 and 15-12 may be slightly higher (3–5 percent) in the concentration of ME for camelids than is listed.

Important Considerations in Management of Camelids

Critical periods in the nutrition of camelids relate to the physiological development of the cria and the annual production cycle. Developing females may reach puberty by 6 months of age, but many breeders prefer to delay breeding until up to 2 years of age to allow for sufficient body development. Twelve months of age could be considered an appropriate breeding age if special care and nutrition are provided up to and subsequent to breeding. Body weight at first breeding should approximate 60 percent of mature weight and should continue to increase during first pregnancy. In adult animals, the critical period surrounds parturition. The gestation period in camelids varies but averages about 11 months (340 days). Therefore, rebreeding must occur quickly after parturition if a 12-month reproductive cycle is to occur. The elevated requirements recommended for camelid females during late gestation and early lactation account for demands of rapid fetal growth, onset of lactation, and proper recovery from parturition in preparation for breeding. Poor nutrition during this perinatal period can result in embryo loss, abortion, stillbirth, low survival of live cria, and delayed breeding.

Camelids should not be allowed to become obese during the nonproductive period. After weaning of the cria at 4–6 months of age, feeding levels should be held at maintenance or only slightly higher only to regain body condition that was lost during the lactation phase. Obesity predisposes the animals to **hepatic lipidosis** that can occur under stressful conditions when feed intake decreases rapidly and body weight plummets. A low feeding level during the postweaning period followed by elevated nutrition as parturition nears is most appropriate. Underfeeding during late gestation increases the risk of **pregnancy toxemia**, a fatal condition caused by rapid breakdown of fat. Excessively low nutrition during early and mid-pregnancy can cause **embryo death**.

Other nutrition-related health concerns include lactic acidosis, urolithiasis, and rickets (Chapter 13). **Lactic acidosis** occurs when large amounts of starchy feeds (e.g., corn, sorghum grain, and wheat) are fed to animals that are adapted to more fibrous diets. The microbial population in the forestomach ferments the starch rapidly, producing an accumulation of lactic that is not properly metabolized. Diet changes should occur gradually, a series of small increases in grain feeding over several days or weeks. **Urinary calculi** (urolithiasis, kidney stones) is common in both intact and castrated males and usually results from a mineral imbalance in the diet over an extended period. Maintaining a relatively wide Ca:P ratio (> 2) and/or including a urine-acidifying agent (e.g., ammonium chloride) will prevent or greatly reduce the incidence of this malady. **Rickets**, a condition of poor mineralization and weakness of bone, occurs in growing animals restricted in vitamin D and is particularly prevalent in NWC (Chapter 13). Vitamin D deficiencies can occur during extended cloudy or housed conditions that limit exposure to sunlight. In such cases, vitamin D should be supplied in the feed or, in some cases, can be injected.

NUTRIENT CONTENTS OF FORAGES RELATED TO GROWTH FORM AND PHENOLOGICAL STAGE

The broad concept of forage includes plant materials that accumulate above ground, usually not including excessively woody stems or seeds with quantitatively high amounts of starch. At the extremes, neither tree trunks nor grains from cereal plants (such as wheat or barley) are considered forage, but leaves and twigs that attach to trees and the bodies of the plants that produce grain are considered forage. Stems of lesser gigantic structure (compared with tree trunks) such as in grasses, some vines and shrubs, and much of the other herbaceous materials are classified as forage. Also, seeds having less prominence and practically inseparable from other plant parts are grouped into the forage portion. Therefore, forage is a classification of a food resource for animals, particularly ruminant animals, and is available for consumption at or near its site of growth. It varies in growth form (trees, shrubs, vines, grasses, other herbaceous materials), season of growth, resilience to defoliation, reproductive process, and nutrient concentrations (Chapter 10).

Small ruminants consume from a wide variety of plant species, parts, and forms (Chapters 3, 10, and 11). Sheep are classified as **grazers** but overlap in diet preference with intermediate and concentrate selectors under certain circumstances. Their unique characteristic in diet selection is the cleft lower lip that enables them to grip and ingest very short plant parts that are unattainable to other grazers. Compared with the larger grazers, sheep exhibit the ability to select the higher quality parts of grasses, other monocotyledons, and various herbaceous dicotyledons and satisfy their higher nutrient requirements. They are particularly drawn to short regrowth that appears quickly when good growing conditions follow the defoliation of the more mature parts of the forage. Goats are classified as **intermediate feeders**, adept at adjusting feeding behavior to take advantage of the dynamic offerings associated with seasonal and climatic changes. Using mobile lips and tongue, goats discriminate efficiently from a close mix of components whether from growing vegetation or mixtures in the feed trough. Compared with the larger grazers such as cattle, buffalo, and even sheep, concentrate selectors such as the various cervids and goats show diversity in diet selection, thereby reducing direct competition with other species with which they share grazing space. The white-tailed deer belongs to the third morphological classification, known as the **concentrate selector**. Species in this group select diets that are highly digestible and avoid plant components high in fiber. Their narrow mouth and long tongue equip them to be highly discriminating for plant components high in starch, proteins, and oils. The other cervids considered (wapiti, reindeer, and caribou) are classified as intermediate feeders but, like the goat, overlap with both grazers and concentrate selectors. Camelids are intermediate feeders tending toward the grazer end of the continuum.

Plants within a type (e.g., grasses) vary predictably in nutrient content. Leaves are more tender and digestible than stems. Annuals are more nutritious than perennials. Early growth contains greater soluble carbohydrates and protein and less fiber than mature forage. Cool-season (C_3) plants are higher in nutritional value than warm-season (C_4) plants. Many exceptions to these general statements occur. Also, comparisons of individual forages between plant types often do not follow these rules. For example, foliage grazed from a mature herbaceous legume may be of greater nutritional value compared with that selected from a less mature perennial grass. Table 15-12 lists nutrient contents of an array of plants at different stages of maturity and within each forage type that commonly appear in small ruminant diets.

NUTRIENT CONTENTS OF ROUGHAGES, GRAINS, CONCENTRATES, AND MINOR FEED ADDITIVES

Nutrient concentrations in preserved forages (e.g., hay and silage), high-energy sources, protein concentrates, and other potential feed ingredients are listed in Table 15-11. The values listed are typical values derived from numerous analyses of samples of the particular feedstuff, but may not represent the actual value of the ingredient available. Laboratory analyses of ingredients to be used are recommended when practical. However, the values presented are considered safe estimates for appropriate use in most situations.

MATCHING NUTRIENT INTAKE TO NUTRIENT REQUIREMENTS IN SMALL RUMINANTS

Small ruminant and ruminant-like species derive nutrients from a variety of feed sources including protein, fat, and both structural and nonstructural carbohydrates. The free-ranging animal possesses an enterprising nature in diet selection, taking small portions from many sources and thereby increasing the likelihood that the complex diet will satisfy its nutrient requirements. The structural carbohydrate component of feeds, often defined as fiber (Chapter 10), is a primary key in nutrition management. Consumed materials undergo a period of fermentation within the reticulo-rumen, where certain products of fermentation are extracted from the liquid pool and the mass of residue that pass to the lower gastrointestinal tract for further digestion and passage of undigested materials (Chapter 2). Successful management manipulates the forms and amounts of consumed materials while targeting the forms and amounts of nutrients reaching the sites of digestion. The most common means of manipulation of diet is in varying the proportion of fiber in the diet. Fiber can be fermented and contribute to the energy portion of the requirements, but also serves to limit total consumption as well as consumption of other required nutrients. In general, high-fiber diets equate to low nutrient intake and are good for animals in low stages of productivity (e.g., nonpregnant, nonlactating; early gestation) but inadequate for animals in stages of elevated requirements. Low-fiber diets, if properly balanced to supply all nutrients, are suited to animals of high genetic potential and in stages of high productivity. A useful perspective is that diets are available in a continuum in fiber content from low to high, and animals in various states of productivity and having varying levels of requirements distribute appropriately along that continuum. Note the simplified example below for sheep having increasing specific energy requirements supplied by a mixture of alfalfa and corn (values taken from Tables 15-1, 15-2, and 15-11). As the energy requirements increase, the proportion of alfalfa must decrease to yield appropriate mixtures having decreasing fiber.

Stage of Production	Adult Ewe Maintenance (70 kg)	Late Pregnant Ewe (twins) (70 kg)	4-month lamb Growing (40 kg)
ME requirement, Mcal	2.25	4.37	4.76
DM Intake, kg/d	1.18	1.83	1.66
Mcal ME/kg diet	1.91	2.39	2.87
Alfalfa/corn mixtures			
Alfalfa, %	93	57	24
Corn, %	7	43	76
Fiber, %	35	23	12
Example grasses	Bluestem	Bromegrass	Wheat pasture
CF, %	34	28	18

Similarly, grasses appropriate to satisfy these increasing requirements are those having decreasing levels of fiber and corresponding increasing amounts of soluble carbohydrates (Chapter 10).

USE OF THE TABLES IN MEETING NUTRIENT REQUIREMENTS OF SMALL RUMINANTS

There is a host of factors to be considered in developing strategies for appropriately feeding animals. The most important ones are nutrient requirements, including attention to minimum and maximum tolerable levels (some minerals and vitamins), and available feedstuffs relative to their nutrient concentrations, interactions and complementarities with others, and cost. Greater details concerning these factors are presented in previous chapters. This section is devoted to defining nutrient requirements of individuals or groups of animals and strategies for supplying those nutrients in the diet.

Nutrient Requirements

Nutrient requirement expressions are appropriate for animals within the midrange of a population. This may result in slightly greater or lesser than expected performance in animals that deviate from the average in production potential and characteristics. Also, present and past nutritional planes may raise or lower requirements for certain nutrients, thereby influencing performance during a subsequent period. Many production systems by design have periods of relatively low nutrient intake followed by higher planes to take advantage of compensatory growth in accordance with seasonal change in forage conditions. Hence, for example, not in all instances would a level of feeding for body weight or energy stasis of a mature animal be used or be most economical.

Although energy and protein are quantitatively the most targeted nutrients as animal feeds are developed and evaluated, all nutrients are critical and must not be ignored as ingredients are combined to provide animal diets. The absence or severe deficiency of any nutrient can render the diet totally inadequate even if all other nutrients are provided in correct proportions. However, some nutrients, such as many of the macro- and microminerals, are almost always present in adequate amounts in the common feedstuffs or in grazed or browsed plant material. Most of the water-soluble vitamins and some of the fat-soluble vitamins are synthesized in adequate amounts by the microbial population in the rumen and, thus, are not required in the diet. Other nutrients are dietary essentials but are highly variable in feedstuffs and grazed or browsed materials in respect to dietary requirements. In some cases, a diet may be adequate for a class of animals at one stage of production, but inadequate under another circumstance. Discussions in the preceding section identified the nutrient deficiency symptoms most likely to occur for the different small ruminant species (sheep, goats, cervids, and camelids). The most common deficiencies, excesses, or imbalances involve energy (ME), protein (MP), calcium (Ca), phosphorus (P), vitamin A, and vitamin E. The requirements of these nutrients are presented in Tables 15-1 and 15-2 for sheep, 15-4 and 15-5 for goats, 15-9 for cervids, and 15-10 for camelids. In each table, requirements are specified for animals of different body size, physiological stage, and expected level of production. Other nutrients are less likely to be outside of the optimal ranges of concentration, but any nutrient may require primary attention in certain local areas and with certain combinations of dietary ingredients. Discussions presented in Chapter 2 are recommended if deficient or toxic levels of these nutrients are suspected.

Available Feedstuffs

Ingredients included in small ruminant diets are varied, especially when wild ruminants are included. Grazing/browsing animals consume diets comprised of various parts of large numbers of grasses, sedges, other herbaceous plants (both leguminous and nonleguminous), shrubs, trees, mosses, and lichens; animal refuge and other animal forms; and soil or mineral deposits. Conventional feedstuffs include hays and other dry roughages, grains and other high-energy feeds, high-protein feeds (oilseed meals and other byproduct concentrates), harvested green forages and silages, mineral concentrates and premixes, vitamin premixes, and various feed additives (such as medications and growth promotants). Managers of animal populations should become familiar with available feedstuffs and their composition and price. For those managing grazing populations, familiarity with dietary preferences and nutritive values of dietary ingredients is essential for developing strategies for nutrition management.

Tables 15-11 and 15-12 describe the nutrient contents of conventional feedstuffs and many of the plants or plant parts that are grazed, browsed, or scavenged from the landscape. The various expressions of energy and protein can be converted one to another as footnoted and are included for the convenience of the user. Table 15-12 includes extensive listings of novel feedstuffs that are rarely considered in other data sources. For certain entries, values are not included for all nutrients because they were not reported in the original source of the composition data. No assumptions should be drawn from these missing values, and other sources should be sought for estimating the contents for these nutrients.

Use of Requirements Tables

The requirements tables (Tables 15-1 and 15-2 for sheep; 15-4, 15-5, and 15-6 for goats; 15-9 for cervids; and 15-10 for camelids) show the nutrients required by animals of different body sizes (weights) that are in different physiological stages and levels of productivity (litter size, milk production, daily weight gain, etc). To identify the animal(s) for which requirements are being determined, search down the left margin of a table to select the correct major group heading (e.g., Ewes). Under this main heading are subheadings defining the physiological state such as Maintenance, Late Gestation, and Early Lactation. Under each subheading is a column of body weights. These body weights for adult animals are indicators of mature body size and approximate weight of the respective animal if not pregnant or during early pregnancy and in average body condition (BCS = 2.5). Therefore, the weight selected may be lower or greater than the current weight that is influenced by physiological state (late pregnancy, heavy lactation, or other state). For immature animals, these weights usually represent current weights if their development is similar to the normal growth curve for their respective genotype. This selection of body weight identifies the line in the table that extends across to the right and contains entries of requirements that are defined in the heading at the top of the table. For example, a ewe in late gestation carrying twin fetuses and weighing 60 kg should receive daily 3.94 Mcal ME, 116 g MP, 8.1 g Ca, 4.8 g P, and 2,730 international units (IU) of vitamin A. These amounts of nutrients could be supplied in relatively high concentrations and require a lower intake of total diet or in lower concentrations in a diet that allowed a higher level of intake.

Use of Feed Composition Table

Table 15-11 contains nutritional descriptions of common feedstuffs that can be used in feeding programs for small ruminants. The individual feeds are listed alphabetically in the left column with some having multiple entries representing different stages of harvest, processing methods, or anatomical parts. The column headings across the top of the table identify the numerical characteristics that are entered on the lines corresponding to the feedstuffs listed in the first column along the left margin. The feedstuff characteristics include dry matter content (percent of weight retained after water is removed), various chemical components (including fiber), expressions of energy and protein content, concentrations of vitamins A and E activity, and composition of various minerals. To determine the nutritional value of a selected feedstuff using cottonseed as an example, move down the left margin feedstuffs beginning with "C," follow the alphabetical order to Cottonseed meal (there may be multiple entries from which to select), and then inspect entries along the line in the columns to the right to describe the composition as desired. Entries for Cottonseed Meal, Solvent 41 percent CP include 2.80 Mcal/kg ME, 33.6 percent MP, 0.22 percent Ca, and 1.25 percent P along with concentrations for several other chemical or nutritional components.

METHODS OF FORMULATING BALANCED DIETS

The term "ration" denotes a daily amount, whereas diet refers to feed consumed regardless of time. Animals require absolute amounts of energy and nutrients rather than concentrations. Hence, to balance a ration it is necessary to have an estimate of daily feed intake and express requirements as concentrations thereof. This intake estimate can be based on experience or established methods of prediction that rely heavily on fiber content. Ration balancing must consider factors in addition to energy and protein, most notably minerals and vitamins. A deficiency in any of these constituents can make supplying appropriate amounts of energy and protein irrelevant. Supplying nutrients to animals in proper proportions is the practical application of the extensive information contained in the Nutrient Requirements and Feed Composition tables.

Example 1. Simultaneous Equations Method for three ingredients

A simple exercise in balancing a ration could be using three common feedstuffs (meadow hay, corn, and cottonseed meal) to prepare a diet for the ewe described above that required 3.94 Mcal ME, 116 g MP, 8.1 g Ca, and 4.8 g P per day. Actual composition of feed ingredients determined by laboratory analyses gives accurate values for formulating diets. In the absence of actual nutrient composition, Tables 15-11, 15-12, and 15-13 give estimates that can be used in approximating the nutrient composition of diets. Information in the feed composition table (Table 15-11) shows the following estimates of nutrient concentrations.

	ME Mcal/kg	MP %	Ca %	P %
Meadow hay	1.8	4.9	0.61	0.18
Corn (grain whole)	3.2	6.3	0.02	0.30
Cottonseed meal (41% solvent)	2.8	33.6	0.22	1.25

The ewe would be expected to consume approximately 1.65 kg (2.75 percent of body weight; Table 15-1) per day.

An individual determines from experience that the ration should contain 50–60 percent hay (approximates the energy content of the ration). If the hay were included at 55 percent (907.5 g), then it would supply the following amount of the indicated nutrients:

1.63 Mcal of the ME
44.5 g of the MP
5.5 g of the Ca
1.6 g of the P

The remainder of the required nutrients must be supplied from the remaining 45 percent of the ration (742.5 g) made from a mixture of corn and cottonseed meal (CSM). Thus, the mixture of corn and cottonseed meal must contain the following:

$$3.94 \text{ Mcal} - 1.63 \text{ Mcal} = 2.31 \text{ Mcal ME}$$
$$116 \text{ g} - 44.5 \text{ g} = 71.5 \text{ g MP}$$

The mixture of corn and cottonseed meal (742.5 g) that contains 71.5 g MP can be obtained using simultaneous equations as follows:

$$0.063\,X + 0.336\,Y = 71.5 \text{ g}$$
$$X + Y = 742.5 \text{ g}$$

where X = amount (g) of corn and Y = amount (g) of CSM, which contain 6.3 percent (0.063) and 33.6 percent (0.336) MP, respectively.

The second equation is multiplied by –0.063 to eliminate the X factor.

$$0.063\,X + 0.336\,Y = 71.5 \text{ g}$$
$$-0.063\,X - 0.063\,Y = -46.8 \text{ g}$$
$$0.273\,Y = 24.7 \text{ g}$$
$$Y = 90.5 \text{ g } (12.2\%)$$

Thus, 90.5 g (12.2 percent) of the mixture is CSM and the remaining 652 g (87.8 percent) is corn. The complete ration becomes as below.

Meadow hay	=	55%
Corn (45 × 0.878)		=39.5%
CSM (45 × 0.122)		=5.5%

Concentrations of nutrients in ration can be calculated.

Energy	=	2.41 Mcal/kg
Protein	=	7.0% MP
Calcium	=	0.36% Ca
Phosphorus	=	0.29% P

Nutrients supplied at 1,650 g/day consumption are similar to the requirements listed in parentheses.

Energy (ME)	=	3.98Mcal/d (3.94)
Protein (MP)	=	116g/d (116)
Calcium	=	5.9g/d (8.1)
Phosphorus	=	4.8g/d (4.8)

The ration is balanced for energy and protein. It supplies adequate P but is deficient in Ca, a nutrient that may be very important for a ewe about to begin lactation. This imbalance can be corrected by replacing 0.5 percent of the corn portion with calcium carbonate without detectable changes in the other nutrients. The actual feeding level should be adjusted to account for moisture content to an as-fed basis usually by a 10 to 12 percent moisture factor (1,650 × 100/90 = 1,833 g/day).

Example 2. Simultaneous Equation (Substitution) Method for two ingredients

Drought conditions suggest that a deer herd is suffering from a protein deficiency during the winter season. A supplement to provide one-half of the protein requirements and one-third of the energy requirements for pregnant does is desired. This supplement could be prepared with the proper combination of corn and cottonseed meal. A 50 kg pregnant doe during late gestation and carrying a single fetus requires daily 3.4 Mcal ME and 150 g MP (Table 15-9). One-third and one-half daily requirements of energy and protein are 1.13 Mcal ME and 75 g MP, respectively. The quantities of corn and cottonseed meal in a mixture to supply these amounts can be calculated from the nutrient requirements and the composition of the feed ingredients shown in Example 1 above. Assume that X and Y equal the amounts (kg) of corn and cottonseed meal needed.

First set the equations for the concentrations of energy (3.2 and 2.8) and amounts (X and Y) of corn and cottonseed meal to supply the desired energy (1.13 Mcal). Then do the same for protein (concentrations shown as g/kg):

$$3.2\ X + 2.8\ Y = 1.13$$
$$63\ X + 336\ Y = 75$$

Solve the simultaneous equations by substitution.

$$336\ Y = 75 - 63\ X$$
$$Y = 0.223 - 0.188\ X$$
$$3.2\ X + 2.8\ (0.223 - 0.188\ X) = 1.13$$
$$3.2\ X + 0.624 - 0.526\ X = 1.13$$
$$2.68\ X = 0.506$$
$$X = 0.190\ \text{kg}$$
$$Y = 0.187\ \text{kg}$$

Feeding 190 g corn and 187 g cottonseed meal (377 g of a 50.4 percent corn:49.6 percent CSM mixture) would provide 1.13 Mcal of ME and 75 g MP daily. Adjusted to an as-fed basis, feeding level of the mixture would be 419 g/day, about 0.84 percent of body weight.

These examples illustrate a simple, eight-step method to develop a ration:

1. Identify the nutrient requirements using the tables.
2. Determine the energy content of the diet to be fed (estimated by roughage/fiber level of the diet or by other means) and expected level of intake.
3. Identify the feed ingredients to be used and determine their nutrient contents from the feed composition tables.
4. Set the levels of all but two ingredients according to knowledge and experience (the roughage level in simple three-ingredient diets). The two remaining ingredients should be similar in all but one major nutrient (e.g., protein).
5. Determine the proportion of the required nutrients supplied by the set ingredients and the required concentration of the major nutrient (usually protein) in the mixture of the remaining two ingredients.
6. Use simultaneous equations (or Pearson's Square or other simple mathematical methods) to determine the proper proportion of the two ingredients.
7. Calculate the nutrients supplied by the formulated ration and compare with requirements.
8. Make adjustments to eliminate imbalances and for moisture contents.

There are many different methods of balancing rations. This can be done in a very simplistic fashion, such as with a hand calculator as illustrated. Spreadsheets are often used as well, which greatly increases the speed with which formations can be changed. Typically, effectiveness of these methods is dependent on the knowledge of the balancer. Alternatively, there are software packages available that have incorporated requirements. Some such packages have capabilities of determining least-cost rations; however, factors such as feedstuff availability, ease of handling, and minimum fiber levels still need consideration. Regardless of the method used, most appropriate requirement expressions and feedstuff composition values are usually deemed of relatively greater importance.

As the number of animals in the herd or flock increases, the desired sophistication of ration formulation and feeding management also increases because of the greater importance of small differences in unit cost and return. Greater attention to minor nutrient concentrations, feed processing methods, differences in nutrient form and solubility, associative effects of feed ingredients, and other factors is recommended for these management systems. The earlier chapters in this document are filled with the latest scientific information on all aspects of the nutrition of small ruminants and are recommended to supply related discussions and any known solutions.

NUTRIENT REQUIREMENTS OF SHEEP TABLES

Energy and protein requirements of sheep were projected as described earlier in the Energy and Protein sections (Chapters 4 and 5). Energy requirements are influenced by age and stage of maturity in the CNCPS-S method, in addition to effects of BW and ADG (Cannas et al., 2004). Because the efficiency of energy utilization for gain in CNCPS-S varies with diet metabolizability, values are given for three dietary ME concentrations: 1.91, 2.39, and 2.87 Mcal/kg DM (i.e., 8, 10, and 12 MJ/kg DM, respectively). The visceral organ adjustment (VO) of the ME requirement for maintenance of CNCPS-S, which is based on ME intake, was included. VO was determined from and added to ME intake estimated without the adjustment. Listed DM intakes are needed to supply required energy from the indicated energy concentrations of the diets. Selections were made from the three example diets based on an expected range of intake on a percent of body weight. In some instances, selections of other diets may be more appropriate. The protein requirement for fiber growth was based on the method of SCA (1990), assuming a ratio of standard fleece weight (greasy fiber produced by a mature sheep per year) to mature BW at BCS of 3.0 (scale of 0 to 5) of 0.1, along with an adjustment for age when less than 2 years. The metabolic fecal protein requirement, which is a component of the maintenance need, was based on the estimate of DM intake required to supply needed energy for a given BW to achieved the specified level of production. Because the relationship between MP and CP requirements varies with the nature of the diet, the aforementioned conversion of CP to MP of NRC (2000) was applied for diets with rumen undegraded intake (UIP) concentrations of 20, 40, and 60 percent of total CP. The requirement for DIP is given as well. It is important to note that in some instances the DIP needed is greater than required amounts of CP. For example, an 80 kg ewe (at maintenance) consuming a diet with an ME concentration of 1.91 Mcal/kg would require 98 g of CP with diet having a UIP concentration of 20 percent of CP. Under these conditions, DIP intake is 78 g (i.e., 98 g × 80 percent DIP), but the estimated DIP requirement is 90. Hence, to satisfy the DIP requirement, intake of CP with this diet would be 112 g, with a corresponding greater dietary CP requirement on a concentration basis (i.e., 8.7 vs. 7.5 percent). Also, the DIP requirements often exceed the estimates of MP requirements and are partially supplied by recycled nitrogen. Because BCS is an input to determine the energy concentration in tissue being accreted or mobilized in mature sheep in the CNCPS-S method, for mature animals and yearlings a concentration of 5.7 Mcal/kg was assumed. Assumptions used to derive the recommended requirements presented in Tables 15-1 and 15-2 are given below.

Requirements for mature ewes were determined assuming an age of 3 years and a 100 percent stage of maturity. Requirements for early, mid-, and late lactation are given with assumptions of BW change. Because CNCPS-S assumes that efficiencies of energy utilization for maintenance and lactation are the same, requirements for ME and TDN do not differ among dietary ME concentrations with negative and 0 ADG (Table 15-1). Requirements for all classes in which weight gain is attached (other than recovery weight gain) are presented in Table 15-2. These classes include growing lambs and yearlings and yearling ewes at maintenance (plus growth), gestation, and lactation. Requirements are presented for "Farm" and "Range" yearlings for common production systems and practices, which include typical ages and stages of maturity in the various stages of production. An age of 3 years and stage of maturity of 100 percent were assumed for rams. Energy and protein requirements in the breeding period were increased by 10 percent of maintenance energy and protein needs for mature ewes, yearlings, and rams.

Pregnancy requirements are presented for early and late gestation, with input of day 105 and 133, respectively. Yearlings were assumed to be growing during gestation. Live weight gain values given for gestating animals are for both pregnancy and nonpregnancy tissues of yearlings. The maintenance requirement for nonpregnancy tissues should, however, be based on weight of nonpregnancy tissues alone or weight of the animal before days 80–90 of pregnancy.

For growing/finishing sheep, values are presented for two ages, 4 and 8 months, which affect the maintenance energy requirement. Stage of maturity, affecting the energy concentration in tissue being gained, is 30 and 60 percent for 4-month-old lambs and 40 and 80 percent for 8-month-old lambs. These combinations should provide values applicable to many production practices. For example, a 4-month-old wether with a BW 30 percent of that when mature at a BCS of 3.0 (5-point scale) is at an early stage of maturity and possibly of a late-maturing breed; hence, a considerable portion of tissue being gained would be lean. On the other extreme, a wether 8 months of age with a BW 80 percent of that when mature would be at a late stage of maturity and most likely of an early maturing breed accreting considerable fat. In addition to values for wether and ewe lambs, values are presented for ram lambs, which differ because of a greater energy requirement for maintenance.

Tables 15-1 and 15-2 include estimates of requirements of Ca and P and vitamins A and E. Requirements for the remaining essential minerals are included in Table 15-3. Details of the requirements of minerals and vitamins are discussed in Chapters 7 and 8, respectively.

REFERENCES

Cannas, A., L. O. Tedeschi, D. G. Fox, A. N. Pell, and P. J. Van Soest. 2004. A mechanistic model for predicting the nutrient requirements and feed biological values for sheep. J. Anim. Sci. 82:149–169.

NRC. 2000. Nutrient Requirements of Beef Cattle (Update 2000). Washington, DC: National Academy Press.

SCA (Standing Committee on Agriculture). 1990. Feeding Standards for Australian Livestock. Ruminants. East Melbourne, Australia: CSIRO Publications.

TABLE 15-1 Nutrient Requirements of Sheep (mature ewes and rams and yearlings maintenance and lactation)

Class/Age/Other	Body Weight[a] kg	Birth Weight or Milk Yield[b] kg	Body Weight Gain[c] g/d	Energy Concentration in Diet[d] kcal/kg	Daily Dry Matter Intake[e] kg	Daily Dry Matter Intake[e] % BW	Energy Requirements[f] TDN kg/d	Energy Requirements[f] ME Mcal/d	Protein Requirements[g] CP @20% UIP g/d	CP @40% UIP g/d	CP @60% UIP g/d	MP g/d	DIP g/d	Mineral Requirements[h] Ca g/d	Mineral Requirements[h] P g/d	Vitamin Requirements[i] A RE/d	Vitamin Requirements[i] E IU/d
Mature Ewes																	
Maintenance only																	
	40		0	1.91	0.77	1.93	0.41	1.48	59	56	54	40	53	1.8	1.3	1,256	212
	50		0	1.91	0.91	1.83	0.49	1.75	69	66	63	47	63	2.0	1.5	1,570	265
	60		0	1.91	1.05	1.75	0.56	2.01	79	76	72	53	72	2.2	1.8	1,884	318
	70		0	1.91	1.18	1.68	0.62	2.25	89	85	81	60	81	2.4	2.0	2,198	371
	80		0	1.91	1.30	1.63	0.69	2.49	98	94	90	66	90	2.6	2.2	2,512	424
	90		0	1.91	1.42	1.58	0.75	2.72	107	103	98	72	98	2.8	2.5	2,826	477
	100		0	1.91	1.54	1.54	0.82	2.94	116	111	106	78	106	3.0	2.7	3,140	530
	120		0	1.91	1.76	1.47	0.94	3.37	134	128	123	90	122	3.3	3.1	3,768	636
	140		0	1.91	1.98	1.41	1.05	3.79	151	145	138	102	136	3.7	3.5	4,396	742
Breeding																	
	40		20	1.91	0.85	2.13	0.45	1.63	69	66	63	46	59	2.1	1.5	1,256	212
	50		23	1.91	1.01	2.01	0.53	1.92	81	77	74	55	69	2.4	1.8	1,570	265
	60		26	1.91	1.15	1.92	0.61	2.21	93	89	85	62	80	2.6	2.1	1,884	318
	70		29	1.91	1.30	1.85	0.69	2.48	104	99	95	70	89	2.9	2.4	2,198	371
	80		32	1.91	1.43	1.79	0.76	2.74	115	110	105	77	99	3.1	2.7	2,512	424
	90		35	1.91	1.56	1.74	0.83	2.99	126	120	115	85	108	3.4	2.9	2,826	477
	100		38	1.91	1.69	1.69	0.90	3.24	137	130	125	92	117	3.6	3.2	3,140	530
	120		44	1.91	1.94	1.62	1.03	3.71	157	150	144	106	134	4.0	3.7	3,768	636
	140		50	1.91	2.18	1.56	1.15	4.16	177	169	162	119	150	4.5	4.2	4,396	742
Early gestation (Single lamb; BW = 3.9 to 7.5 kg)																	
	40	3.9	18	1.91	0.99	2.47	0.52	1.89	82	79	75	55	68	3.4	2.4	1,256	212
	50	4.4	21	1.91	1.16	2.32	0.61	2.21	96	91	87	64	80	3.8	2.8	1,570	265
	60	4.8	24	1.91	1.31	2.19	0.70	2.51	108	103	99	73	91	4.2	3.2	1,884	318
	70	5.2	27	1.91	1.46	2.09	0.78	2.80	120	114	110	81	101	4.5	3.5	2,198	371
	80	5.6	30	1.91	1.61	2.01	0.85	3.08	132	126	120	89	111	4.9	3.9	2,512	424
	90	6.0	33	1.91	1.75	1.95	0.93	3.35	143	137	131	96	121	5.2	4.2	2,826	477
	100	6.3	35	1.91	1.89	1.89	1.00	3.61	154	147	141	104	130	5.5	4.5	3,140	530
	120	7.0	41	1.91	2.15	1.79	1.14	4.11	176	168	161	118	148	6.1	5.1	3,768	636
	140	7.5	46	1.91	2.39	1.71	1.27	4.58	196	187	179	132	165	6.7	5.7	4,396	742
Early gestation (Twin lambs; BW = 3.4 to 6.6 kg)																	
	40	3.4	30	1.91	1.15	2.87	0.61	2.20	100	95	91	67	79	4.8	3.2	1,256	212
	50	3.8	35	1.91	1.31	2.62	0.70	2.51	112	107	103	76	90	5.4	3.7	1,570	265
	60	4.2	40	1.91	1.51	2.52	0.80	2.89	129	124	118	87	104	5.9	4.2	1,884	318
	70	4.6	45	1.91	1.69	2.41	0.89	3.22	144	137	131	97	116	6.5	4.6	2,198	371
	80	4.9	50	1.91	1.84	2.30	0.98	3.52	157	150	143	105	127	7.0	5.1	2,512	424
	90	5.2	55	1.91	2.00	2.22	1.06	3.82	170	162	155	114	138	7.4	5.5	2,826	477
	100	5.5	59	1.91	2.15	2.15	1.14	4.10	182	174	167	123	148	7.9	5.9	3,140	530
	120	6.1	68	1.91	2.44	2.03	1.29	4.66	207	198	189	139	168	8.7	6.6	3,768	636
	140	6.6	76	1.91	2.71	1.94	1.44	5.18	231	220	211	155	187	9.5	7.3	4,396	742

Early gestation (Three lambs; BW = 2.9 to 5.7 kg)																	
40	2.9	39	2.39	1.00	2.51	0.67	2.40	103	98	94	69	86	5.4	3.3	1,256	212
50	3.3	46	1.91	1.46	2.92	0.77	2.79	129	123	117	86	101	6.5	4.4	1,570	265
60	3.6	52	1.91	1.65	2.74	0.87	3.15	144	137	131	97	113	7.1	4.9	1,884	318
70	3.9	59	1.91	1.82	2.61	0.97	3.49	159	152	145	107	126	7.8	5.4	2,198	371
80	4.2	65	1.91	2.00	2.50	1.06	3.82	174	166	159	117	138	8.3	5.9	2,512	424
90	4.5	71	1.91	2.17	2.41	1.15	4.14	188	180	172	127	149	8.9	6.3	2,826	477
100	4.7	77	1.91	2.32	2.32	1.23	4.43	201	192	183	135	160	9.4	6.7	3,140	530
120	5.2	88	1.91	2.63	2.19	1.39	5.02	228	217	208	153	181	10.4	7.6	3,768	636
140	5.7	99	1.91	2.92	2.09	1.55	5.59	254	242	232	171	202	11.4	8.4	4,396	742
Late gestation (Single lamb; BW = 3.9 to 7.5 kg)																	
40	3.9	71	2.39	1.00	2.49	0.66	2.38	101	96	92	68	86	4.3	2.6	1,820	224
50	4.4	84	1.91	1.45	2.89	0.77	2.76	126	120	115	85	100	5.1	3.5	2,275	280
60	4.8	97	1.91	1.63	2.71	0.86	3.11	141	134	129	95	112	5.7	4.0	2,730	336
70	5.2	109	1.91	1.80	2.58	0.96	3.45	156	149	142	105	124	6.1	4.4	3,185	392
80	5.6	120	1.91	1.98	2.47	1.05	3.78	170	163	155	114	136	6.6	4.8	3,640	448
90	6.0	131	1.91	2.15	2.38	1.14	4.10	185	176	169	124	148	7.1	5.2	4,095	504
100	6.3	142	1.91	2.30	2.30	1.22	4.40	198	189	180	133	158	7.5	5.5	4,550	560
120	7.0	163	1.91	2.61	2.17	1.38	4.99	224	214	205	151	180	8.3	6.3	5,460	672
140	7.5	183	1.91	2.89	2.06	1.53	5.52	248	237	226	167	199	9.0	6.9	6,370	784
Late gestation (Twin lambs; BW = 3.4 to 6.6 kg)																	
40	3.4	119	2.87	1.06	2.66	0.85	3.05	128	123	117	86	110	6.3	3.4	1,820	224
50	3.8	141	2.39	1.47	2.93	0.97	3.50	155	148	141	104	126	7.3	4.3	2,275	280
60	4.2	161	2.39	1.65	2.75	1.09	3.94	173	165	158	116	142	8.1	4.8	2,730	336
70	4.6	181	2.39	1.83	2.61	1.21	4.37	192	183	175	129	158	8.8	5.3	3,185	392
80	4.9	200	2.39	1.99	2.48	1.32	4.75	208	198	189	139	171	9.4	5.8	3,640	448
90	5.2	218	1.91	2.68	2.97	1.42	5.12	241	230	220	162	185	10.7	7.2	4,095	504
100	5.5	236	1.91	2.87	2.87	1.52	5.48	258	246	236	173	198	11.3	7.7	4,550	560
120	6.1	271	1.91	3.24	2.70	1.72	6.19	291	278	266	196	223	12.5	8.6	5,460	672
140	6.6	304	1.91	3.57	2.55	1.89	6.83	321	307	293	216	246	13.6	9.5	6,370	784
Late gestation (Three or more lambs; BW = 2.9 to 5.7 kg)																	
40	2.9	155	2.87	1.22	3.04	0.97	3.49	150	144	137	101	126	7.7	4.1	1,820	224
50	3.3	183	2.87	1.41	2.81	1.12	4.03	173	165	158	116	145	8.7	4.7	2,275	280
60	3.6	210	2.87	1.57	2.61	1.25	4.50	192	183	175	129	162	9.5	5.2	2,730	336
70	3.9	235	2.39	2.07	2.96	1.37	4.95	222	212	203	149	178	10.8	6.4	3,185	392
80	4.2	260	2.39	2.26	2.82	1.50	5.40	241	230	220	162	195	11.6	6.9	3,640	448
90	4.5	284	2.39	2.44	2.71	1.62	5.83	261	249	238	175	210	12.3	7.4	4,095	504
100	4.7	307	2.39	2.59	2.59	1.72	6.20	276	263	252	185	223	13.0	7.9	4,550	560
120	5.2	352	2.39	2.92	2.43	1.93	6.97	310	296	283	209	251	14.4	8.8	5,460	672
140	5.7	396	1.91	4.04	2.89	2.14	7.73	371	355	339	250	279	16.7	11.2	6,370	784
Early lactation (Single lamb; milk yield = 0.71 to 1.32 kg/d)																	
40	0.71	–14	2.39	1.09	2.73	0.72	2.61	156	149	143	105	94	4.1	3.4	1,820	224
50	0.79	–16	2.39	1.26	2.51	0.83	3.00	177	169	161	119	108	4.6	3.9	2,275	280
60	0.87	–17	1.91	1.77	2.96	0.94	3.39	210	200	191	141	122	5.4	5.0	2,730	336
70	0.94	–19	1.91	1.96	2.80	1.04	3.75	229	219	209	154	135	5.9	5.5	3,185	392
80	1.00	–20	1.91	2.13	2.67	1.13	4.08	248	237	226	167	147	6.3	5.9	3,640	448

TABLE 15-1 continued

Class/Age/Other	Body Weight[a] kg	Birth Weight or Milk Yield[b] kg	Body Weight Gain[c] g/d	Energy Concentration in Diet[d] kcal/kg	Daily Dry Matter Intake[e] kg	Daily Dry Matter Intake[e] % BW	Energy Requirements[f] TDN kg/d	Energy Requirements[f] ME Mcal/d	Protein Requirements[g] CP @20% UIP g/d	CP @40% UIP g/d	CP @60% UIP g/d	MP g/d	DIP g/d	Mineral Requirements[h] Ca g/d	Mineral Requirements[h] P g/d	Vitamin Requirements[i] A RE/d	Vitamin Requirements[i] E IU/d
	90	1.06	–21	1.91	2.30	2.56	1.22	4.41	266	254	243	179	159	6.7	6.4	4,095	504
	100	1.12	–22	1.91	2.47	2.47	1.31	4.73	284	272	260	191	170	7.1	6.8	4,550	560
	120	1.22	–24	1.91	2.78	2.32	1.47	5.32	317	303	290	213	192	7.8	7.6	5,460	672
	140	1.32	–26	1.91	3.08	2.20	1.63	5.89	349	333	319	235	212	8.5	8.4	6,370	784
Early lactation (Twin lambs; milk yield = 1.18 to 2.21 kg/d)																	
	40	1.18	–24	2.39	1.40	3.51	0.93	3.35	224	213	204	150	121	6.0	5.0	2,140	224
	50	1.32	–26	2.39	1.61	3.22	1.07	3.85	254	242	231	170	139	6.7	5.7	2,675	280
	60	1.45	–29	2.39	1.80	3.01	1.20	4.31	281	268	257	189	155	7.3	6.3	3,210	336
	70	1.56	–31	2.39	1.98	2.83	1.31	4.73	306	292	279	205	171	7.9	6.9	3,745	392
	80	1.67	–33	2.39	2.15	2.69	1.43	5.15	330	315	302	222	186	8.5	7.4	4,280	448
	90	1.77	–35	2.39	2.32	2.57	1.54	5.54	353	337	322	237	200	9.0	8.0	4,815	504
	100	1.87	–37	2.39	2.48	2.48	1.64	5.92	376	359	343	253	213	9.5	8.5	5,350	560
	120	2.05	–41	1.91	3.47	2.89	1.84	6.63	441	421	403	296	239	11.3	10.7	6,420	672
	140	2.21	–44	1.91	3.82	2.73	2.03	7.30	483	461	441	324	263	12.3	11.7	7,490	784
Early lactation (Three or more lambs; milk yield = 1.53 to 2.87 kg/d)																	
	40	1.53	–31	2.87	1.36	3.41	1.08	3.91	265	253	242	178	141	7.1	5.7	2,140	224
	50	1.72	–34	2.39	1.88	3.76	1.24	4.49	311	297	284	209	162	8.3	7.0	2,675	280
	60	1.88	–38	2.39	2.09	3.48	1.38	4.99	343	327	313	230	180	9.1	7.8	3,210	336
	70	2.03	–41	2.39	2.29	3.27	1.52	5.48	373	356	341	251	197	9.8	8.5	3,745	392
	80	2.17	–43	1.91	3.11	3.89	1.65	5.94	423	404	387	285	214	11.3	10.3	4,280	448
	90	2.30	–46	1.91	3.34	3.71	1.77	6.38	452	431	413	304	230	12.0	11.0	4,815	504
	100	2.43	–49	1.91	3.56	3.56	1.89	6.80	480	458	438	323	245	12.7	11.7	5,350	560
	120	2.66	–53	1.91	3.98	3.32	2.11	7.61	533	508	486	358	274	13.9	13.0	6,420	672
	140	2.87	–57	1.91	4.37	3.12	2.32	8.36	581	555	531	391	301	15.1	14.1	7,490	784
Early lactation (Parlor production only; milk yield = 2.37 to 3.97 kg/d)																	
	50	2.37	–47	2.87	1.93	3.85	1.53	5.52	392	374	358	263	199	10.4	8.5	2,675	280
	60	2.60	–52	2.87	2.14	3.57	1.70	6.14	432	413	395	291	221	11.4	9.4	3,210	336
	70	2.81	–56	2.87	2.34	3.35	1.86	6.72	470	449	429	316	242	12.4	10.3	3,745	392
	80	3.00	–60	2.39	3.04	3.80	2.01	7.26	522	498	476	351	262	13.8	12.0	4,280	448
	90	3.18	–64	2.39	3.25	3.61	2.16	7.77	556	531	508	374	280	14.7	12.7	4,815	504
	100	3.35	–67	2.39	3.46	3.46	2.29	8.27	589	562	538	396	298	15.5	13.5	5,350	560
	120	3.67	–73	2.39	3.86	3.21	2.56	9.22	651	622	595	438	332	17.0	14.9	6,420	672
	140	3.97	–79	1.91	5.29	3.78	2.80	10.11	746	712	681	501	364	19.7	18.2	7,490	784
Mid-lactation (Single lamb; milk yield = 0.47 to 0.89 kg/d)																	
	40	0.47	0	1.91	1.20	3.01	0.64	2.30	134	128	123	90	83	3.5	3.1	2,140	224
	50	0.53	0	1.91	1.40	2.80	0.74	2.68	154	147	141	104	96	3.9	3.6	2,675	280
	60	0.58	0	1.91	1.58	2.63	0.84	3.02	172	164	157	116	109	4.3	4.0	3,210	336
	70	0.63	0	1.91	1.75	2.51	0.93	3.35	190	181	173	128	121	4.6	4.4	3,745	392
	80	0.67	0	1.91	1.91	2.39	1.02	3.66	206	196	188	138	132	5.0	4.8	4,280	448

90	0.71	0	1.91	2.07	2.30	1.10	3.96	221	211	202	149	143	5.3	5.2	4,815	504
100	0.75	0	1.91	2.22	2.22	1.18	4.25	237	226	216	159	153	5.6	5.6	5,350	560
120	0.82	0	1.91	2.51	2.10	1.33	4.81	266	254	243	179	173	6.2	6.3	6,420	672
140	0.89	0	1.91	2.79	2.00	1.48	5.34	294	281	269	198	193	6.8	6.9	7,490	784
Mid-lactation (Twin lambs; milk yield = 0.79 to 1.48 kg/d)																
40	0.79	0	1.91	1.50	3.74	0.79	2.86	186	177	170	125	103	4.9	4.3	2,140	224
50	0.88	0	1.91	1.72	3.44	0.91	3.29	210	201	192	141	119	5.4	4.9	2,675	280
60	0.97	0	1.91	1.94	3.23	1.03	3.70	235	224	214	158	133	6.0	5.5	3,210	336
70	1.05	0	1.91	2.14	3.05	1.13	4.09	257	245	235	173	147	6.5	6.1	3,745	392
80	1.12	0	1.91	2.33	2.91	1.23	4.45	278	265	254	187	160	6.9	6.6	4,280	448
90	1.19	0	1.91	2.51	2.79	1.33	4.80	298	285	272	200	173	7.4	7.1	4,815	504
100	1.25	0	1.91	2.68	2.68	1.42	5.13	317	303	289	213	185	7.8	7.5	5,350	560
120	1.37	0	1.91	3.02	2.51	1.60	5.77	354	338	323	238	208	8.6	8.4	6,420	672
140	1.48	0	1.91	3.33	2.38	1.77	6.37	389	371	355	261	230	9.3	9.2	7,490	784
Mid-lactation (Three or more lambs; milk yield = 1.03 to 1.92 kg/d)																
40	1.03	0	2.39	1.37	3.43	0.91	3.28	213	203	194	143	118	5.5	4.6	2,140	224
50	1.15	0	1.91	1.97	3.93	1.04	3.76	254	242	232	170	136	6.6	6.0	2,675	280
60	1.26	0	1.91	2.20	3.67	1.17	4.21	281	268	257	189	152	7.2	6.6	3,210	336
70	1.36	0	1.91	2.42	3.46	1.28	4.63	307	293	280	206	167	7.8	7.3	3,745	392
80	1.45	0	1.91	2.63	3.29	1.39	5.02	331	316	302	222	181	8.4	7.8	4,280	448
90	1.54	0	1.91	2.83	3.15	1.50	5.41	354	338	324	238	195	8.9	8.4	4,815	504
100	1.63	0	1.91	3.03	3.03	1.61	5.79	378	361	345	254	209	9.4	9.0	5,350	560
120	1.78	0	1.91	3.39	2.83	1.80	6.49	420	401	383	282	234	10.4	10.0	6,420	672
140	1.92	0	1.91	3.74	2.67	1.98	7.14	459	439	419	309	258	11.3	10.9	7,490	784
Mid-lactation (Parlor production only; milk yield = 1.59 to 2.66 kg/d)																
50	1.59	0	2.39	1.90	3.79	1.26	4.53	308	294	281	207	163	7.9	6.8	2,675	280
60	1.74	0	2.39	2.11	3.52	1.40	5.05	340	325	311	229	182	8.7	7.5	3,210	336
70	1.88	0	2.39	2.32	3.31	1.54	5.54	371	354	338	249	200	9.4	8.2	3,745	392
80	2.01	0	1.91	3.14	3.93	1.67	6.00	421	401	384	283	216	10.8	10.0	4,280	448
90	2.13	0	1.91	3.37	3.74	1.79	6.44	449	429	410	302	232	11.5	10.7	4,815	504
100	2.25	0	1.91	3.60	3.60	1.91	6.88	477	456	436	321	248	12.1	11.4	5,350	560
120	2.46	0	1.91	4.03	3.36	2.14	7.71	532	508	486	357	278	13.4	12.6	6,420	672
140	2.66	0	1.91	4.41	3.15	2.34	8.44	578	552	528	388	304	14.5	13.8	7,490	784
Late lactation (Single lamb; milk yield = 0.23 to 0.45 kg/d)																
40	0.23	10	1.91	1.09	2.72	0.58	2.08	105	100	96	70	75	2.7	2.3	2,140	224
50	0.25	11	1.91	1.26	2.52	0.67	2.40	119	114	109	80	87	3.0	2.7	2,675	280
60	0.28	12	1.91	1.43	2.38	0.76	2.73	135	129	123	91	99	3.3	3.1	3,210	336
70	0.31	14	1.91	1.61	2.29	0.85	3.07	151	144	138	102	111	3.6	3.5	3,745	392
80	0.33	15	1.91	1.76	2.20	0.93	3.36	165	157	150	111	121	3.9	3.8	4,280	448
90	0.35	16	1.91	1.91	2.12	1.01	3.65	178	170	163	120	132	4.2	4.1	4,815	504
100	0.37	17	1.91	2.05	2.05	1.09	3.93	191	182	175	128	142	4.4	4.4	5,350	560
120	0.41	18	1.91	2.33	1.94	1.23	4.45	216	206	197	145	160	4.9	5.0	6,420	672
140	0.45	20	1.91	2.60	1.86	1.38	4.97	242	231	221	162	179	5.4	5.6	7,490	784
Late lactation (Twin lambs; milk yield = 0.38 to 0.75 kg/d)																
40	0.38	25	1.91	1.38	3.45	0.73	2.64	142	136	130	96	95	3.7	3.2	2,140	224
50	0.43	28	1.91	1.60	3.20	0.85	3.06	163	156	149	110	110	4.2	3.7	2,675	280

TABLE 15-1 continued

Class/Age/Other	Body Weight[a] kg	Birth Weight or Milk Yield[b] kg	Body Weight Gain[c] g/d	Energy Concentration in Diet[d] kcal/kg	Daily Dry Matter Intake[e] kg	Daily Dry Matter Intake[e] % BW	Energy Requirements[f] TDN kg/d	Energy Requirements[f] ME Mcal/d	Protein Requirements[g] CP @20% UIP g/d	CP @40% UIP g/d	CP @60% UIP g/d	MP g/d	DIP g/d	Mineral Requirements[h] Ca g/d	P g/d	Vitamin Requirements[i] A RE/d	E IU/d
	60	0.47	31	1.91	1.80	3.00	0.95	3.44	182	174	167	123	124	4.6	4.2	3,210	336
	70	0.51	34	1.91	2.00	2.85	1.06	3.82	201	192	184	135	138	5.0	4.6	3,745	392
	80	0.55	37	1.91	2.19	2.74	1.16	4.18	220	210	201	148	151	5.4	5.1	4,280	448
	90	0.59	39	1.91	2.37	2.63	1.25	4.52	237	226	217	159	163	5.8	5.5	4,815	504
	100	0.62	41	1.91	2.53	2.53	1.34	4.84	253	241	231	170	174	6.2	5.9	5,350	560
	120	0.69	46	1.91	2.87	2.39	1.52	5.49	286	273	261	192	198	6.9	6.6	6,420	672
	140	0.75	50	1.91	3.19	2.28	1.69	6.09	317	302	289	213	220	7.5	7.4	7,490	784
Late lactation (Three or more lambs; milk yield = 0.55 to 0.97 kg/d)																	
	50	0.55	40	1.91	1.83	3.67	0.97	3.51	193	185	177	130	126	5.0	4.4	2,675	280
	60	0.61	44	1.91	2.06	3.44	1.09	3.95	217	207	198	146	142	5.6	5.0	3,210	336
	70	0.67	48	1.91	2.29	3.27	1.21	4.38	239	229	219	161	158	6.1	5.5	3,745	392
	80	0.72	52	1.91	2.50	3.13	1.33	4.78	261	249	238	175	172	6.6	6.0	4,280	448
	90	0.76	55	1.91	2.69	2.99	1.43	5.14	279	266	255	187	185	7.0	6.5	4,815	504
	100	0.81	59	1.91	2.89	2.89	1.53	5.53	300	286	274	201	199	7.4	6.9	5,350	560
	120	0.90	65	1.91	3.26	2.72	1.73	6.24	337	322	308	227	225	8.3	7.8	6,420	672
	140	0.97	70	1.91	3.59	2.57	1.91	6.87	370	353	338	249	248	9.0	8.6	7,490	784
Late lactation (Parlor production only; milk yield = 0.85 to 1.35 kg/d)																	
	60	0.85	50	1.91	2.35	3.91	1.24	4.48	261	249	238	175	162	6.8	6.0	3,210	336
	70	0.92	54	1.91	2.58	3.69	1.37	4.93	285	272	260	192	178	7.3	6.6	3,745	392
	80	0.99	59	1.91	2.82	3.52	1.50	5.39	310	296	283	208	194	7.9	7.2	4,280	448
	90	1.06	62	1.91	3.04	3.37	1.61	5.80	333	318	304	224	209	8.5	7.7	4,815	504
	100	1.12	66	1.91	3.25	3.25	1.72	6.21	356	339	325	239	224	9.0	8.3	5,350	560
	120	1.24	73	1.91	3.66	3.05	1.94	6.99	399	381	364	268	252	10.0	9.3	6,420	672
	140	1.35	80	1.91	4.05	2.89	2.15	7.74	440	420	402	296	279	10.9	10.2	7,490	784
Yearling Farm Ewes																	
Maintenance only																	
	40		0	1.91	0.8216	2.05	0.44	1.57	60	58	55	41	57	1.8	1.4	1,256	212
	50		0	1.91	0.9713	1.94	0.51	1.86	71	68	65	48	67	2.1	1.6	1,570	265
	60		0	1.91	1.1136	1.86	0.59	2.13	81	77	74	54	77	2.3	1.9	1,884	318
	70		0	1.91	1.2501	1.79	0.66	2.39	91	87	83	61	86	2.5	2.2	2,198	371
	80		0	1.91	1.3818	1.73	0.73	2.64	101	96	92	68	95	2.7	2.4	2,512	424
	90		0	1.91	1.5094	1.68	0.80	2.89	110	105	101	74	104	2.9	2.6	2,826	477
	100		0	1.91	1.6335	1.63	0.87	3.12	119	114	109	80	113	3.1	2.9	3,140	530
	120		0	1.91	1.8729	1.56	0.99	3.58	137	131	126	92	129	3.5	3.3	3,768	636

Values for maintenance plus growth, breeding, and pregnancy plus growth in yearling ewes are included in Table 15-2.

Early lactation (Single lamb; milk yield = 0.71 to 1.22 kg/d)																	
40	0.71	−14	1.91	1.41	3.53	0.75	2.70	167	159	152	112	97	4.5	4.0	2,140	224
50	0.79	−16	1.91	1.63	3.25	0.86	3.11	189	180	172	127	112	5.0	4.6	2,675	280
60	0.87	−17	1.91	1.84	3.06	0.97	3.51	211	202	193	142	127	5.5	5.1	3,210	336
70	0.94	−19	1.91	2.03	2.90	1.08	3.88	231	221	211	155	140	6.0	5.6	3,745	392
80	1.00	−20	1.91	2.21	2.76	1.17	4.23	250	239	228	168	152	6.4	6.1	4,280	448
90	1.06	−21	1.91	2.39	2.65	1.27	4.57	268	256	245	180	165	6.8	6.6	4,815	504
100	1.12	−22	1.91	2.56	2.56	1.36	4.90	287	274	262	193	177	7.2	7.0	5,350	560
120	1.22	−24	1.91	2.88	2.40	1.53	5.51	320	305	292	215	199	8.0	7.8	6,420	672
Early lactation (Twin lambs; milk yield = 1.18 to 2.05 kg/d)																	
40	1.18	−24	2.39	1.44	3.60	0.95	3.44	224	214	205	151	124	6.0	5.1	2,140	224
50	1.32	−26	2.39	1.65	3.31	1.10	3.96	255	243	232	171	143	6.7	5.8	2,675	280
60	1.45	−29	1.91	2.32	3.86	1.23	4.43	298	284	272	200	160	8.0	7.3	3,210	336
70	1.56	−31	1.91	2.55	3.64	1.35	4.87	324	310	296	218	175	8.6	7.9	3,745	392
80	1.67	−33	1.91	2.77	3.46	1.47	5.29	350	335	320	236	191	9.3	8.6	4,280	448
90	1.77	−35	1.91	2.98	3.31	1.58	5.70	375	358	342	252	205	9.8	9.2	4,815	504
100	1.87	−37	1.91	3.19	3.19	1.69	6.09	399	381	364	268	220	10.4	9.8	5,350	560
120	2.05	−41	1.91	3.57	2.98	1.89	6.83	444	424	405	298	246	11.5	10.9	6,420	672
Early lactation (Three or more lambs; milk yield = 1.53 to 2.66 kg/d)																	
40	1.53	−31	2.87	1.39	3.48	1.11	4.00	265	253	242	178	144	7.1	5.7	2,140	224
50	1.72	−34	2.39	1.92	3.84	1.27	4.59	312	298	285	210	166	8.3	7.1	2,675	280
60	1.88	−38	2.39	2.14	3.56	1.42	5.11	344	328	314	231	184	9.1	7.9	3,210	336
70	2.03	−41	2.39	2.35	3.35	1.56	5.61	374	357	342	252	202	9.9	8.6	3,745	392
80	2.17	−43	1.91	3.19	3.98	1.69	6.09	425	406	388	286	220	11.4	10.4	4,280	448
90	2.30	−46	1.91	3.42	3.80	1.81	6.54	454	433	414	305	236	12.1	11.1	4,815	504
100	2.43	−49	1.91	3.65	3.65	1.93	6.98	482	461	441	324	252	12.8	11.8	5,350	560
120	2.66	−53	1.91	4.08	3.40	2.16	7.80	535	511	489	360	281	14.0	13.1	6,420	672
Mid-lactation (Single lamb; milk yield = 0.47 to 0.82 kg/d)																	
40	0.47	0	1.91	1.25	3.12	0.66	2.38	135	129	124	91	86	3.5	3.2	2,140	224
50	0.53	0	1.91	1.45	2.90	0.77	2.77	156	148	142	105	100	4.0	3.7	2,675	280
60	0.58	0	1.91	1.64	2.73	0.87	3.13	174	166	159	117	113	4.4	4.1	3,210	336
70	0.63	0	1.91	1.82	2.60	0.96	3.48	192	183	175	129	125	4.7	4.6	3,745	392
80	0.67	0	1.91	1.99	2.48	1.05	3.80	208	198	190	139	137	5.1	5.0	4,280	448
90	0.71	0	1.91	2.15	2.39	1.14	4.11	223	213	204	150	148	5.4	5.4	4,815	504
100	0.75	0	1.91	2.31	2.31	1.22	4.42	239	228	218	161	159	5.7	5.7	5,350	560
120	0.82	0	1.91	2.61	2.18	1.38	4.99	268	256	245	180	180	6.3	6.4	6,420	672
Mid-lactation (Twin lambs; milk yield = 0.79 to 1.37 kg/d)																	
40	0.79	0	1.91	1.54	3.85	0.82	2.94	187	178	171	125	106	4.9	4.4	2,140	224
50	0.89	0	1.91	1.78	3.56	0.94	3.40	213	204	195	143	123	5.5	5.0	2,675	280
60	0.97	0	1.91	1.99	3.32	1.06	3.81	236	225	216	159	137	6.0	5.6	3,210	336
70	1.05	0	1.91	2.20	3.15	1.17	4.21	259	247	236	174	152	6.6	6.2	3,745	392
80	1.12	0	1.91	2.40	3.00	1.27	4.59	280	267	255	188	165	7.0	6.7	4,280	448
90	1.19	0	1.91	2.59	2.88	1.37	4.95	300	287	274	202	178	7.5	7.2	4,815	504
100	1.25	0	1.91	2.77	2.77	1.47	5.29	319	305	291	214	191	7.9	7.7	5,350	560
120	1.37	0	1.91	3.12	2.60	1.65	5.96	356	340	325	240	215	8.7	8.6	6,420	672

TABLE 15-1 continued

Class/Age/Other	Body Weight[a] kg	Birth Weight or Milk Yield[b] kg	Body Weight Gain[c] g/d	Energy Concentration in Diet[d] kcal/kg	Daily Dry Matter Intake[e] kg	Daily Dry Matter Intake[e] % BW	Energy Requirements[f] TDN kg/d	Energy Requirements[f] ME Mcal/d	Protein Requirements[g] CP @20% UIP g/d	Protein Requirements[g] CP @40% UIP g/d	Protein Requirements[g] CP @60% UIP g/d	Protein Requirements[g] MP g/d	Protein Requirements[g] DIP g/d	Mineral Requirements[h] Ca g/d	Mineral Requirements[h] P g/d	Vitamin Requirements[i] A RE/d	Vitamin Requirements[i] E IU/d
Mid-lactation (Three or more lambs; milk yield = 1.03 to 1.78 kg/d)																	
	40	1.03	0	2.39	1.41	3.52	0.93	3.36	213	204	195	143	121	5.5	4.7	2,140	224
	50	1.15	0	2.39	1.61	3.23	1.07	3.86	241	230	220	162	139	6.1	5.3	2,675	280
	60	1.26	0	1.91	2.26	3.77	1.20	4.32	283	270	258	190	156	7.3	6.7	3,210	336
	70	1.36	0	1.91	2.49	3.55	1.32	4.76	309	295	282	207	171	7.9	7.4	3,745	392
	80	1.45	0	1.91	2.70	3.38	1.43	5.16	333	317	304	223	186	8.5	8.0	4,280	448
	90	1.54	0	1.91	2.91	3.23	1.54	5.56	356	340	325	240	201	9.0	8.5	4,815	504
	100	1.62	0	1.91	3.11	3.11	1.65	5.94	378	361	346	254	214	9.5	9.1	5,350	560
	120	1.78	0	1.91	3.49	2.91	1.85	6.67	422	403	385	284	241	10.5	10.1	6,420	672
Late lactation (Single lamb; milk yield = 0.23 to 0.41 kg/d)																	
	40	0.23	60	1.91	1.55	3.86	0.82	2.95	142	135	129	95	107	3.9	2.5	2,140	224
	50	0.25	61	1.91	1.83	3.65	0.97	3.49	165	158	151	111	126	4.4	2.9	2,675	280
	60	0.28	72	1.91	2.11	3.52	1.12	4.03	190	181	173	128	145	5.0	3.4	3,210	336
	70	0.31	84	1.91	2.40	3.42	1.27	4.58	215	205	197	145	165	5.6	3.8	3,745	392
	80	0.33	95	1.91	2.66	3.32	1.41	5.09	238	227	217	160	183	6.1	4.3	4,280	448
	90	0.35	106	1.91	2.92	3.24	1.55	5.58	260	248	238	175	201	6.6	4.7	4,815	504
	100	0.37	117	1.91	3.17	3.17	1.68	6.07	283	270	258	190	219	7.2	5.1	5,350	560
	120	0.41	138	1.91	3.67	3.06	1.94	7.01	326	311	297	219	253	8.2	5.9	6,420	672
Late lactation (Twin lambs; milk yield = 0.38 to 0.69 kg/d)																	
	40	0.38	65	2.39	1.47	3.68	0.97	3.51	167	159	152	112	127	4.4	2.8	2,140	224
	50	0.43	78	2.39	1.73	3.47	1.15	4.14	195	186	178	131	149	5.0	3.3	2,675	280
	60	0.47	91	2.39	1.98	3.31	1.32	4.74	221	211	201	148	171	5.7	3.8	3,210	336
	70	0.51	104	1.91	2.79	3.98	1.48	5.33	265	253	242	178	192	7.0	4.8	3,745	392
	80	0.55	117	1.91	3.09	3.86	1.64	5.91	293	279	267	197	213	7.6	5.4	4,280	448
	90	0.59	129	1.91	3.38	3.75	1.79	6.46	319	305	292	215	233	8.3	5.8	4,815	504
	100	0.62	141	1.91	3.65	3.65	1.94	6.98	344	328	314	231	252	8.9	6.3	5,350	560
	120	0.69	166	1.91	4.21	3.51	2.23	8.06	396	378	361	266	290	10.1	7.2	6,420	672
Late lactation (Three or more lambs; milk yield = 0.55 to 0.90 kg/d)																	
	50	0.55	90	2.39	1.92	3.84	1.27	4.59	223	213	203	150	166	5.8	3.9	2,675	280
	60	0.61	104	2.39	2.19	3.66	1.45	5.25	253	241	231	170	189	6.6	4.4	3,210	336
	70	0.67	118	2.39	2.46	3.52	1.63	5.89	282	270	258	190	212	7.2	4.9	3,745	392
	80	0.72	132	2.39	2.72	3.40	1.80	6.50	310	296	283	209	234	7.9	5.4	4,280	448
	90	0.76	145	2.39	2.96	3.29	1.96	7.07	336	321	307	226	255	8.5	5.8	4,815	504
	100	0.81	159	2.39	3.21	3.21	2.13	7.67	363	347	332	244	277	9.2	6.3	5,350	560
	120	0.90	185	1.91	4.60	3.84	2.44	8.80	446	426	407	300	317	11.5	8.3	6,420	672
Yearling Range Ewes																	
Maintenance only																	
	40		0	1.91	0.80	1.99	0.42	1.52	60	57	55	40	55	1.8	1.3	1,256	212
	50		0	1.91	0.94	1.89	0.50	1.80	70	67	64	47	65	2.0	1.6	1,570	265

60		0	1.91	1.08	1.80	0.57	2.07	80	77	73	54	74	2.3	1.8	1,884	318
70		0	1.91	1.21	1.73	0.64	2.32	90	86	82	60	84	2.5	2.1	2,198	371
80		0	1.91	1.34	1.68	0.71	2.56	99	95	91	67	92	2.7	2.3	2,512	424
90		0	1.91	1.46	1.63	0.78	2.80	109	104	99	73	101	2.9	2.5	2,826	477
100		0	1.91	1.59	1.59	0.84	3.03	118	113	108	79	109	3.0	2.8	3,140	530
120		0	1.91	1.82	1.51	0.96	3.48	136	130	124	91	125	3.4	3.2	3,768	636
Values for maintenance plus growth, breeding, and pregnancy plus growth in yearling ewes are included in Table 15-2.																
Early lactation (Single lamb; milk yield = 0.71 to 1.22 kg/d)																
40	0.71	–14	1.91	1.39	3.47	0.74	2.66	166	159	152	112	96	4.4	3.9	2,140	224
50	0.79	–16	1.91	1.60	3.20	0.85	3.06	188	180	172	127	110	5.0	4.5	2,675	280
60	0.87	–17	1.91	1.81	3.01	0.96	3.45	211	201	192	142	125	5.5	5.1	3,210	336
70	0.94	–19	1.91	1.99	2.85	1.06	3.81	231	220	211	155	137	5.9	5.6	3,745	392
80	1.00	–20	1.91	2.17	2.72	1.15	4.16	249	238	228	167	150	6.4	6.0	4,280	448
90	1.06	–21	1.91	2.35	2.61	1.24	4.49	268	255	244	180	162	6.8	6.5	4,815	504
100	1.12	–22	1.91	2.52	2.52	1.34	4.82	286	273	261	192	174	7.2	6.9	5,350	560
120	1.22	–24	1.91	2.83	2.36	1.50	5.42	319	304	291	214	195	7.9	7.7	6,420	672
Early lactation (Twin lambs; milk yield = 1.18 to 2.05 kg/d)																
40	1.18	–24	2.39	1.42	3.56	0.94	3.40	224	214	205	151	123	6.0	5.0	2,140	224
50	1.32	–26	2.39	1.63	3.27	1.08	3.91	254	243	232	171	141	6.7	5.7	2,675	280
60	1.45	–29	1.91	2.29	3.81	1.21	4.37	297	284	271	200	158	7.9	7.2	3,210	336
70	1.56	–31	1.91	2.51	3.59	1.33	4.80	324	309	295	217	173	8.6	7.9	3,745	392
80	1.67	–33	1.91	2.73	3.42	1.45	5.22	350	334	319	235	188	9.2	8.5	4,280	448
90	1.77	–35	1.91	2.94	3.27	1.56	5.62	374	357	341	251	203	9.8	9.1	4,815	504
100	1.87	–37	1.91	3.14	3.14	1.67	6.01	398	380	364	268	217	10.3	9.7	5,350	560
120	2.05	–41	1.91	3.52	2.94	1.87	6.74	443	423	404	298	243	11.4	10.8	6,420	672
Early lactation (Three or more lambs; milk yield = 1.53 to 2.66 kg/d)																
40	1.53	–31	2.87	1.38	3.45	1.10	3.96	265	253	242	178	143	7.1	5.7	2,140	224
50	1.72	–34	2.39	1.90	3.80	1.26	4.54	312	298	285	210	164	8.3	7.1	2,675	280
60	1.88	–38	2.39	2.11	3.52	1.40	5.05	344	328	314	231	182	9.1	7.8	3,210	336
70	2.03	–41	2.39	2.32	3.32	1.54	5.55	374	357	342	251	200	9.8	8.5	3,745	392
80	2.17	–43	1.91	3.15	3.94	1.67	6.02	425	405	388	285	217	11.3	10.4	4,280	448
90	2.30	–46	1.91	3.38	3.75	1.79	6.46	453	433	414	305	233	12.0	11.1	4,815	504
100	2.43	–49	1.91	3.61	3.61	1.91	6.89	482	460	440	324	249	12.7	11.8	5,350	560
120	2.66	–53	1.91	4.03	3.36	2.14	7.71	534	510	488	359	278	14.0	13.0	6,420	672
Mid-lactation (Single lamb; milk yield = 0.47 to 0.82 kg/d)																
40	0.47	0	1.91	1.22	3.06	0.65	2.34	135	129	123	91	84	3.5	3.1	2,140	224
50	0.53	0	1.91	1.42	2.85	0.76	2.72	155	148	142	104	98	3.9	3.6	2,675	280
60	0.58	0	1.91	1.61	2.68	0.85	3.07	173	165	158	116	111	4.3	4.1	3,210	336
70	0.63	0	1.91	1.79	2.55	0.95	3.41	191	182	174	128	123	4.7	4.5	3,745	392
80	0.67	0	1.91	1.95	2.44	1.03	3.73	207	197	189	139	134	5.0	4.9	4,280	448
90	0.71	0	1.91	2.11	2.34	1.12	4.03	223	212	203	150	145	5.4	5.3	4,815	504
100	0.75	0	1.91	2.27	2.27	1.20	4.33	238	227	217	160	156	5.7	5.7	5,350	560
120	0.82	0	1.91	2.56	2.14	1.36	4.90	267	255	244	180	177	6.3	6.4	6,420	672

TABLE 15-1 continued

Class/Age/Other	Body Weight[a] kg	Birth Weight or Milk Yield[b] kg	Body Weight Gain[c] g/d	Energy Concentration in Diet[d] kcal/kg	Daily Dry Matter Intake[e] kg	Daily Dry Matter Intake[e] % BW	Energy Requirements[f] TDN kg/d	Energy Requirements[f] ME Mcal/d	Protein Requirements[g] CP @20% UIP g/d	CP @40% UIP g/d	CP @60% UIP g/d	MP g/d	DIP g/d	Mineral Requirements[h] Ca g/d	P g/d	Vitamin Requirements[i] A RE/d	E IU/d
Mid-lactation (Twin lambs; milk yield = 0.79 to 1.37 kg/d)																	
	40	0.79	0	1.91	1.52	3.79	0.80	2.90	186	178	170	125	105	4.9	4.4	2,140	224
	50	0.89	0	1.91	1.75	3.51	0.93	3.35	213	203	194	143	121	5.5	5.0	2,675	280
	60	0.97	0	1.91	1.96	3.27	1.04	3.76	236	225	215	158	135	6.0	5.6	3,210	336
	70	1.05	0	1.91	2.17	3.10	1.15	4.15	258	246	236	174	150	6.5	6.1	3,745	392
	80	1.12	0	1.91	2.36	2.95	1.25	4.52	279	266	255	187	163	7.0	6.6	4,280	448
	90	1.19	0	1.91	2.55	2.83	1.35	4.87	300	286	274	201	176	7.4	7.1	4,815	504
	100	1.25	0	1.91	2.72	2.72	1.44	5.21	318	304	291	214	188	7.9	7.6	5,350	560
	120	1.37	0	1.91	3.07	2.55	1.63	5.86	356	339	325	239	211	8.7	8.5	6,420	672
Mid-lactation (Three or more lambs; milk yield = 1.03 to 1.78 kg/d)																	
	40	1.03	0	2.39	1.39	3.47	0.92	3.32	213	203	195	143	120	5.5	4.6	2,140	224
	50	1.15	0	1.91	1.99	3.98	1.06	3.81	254	243	232	171	137	6.6	6.0	2,675	280
	60	1.26	0	1.91	2.23	3.72	1.18	4.26	282	269	258	190	154	7.3	6.7	3,210	336
	70	1.36	0	1.91	2.45	3.51	1.30	4.69	308	294	281	207	169	7.9	7.3	3,745	392
	80	1.45	0	1.91	2.66	3.33	1.41	5.09	332	317	303	223	184	8.4	7.9	4,280	448
	90	1.54	0	1.91	2.87	3.19	1.52	5.49	356	340	325	239	198	9.0	8.5	4,815	504
	100	1.62	0	1.91	3.06	3.06	1.62	5.86	378	361	345	254	211	9.5	9.0	5,350	560
	120	1.78	0	1.91	3.44	2.87	1.82	6.58	421	402	385	283	237	10.4	10.0	6,420	672
Late lactation (Single lamb; milk yield = 0.23 to 0.41 kg/d)																	
	40	0.23	50	1.91	1.52	3.81	0.81	2.91	141	135	129	95	105	3.7	2.4	2,140	224
	50	0.25	61	1.91	1.80	3.60	0.95	3.44	165	157	150	111	124	4.3	2.9	2,675	280
	60	0.28	72	1.91	2.08	3.46	1.10	3.97	189	181	173	127	143	4.9	3.3	3,210	336
	70	0.31	84	1.91	2.36	3.37	1.25	4.52	215	205	196	144	163	5.5	3.8	3,745	392
	80	0.33	95	1.91	2.62	3.28	1.39	5.01	237	227	217	159	181	6.1	4.2	4,280	448
	90	0.35	106	1.91	2.88	3.20	1.53	5.50	260	248	237	175	198	6.6	4.6	4,815	504
	100	0.37	117	1.91	3.13	3.13	1.66	5.98	282	269	257	189	216	7.1	5.0	5,350	560
	120	0.41	138	1.91	3.61	3.01	1.92	6.91	325	310	297	218	249	8.1	5.8	6,420	672
Late lactation (Twin lambs; milk yield = 0.38 to 0.69 kg/d)																	
	40	0.38	65	2.39	1.45	3.63	0.96	3.47	167	159	152	112	125	4.3	2.8	2,140	224
	50	0.43	78	2.39	1.71	3.42	1.13	4.09	194	186	177	131	148	5.0	3.3	2,675	280
	60	0.47	91	2.39	1.96	3.27	1.30	4.68	220	210	201	148	169	5.6	3.7	3,210	336
	70	0.51	104	1.91	2.75	3.93	1.46	5.26	265	253	242	178	190	6.9	4.8	3,745	392
	80	0.55	117	1.91	3.05	3.81	1.62	5.83	292	279	267	196	210	7.6	5.3	4,280	448
	90	0.59	129	1.91	3.34	3.71	1.77	6.38	319	304	291	214	230	8.2	5.8	4,815	504
	100	0.62	141	1.91	3.61	3.61	1.91	6.90	344	328	314	231	249	8.9	6.3	5,350	560
	120	0.69	166	1.91	4.16	3.47	2.21	7.96	395	377	361	265	287	10.1	7.2	6,420	672
Late lactation (Three or more lambs; milk yield = 0.55 to 0.90 kg/d)																	
	50	0.55	90	2.39	1.90	3.80	1.26	4.54	223	213	203	150	164	5.8	3.8	2,675	280
	60	0.61	104	2.39	2.17	3.62	1.44	5.19	253	241	231	170	187	6.5	4.4	3,210	336

	70	0.67	118	2.39	2.44	3.48	1.61	5.82	282	270	258	190	210	7.2	4.9	3,745	392
	80	0.72	132	2.39	2.69	3.36	1.78	6.43	310	296	283	209	232	7.9	5.3	4,280	448
	90	0.76	145	2.39	2.93	3.25	1.94	6.99	336	320	307	226	252	8.5	5.8	4,815	504
	100	0.81	159	1.91	3.97	3.97	2.10	7.59	390	372	356	262	274	10.1	7.2	5,350	560
	120	0.90	185	1.91	4.55	3.79	2.41	8.70	446	425	407	300	314	11.5	8.2	6,420	672
Rams																	
Maintenance	100		0	1.91	1.77	1.77	0.94	3.38	128	122	117	86	122	3.3	3.1	3,140	530
	125		0	1.91	2.09	1.67	1.11	4.00	152	145	139	102	144	3.8	3.7	3,925	663
	150		0	1.91	2.40	1.60	1.27	4.58	175	168	160	118	165	4.3	4.3	4,710	795
	200		0	1.91	2.98	1.49	1.58	5.69	220	210	201	148	205	5.2	5.3	6,280	1,060
Prebreeding	100		47	1.91	1.95	1.95	1.03	3.72	150	144	137	101	134	3.6	3.4	4,550	560
	125		56	1.91	2.30	1.84	1.22	4.40	179	171	163	120	159	4.2	4.1	5,688	700
	150		64	1.91	2.64	1.76	1.40	5.04	206	197	188	139	182	4.7	4.7	6,825	840
	200		79	1.91	3.27	1.64	1.74	6.26	259	247	236	174	226	5.7	5.9	9,100	1,120

[a]Body weight used in estimating requirements is the determined or estimated weight in kilograms (kg) average for the period during which these requirements will be applied.
[b]Birth weight (kg) of single and average of multiple lambs or liquid milk yield (kg/d).
[c]Average change in body weight over a 24-hour period.
[d]Three hypothetical diets with increasing energy concentrations (1.91, 2.34, and 2.87 kcal/kg) were used in the calculations of intake and nutrient requirements. For each line entry, a diet was selected to represent the level of energy concentration that approximates that needed by the animal to achieve adequate intake to satisfy its energy requirement.
[e]The daily dry matter intake, expressed as kg or as percentage of body weight, of a diet having the indicated energy concentration (previous column) that is required to meet energy requirements. These energy concentrations should be viewed only as examples. In some cases, diets having greater or lesser concentrations of energy would be more appropriate.
[f]Energy requirements expressed as total digestible nutrients (TDN) in kg/d and metabolizable energy (ME) as kcal/d.
[g]Protein requirements expressed as crude protein (CP), metabolizable protein (MP), and degradable intake protein (DIP). The CP requirement differs with the proportion of undegradable intake protein (UIP) because of the required minimal DIP.
[h]Two macro minerals, calcium (Ca) and phosphorus (P), commonly considered in balancing diets are included. Often, the balance (ratio) of the two minerals also is of concern.
[i]Two fat-soluble vitamins, A and E, that often are deficient in animal diets are expressed as retinol equivalents (RE) and international units (IU) for vitamins A and E, respectively. RE = 1.0 μg of all-trans retinol, 5.0 μg of all-trans betacarotene, and 7.6 μg of other carotenoids.

TABLE 15-2 Nutrient Requirements of Sheep (growing, finishing lambs, and yearlings during growth/gestation)

Class/Age/Other	Body Weight[a] kg	Birth Weight or Milk Yield[b] kg	Body Weight Gain[c,d] g/d	Energy Concentration in Diet[e] kcal/kg	Daily Dry Matter Intake[f] kg	Daily Dry Matter Intake[f] % BW	Energy Requirements[g] TDN kg/d	ME Mcal/d	NEm Mcal/d	NEg Mcal/d	Protein Requirements[h] CP @20% UIP g/d	CP @40% UIP g/d	CP @60% UIP g/d	MP g/d	DIP g/d	Mineral Requirements[i] Ca g/d	P g/d	Vitamin Requirements[j] A RE/d	E IU/d
Growing Lambs and Yearlings																			
	20		100	1.91	0.57	2.86	0.30	1.09	0.20	0.21	76	73	69	51	39	2.3	1.5	2,000	200
Age = 4 months	20		150	1.91	0.78	3.91	0.41	1.50	0.21	0.32	104	99	95	70	54	3.1	2.2	2,000	200
Maturity = 0.3	20		200	2.39	0.59	2.97	0.39	1.42	0.21	0.42	116	111	106	78	51	3.7	2.5	2,000	200
(late maturing)	20		300	2.87	0.61	3.04	0.48	1.74	0.21	0.63	155	148	142	104	63	5.1	3.5	2,000	200
	30		200	1.91	1.05	3.51	0.56	2.02	0.29	0.42	137	131	125	92	73	4.1	2.9	3,000	300
	30		250	2.39	0.76	2.53	0.50	1.82	0.29	0.53	145	139	133	98	65	4.5	3.2	3,000	300
	30		300	2.39	0.88	2.93	0.58	2.10	0.29	0.63	169	162	155	114	76	5.3	3.8	3,000	300
	30		400	2.39	1.12	3.72	0.74	2.67	0.30	0.84	218	208	199	146	96	6.9	5.0	3,000	300
	40		250	1.91	1.32	3.31	0.70	2.53	0.37	0.53	171	163	156	115	91	5.0	3.7	4,000	400
	40		300	1.91	1.54	3.84	0.82	2.94	0.38	0.63	199	190	182	134	106	5.9	4.4	4,000	400
	40		400	2.39	1.16	2.91	0.77	2.78	0.38	0.84	223	213	204	150	100	7.0	5.1	4,000	400
	40		500	2.39	1.40	3.51	0.93	3.35	0.39	1.05	271	259	248	182	121	8.6	6.3	4,000	400
	50		250	1.91	1.38	2.76	0.73	2.64	0.44	0.53	177	169	161	119	95	5.1	3.8	5,000	500
	50		300	1.91	1.59	3.19	0.85	3.05	0.45	0.63	205	195	187	137	110	6.0	4.5	5,000	500
	50		400	2.39	1.21	2.42	0.80	2.89	0.45	0.84	228	218	208	153	104	7.0	5.1	5,000	500
	50		500	2.39	1.45	2.90	0.96	3.47	0.47	1.05	277	264	253	186	125	8.6	6.3	5,000	500
	50		600	2.39	1.69	3.38	1.12	4.04	0.48	1.26	325	310	297	219	146	10.2	7.6	5,000	500
	60		250	1.91	1.43	2.39	0.76	2.74	0.50	0.53	182	174	166	122	99	5.1	3.8	6,000	600
	60		300	1.91	1.65	2.75	0.87	3.15	0.52	0.63	210	201	192	141	114	6.0	4.5	6,000	600
	60		400	1.91	2.08	3.47	1.10	3.98	0.55	0.84	266	254	243	179	143	7.8	5.9	6,000	600
	60		500	2.39	1.49	2.49	0.99	3.57	0.53	1.05	282	269	257	190	129	8.7	6.4	6,000	600
	60		600	2.39	1.74	2.90	1.15	4.15	0.55	1.26	330	315	302	222	150	10.3	7.6	6,000	600
	70		150	1.91	1.04	1.49	0.55	2.00	0.53	0.32	131	125	120	88	72	3.4	2.4	7,000	700
	70		200	1.91	1.26	1.80	0.67	2.42	0.55	0.42	159	152	146	107	87	4.3	3.1	7,000	700
	70		300	1.91	1.70	2.43	0.90	3.25	0.58	0.63	216	206	197	145	117	6.1	4.6	7,000	700
	70		400	1.91	2.14	3.05	1.13	4.08	0.62	0.84	272	259	248	183	147	7.9	6.0	7,000	700
	70		500	1.91	2.57	3.68	1.36	4.92	0.65	1.05	328	313	300	220	177	9.6	7.4	7,000	700
	80		150	1.91	1.09	1.36	0.58	2.08	0.59	0.32	137	130	125	92	75	3.4	2.5	8,000	800
	80		200	1.91	1.31	1.64	0.69	2.50	0.61	0.42	165	157	150	111	90	4.3	3.2	8,000	800
	80		300	1.91	1.75	2.19	0.93	3.34	0.64	0.63	221	211	202	149	121	6.1	4.6	8,000	800
	80		400	1.91	2.19	2.74	1.16	4.19	0.68	0.84	277	265	253	186	151	7.9	6.0	8,000	800
	80		500	1.91	2.63	3.29	1.39	5.03	0.72	1.05	334	318	305	224	181	9.7	7.5	8,000	800
	20		100	2.39	0.63	3.16	0.42	1.51	0.21	0.46	70	66	64	47	55	2.1	1.5	2,000	200
Age = 4 months	20		150	2.87	0.65	3.25	0.52	1.87	0.21	0.68	84	80	77	57	67	2.6	2.0	2,000	200
Maturity = 0.6	20		200	2.87	0.83	4.17	0.66	2.39	0.22	0.91	106	101	97	71	86	3.4	2.7	2,000	200
(early maturing)	20		300	2.87	1.20	6.00	0.95	3.44	0.24	1.37	149	142	136	100	124	4.9	4.0	2,000	200
	30		200	2.39	1.20	3.99	0.79	2.86	0.31	0.91	125	119	114	84	103	3.7	3.0	3,000	300
	30		250	2.87	1.06	3.54	0.84	3.04	0.31	1.14	133	127	122	89	110	4.2	3.4	3,000	300
	30		300	2.87	1.25	4.15	0.99	3.57	0.32	1.37	155	148	141	104	129	4.9	4.0	3,000	300
	30		400	2.87	1.62	5.38	1.28	4.63	0.35	1.83	198	189	181	133	167	6.4	5.4	3,000	300
	40		250	2.39	1.50	3.76	1.00	3.60	0.40	1.14	155	148	142	104	130	4.6	3.8	4,000	400

	40	300	2.87	1.29	3.22	1.02	3.69	0.40	1.37	160	153	146	108	133	5.0	4.1	4,000	400
	40	400	2.87	1.66	4.15	1.32	4.76	0.43	1.83	204	195	186	137	172	6.4	5.4	4,000	400
	40	500	2.87	2.03	5.08	1.62	5.83	0.46	2.28	247	236	226	166	210	7.9	6.7	4,000	400
	50	250	2.39	1.55	3.10	1.03	3.71	0.47	1.14	161	154	147	108	134	4.6	3.8	5,000	500
	50	300	2.39	1.81	3.63	1.20	4.34	0.49	1.37	186	178	170	125	156	5.4	4.6	5,000	500
	50	400	2.87	1.70	3.41	1.35	4.88	0.51	1.83	209	200	191	141	176	6.5	5.4	5,000	500
	50	500	2.87	2.08	4.16	1.65	5.96	0.54	2.28	253	242	231	170	215	8.0	6.8	5,000	500
	50	600	2.87	2.45	4.91	1.95	7.04	0.58	2.74	297	283	271	199	254	9.5	8.1	5,000	500
	60	250	2.39	1.60	2.66	1.06	3.82	0.54	1.14	167	159	152	112	138	4.7	3.9	6,000	600
	60	300	2.39	1.86	3.10	1.23	4.45	0.57	1.37	192	183	175	129	160	5.5	4.6	6,000	600
	60	400	2.39	2.39	3.98	1.58	5.71	0.61	1.83	242	231	221	163	206	7.1	6.1	6,000	600
	60	500	2.87	2.12	3.54	1.69	6.08	0.62	2.28	259	247	236	174	219	8.0	6.8	6,000	600
	60	600	2.87	2.50	4.17	1.99	7.17	0.66	2.74	302	289	276	203	258	9.5	8.1	6,000	600
	70	150	1.91	1.81	2.59	0.96	3.46	0.59	0.68	152	145	139	102	125	3.7	3.1	7,000	700
	70	200	1.91	2.28	3.26	1.21	4.37	0.63	0.91	186	177	170	125	157	4.7	4.1	7,000	700
	70	300	2.39	1.91	2.72	1.26	4.55	0.63	1.37	197	188	180	133	164	5.5	4.7	7,000	700
	70	400	2.39	2.44	3.48	1.62	5.82	0.69	1.83	248	237	226	167	210	7.1	6.1	7,000	700
	70	500	2.87	2.16	3.09	1.72	6.20	0.70	2.28	264	252	241	178	224	8.0	6.8	7,000	700
	80	150	1.91	1.86	2.33	0.99	3.56	0.65	0.68	157	150	144	106	128	3.8	3.2	8,000	800
	80	200	1.91	2.34	2.92	1.24	4.47	0.69	0.91	192	183	175	129	161	4.8	4.1	8,000	800
	80	300	2.39	1.95	2.44	1.29	4.66	0.70	1.37	203	194	185	136	168	5.6	4.7	8,000	800
	80	400	2.39	2.48	3.10	1.65	5.94	0.76	1.83	253	242	231	170	214	7.2	6.2	8,000	800
	80	500	2.39	3.02	3.77	2.00	7.21	0.82	2.28	304	290	278	204	260	8.8	7.7	8,000	800
	20	100	2.39	0.59	2.94	0.39	1.41	0.41	0.30	73	70	67	49	51	2.2	1.5	2,000	200
Age = 8 months	20	150	2.39	0.76	3.80	0.50	1.81	0.42	0.45	97	93	89	65	65	3.0	2.1	2,000	200
Maturity = 0.4	20	200	2.87	0.70	3.48	0.55	1.99	0.43	0.59	112	107	102	75	72	3.5	2.6	2,000	200
(late maturing)	20	300	2.87	0.94	4.70	0.75	2.69	0.45	0.89	156	149	142	105	97	5.0	3.8	2,000	200
	30	200	2.39	1.03	3.43	0.68	2.46	0.59	0.59	129	123	117	86	89	3.8	2.9	3,000	300
	30	250	2.87	0.90	3.01	0.72	2.59	0.59	0.74	141	135	129	95	93	4.4	3.3	3,000	300
	30	300	2.87	1.03	3.42	0.82	2.94	0.61	0.89	163	156	149	110	106	5.1	3.9	3,000	300
	30	400	2.87	1.27	4.25	1.01	3.66	0.64	1.19	207	198	189	139	132	6.6	5.1	3,000	300
	40	250	2.39	1.30	3.25	0.86	3.10	0.75	0.74	160	153	146	108	112	4.7	3.6	4,000	400
	40	300	2.39	1.48	3.69	0.98	3.53	0.77	0.89	184	176	168	124	127	5.5	4.3	4,000	400
	40	400	2.87	1.36	3.40	1.08	3.90	0.79	1.19	215	205	196	144	140	6.7	5.2	4,000	400
	40	500	2.87	1.61	4.03	1.28	4.62	0.83	1.48	259	247	237	174	167	8.2	6.4	4,000	400
	50	250	2.39	1.39	2.78	0.92	3.32	0.89	0.74	168	160	153	113	120	4.8	3.7	5,000	500
	50	300	2.39	1.57	3.13	1.04	3.74	0.92	0.89	192	183	175	129	135	5.6	4.4	5,000	500
	50	400	2.39	1.92	3.85	1.28	4.60	0.97	1.19	240	230	220	162	166	7.2	5.7	5,000	500
	50	500	2.87	1.69	3.39	1.35	4.86	0.98	1.48	266	254	243	179	175	8.3	6.5	5,000	500
	50	600	2.87	1.95	3.90	1.55	5.59	1.03	1.78	311	297	284	209	202	9.8	7.7	5,000	500
	60	250	1.91	2.32	3.87	1.23	4.44	1.08	0.74	208	198	190	140	160	5.7	4.6	6,000	600
	60	300	2.39	1.65	2.76	1.10	3.95	1.05	0.89	199	190	182	134	143	5.7	4.5	6,000	600
	60	400	2.39	2.02	3.36	1.34	4.82	1.11	1.19	248	237	226	167	174	7.3	5.8	6,000	600
	60	500	2.39	2.38	3.97	1.58	5.69	1.17	1.48	297	283	271	199	205	8.9	7.2	6,000	600
	60	600	2.87	2.03	3.39	1.62	5.83	1.18	1.78	318	304	290	214	210	9.9	7.8	6,000	600
	70	150	1.91	1.78	2.54	0.94	3.40	1.12	0.45	155	148	142	104	122	3.9	3.1	7,000	700
	70	200	1.91	2.10	3.01	1.12	4.02	1.17	0.59	185	177	169	125	145	4.8	3.9	7,000	700
	70	300	1.91	2.76	3.94	1.46	5.28	1.27	0.89	246	235	225	165	190	6.7	5.5	7,000	700
	70	400	2.39	2.11	3.01	1.40	5.03	1.25	1.19	255	244	233	171	181	7.4	5.9	7,000	700

TABLE 15-2 continued

Class/Age/Other	Body Weight[a] kg	Weight or Milk Yield[b] kg	Body Weight Gain[c,d] g/d	Energy Concentration in Diet[e] kcal/kg	Daily Dry Matter Intake[f] kg	Daily Dry Matter Intake[f] % BW	Energy Requirements[g] TDN kg/d	Energy Requirements[g] ME Mcal/d	Energy Requirements[g] NEm Mcal/d	Energy Requirements[g] NEg Mcal/d	Protein Requirements[h] CP @20% UIP g/d	Protein Requirements[h] CP @40% UIP g/d	Protein Requirements[h] CP @60% UIP g/d	Protein Requirements[h] MP g/d	Protein Requirements[h] DIP g/d	Mineral Requirements[i] Ca g/d	Mineral Requirements[i] P g/d	Vitamin Requirements[j] A RE/d	Vitamin Requirements[j] E IU/d
	70		500	2.39	2.47	3.53	1.64	5.91	1.31	1.48	304	290	278	204	213	9.0	7.2	7,000	700
	80		150	1.91	1.87	2.34	0.99	3.58	1.24	0.45	163	155	148	109	129	4.0	3.2	8,000	800
	80		200	1.91	2.20	2.75	1.17	4.21	1.29	0.59	193	184	176	130	152	4.9	4.0	8,000	800
	80		300	1.91	2.87	3.58	1.52	5.48	1.40	0.89	254	242	232	171	198	6.8	5.6	8,000	800
	80		400	2.39	2.19	2.74	1.45	5.24	1.38	1.19	262	250	239	176	189	7.5	6.0	8,000	800
	80		500	2.39	2.56	3.20	1.70	6.13	1.45	1.48	312	297	284	209	221	9.1	7.3	8,000	800
	20		100	2.87	0.65	3.27	0.52	1.88	0.45	0.54	68	65	62	46	68	2.0	1.5	2,000	200
Age = 8 months	20		150	2.87	0.88	4.39	0.70	2.52	0.49	0.82	89	85	82	60	91	2.7	2.2	2,000	200
Maturity = 0.8	20		200	2.87	1.10	5.51	0.88	3.16	0.52	1.09	111	106	101	74	114	3.5	2.9	2,000	200
(early maturing)	20		300	2.87	1.55	7.75	1.23	4.45	0.59	1.63	153	146	140	103	160	4.9	4.3	2,000	200
	30		200	2.87	1.19	3.97	0.95	3.42	0.70	1.09	119	114	109	80	123	3.5	3.0	3,000	300
	30		250	2.87	1.42	4.73	1.13	4.07	0.75	1.36	140	134	128	94	147	4.3	3.7	3,000	300
	30		300	2.87	1.65	5.49	1.31	4.73	0.80	1.63	162	155	148	109	170	5.0	4.4	3,000	300
	30		400	2.87	2.10	7.02	1.67	6.04	0.89	2.18	205	196	187	138	218	6.5	5.8	3,000	300
	40		250	2.87	1.51	3.77	1.20	4.32	0.93	1.36	149	142	136	100	156	4.4	3.8	4,000	400
	40		300	2.87	1.74	4.34	1.38	4.98	0.99	1.63	170	163	155	114	180	5.1	4.5	4,000	400
	40		400	2.87	2.20	5.50	1.75	6.31	1.11	2.18	214	204	195	144	228	6.6	5.9	4,000	400
	40		500	2.87	2.67	6.66	2.12	7.64	1.22	2.72	257	245	235	173	276	8.1	7.3	4,000	400
	50		250	2.87	1.59	3.17	1.26	4.55	1.10	1.36	156	149	143	105	164	4.4	3.8	5,000	500
	50		300	2.87	1.82	3.64	1.45	5.23	1.17	1.63	178	170	163	120	188	5.2	4.5	5,000	500
	50		400	2.87	2.29	4.58	1.82	6.57	1.31	2.18	222	212	203	149	237	6.7	6.0	5,000	500
	50		500	2.87	2.76	5.53	2.20	7.92	1.45	2.72	266	254	243	179	286	8.1	7.4	5,000	500
	50		600	2.87	3.23	6.47	2.57	9.27	1.59	3.27	310	296	283	208	334	9.6	8.8	5,000	500
	60		250	2.39	2.23	3.72	1.48	5.33	1.26	1.36	164	156	150	110	192	5.0	4.5	6,000	600
	60		300	2.87	1.90	3.17	1.51	5.45	1.34	1.63	186	177	170	125	197	5.2	4.6	6,000	600
	60		400	2.87	2.38	3.96	1.89	6.82	1.50	2.18	230	220	210	155	246	6.7	6.0	6,000	600
	60		500	2.87	2.86	4.76	2.27	8.19	1.66	2.72	274	262	250	184	295	8.2	7.5	6,000	600
	60		600	2.87	3.33	5.56	2.65	9.56	1.82	3.27	319	304	291	214	345	9.7	8.9	6,000	600
	70		150	1.91	2.60	3.71	1.38	4.96	1.24	0.82	182	174	167	123	179	4.3	3.9	7,000	700
	70		200	2.39	1.98	2.83	1.31	4.74	1.33	1.09	169	161	154	113	171	4.3	3.7	7,000	700
	70		300	2.39	2.66	3.80	1.76	6.35	1.51	1.63	222	212	202	149	229	5.9	5.3	7,000	700
	70		400	2.87	2.46	3.52	1.96	7.06	1.69	2.18	238	227	217	160	255	6.8	6.1	7,000	700
	70		500	2.87	2.95	4.21	2.34	8.45	1.86	2.72	283	270	258	190	305	8.3	7.5	7,000	700
	80		150	1.91	2.70	3.38	1.43	5.17	1.37	0.82	191	182	174	128	186	4.4	4.0	8,000	800
	80		200	2.39	2.07	2.58	1.37	4.94	1.47	1.09	176	168	161	119	178	4.3	3.8	8,000	800
	80		300	2.39	2.75	3.44	1.82	6.57	1.67	1.63	230	219	210	154	237	6.0	5.4	8,000	800
	80		400	2.87	2.54	3.18	2.02	7.29	1.86	2.18	246	235	224	165	263	6.9	6.2	8,000	800
	80		500	2.87	3.03	3.79	2.41	8.69	2.06	2.72	291	277	265	195	313	8.4	7.6	8,000	800
Growing Rams																			
	20		100	1.91	0.60	2.98	0.32	1.14	0.23	0.21	77	74	70	52	41	2.3	1.5	2,000	200
Age = 4 months	20		150	2.39	0.49	2.47	0.33	1.18	0.23	0.32	93	88	85	62	43	2.9	1.9	2,000	200
Maturity = 0.3	20		200	2.39	0.61	3.07	0.41	1.47	0.24	0.42	117	111	107	78	53	3.7	2.5	2,000	200
(late maturing)	20		300	2.87	0.63	3.13	0.50	1.79	0.24	0.63	156	149	143	105	65	5.1	3.5	2,000	200

	30	200	1.91	1.09	3.63	0.58	2.08	0.33	0.42	139	133	127	93	75	4.1	3.0	3,000	300
	30	250	2.39	0.79	2.62	0.52	1.88	0.33	0.53	147	140	134	98	68	4.5	3.2	3,000	300
	30	300	2.39	0.91	3.02	0.60	2.17	0.34	0.63	171	163	156	115	78	5.3	3.8	3,000	300
	30	400	2.39	1.15	3.82	0.76	2.74	0.35	0.84	219	209	200	147	99	6.9	5.0	3,000	300
	40	250	1.91	1.37	3.42	0.73	2.62	0.43	0.53	173	165	158	116	94	5.1	3.7	4,000	400
	40	300	1.91	1.58	3.96	0.84	3.03	0.44	0.63	201	192	183	135	109	6.0	4.5	4,000	400
	40	400	2.39	1.20	3.00	0.80	2.87	0.43	0.84	225	215	205	151	103	7.0	5.1	4,000	400
	40	500	2.39	1.44	3.60	0.96	3.45	0.45	1.05	273	261	249	184	124	8.6	6.3	4,000	400
	50	250	1.91	1.43	2.87	0.76	2.74	0.50	0.53	179	171	163	120	99	5.1	3.8	5,000	500
	50	300	1.91	1.65	3.30	0.87	3.15	0.52	0.63	207	198	189	139	114	6.0	4.5	5,000	500
	50	400	2.39	1.25	2.50	0.83	2.99	0.51	0.84	230	220	210	155	108	7.0	5.1	5,000	500
	50	500	2.39	1.50	2.99	0.99	3.57	0.54	1.05	279	266	255	187	129	8.7	6.4	5,000	500
	50	600	2.39	1.74	3.48	1.15	4.16	0.56	1.26	327	312	299	220	150	10.3	7.6	5,000	500
	60	250	1.91	1.49	2.49	0.79	2.85	0.58	0.53	185	176	169	124	103	5.2	3.9	6,000	600
	60	300	1.91	1.71	2.85	0.91	3.27	0.60	0.63	213	203	194	143	118	6.1	4.6	6,000	600
	60	400	1.91	2.15	3.58	1.14	4.11	0.63	0.84	269	257	246	181	148	7.9	6.0	6,000	600
	60	500	2.39	1.55	2.58	1.02	3.70	0.61	1.05	284	271	260	191	133	8.7	6.4	6,000	600
	60	600	2.39	1.79	2.99	1.19	4.28	0.64	1.26	333	318	304	224	154	10.3	7.7	6,000	600
	70	150	1.91	1.11	1.59	0.59	2.12	0.61	0.32	134	128	122	90	76	3.4	2.5	7,000	700
	70	200	1.91	1.33	1.90	0.71	2.54	0.63	0.42	162	155	148	109	92	4.3	3.2	7,000	700
	70	300	1.91	1.77	2.53	0.94	3.39	0.67	0.63	219	209	200	147	122	6.1	4.6	7,000	700
	70	400	1.91	2.21	3.16	1.17	4.23	0.71	0.84	275	263	251	185	152	7.9	6.1	7,000	700
	70	500	1.91	2.65	3.79	1.41	5.07	0.75	1.05	331	316	303	223	183	9.7	7.5	7,000	700
	80	150	1.91	1.16	1.45	0.62	2.22	0.67	0.32	140	133	127	94	80	3.5	2.5	8,000	800
	80	200	1.91	1.38	1.73	0.73	2.65	0.70	0.42	168	160	153	113	95	4.4	3.3	8,000	800
	80	300	1.91	1.83	2.28	0.97	3.49	0.74	0.63	224	214	205	151	126	6.2	4.7	8,000	800
	80	400	1.91	2.27	2.84	1.20	4.34	0.78	0.84	281	268	256	189	157	8.0	6.1	8,000	800
	80	500	1.91	2.72	3.39	1.44	5.19	0.83	1.05	337	322	308	227	187	9.8	7.6	8,000	800
	20	100	2.39	0.65	3.27	0.43	1.56	0.24	0.46	71	67	65	47	56	2.1	1.5	2,000	200
Age = 4 months	20	150	2.87	0.67	3.34	0.53	1.92	0.25	0.68	85	81	78	57	69	2.7	2.0	2,000	200
Maturity = 0.6	20	200	2.87	0.85	4.26	0.68	2.44	0.26	0.91	107	102	98	72	88	3.4	2.7	2,000	200
(early maturing)	20	300	2.87	1.22	6.10	0.97	3.50	0.28	1.37	150	143	137	101	126	4.9	4.0	2,000	200
	30	200	2.87	0.90	3.00	0.72	2.58	0.35	0.91	113	108	103	76	93	3.5	2.7	3,000	300
	30	250	2.87	1.09	3.62	0.86	3.12	0.36	1.14	135	128	123	90	112	4.2	3.4	3,000	300
	30	300	2.87	1.27	4.24	1.01	3.65	0.37	1.37	156	149	143	105	132	4.9	4.1	3,000	300
	30	400	2.87	1.64	5.48	1.31	4.71	0.40	1.83	200	191	182	134	170	6.4	5.4	3,000	300
	40	250	2.39	1.54	3.86	1.02	3.69	0.46	1.14	157	150	144	106	133	4.6	3.8	4,000	400
	40	300	2.87	1.32	3.30	1.05	3.79	0.46	1.37	162	155	148	109	137	5.0	4.1	4,000	400
	40	400	2.87	1.70	4.24	1.35	4.86	0.50	1.83	206	196	188	138	175	6.5	5.4	4,000	400
	40	500	2.87	2.07	5.18	1.65	5.94	0.53	2.28	249	238	228	168	214	8.0	6.8	4,000	400
	50	250	2.39	1.60	3.20	1.06	3.82	0.54	1.14	164	156	149	110	138	4.7	3.9	5,000	500
	50	300	2.39	1.86	3.72	1.23	4.45	0.57	1.37	189	180	172	127	160	5.5	4.6	5,000	500
	50	400	2.87	1.74	3.49	1.39	5.00	0.59	1.83	212	202	193	142	180	6.5	5.5	5,000	500
	50	500	2.87	2.12	4.25	1.69	6.09	0.63	2.28	255	244	233	172	219	8.0	6.8	5,000	500
	50	600	2.87	2.50	5.00	1.99	7.17	0.67	2.74	299	286	273	201	259	9.5	8.1	5,000	500
	60	250	2.39	1.65	2.75	1.09	3.94	0.62	1.14	170	162	155	114	142	4.7	3.9	6,000	600
	60	300	2.39	1.92	3.19	1.27	4.58	0.65	1.37	195	186	178	131	165	5.5	4.7	6,000	600
	60	400	2.87	1.79	2.99	1.42	5.14	0.67	1.83	218	208	199	146	185	6.6	5.5	6,000	600
	60	500	2.87	2.17	3.62	1.73	6.23	0.72	2.28	261	250	239	176	225	8.1	6.9	6,000	600

TABLE 15-2 continued

Class/Age/Other	Body Weight[a] kg	Weight or Milk Yield[b] kg	Body Weight Gain[c,d] g/d	Energy Concentration in Diet[e] kcal/kg	Daily Dry Matter Intake[f] kg	Daily Dry Matter Intake[f] % BW	Energy Requirements[g] TDN kg/d	Energy Requirements[g] ME Mcal/d	Energy Requirements[g] NEm Mcal/d	Energy Requirements[g] NEg Mcal/d	Protein Requirements[h] CP @20% UIP g/d	Protein Requirements[h] CP @40% UIP g/d	Protein Requirements[h] CP @60% UIP g/d	Protein Requirements[h] MP g/d	Protein Requirements[h] DIP g/d	Mineral Requirements[i] Ca g/d	Mineral Requirements[i] P g/d	Vitamin Requirements[j] A RE/d	Vitamin Requirements[j] E IU/d
	60		600	2.87	2.55	4.26	2.03	7.32	0.76	2.74	305	292	279	205	264	9.5	8.2	6,000	600
	70		150	1.91	1.88	2.69	1.00	3.60	0.68	0.68	155	148	142	104	130	3.8	3.2	7,000	700
	70		200	1.91	2.36	3.37	1.25	4.51	0.72	0.91	190	181	173	127	163	4.8	4.1	7,000	700
	70		300	2.39	1.97	2.81	1.30	4.70	0.73	1.37	201	192	183	135	170	5.6	4.7	7,000	700
	70		400	2.39	2.50	3.58	1.66	5.98	0.79	1.83	251	240	229	169	216	7.2	6.2	7,000	700
	70		500	2.87	2.22	3.17	1.77	6.37	0.81	2.28	267	255	244	180	230	8.1	6.9	7,000	700
	80		150	1.91	1.94	2.43	1.03	3.71	0.75	0.68	161	154	147	108	134	3.8	3.2	8,000	800
	80		200	1.91	2.42	3.03	1.28	4.63	0.80	0.91	196	187	179	132	167	4.8	4.2	8,000	800
	80		300	2.39	2.02	2.52	1.34	4.82	0.81	1.37	206	197	189	139	174	5.6	4.8	8,000	800
	80		400	2.39	2.56	3.20	1.70	6.11	0.87	1.83	257	246	235	173	220	7.3	6.3	8,000	800
	80		500	2.39	3.10	3.87	2.05	7.40	0.94	2.28	308	294	281	207	267	8.9	7.8	8,000	800
	20		100	2.39	0.63	3.14	0.42	1.50	0.47	0.30	75	71	68	50	54	2.2	1.5	2,000	200
Age = 8 months	20		150	2.39	0.80	4.00	0.53	1.91	0.48	0.45	99	94	90	66	69	3.0	2.2	2,000	200
Maturity = 0.4	20		200	2.87	0.73	3.65	0.58	2.09	0.49	0.59	113	108	104	76	75	3.6	2.6	2,000	200
(late maturing)	20		300	2.87	0.98	4.88	0.78	2.80	0.52	0.89	158	150	144	106	101	5.1	3.8	2,000	200
	30		200	2.39	1.09	3.62	0.72	2.60	0.68	0.59	131	125	120	88	94	3.9	2.9	3,000	300
	30		250	2.87	0.95	3.17	0.76	2.72	0.68	0.74	143	137	131	96	98	4.4	3.3	3,000	300
	30		300	2.87	1.08	3.59	0.86	3.08	0.70	0.89	166	158	151	111	111	5.2	3.9	3,000	300
	30		400	2.87	1.33	4.42	1.06	3.81	0.74	1.19	210	200	192	141	137	6.7	5.2	3,000	300
	40		250	2.39	1.37	3.43	0.91	3.28	0.87	0.74	164	156	149	110	118	4.8	3.7	4,000	400
	40		300	2.39	1.55	3.88	1.03	3.71	0.89	0.89	188	179	172	126	134	5.6	4.4	4,000	400
	40		400	2.87	1.42	3.56	1.13	4.08	0.91	1.19	218	208	199	146	147	6.8	5.2	4,000	400
	40		500	2.87	1.68	4.20	1.34	4.81	0.96	1.48	262	250	239	176	174	8.3	6.5	4,000	400
	50		250	2.39	1.47	2.95	0.98	3.52	1.02	0.74	171	164	157	115	127	4.9	3.8	5,000	500
	50		300	2.39	1.66	3.31	1.10	3.96	1.05	0.89	196	187	179	132	143	5.7	4.5	5,000	500
	50		400	2.87	1.51	3.03	1.20	4.34	1.08	1.19	225	215	206	151	156	6.9	5.3	5,000	500
	50		500	2.87	1.77	3.55	1.41	5.09	1.13	1.48	270	258	247	181	183	8.4	6.6	5,000	500
	50		600	2.87	2.03	4.07	1.62	5.83	1.18	1.78	315	300	287	212	210	9.9	7.8	5,000	500
	60		250	2.39	1.57	2.62	1.04	3.76	1.17	0.74	179	171	164	120	135	5.0	3.9	6,000	600
	60		300	2.39	1.76	2.93	1.16	4.20	1.21	0.89	204	194	186	137	151	5.8	4.6	6,000	600
	60		400	2.39	2.13	3.54	1.41	5.08	1.28	1.19	253	241	231	170	183	7.4	5.9	6,000	600
	60		500	2.87	1.86	3.11	1.48	5.34	1.30	1.48	278	265	253	187	193	8.5	6.7	6,000	600
	60		600	2.87	2.13	3.55	1.69	6.10	1.36	1.78	323	308	294	217	220	10.0	7.9	6,000	600
	70		150	1.91	1.91	2.73	1.01	3.66	1.29	0.45	161	154	147	108	132	4.0	3.2	7,000	700
	70		200	1.91	2.25	3.21	1.19	4.29	1.34	0.59	192	183	175	129	155	5.0	4.1	7,000	700
	70		300	2.39	1.85	2.65	1.23	4.43	1.36	0.89	211	202	193	142	160	5.9	4.7	7,000	700
	70		400	2.39	2.23	3.18	1.48	5.32	1.43	1.19	261	249	238	175	192	7.5	6.0	7,000	700
	70		500	2.39	2.60	3.72	1.72	6.22	1.51	1.48	310	296	283	208	224	9.1	7.4	7,000	700
	80		150	1.91	2.02	2.53	1.07	3.87	1.42	0.45	169	161	154	114	139	4.1	3.3	8,000	800
	80		200	1.91	2.36	2.95	1.25	4.51	1.49	0.59	200	191	182	134	163	5.1	4.2	8,000	800
	80		300	1.91	3.04	3.80	1.61	5.81	1.61	0.89	261	249	239	176	209	7.0	5.8	8,000	800
	80		400	2.39	2.33	2.91	1.54	5.56	1.58	1.19	268	256	245	180	200	7.6	6.1	8,000	800
	80		500	2.39	2.71	3.38	1.79	6.47	1.67	1.48	318	303	290	214	233	9.2	7.5	8,000	800

	20	100	2.87	0.69	3.44	0.55	1.98	0.49	0.54	70	67	64	47	71	2.0	1.5	2,000	200
Age = 8 months	20	150	2.87	0.91	4.57	0.73	2.62	0.51	0.82	91	87	83	61	95	2.8	2.2	2,000	200
Maturity = 0.8	20	200	2.87	1.14	5.70	0.91	3.27	0.53	1.09	113	108	103	76	118	3.5	2.9	2,000	200
(early maturing)	20	300	2.87	1.59	7.96	1.27	4.57	0.58	1.63	156	149	142	105	165	5.0	4.3	2,000	200
	30	200	2.87	1.24	4.14	0.99	3.57	0.72	1.09	122	116	111	82	129	3.6	3.0	3,000	300
	30	250	2.87	1.47	4.91	1.17	4.23	0.76	1.36	143	137	131	96	152	4.3	3.7	3,000	300
	30	300	2.87	1.70	5.68	1.36	4.89	0.79	1.63	165	158	151	111	176	5.1	4.4	3,000	300
	30	400	2.87	2.16	7.22	1.72	6.21	0.85	2.18	208	199	190	140	224	6.5	5.8	3,000	300
	40	250	2.87	1.57	3.93	1.25	4.51	0.94	1.36	152	145	139	102	163	4.4	3.8	4,000	400
	40	300	2.87	1.81	4.52	1.44	5.18	0.98	1.63	174	166	159	117	187	5.2	4.5	4,000	400
	40	400	2.87	2.28	5.69	1.81	6.53	1.06	2.18	218	208	199	146	235	6.6	5.9	4,000	400
	40	500	2.87	2.75	6.86	2.18	7.87	1.14	2.72	262	250	239	176	284	8.1	7.4	4,000	400
	50	250	2.87	1.66	3.33	1.32	4.78	1.11	1.36	161	153	147	108	172	4.5	3.9	5,000	500
	50	300	2.87	1.90	3.81	1.51	5.46	1.16	1.63	183	174	167	123	197	5.2	4.6	5,000	500
	50	400	2.87	2.38	4.76	1.89	6.83	1.25	2.18	227	217	207	153	246	6.7	6.0	5,000	500
	50	500	2.87	2.86	5.72	2.27	8.20	1.35	2.72	271	259	248	182	296	8.2	7.5	5,000	500
	50	600	2.87	3.34	6.67	2.65	9.57	1.45	3.27	315	301	288	212	345	9.7	8.9	5,000	500
	60	250	2.39	2.34	3.90	1.55	5.60	1.32	1.36	169	161	154	113	202	5.1	4.6	6,000	600
	60	300	2.87	2.00	3.33	1.59	5.72	1.33	1.63	191	182	175	128	206	5.3	4.7	6,000	600
	60	400	2.87	2.48	4.13	1.97	7.11	1.44	2.18	236	225	215	158	256	6.8	6.1	6,000	600
	60	500	2.87	2.97	4.94	2.36	8.50	1.55	2.72	280	268	256	188	307	8.3	7.6	6,000	600
	60	600	2.87	3.45	5.75	2.74	9.90	1.66	3.27	325	310	297	218	357	9.8	9.0	6,000	600
	70	150	1.91	2.75	3.92	1.46	5.25	1.43	0.82	190	181	173	128	189	4.4	4.0	7,000	700
	70	200	2.39	2.10	3.00	1.39	5.02	1.41	1.09	175	167	160	118	181	4.4	3.9	7,000	700
	70	300	2.39	2.79	3.98	1.85	6.67	1.55	1.63	228	218	209	154	240	6.1	5.5	7,000	700
	70	400	2.87	2.58	3.68	2.05	7.39	1.61	2.18	244	233	223	164	266	6.9	6.2	7,000	700
	70	500	2.87	3.07	4.38	2.44	8.80	1.74	2.72	289	276	264	194	317	8.4	7.7	7,000	700
	80	150	1.91	2.87	3.59	1.52	5.49	1.58	0.82	199	190	182	134	198	4.5	4.1	8,000	800
	80	200	2.39	2.20	2.75	1.46	5.26	1.56	1.09	183	175	167	123	189	4.5	3.9	8,000	800
	80	300	2.39	2.90	3.62	1.92	6.92	1.71	1.63	237	226	217	159	249	6.2	5.6	8,000	800
	80	400	2.87	2.67	3.33	2.12	7.65	1.78	2.18	253	241	231	170	276	7.0	6.3	8,000	800
	80	500	2.87	3.17	3.96	2.52	9.08	1.92	2.72	298	285	272	200	327	8.5	7.8	8,000	800
Yearling Farm Ewes																		
Maintenance plus growth	40	40	2.39	1.18	2.94	0.78	2.81	1.43	0.23	97	93	89	65	101	3.1	1.7	2,140	224
Age = 1.0 year	50	50	2.39	1.43	2.85	0.95	3.41	1.72	0.29	117	112	107	79	123	3.7	2.1	2,675	280
Maturity = 0.87	60	60	2.39	1.67	2.78	1.11	3.99	2.00	0.34	137	131	125	92	144	4.2	2.5	3,210	336
	70	70	2.39	1.91	2.73	1.27	4.56	2.27	0.40	156	149	143	105	165	4.8	2.9	3,745	392
	80	80	2.39	2.15	2.68	1.42	5.13	2.54	0.46	176	168	161	118	185	5.3	3.3	4,280	448
	90	90	2.39	2.38	2.64	1.58	5.68	2.80	0.51	195	186	178	131	205	5.9	3.7	4,815	504
	100	100	2.39	2.61	2.61	1.73	6.23	3.05	0.57	214	204	195	144	225	6.4	4.1	5,350	560
	120	120	2.39	3.06	2.55	2.03	7.31	3.56	0.68	252	240	230	169	263	7.4	4.8	6,420	672
Breeding																		
	40	60	2.39	1.28	3.20	0.85	3.06	1.59	0.23	110	105	100	74	110	3.6	2.1	2,140	224
Age = 0.6 year	50	74	2.39	1.55	3.10	1.03	3.70	1.91	0.29	132	126	121	89	133	4.3	2.5	2,675	280
Maturity = 0.7	60	88	2.39	1.81	3.02	1.20	4.33	2.22	0.34	154	147	141	104	156	4.9	3.0	3,210	336
	70	101	2.39	2.07	2.96	1.37	4.95	2.52	0.40	176	168	161	118	178	5.6	3.4	3,745	392
	80	115	2.39	2.32	2.91	1.54	5.56	2.81	0.46	198	189	181	133	200	6.2	3.9	4,280	448
	90	129	2.39	2.58	2.86	1.71	6.15	3.10	0.51	219	209	200	147	222	6.8	4.4	4,815	504

TABLE 15-2 continued

Class/Age/Other	Body Weight[a] kg	Weight or Milk Yield[b] kg	Body Weight Gain[c,d] g/d	Energy Concentration in Diet[e] kcal/kg	Daily Dry Matter Intake[f] kg	Daily Dry Matter Intake[f] % BW	Energy Requirements[g] TDN kg/d	ME Mcal/d	NEm Mcal/d	NEg Mcal/d	Protein Requirements[h] CP @20% UIP g/d	CP @40% UIP g/d	CP @60% UIP g/d	MP g/d	DIP g/d	Mineral Requirements[i] Ca g/d	P g/d	Vitamin Requirements[j] A RE/d	E IU/d
	100		143	2.39	2.82	2.82	1.87	6.75	3.39	0.57	241	230	220	162	243	7.5	4.8	5,350	560
	120		170	2.39	3.31	2.76	2.19	7.91	3.94	0.68	283	270	258	190	285	8.7	5.7	6,420	672
Early gestation (Single lamb; BW = 3.5 to 6.3 kg)																			
	40	3.5	58	2.39	1.33	3.33	0.88	3.19	1.43	0.23	116	111	106	78	115	4.4	2.8	1,256	212
	50	3.9	71	2.39	1.60	3.20	1.06	3.83	1.72	0.29	138	132	126	93	138	5.1	3.3	1,570	265
	60	4.3	84	2.39	1.86	3.11	1.24	4.45	2.00	0.34	160	153	146	108	161	5.8	3.8	1,884	318
	70	4.7	97	2.39	2.12	3.03	1.41	5.07	2.27	0.40	182	174	166	122	183	6.5	4.3	2,198	371
	80	5.0	110	2.39	2.37	2.96	1.57	5.66	2.54	0.46	203	194	185	136	204	7.1	4.8	2,512	424
	90	5.4	123	2.39	2.62	2.91	1.74	6.26	2.80	0.51	224	214	205	151	226	7.8	5.3	2,826	477
	100	5.7	135	2.39	2.86	2.86	1.90	6.84	3.06	0.57	245	234	223	164	247	8.4	5.8	3,140	530
	120	6.3	161	2.39	3.34	2.78	2.21	7.99	3.57	0.68	286	273	261	192	288	9.6	6.8	3,768	636
Early gestation (Twin lambs; BW = 3.1 to 5.5 kg)																			
	40	3.1	70	2.87	1.15	2.88	0.91	3.30	1.37	0.23	120	114	109	81	119	5.5	3.2	1,256	212
	50	3.4	85	2.39	1.73	3.46	1.15	4.13	1.72	0.29	155	148	141	104	149	6.7	4.1	1,570	265
	60	3.8	100	2.39	2.01	3.35	1.33	4.80	2.00	0.34	179	171	163	120	173	7.6	4.8	1,884	318
	70	4.1	146	2.39	2.28	3.25	1.51	5.44	2.27	0.40	202	192	184	135	196	8.9	5.7	2,198	371
	80	4.4	110	2.39	2.54	3.17	1.68	6.06	2.54	0.46	224	214	205	151	219	9.0	5.7	2,512	424
	90	4.7	123	2.39	2.80	3.11	1.85	6.68	2.80	0.51	247	235	225	166	241	9.7	6.3	2,826	477
	100	5.0	135	2.39	3.05	3.05	2.02	7.30	3.06	0.57	269	257	246	181	263	10.5	6.8	3,140	530
	120	5.5	161	2.39	3.55	2.96	2.35	8.48	3.57	0.68	312	298	285	210	306	11.9	7.9	3,768	636
Early gestation (Three lambs; BW = 2.6 to 4.7 kg)																			
	40	2.6	79	2.87	1.21	3.02	0.96	3.47	1.37	0.23	128	123	117	86	125	6.4	3.6	1,256	212
	50	2.9	96	2.87	1.44	2.87	1.14	4.12	1.65	0.29	151	144	138	101	148	7.3	4.3	1,570	265
	60	3.2	112	2.39	2.10	3.50	1.39	5.01	2.00	0.34	190	181	174	128	181	8.8	5.4	1,884	318
	70	3.5	129	2.39	2.38	3.40	1.58	5.68	2.27	0.40	215	205	196	144	205	9.8	6.1	2,198	371
	80	3.8	145	2.39	2.65	3.32	1.76	6.34	2.54	0.46	239	228	218	160	229	10.7	6.7	2,512	424
	90	4.0	161	2.39	2.91	3.23	1.93	6.96	2.80	0.51	261	249	239	176	251	11.5	7.3	2,826	477
	100	4.3	177	2.39	3.18	3.18	2.11	7.60	3.06	0.57	285	272	260	192	274	12.5	8.0	3,140	530
	120	4.7	208	2.39	3.69	3.07	2.44	8.81	3.57	0.68	329	314	301	221	318	14.1	9.2	3,768	636
Late gestation (Single lamb; BW = 3.5 to 6.3 kg)																			
	40	3.5	111	2.87	1.20	3.01	0.96	3.45	1.37	0.23	128	122	117	86	124	5.8	3.4	1,820	224
	50	3.9	134	2.87	1.43	2.86	1.14	4.10	1.65	0.29	150	143	137	101	148	6.7	4.0	2,275	280
	60	4.3	157	2.39	2.09	3.48	1.38	4.99	2.00	0.34	189	181	173	127	180	8.1	5.1	2,730	336
	70	4.7	179	2.39	2.37	3.38	1.57	5.65	2.27	0.40	214	204	195	144	204	9.0	5.8	3,185	392
	80	5.0	200	2.39	2.63	3.29	1.74	6.29	2.54	0.46	237	226	216	159	227	9.8	6.4	3,640	448
	90	5.4	221	2.39	2.90	3.22	1.92	6.93	2.80	0.51	261	249	238	175	250	10.7	7.0	4,095	504
	100	5.7	242	2.39	3.16	3.16	2.09	7.55	3.06	0.57	283	270	259	190	272	11.6	7.6	4,550	560
	120	6.3	283	2.39	3.67	3.06	2.43	8.77	3.56	0.68	328	313	300	221	316	13.2	8.8	5,460	672

Late gestation (Twin lambs; BW = 3.1 to 5.5 kg)																		
40	3.1	159	2.87	1.42	3.55	1.13	4.07	1.37	0.23	159	151	145	107	147	8.5	4.8	1,820	224
50	3.4	191	2.87	1.66	3.32	1.32	4.76	1.65	0.29	183	175	168	123	172	9.7	5.6	2,275	280
60	3.8	221	2.87	1.91	3.19	1.52	5.49	1.91	0.34	210	201	192	141	198	11.0	6.4	2,730	336
70	4.1	251	2.87	2.15	3.07	1.71	6.16	2.17	0.40	235	224	214	158	222	12.1	7.1	3,185	392
80	4.4	280	2.87	2.38	2.97	1.89	6.81	2.42	0.46	259	247	236	174	246	13.1	7.9	3,640	448
90	4.7	308	2.87	2.60	2.89	2.07	7.46	2.67	0.51	283	270	258	190	269	14.2	8.6	4,095	504
100	5.0	336	2.87	2.83	2.83	2.25	8.11	2.91	0.57	307	293	280	206	292	15.3	9.3	4,550	560
120	5.5	391	2.39	4.12	3.44	2.73	9.85	3.56	0.68	385	367	352	259	355	18.3	11.7	5,460	672
Late gestation (Three lambs; BW = 2.6 to 4.7 kg)																		
40	2.6	195	2.87	1.55	3.87	1.23	4.44	1.37	0.23	177	169	162	119	160	10.3	5.7	1,820	224
50	2.9	233	2.87	1.81	3.63	1.44	5.20	1.65	0.29	205	196	188	138	188	11.7	6.7	2,275	280
60	3.2	270	2.87	2.07	3.46	1.65	5.95	1.91	0.34	233	223	213	157	215	13.2	7.6	2,730	336
70	3.5	305	2.87	2.33	3.33	1.85	6.69	2.17	0.40	261	249	238	175	241	14.6	8.5	3,185	392
80	3.8	340	2.87	2.58	3.23	2.06	7.41	2.42	0.46	289	276	264	194	267	16.0	9.4	3,640	448
90	4.0	374	2.87	2.81	3.12	2.24	8.06	2.67	0.51	313	298	285	210	291	17.1	10.2	4,095	504
100	4.3	407	2.87	3.06	3.06	2.43	8.78	2.91	0.57	340	324	310	228	316	18.5	11.1	4,550	560
120	4.7	472	2.87	3.50	2.92	2.79	10.05	3.39	0.68	387	370	354	260	362	20.7	12.6	5,460	672
Lactation; early, mid-, and late lactation for yearlings in farm flocks nursing 1, 2, or 3 lambs are in Table 15-1.																		
Yearling Range Ewes																		
Maintenance plus growth																		
Age = 2 years 40		40	2.39	1.18	2.94	0.78	2.81	1.43	0.23	97	93	89	65	101	3.1	1.7	1,256	212
Maturity = 0.94 50		50	2.39	1.43	2.85	0.95	3.41	1.72	0.29	117	112	107	79	123	3.7	2.1	1,570	265
60		60	2.39	1.67	2.78	1.11	3.99	2.00	0.34	137	131	125	92	144	4.2	2.5	1,884	318
70		70	2.39	1.91	2.73	1.27	4.56	2.27	0.40	156	149	143	105	165	4.7	2.9	2,198	371
80		80	2.39	2.15	2.68	1.42	5.13	2.54	0.46	176	168	161	118	185	5.3	3.3	2,512	424
90		90	2.39	2.38	2.64	1.58	5.68	2.80	0.51	195	186	178	131	205	5.8	3.7	2,826	477
100		100	2.39	2.61	2.61	1.73	6.23	3.05	0.57	214	204	195	144	225	6.3	4.1	3,140	530
120		120	2.39	3.06	2.55	2.03	7.31	3.56	0.68	252	240	230	169	263	7.4	4.8	3,768	636
Breeding																		
40		60	2.39	1.26	3.15	0.83	3.01	1.56	0.23	110	105	101	74	109	3.6	2.0	1,256	212
Age = 1.5 years 50		74	2.39	1.53	3.05	1.01	3.65	1.87	0.29	133	127	122	90	131	4.2	2.5	1,570	265
Maturity = 0.9 60		88	2.39	1.79	2.98	1.18	4.27	2.17	0.34	156	149	142	105	154	4.9	3.0	1,884	318
70		101	2.39	2.04	2.92	1.35	4.88	2.47	0.40	178	170	162	119	176	5.5	3.4	2,198	371
80		115	2.39	2.29	2.87	1.52	5.48	2.76	0.46	200	191	182	134	197	6.1	3.9	2,512	424
90		129	2.39	2.54	2.82	1.68	6.07	3.05	0.51	221	211	202	149	219	6.8	4.3	2,826	477
100		143	2.39	2.78	2.78	1.84	6.65	3.33	0.57	243	232	222	163	240	7.4	4.8	3,140	530
120		170	2.39	3.26	2.72	2.16	7.80	3.88	0.68	285	272	261	192	281	8.6	5.6	3,768	636
Early gestation (Single lamb; BW = 3.5 to 6.3 kg)																		
40	3.5	58	2.39	1.32	3.29	0.87	3.15	1.41	0.23	117	112	107	79	113	4.4	2.7	1,256	212
50	3.9	71	2.39	1.58	3.16	1.05	3.78	1.69	0.29	139	133	127	94	136	5.1	3.3	1,570	265
60	4.3	84	2.39	1.84	3.07	1.22	4.40	1.96	0.34	161	154	147	108	159	5.7	3.8	1,884	318
70	4.7	97	2.39	2.09	2.99	1.39	5.00	2.23	0.40	183	175	167	123	180	6.4	4.3	2,198	371
80	5.0	110	2.39	2.34	2.93	1.55	5.59	2.50	0.46	204	195	186	137	202	7.0	4.8	2,512	424
90	5.4	123	2.39	2.59	2.87	1.71	6.18	2.75	0.51	226	215	206	152	223	7.7	5.3	2,826	477
100	5.7	135	2.39	2.83	2.83	1.87	6.76	3.01	0.57	246	235	225	166	244	8.3	5.8	3,140	530
120	6.3	161	2.39	3.30	2.75	2.19	7.89	3.50	0.68	288	274	263	193	284	9.5	6.7	3,768	636

TABLE 15-2 continued

Class/Age/Other	Body Weight[a] kg	Weight or Milk Yield[b] kg	Body Weight Gain[c,d] g/d	Energy Concentration in Diet[e] kcal/kg	Daily Dry Matter Intake[f] kg	Daily Dry Matter Intake[f] % BW	Energy Requirements[g] TDN kg/d	ME Mcal/d	NEm Mcal/d	NEg Mcal/d	Protein Requirements[h] CP @20% UIP g/d	CP @40% UIP g/d	CP @60% UIP g/d	MP g/d	DIP g/d	Mineral Requirements[i] Ca g/d	P g/d	Vitamin Requirements[j] A RE/d	E IU/d
Early gestation (Twin lambs; BW = 3.1 to 5.5 kg)																			
	40	3.1	70	2.87	1.14	2.84	0.90	3.26	1.35	0.23	120	115	110	81	117	5.5	3.2	1,256	212
	50	3.4	85	2.39	1.71	3.42	1.13	4.08	1.69	0.29	156	148	142	104	147	6.7	4.1	1,570	265
	60	3.8	100	2.39	1.99	3.31	1.32	4.75	1.96	0.34	180	172	164	121	171	7.6	4.7	1,884	318
	70	4.1	115	2.39	2.25	3.21	1.49	5.37	2.23	0.40	203	194	185	136	194	8.4	5.3	2,198	371
	80	4.4	130	2.39	2.51	3.14	1.66	5.99	2.50	0.46	226	215	206	152	216	9.1	5.9	2,512	424
	90	4.7	145	2.39	2.76	3.07	1.83	6.61	2.75	0.51	248	237	227	167	238	9.9	6.5	2,826	477
	100	5.0	159	2.39	3.02	3.02	2.00	7.21	3.01	0.57	271	258	247	182	260	10.7	7.1	3,140	530
	120	5.5	188	2.39	3.51	2.92	2.33	8.39	3.50	0.68	314	300	287	211	302	12.1	8.1	3,768	636
Early gestation (Three lambs; BW = 2.6 to 4.7 kg)																			
	40	2.6	79	2.87	1.19	2.99	0.95	3.43	1.35	0.23	129	123	118	87	124	6.4	3.6	1,256	212
	50	2.9	96	2.87	1.42	2.84	1.13	4.07	1.62	0.29	152	145	139	102	147	7.3	4.2	1,570	265
	60	3.2	112	2.39	2.07	3.46	1.37	4.96	1.96	0.34	191	182	174	128	179	8.7	5.4	1,884	318
	70	3.5	129	2.39	2.35	3.36	1.56	5.62	2.23	0.40	216	206	197	145	203	9.7	6.0	2,198	371
	80	3.8	145	2.39	2.62	3.28	1.74	6.27	2.50	0.46	240	229	219	161	226	10.6	6.7	2,512	424
	90	4.0	161	2.39	2.88	3.20	1.91	6.88	2.75	0.51	263	251	240	177	248	11.4	7.3	2,826	477
	100	4.3	177	2.39	3.15	3.15	2.08	7.52	3.01	0.57	287	274	262	193	271	12.3	7.9	3,140	530
	120	4.7	208	2.39	3.65	3.04	2.42	8.71	3.50	0.68	331	316	303	223	314	13.9	9.1	3,768	636
Late gestation (Single lamb; BW = 3.5 to 6.3 kg)																			
	40	3.5	111	2.87	1.19	2.97	0.94	3.41	1.34	0.23	128	122	116	86	123	5.8	3.3	1,820	224
	50	3.9	134	2.87	1.41	2.82	1.12	4.04	1.61	0.29	150	143	137	101	146	6.6	4.0	2,275	280
	60	4.3	157	2.39	2.06	3.44	1.37	4.93	1.96	0.34	189	180	173	127	178	8.0	5.1	2,730	336
	70	4.7	179	2.39	2.34	3.34	1.55	5.59	2.23	0.40	213	204	195	143	201	8.9	5.7	3,185	392
	80	5.0	200	2.39	2.60	3.25	1.72	6.21	2.49	0.46	236	226	216	159	224	9.7	6.3	3,640	448
	90	5.4	221	2.39	2.87	3.19	1.90	6.85	2.75	0.51	261	249	238	175	247	10.6	7.0	4,095	504
	100	5.7	242	2.39	3.12	3.12	2.07	7.46	3.00	0.57	283	270	259	190	269	11.4	7.6	4,550	560
	120	6.3	283	2.39	3.63	3.02	2.40	8.67	3.50	0.68	328	313	300	221	312	13.0	8.8	5,460	672
Late gestation (Twin lambs; BW = 3.1 to 5.5 kg)																			
	40	3.1	159	2.87	1.40	3.51	1.12	4.03	1.34	0.23	159	151	145	107	145	8.5	4.8	1,820	224
	50	3.4	191	2.87	1.64	3.29	1.31	4.71	1.61	0.29	183	175	167	123	170	9.6	5.5	2,275	280
	60	3.8	221	2.87	1.89	3.16	1.51	5.43	1.87	0.34	210	201	192	141	196	10.9	6.4	2,730	336
	70	4.1	251	2.87	2.12	3.03	1.69	6.09	2.13	0.40	235	224	214	158	219	11.9	7.1	3,185	392
	80	4.4	280	2.87	2.35	2.94	1.87	6.74	2.37	0.46	259	247	236	174	243	13.0	7.8	3,640	448
	90	4.7	308	2.87	2.57	2.86	2.05	7.38	2.62	0.51	283	270	258	190	266	14.1	8.6	4,095	504
	100	5.0	336	2.87	2.80	2.80	2.22	8.02	2.85	0.57	307	293	280	206	289	15.1	9.3	4,550	560
	120	5.5	391	2.39	4.08	3.40	2.70	9.75	3.50	0.68	385	367	31	259	352	18.1	11.6	5,460	672

Late gestation (Three lambs; BW = 2.6 to 4.7 kg)																		
40	2.6	195	2.87	1.53	3.83	1.22	4.40	1.34	0.23	177	169	162	119	159	10.2	5.7	1,820	224
50	2.9	233	2.87	1.80	3.59	1.43	5.15	1.61	0.29	205	196	187	138	186	11.6	6.6	2,275	280
60	3.2	270	2.87	2.05	3.42	1.63	5.89	1.87	0.34	233	223	213	157	212	13.0	7.6	2,730	336
70	3.5	305	2.87	2.31	3.30	1.84	6.62	2.13	0.40	261	249	238	175	239	14.4	8.5	3,185	392
80	3.8	340	2.87	2.56	3.20	2.04	7.34	2.37	0.46	289	275	263	194	265	15.8	9.4	3,640	448
90	4.0	374	2.87	2.78	3.09	2.21	7.98	2.62	0.51	313	298	285	210	288	17.0	10.1	4,095	504
100	4.3	407	2.87	3.03	3.03	2.41	8.69	2.85	0.57	340	324	310	228	313	18.3	11.0	4,550	560
120	4.7	472	2.87	3.47	2.89	2.76	9.94	3.32	0.68	387	370	354	260	359	20.5	12.5	5,460	672

Lactation; early, mid-, and late lactation for yearlings in range flocks nursing 1, 2, or 3 lambs are in Table 15-1.

[a]Body weight used in estimating requirements is the determined or estimated weight in kilograms (kg) average for the period during which these requirements will be applied.

[b]Birth weight (kg) of single and average of multiple lambs or liquid milk yield (kg/d).

[c]Average change in body weight over a 24-hour period.

[d]Body weight change in yearling ewes includes both weight gain associated with growth toward maturity and weight change related to breeding, pregnancy, and lactation.

[e]Three hypothetical diets with increasing energy concentrations (1.91, 2.34, and 2.87 kcal/kg) were used in the calculations of intake and nutrient requirements. For each line entry, a diet was selected to represent the level of energy concentration that approximates that needed by the animal to achieve adequate intake to satisfy its energy requirement.

[f]The daily dry matter intake, expressed as kg or as percentage of body weight, of a diet having the indicated energy concentration (previous column) that is required to meet energy requirements. These energy concentrations should be viewed only as examples. In some cases, diets having greater or lesser concentrations of energy would be more appropriate.

[g]Energy requirements expressed as total digestible nutrients (TDN) in kg/d and metabolizable energy (ME), net energy for maintenance (NE_m), and net energy for gain (NE_g) as kcal/d.

[h]Protein requirements expressed as crude protein (CP), metabolizable protein (MP), and degradable intake protein (DIP). The CP requirement differs with the proportion of undegradable intake protein (UIP) because of the required minimal DIP.

[i]Two macro minerals, calcium (Ca) and phosphorus (P), commonly considered in balancing diets are included. Often, the balance (ratio) of the two minerals also is of concern.

[j]Two fat-soluble vitamins, A and E, that often are deficient in animal diets are expressed as retinol equivalents (RE) and international units (IU) for vitamins A and E, respectively. RE = 1.0 μg of all-trans retinol, 5.0 μg of all-trans betacarotene, and 7.6 μg of other carotenoids.

TABLE 15-3 Mineral Requirements of Sheep[a]

Class/Stage/Other	Body Weight[b] kg	Body Weight Gain[c] g/d	Dry Matter Intake[d] kg/d	Na g/d	Cl g/d	K g/d	Mg g/d	S g/d	Co mg/d	Cu[e] mg/d	I mg/d	Fe mg/d	Mn mg/d	Se[f] mg/d	Se[g] mg/d	Zn[h] mg/d
Growing Lambs and Yearlings																
(Rams, ewes, castrates)																
	20	100	0.63	0.4	0.3	2.9	0.6	1.1	0.13	3.1	0.3	32	12	0.09	0.18	13
	20	150	0.74	0.4	0.3	3.3	0.7	1.3	0.15	4.0	0.4	46	15	0.13	0.27	17
	20	200	0.82	0.5	0.4	3.6	0.8	1.5	0.16	4.9	0.4	61	18	0.18	0.35	21
	20	300	1.09	0.6	0.5	4.6	1.1	2.0	0.22	6.6	0.5	90	24	0.26	0.52	29
	30	200	1.10	0.6	0.5	4.8	1.0	2.0	0.22	5.5	0.5	62	21	0.18	0.36	24
	30	250	1.05	0.7	0.5	4.8	1.1	1.9	0.21	6.4	0.5	77	24	0.22	0.44	28
	30	300	1.22	0.7	0.6	5.4	1.3	2.2	0.24	7.3	0.6	91	27	0.26	0.53	32
	30	400	1.55	0.8	0.7	6.5	1.5	2.8	0.31	9.1	0.8	120	33	0.35	0.69	40
	40	250	1.44	0.8	0.6	6.3	1.3	2.6	0.29	7.1	0.7	78	26	0.23	0.45	45
	40	300	1.54	0.8	0.7	6.7	1.4	2.8	0.31	8.0	0.8	92	29	0.27	0.53	51
	40	400	1.62	1.0	0.7	7.2	1.7	2.9	0.32	9.7	0.8	121	36	0.35	0.70	63
	40	500	1.96	1.1	0.8	8.3	1.9	3.5	0.39	11.5	1.0	150	42	0.43	0.87	75
	50	250	1.51	0.9	0.7	7.0	1.5	2.7	0.30	7.8	0.8	79	29	0.23	0.46	49
	50	300	1.73	1.0	0.7	7.7	1.6	3.1	0.35	8.6	0.9	94	32	0.27	0.54	55
	50	400	1.75	1.1	0.8	8.0	1.8	3.2	0.35	10.4	0.9	123	38	0.35	0.71	67
	50	500	2.03	1.2	0.9	9.0	2.1	3.7	0.41	12.2	1.0	152	45	0.44	0.88	79
	50	600	2.37	1.3	1.0	10.1	2.3	4.3	0.47	13.9	1.2	181	51	0.52	1.04	91
	60	250	1.83	1.0	0.8	8.3	1.7	3.3	0.37	8.4	0.9	81	32	0.23	0.47	53
	60	300	1.81	1.1	0.8	8.3	1.8	3.2	0.36	9.3	0.9	95	35	0.28	0.55	59
	60	400	2.18	1.2	0.9	9.6	2.0	3.9	0.44	11.1	1.1	124	41	0.36	0.72	71
	60	500	2.17	1.3	1.0	9.8	2.3	3.9	0.43	12.8	1.1	153	47	0.44	0.88	83
	60	600	2.44	1.4	1.1	10.8	2.5	4.4	0.49	14.6	1.2	182	54	0.53	1.05	95
	70	150	1.86	1.0	0.8	8.6	1.6	3.3	0.37	7.3	0.9	53	28	0.15	0.31	45
	70	200	1.96	1.1	0.8	9.0	1.7	3.5	0.39	8.2	1.0	68	31	0.20	0.39	51
	70	300	2.18	1.2	0.9	9.8	2.0	3.9	0.44	10.0	1.1	97	37	0.28	0.56	63
	70	400	2.33	1.3	1.0	10.5	2.2	4.2	0.47	11.7	1.2	126	44	0.36	0.73	75
	70	500	2.59	1.4	1.1	11.4	2.4	4.7	0.52	13.5	1.3	155	50	0.45	0.89	87
	80	150	1.94	1.1	0.9	9.3	1.8	3.5	0.39	8.0	1.0	55	31	0.16	0.32	48
	80	200	2.04	1.2	0.9	9.7	1.9	3.7	0.41	8.9	1.0	69	34	0.20	0.40	54
	80	300	2.39	1.3	1.0	10.9	2.1	4.3	0.48	10.6	1.2	98	40	0.28	0.57	66
	80	400	2.40	1.4	1.1	11.1	2.4	4.3	0.48	12.4	1.2	127	46	0.37	0.73	78
	80	500	2.87	1.6	1.2	12.7	2.6	5.2	0.57	14.2	1.4	156	53	0.45	0.90	90
Yearling Ewes (Farm and range flocks)																
Maintenance only																
	40	0	0.81	0.5	0.4	4.0	0.7	1.3	0.08	2.7	0.4	6	11	0.02	0.03	20
	60	0	1.10	0.7	0.6	5.7	1.1	1.8	0.11	4.0	0.5	8	16	0.03	0.05	30
	80	0	1.36	0.9	0.7	7.3	1.4	2.2	0.14	5.3	0.7	11	21	0.03	0.07	41
	100	0	1.61	1.2	0.9	8.9	1.8	2.6	0.16	6.7	0.8	14	27	0.04	0.08	51
	120	0	1.85	1.4	1.1	10.4	2.1	3.0	0.18	8.0	0.9	17	32	0.05	0.10	61
Maintenance plus growth																
	40	40	1.18	0.5	0.4	5.2	0.8	2.1	0.12	3.4	0.6	17	13	0.05	0.10	27
	60	60	1.67	0.8	0.6	7.5	1.2	3.0	0.17	5.1	0.8	26	20	0.08	0.15	40
	80	80	2.15	1.0	0.8	9.7	1.6	3.9	0.21	6.7	1.1	34	26	0.10	0.20	53
	100	100	2.61	1.3	1.0	12.0	2.0	4.7	0.26	8.4	1.3	43	33	0.13	0.25	67
	120	120	3.06	1.6	1.2	14.1	2.4	5.5	0.31	10.1	1.5	52	40	0.15	0.30	80
Breeding																
	40	60	1.27	0.5	0.4	5.5	0.9	2.3	0.13	3.7	0.6	23	14	0.07	0.13	30
	60	88	1.80	0.8	0.6	7.9	1.3	3.2	0.18	5.6	0.9	34	22	0.10	0.20	44
	80	115	2.31	1.1	0.9	10.3	1.7	4.2	0.23	7.4	1.2	44	29	0.13	0.26	59
	100	143	2.80	1.4	1.1	12.6	2.1	5.0	0.28	9.2	1.4	55	36	0.16	0.32	74
	120	170	3.29	1.6	1.3	14.9	2.5	5.9	0.33	11.0	1.6	66	43	0.19	0.38	88
Early gestation (Single lamb)																
	40	40	1.33	0.6	0.5	5.7	1.0	2.4	0.13	6.3	0.7	35	23	0.06	0.13	35
	60	60	1.85	0.9	0.7	8.1	1.4	3.3	0.19	8.6	0.9	47	31	0.09	0.19	51
	80	80	2.35	1.2	0.9	10.5	1.9	4.2	0.24	10.9	1.2	59	40	0.12	0.24	66
	100	100	2.85	1.4	1.1	12.8	2.3	5.1	0.28	13.2	1.4	71	48	0.15	0.30	81
	120	120	3.32	1.7	1.3	15.1	2.7	6.0	0.33	15.4	1.7	83	56	0.18	0.35	96

TABLE 15-3 continued

Class/Stage/Other	Body Weight[b] kg	Body Weight Gain[c] g/d	Dry Matter Intake[d] kg/d	Na g/d	Cl g/d	K g/d	Mg g/d	S g/d	Co mg/d	Cu[e] mg/d	I mg/d	Fe mg/d	Mn mg/d	Se[f] mg/d	Se[g] mg/d	Zn[h] mg/d
Early gestation (Twin lambs)																
	40	40	1.14	0.7	0.5	5.3	1.1	2.1	0.11	8.5	0.6	48	30	0.08	0.15	42
	60	60	2.00	1.0	0.7	8.7	1.6	3.6	0.20	11.4	1.0	64	40	0.11	0.21	59
	80	80	2.52	1.2	1.0	11.1	2.1	4.5	0.25	14.1	1.3	78	50	0.14	0.27	75
	100	100	3.04	1.5	1.2	13.5	2.5	5.5	0.30	16.8	1.5	93	60	0.17	0.33	92
	120	120	3.53	1.8	1.4	15.9	3.0	6.4	0.35	19.3	1.8	107	69	0.20	0.39	108
Early gestation (Three lambs)																
	40	40	1.20	0.7	0.5	5.5	1.2	2.2	0.12	9.9	0.6	56	34	0.08	0.17	46
	60	60	2.09	1.0	0.8	9.0	1.7	3.8	0.21	13.1	1.0	74	45	0.12	0.23	64
	80	80	2.64	1.3	1.0	11.5	2.2	4.7	0.26	16.2	1.3	91	57	0.15	0.30	82
	100	100	3.16	1.6	1.3	14.0	2.7	5.7	0.32	19.2	1.6	107	67	0.18	0.36	99
	120	120	3.67	1.9	1.5	16.4	3.2	6.6	0.37	21.9	1.8	122	77	0.21	0.42	115
Late gestation (Single lamb)																
	40	40	1.20	0.6	0.4	5.3	1.1	2.2	0.12	6.3	0.6	35	23	0.06	0.13	35
	60	60	2.07	0.8	0.7	8.8	1.5	3.7	0.21	8.6	1.0	47	31	0.09	0.19	51
	80	80	2.61	1.1	0.9	11.2	2.0	4.7	0.26	10.9	1.3	59	40	0.12	0.24	66
	100	100	3.14	1.4	1.1	13.6	2.4	5.7	0.31	13.2	1.6	71	48	0.15	0.30	81
	120	120	3.65	1.7	1.3	16.0	2.9	6.6	0.36	15.4	1.8	83	56	0.18	0.35	96
Late gestation (Twin lambs)																
	40	40	1.41	0.6	0.5	6.0	1.3	2.5	0.14	8.5	0.7	48	30	0.08	0.15	42
	60	60	1.90	0.9	0.7	8.3	1.8	3.4	0.19	11.4	1.0	64	40	0.11	0.21	59
	80	80	2.36	1.2	0.9	10.6	2.3	4.3	0.24	14.1	1.2	78	50	0.14	0.27	75
	100	100	2.81	1.5	1.1	12.8	2.8	5.1	0.28	16.8	1.4	93	60	0.17	0.33	92
	120	120	4.10	1.7	1.3	17.4	3.2	7.4	0.41	19.3	2.1	107	69	0.20	0.39	108
Late gestation (Three lambs)																
	40	40	1.54	0.6	0.5	6.4	1.4	2.8	0.15	9.9	0.8	56	34	0.08	0.17	46
	60	60	2.06	0.9	0.7	8.9	1.9	3.7	0.21	13.1	1.0	74	45	0.12	0.23	64
	80	80	2.57	1.2	0.9	11.3	2.5	4.6	0.26	16.2	1.3	91	57	0.15	0.30	82
	100	100	3.04	1.5	1.2	13.5	3.0	5.5	0.30	19.2	1.5	107	67	0.18	0.36	99
	120	120	3.49	1.8	1.4	15.7	3.5	6.3	0.35	21.9	1.7	122	77	0.21	0.42	115
Early lactation (Single lamb)																
	40	–14	1.40	0.8	1.3	6.8	1.4	2.2	0.28	6.4	1.1	8	15	0.17	0.34	44
	60	–17	1.82	1.1	1.7	9.1	1.9	2.9	0.36	8.8	1.5	11	21	0.21	0.43	59
	80	–20	2.19	1.4	2.0	11.2	2.4	3.5	0.44	11.1	1.8	14	27	0.25	0.50	74
	100	–22	2.54	1.7	2.4	13.3	2.8	4.1	0.51	13.3	2.0	18	33	0.28	0.57	88
	120	–24	2.86	1.9	2.7	15.2	3.3	4.6	0.57	15.5	2.3	21	39	0.32	0.63	102
Early lactation (Twin lambs)																
	40	–24	1.43	1.0	1.9	7.6	1.8	2.3	0.29	8.2	1.1	9	18	0.27	0.55	60
	60	–29	2.30	1.3	2.4	11.4	2.4	3.7	0.46	11.1	1.8	13	25	0.34	0.68	79
	80	–33	2.75	1.6	2.9	13.9	3.0	4.4	0.55	13.7	2.2	17	31	0.40	0.79	96
	100	–37	3.16	2.0	3.3	16.2	3.5	5.1	0.63	16.3	2.5	20	38	0.45	0.89	113
	120	–41	3.55	2.3	3.7	18.4	4.1	5.7	0.71	18.8	2.8	23	44	0.49	0.99	129
Early lactation (Three or more lambs)																
	40	–31	1.39	1.1	2.3	8.0	2.2	2.2	0.28	9.7	1.1	11	20	0.35	0.70	72
	60	–38	2.13	1.5	3.0	11.5	2.8	3.4	0.43	12.8	1.7	14	27	0.43	0.86	93
	80	–43	3.17	1.9	3.5	15.8	3.5	5.1	0.63	15.7	2.5	18	35	0.50	1.01	113
	100	–49	3.63	2.2	4.0	18.4	4.1	5.8	0.73	18.5	2.9	22	41	0.57	1.13	132
	120	–53	4.06	2.5	4.5	20.8	4.6	6.5	0.81	21.2	3.2	25	48	0.63	1.25	150
Late lactation (Single lamb)																
	40	55	1.53	0.6	0.7	6.6	1.1	2.5	0.31	5.9	1.2	24	16	0.12	0.23	37
	60	72	2.09	0.9	1.0	9.2	1.5	3.3	0.42	8.3	1.7	32	23	0.15	0.30	52
	80	95	2.64	1.2	1.3	11.7	2.0	4.2	0.53	10.8	2.1	42	30	0.19	0.38	68
	100	117	3.15	1.5	1.5	14.1	2.4	5.0	0.63	13.3	2.5	51	37	0.23	0.45	83
	120	138	3.64	1.8	1.8	16.5	2.9	5.8	0.73	15.8	2.9	61	44	0.26	0.52	98
Late lactation (Twin lambs)																
	40	65	1.46	0.7	0.9	6.6	1.2	2.3	0.29	6.8	1.2	28	18	0.16	0.32	44
	60	91	1.97	1.0	1.3	9.1	1.7	3.2	0.39	9.6	1.6	39	25	0.21	0.42	62
	80	117	3.07	1.3	1.6	13.3	2.2	4.9	0.61	12.3	2.5	50	33	0.26	0.52	79
	100	141	3.63	1.6	1.9	16.0	2.7	5.8	0.73	15.0	2.9	61	40	0.30	0.61	96
	120	166	4.19	1.9	2.2	18.6	3.2	6.7	0.84	17.6	3.4	71	47	0.35	0.70	113

TABLE 15-3 continued

Class/Stage/Other	Body Weight[b] kg	Body Weight Gain[c] g/d	Dry Matter Intake[d] kg/d	Na g/d	Cl g/d	K g/d	Mg g/d	S g/d	Co mg/d	Cu[e] mg/d	I mg/d	Fe mg/d	Mn mg/d	Se[f] mg/d	Se[g] mg/d	Zn[h] mg/d
Late lactation (Three or more lambs)																
	60	104	2.18	1.1	1.4	10.0	1.9	3.5	0.44	10.5	1.7	44	27	0.25	0.51	69
	80	132	2.71	1.4	1.8	12.6	2.4	4.3	0.54	13.4	2.2	56	35	0.31	0.62	88
	100	159	3.59	1.7	2.1	16.2	3.0	5.7	0.72	16.2	2.9	67	43	0.36	0.73	106
	120	185	4.58	2.0	2.4	20.1	3.5	7.3	0.92	19.0	3.7	78	50	0.41	0.83	123
Mature ewes																
Maintenance only																
	40	0	0.77	0.5	0.4	3.9	0.7	1.2	0.08	2.7	0.4	6	11	0.02	0.03	20
	60	0	1.05	0.7	0.6	5.6	1.1	1.7	0.10	4.0	0.5	8	16	0.03	0.05	30
	80	0	1.30	0.9	0.7	7.1	1.4	2.1	0.13	5.3	0.7	11	21	0.03	0.07	41
	100	0	1.54	1.2	0.9	8.7	1.8	2.5	0.15	6.7	0.8	14	27	0.04	0.08	51
	120	0	1.76	1.4	1.1	10.2	2.1	2.8	0.18	8.0	0.9	17	32	0.05	0.10	61
	140	0	1.98	1.7	1.3	11.6	2.5	3.2	0.20	9.3	1.0	20	37	0.06	0.12	71
Breeding																
	40	20	0.85	0.5	0.4	4.2	0.8	1.4	0.09	3.0	0.4	11	12	0.03	0.07	23
	60	26	1.15	0.7	0.6	5.9	1.1	1.8	0.12	4.5	0.6	16	18	0.05	0.09	35
	80	32	1.43	1.0	0.8	7.6	1.5	2.3	0.14	5.9	0.7	20	23	0.06	0.12	46
	100	38	1.69	1.2	1.0	9.2	1.9	2.7	0.17	7.3	0.8	25	29	0.07	0.15	57
	120	44	1.94	1.5	1.2	10.8	2.2	3.1	0.19	8.8	1.0	30	35	0.09	0.17	68
	140	50	2.18	1.7	1.3	12.3	2.6	3.5	0.22	10.2	1.1	34	40	0.10	0.20	79
Early gestation (Single lamb)																
	40	18	0.99	0.6	0.4	4.7	0.9	1.6	0.10	5.9	0.5	25	21	0.03	0.07	30
	60	24	1.31	0.8	0.6	6.5	1.3	2.1	0.13	8.0	0.7	32	29	0.05	0.09	42
	80	30	1.61	1.1	0.8	8.2	1.7	2.6	0.16	10.0	0.8	39	36	0.06	0.11	55
	100	35	1.89	1.3	1.0	9.9	2.1	3.0	0.19	11.9	0.9	46	44	0.07	0.14	66
	120	41	2.15	1.6	1.2	11.5	2.5	3.4	0.22	13.8	1.1	52	51	0.08	0.16	78
	140	46	2.39	1.8	1.4	13.1	2.9	3.8	0.24	15.6	1.2	57	57	0.09	0.18	90
Early gestation (Twin lambs)																
	40	30	1.15	0.6	0.5	5.2	1.1	1.8	0.11	8.3	0.6	40	29	0.04	0.09	37
	60	40	1.51	0.9	0.7	7.2	1.5	2.4	0.15	11.0	0.8	51	38	0.06	0.12	51
	80	50	1.84	1.2	0.9	9.0	1.9	2.9	0.18	13.5	0.9	60	48	0.07	0.15	65
	100	59	2.15	1.4	1.1	10.8	2.3	3.4	0.21	15.9	1.1	69	56	0.09	0.18	78
	120	68	2.44	1.7	1.3	12.5	2.8	3.9	0.24	18.1	1.2	78	64	0.10	0.20	91
	140	76	2.71	2.0	1.5	14.2	3.2	4.3	0.27	20.3	1.4	86	73	0.11	0.23	104
Early gestation (Three lambs)																
	40	39	1.00	0.7	0.5	4.9	1.2	1.6	0.10	9.9	0.5	49	34	0.05	0.11	42
	60	52	1.65	1.0	0.7	7.6	1.6	2.6	0.16	13.0	0.8	63	45	0.07	0.14	57
	80	65	2.00	1.2	1.0	9.6	2.1	3.2	0.20	15.8	1.0	74	55	0.09	0.17	72
	100	77	2.32	1.5	1.2	11.4	2.5	3.7	0.23	18.5	1.2	85	65	0.10	0.20	86
	120	88	2.63	1.8	1.4	13.2	2.9	4.2	0.26	21.0	1.3	95	74	0.12	0.23	100
	140	99	2.92	2.1	1.6	14.9	3.4	4.7	0.29	23.5	1.5	104	83	0.13	0.26	113
Late gestation (Single lamb)																
	40	71	1.00	0.5	0.4	4.7	1.0	1.6	0.10	5.9	0.5	25	21	0.03	0.07	30
	60	97	1.63	0.8	0.6	7.4	1.4	2.6	0.16	8.0	0.8	32	29	0.05	0.09	42
	80	120	1.98	1.0	0.8	9.2	1.8	3.2	0.20	10.0	1.0	39	36	0.06	0.11	55
	100	142	2.30	1.3	1.0	11.0	2.2	3.7	0.23	11.9	1.1	46	44	0.07	0.14	66
	120	163	2.61	1.5	1.2	12.8	2.6	4.2	0.26	13.8	1.3	52	51	0.08	0.16	78
	140	183	2.89	1.8	1.4	14.4	3.0	4.6	0.29	15.6	1.4	57	57	0.09	0.18	90
Late gestation (Twin lambs)																
	40	119	1.06	0.6	0.4	4.9	1.2	1.7	0.11	8.3	0.5	40	29	0.04	0.09	37
	60	161	1.65	0.8	0.6	7.5	1.7	2.6	0.17	11.0	0.8	51	38	0.06	0.12	51
	80	200	1.99	1.1	0.8	9.4	2.2	3.2	0.20	13.5	1.0	60	48	0.07	0.15	65
	100	236	2.87	1.3	1.0	12.8	2.6	4.6	0.29	15.9	1.4	69	56	0.09	0.18	78
	120	271	3.24	1.6	1.2	14.7	3.0	5.2	0.32	18.1	1.6	78	64	0.10	0.20	91
	140	304	3.57	1.9	1.4	16.6	3.5	5.7	0.36	20.3	1.8	86	73	0.11	0.23	104
Late gestation (Three or more lambs)																
	40	155	1.22	0.6	0.5	5.4	1.4	1.9	0.12	9.9	0.6	49	34	0.05	0.11	42
	60	210	1.57	0.9	0.7	7.3	1.9	2.5	0.16	13.0	0.8	63	45	0.07	0.14	57
	80	260	2.26	1.1	0.9	10.2	2.4	3.6	0.23	15.8	1.1	74	55	0.09	0.17	72
	100	307	2.59	1.4	1.1	12.1	2.8	4.1	0.26	18.5	1.3	85	65	0.10	0.20	86

TABLE 15-3 continued

Class/Stage/Other	Body Weight[b] kg	Body Weight Gain[c] g/d	Dry Matter Intake[d] kg/d	Na g/d	Cl g/d	K g/d	Mg g/d	S g/d	Co mg/d	Cu[e] mg/d	I mg/d	Fe mg/d	Mn mg/d	Se[f] mg/d	Se[g] mg/d	Zn[h] mg/d
	120	352	2.92	1.6	1.3	13.9	3.3	4.7	0.29	21.0	1.5	95	74	0.12	0.23	100
	140	396	4.04	1.9	1.5	18.0	3.8	6.5	0.40	23.5	2.0	104	83	0.13	0.26	113
Early lactation (Single lamb)																
	40	–14	1.09	0.8	1.3	5.9	1.4	1.7	0.22	6.4	0.9	8	15	0.17	0.34	44
	60	–17	1.77	1.1	1.7	9.0	1.9	2.8	0.35	8.8	1.4	11	21	0.21	0.43	59
	80	–20	2.13	1.4	2.0	11.1	2.4	3.4	0.43	11.1	1.7	14	27	0.25	0.50	74
	100	–22	2.47	1.7	2.4	13.1	2.8	4.0	0.49	13.3	2.0	18	33	0.28	0.57	88
	120	–24	2.78	1.9	2.7	15.0	3.3	4.4	0.56	15.5	2.2	21	39	0.32	0.63	102
	140	–26	3.08	2.2	3.0	16.8	3.7	4.9	0.62	17.7	2.5	24	45	0.34	0.69	115
Early lactation (Twin lambs)																
	40	–24	1.40	1.0	1.9	7.5	1.8	2.2	0.28	8.2	1.1	9	18	0.27	0.55	60
	60	–29	1.80	1.3	2.4	9.9	2.4	2.9	0.36	11.1	1.4	13	25	0.34	0.68	79
	80	–33	2.15	1.6	2.9	12.1	3.0	3.4	0.43	13.7	1.7	17	31	0.40	0.79	96
	100	–37	2.48	2.0	3.3	14.2	3.5	4.0	0.50	16.3	2.0	20	38	0.45	0.89	113
	120	–41	3.47	2.3	3.7	18.2	4.1	5.6	0.69	18.8	2.8	23	44	0.49	0.99	129
	140	–44	3.82	2.6	4.1	20.3	4.6	6.1	0.76	21.2	3.1	27	51	0.54	1.07	145
Early lactation (Three or more lambs)																
	40	–31	1.36	1.1	2.3	8.0	2.2	2.2	0.27	9.7	1.1	11	20	0.35	0.70	72
	60	–38	2.09	1.5	3.0	11.4	2.8	3.3	0.42	12.8	1.7	14	27	0.43	0.86	93
	80	–43	3.11	1.9	3.5	15.6	3.5	5.0	0.62	15.7	2.5	18	35	0.50	1.01	113
	100	–49	3.56	2.2	4.0	18.2	4.1	5.7	0.71	18.5	2.8	22	41	0.57	1.13	132
	120	–53	3.98	2.5	4.5	20.6	4.6	6.4	0.80	21.2	3.2	25	48	0.63	1.25	150
	140	–57	4.37	2.9	5.0	22.9	5.2	7.0	0.87	23.9	3.5	29	55	0.68	1.36	167
Early lactation (Parlor production only)																
	60	–52	2.14	1.8	3.9	12.7	3.5	3.4	0.43	15.7	1.7	17	32	0.59	1.18	117
	80	–60	3.04	2.2	4.6	16.7	4.3	4.9	0.61	19.0	2.4	21	40	0.68	1.37	141
	100	–67	3.46	2.6	5.2	19.3	5.0	5.5	0.69	22.2	2.8	25	47	0.77	1.54	163
	120	–73	3.86	3.0	5.8	21.8	5.6	6.2	0.77	25.3	3.1	29	54	0.85	1.69	184
	140	–79	5.29	3.3	6.4	27.2	6.2	8.5	1.06	28.2	4.2	32	61	0.92	1.84	204
Late lactation (Single lamb)																
	40	10	1.09	0.6	0.7	5.2	1.0	1.7	0.22	4.8	0.9	11	13	0.08	0.16	30
	60	12	1.43	0.9	0.9	7.1	1.4	2.3	0.29	6.9	1.1	15	19	0.10	0.20	43
	80	15	1.76	1.1	1.2	9.0	1.8	2.8	0.35	8.9	1.4	18	25	0.12	0.25	55
	100	17	2.05	1.4	1.4	10.8	2.2	3.3	0.41	10.9	1.6	22	30	0.14	0.29	67
	120	18	2.33	1.6	1.7	12.5	2.6	3.7	0.47	12.9	1.9	26	36	0.16	0.32	79
	140	20	2.60	1.9	1.9	14.2	3.0	4.2	0.52	14.9	2.1	29	42	0.18	0.36	91
Late lactation (Twin lambs)																
	40	25	1.38	0.7	0.9	6.3	1.1	2.2	0.28	5.8	1.1	16	15	0.13	0.25	38
	60	31	1.80	1.0	1.2	8.5	1.6	2.9	0.36	8.2	1.4	22	21	0.16	0.32	53
	80	37	2.19	1.2	1.5	10.6	2.1	3.5	0.44	10.4	1.8	27	28	0.19	0.38	67
	100	41	2.53	1.5	1.8	12.6	2.5	4.1	0.51	12.6	2.0	32	34	0.22	0.44	80
	120	46	2.87	1.8	2.0	14.5	2.9	4.6	0.57	14.8	2.3	36	40	0.25	0.50	93
	140	50	3.19	2.1	2.3	16.4	3.3	5.1	0.64	16.9	2.5	41	46	0.27	0.55	106
Late lactation (Three or more lambs)																
	60	44	2.06	1.0	1.4	9.5	1.8	3.3	0.41	9.1	1.7	27	23	0.20	0.41	60
	80	52	2.50	1.3	1.7	11.8	2.3	4.0	0.50	11.5	2.0	33	30	0.24	0.49	75
	100	59	2.89	1.6	2.0	14.0	2.7	4.6	0.58	13.9	2.3	38	36	0.28	0.56	90
	120	65	3.26	1.9	2.3	16.0	3.2	5.2	0.65	16.2	2.6	44	43	0.31	0.63	104
	140	70	3.59	2.2	2.6	18.0	3.6	5.8	0.72	18.4	2.9	49	49	0.34	0.69	118
Late lactation (Parlor production only)																
	60	50	2.35	1.1	1.7	10.7	2.0	3.8	0.47	10.3	1.9	30	25	0.26	0.53	69
	80	59	2.82	1.5	2.1	13.2	2.5	4.5	0.56	12.9	2.3	37	32	0.31	0.63	86
	100	66	3.25	1.8	2.4	15.5	3.0	5.2	0.65	15.4	2.6	43	39	0.36	0.72	102
	120	73	3.66	2.1	2.8	17.7	3.5	5.9	0.73	17.9	2.9	49	46	0.40	0.80	118
	140	80	4.05	2.3	3.1	19.9	4.0	6.5	0.81	20.3	3.2	55	52	0.44	0.88	133
Rams																
Maintenance only																
	100	0	1.77	1.2	0.9	9.3	1.8	2.8	0.18	6.7	0.9	14	27	0.04	0.08	51
	125	0	2.09	1.5	1.2	11.3	2.2	3.3	0.21	8.3	1.0	18	33	0.05	0.10	63
	150	0	2.40	1.8	1.4	13.3	2.6	3.8	0.24	10.0	1.2	21	40	0.06	0.13	76
	200	0	2.98	2.4	1.9	17.0	3.5	4.8	0.30	13.3	1.5	28	53	0.08	0.17	101

TABLE 15-3 continued

Class/Stage/Other	Body Weight[b] kg	Body Weight Gain[c] g/d	Dry Matter Intake[d] kg/d	Na g/d	Cl g/d	K g/d	Mg g/d	S g/d	Co mg/d	Cu[e] mg/d	I mg/d	Fe mg/d	Mn mg/d	Se[f] mg/d	Se[g] mg/d	Zn[h] mg/d
Prebreeding																
	100	47	1.95	1.2	1.0	9.9	1.9	3.1	0.39	7.5	1.0	28	30	0.08	0.16	58
	125	56	2.30	1.6	1.2	12.0	2.3	3.7	0.46	9.3	1.2	34	37	0.10	0.20	72
	150	64	2.64	1.9	1.5	14.1	2.8	4.2	0.53	11.1	1.3	40	44	0.12	0.23	86
	200	79	3.27	2.5	1.9	18.1	3.7	5.2	0.65	14.7	1.6	51	58	0.15	0.30	114

[a]Calcium and phosphorus requirements for sheep are listed in Tables 15-1 and 15-2.
[b]Body weight used in estimating requirements is the determined or estimated weight in kilograms (kg) average for the period during which these requirements will be applied.
[c]Average change in body weight over a 24-hour period.
[d]Estimate of dry matter intake of a feed of appropriate energy density to meet energy requirements.
[e]Copper absorption coefficients used were 0.06 for maintenance and gestation, and 0.045 for lactation.
[f]Selenium absorption coefficient used was 0.60 applicable to concentrate diets.
[g]Selenium absorption coefficient used was 0.30 applicable to forage diets.
[h]Zinc absorption coefficient used was 0.15.

NUTRIENT REQUIREMENTS OF GOAT TABLES

Energy and protein requirements of goats (Tables 15-4, 15-5, and 15-6) were projected as described earlier in the Energy and Protein sections (Chapters 4 and 5). The four biotypes of goats are dairy (goats selected for milk production, such as Saanen, Nubian, and Alpine), Boer (50 percent or more Boer breeding), Angora, and all others, termed indigenous or local. The "nondairy" classification applies to Boer and indigenous, with requirements for Angora goats listed separately. Growing non-Angora goats are ones post-weaning to 1.5 years of age.

Listed DM intakes are required to supply required energy from the example diets (containing either 1.91, 2.39, or 2.87 Mcal/kg ME) and were selected based on an expected range of intake considering body weight. In some cases, energy densities above or below those selected would be more appropriate. The metabolic fecal protein requirement for mature and lactating goats, which is a component of the maintenance need, was based on the estimate of DM intake required to supply needed energy for a given BW to achieved the specified level of production. However, protein requirements for other goats are relative to $BW^{0.75}$ and, thus, do not vary with the dietary concentration of ME. Because the relationship between MP and CP requirements varies with the nature of the diet, the aforementioned conversion of CP to MP of NRC (2000) was applied for diets with rumen undegraded intake (UIP) concentrations of 20, 40, and 60 percent of total CP.

Energy requirements are for ME; however, the efficiency of energy utilization varies with diet metabolizability. Therefore, for growing and Angora goats, DM intake for the selected diet (ME concentration of either 1.91, 2.39, or 2.87 Mcal/kg DM), which is necessary to provide required ME, is presented based on the adjustment of Sahlu et al. (2004). These intakes should be comparable to ones based on an NE system, although without encompassing effects of variation in the composition of tissue being accreted. The energy and protein requirements presented are directly applicable to goats in confinement and without an appreciable parasite burden. Hence, adjustments would be desirable for goats expending a great deal of energy in activity and for significant parasitism.

Energy and protein requirements of mature does during breeding and rams pre-breeding are 10 percent greater than at other times. Requirements in early and late gestation were determined for day 105 and 133 of gestation, respectively, and varied with expected birth weights of single, twin, and triplet kids (singles and twins for Angoras) as estimated from mature body weights of the female. Lactation requirements are estimated for early, mid-, and/or late phases for different levels of milk production. The assumed milk fat and protein concentrations are 4 percent (approximately 0.74 Mcal/kg) for goats other than Angora. For Angoras, milk fat and protein concentrations were assumed as 5 and 4 percent, respectively. Change in BW obviously can vary greatly with genotype, body condition, dietary conditions, and other characteristics. The simplest means to address requirements of lactating animals in tabular form would have been to simply assume 0 BW change, with requirements dictated solely by level of milk production and biotype. However, assumptions of BW change varying in accordance with level of production and stage of lactation were provided. Requirements for Angora goats are listed for intact males and females/male castrates. For growing animals, tissue gain listings are 0, 20, and 40 g/d and clean fiber growth rate is 4, 8, and 12 g/d. For mature Angoras, tissue gain is assumed 0 and clean fiber growth rate is 5, 10, 15, and 20 g/d.

Mineral requirements of goats are listed in Tables 15-7 and 15-8.

REFERENCES

NRC (National Research Council). 2000. Nutrient Requirements of Beef Cattle (Update 2000). Washington, DC: National Academy Press.

Sahlu, T., A. L. Goetsch, J. Luo, I. V. Nsahlai, J. E. Moore, M. L. Galyean, F. N. Owens, C. L. Ferrell, and Z. B. Johnson. 2004. Energy and protein requirements of goats: Developed equations, other considerations and future research to improve them. Small Ruminant Res. 53:191–220.

TABLE 15-4 Nutrient Requirements of Meat and Milk Goats (maintenance-gestation-lactation)

Class/Age/Other	Body Weight[a] kg	Birth Weight or Milk Yield[b] kg	Body Weight Gain[c] g/d	Energy Concentration in Diet[d] kcal/kg	Daily Dry Matter Intake[e] kg	Daily Dry Matter Intake[e] % BW	Energy Requirements[f] TDN kg/d	Energy Requirements[f] ME Mcal/d	Protein Requirements[g] CP @20% UIP g/d	CP @40% UIP g/d	CP @60% UIP g/d	MP g/d	DIP g/d	Mineral Requirements[h] Ca g/d	P g/d	Vitamin Requirements[i] A RE/d	E IU/d
Mature does (Dairy) Maintenance only																	
	20			1.91	0.59	2.96	0.31	1.13	40	38	36	27	28	1.3	0.9	628	106
	30			1.91	0.80	2.68	0.43	1.54	54	51	49	36	38	1.6	1.2	942	159
	40			1.91	1.00	2.49	0.53	1.91	67	64	61	45	48	1.9	1.5	1,256	212
	50			1.91	1.18	2.36	0.62	2.25	79	75	72	53	56	2.1	1.7	1,570	265
	60			1.91	1.35	2.25	0.72	2.58	90	86	82	61	64	2.4	2.0	1,884	318
	70			1.91	1.52	2.17	0.80	2.90	101	97	92	68	72	2.6	2.2	2,198	371
	80			1.91	1.68	2.10	0.89	3.20	112	107	102	75	80	2.8	2.4	2,512	424
	90			1.91	1.83	2.03	0.97	3.50	122	116	111	82	87	3.0	2.6	2,826	477
Mature does (Nondairy) Maintenance only																	
	20			1.91	0.50	2.50	0.26	0.96	36	35	33	24	24	1.2	0.8	628	106
	30			1.91	0.68	2.26	0.36	1.30	49	47	45	33	32	1.4	1.0	942	159
	40			1.91	0.84	2.10	0.45	1.61	61	58	55	41	40	1.7	1.3	1,256	212
	50			1.91	0.99	1.99	0.53	1.90	71	68	65	48	47	1.9	1.5	1,570	265
	60			1.91	1.14	1.90	0.60	2.18	82	78	75	55	54	2.1	1.7	1,884	318
	70			1.91	1.28	1.83	0.68	2.44	92	88	84	62	61	2.3	1.9	2,198	371
	80			1.91	1.41	1.77	0.75	2.70	101	97	93	68	67	2.5	2.0	2,512	424
	90			1.91	1.54	1.72	0.82	2.95	111	106	101	74	74	2.6	2.2	2,826	477
Mature does (Dairy) Breeding																	
	20			1.91	0.65	3.26	0.35	1.25	44	42	40	29	31	1.4	1.0	628	106
110% ME_m	30			1.91	0.88	2.95	0.47	1.69	59	57	54	40	42	1.7	1.3	942	159
110% MP_m	40			1.91	1.10	2.74	0.58	2.10	73	70	67	49	52	2.0	1.6	1,256	212
	50			1.91	1.30	2.59	0.69	2.48	87	83	79	58	62	2.3	1.9	1,570	265
	60			1.91	1.49	2.48	0.79	2.84	99	95	91	67	71	2.6	2.1	1,884	318
	70			1.91	1.67	2.38	0.88	3.19	111	106	102	75	80	2.8	2.4	2,198	371
	80			1.91	1.84	2.30	0.98	3.53	123	117	112	83	88	3.1	2.6	2,512	424
	90			1.91	2.01	2.24	1.07	3.85	134	128	123	90	96	3.3	2.9	2,826	477
Mature does (Nondairy) Breeding																	
	20			1.91	0.55	2.75	0.29	1.05	40	38	36	27	26	1.3	0.9	628	106
110% ME_m	30			1.91	0.75	2.48	0.40	1.42	54	51	49	36	36	1.5	1.1	942	159
110% MP_m	40			1.91	0.92	2.31	0.49	1.77	67	64	61	45	44	1.8	1.4	1,256	212
	50			1.91	1.09	2.19	0.58	2.09	79	75	72	53	52	2.0	1.6	1,570	265
	60			1.91	1.25	2.09	0.66	2.40	90	86	82	60	60	2.2	1.8	1,884	318
	70			1.91	1.41	2.01	0.75	2.69	101	96	92	68	67	2.5	2.0	2,198	371
	80			1.91	1.55	1.94	0.82	2.97	111	106	102	75	74	2.7	2.2	2,512	424
	90			1.91	1.70	1.89	0.90	3.25	122	116	111	82	81	2.9	2.4	2,826	477
Mature does (Dairy) Early gestation (Single kid; BW = 2.3 to 5.2 kg)																	
	20	2.3	9	1.91	0.73	3.66	0.39	1.40	63	60	58	42	35	3.5	1.9	628	106
	30	2.9	13	1.91	0.98	3.28	0.52	1.88	83	79	76	56	47	3.8	2.2	942	159

40	3.4	16	1.91	1.21	3.02	0.64	2.31	101	96	92	68	58	4.2	2.5	1,256	212
50	3.8	19	1.91	1.42	2.83	0.75	2.71	117	111	107	78	68	4.4	2.8	1,570	265
60	4.2	21	1.91	1.61	2.69	0.86	3.09	132	126	120	89	77	4.7	3.1	1,884	318
70	4.6	24	1.91	1.81	2.58	0.96	3.46	147	140	134	99	86	5.0	3.3	2,198	371
80	4.9	27	1.91	1.99	2.49	1.06	3.81	161	153	147	108	95	5.2	3.6	2,512	424
90	5.2	29	1.91	2.17	2.41	1.15	4.14	174	166	159	117	103	5.5	3.8	2,826	477

Mature does (Dairy) Early gestation (Twin kids; BW = 2.1 to 4.8 kg)

20	2.1	16	2.39	0.65	3.25	0.43	1.56	68	65	62	46	39	4.9	2.3	628	106
30	2.6	21	1.91	1.08	3.60	0.57	2.06	97	93	89	65	51	5.5	2.9	942	159
40	3	26	1.91	1.32	3.30	0.70	2.52	117	111	106	78	63	5.8	3.2	1,256	212
50	3.4	31	1.91	1.55	3.10	0.82	2.96	135	129	124	91	74	6.2	3.6	1,570	265
60	3.8	36	1.91	1.77	2.95	0.94	3.38	153	146	140	103	84	6.5	3.9	1,884	318
70	4.1	40	1.91	1.97	2.81	1.04	3.77	169	162	155	114	94	6.7	4.1	2,198	371
80	4.5	44	1.91	2.17	2.72	1.15	4.16	187	178	170	125	104	7.0	4.4	2,512	424
90	4.8	49	1.91	2.37	2.63	1.26	4.53	202	193	184	136	113	7.3	4.7	2,826	477

Mature does (Dairy) Early gestation (Three or more kids; BW = 1.8 to 4.1 kg)

30	2.2	28	1.91	1.14	3.81	0.61	2.18	105	101	96	71	55	7.0	3.5	942	159
40	2.6	34	1.91	1.40	3.50	0.74	2.68	127	122	116	86	67	7.3	3.9	1,256	212
50	2.9	41	1.91	1.64	3.27	0.87	3.13	147	140	134	99	78	7.6	4.2	1,570	265
60	3.2	47	1.91	1.86	3.10	0.99	3.56	165	158	151	111	89	8.0	4.5	1,884	318
70	3.5	52	1.91	2.08	2.97	1.10	3.97	183	175	167	123	99	8.2	4.8	2,198	371
80	3.8	58	1.91	2.29	2.86	1.21	4.38	201	192	184	135	109	8.5	5.1	2,512	424
90	4.1	63	1.91	2.49	2.77	1.32	4.77	218	208	199	147	119	8.8	5.4	2,826	477

Mature does (Dairy) Late gestation (Single kid; BW = 2.3 to 5.2 kg)

20	2.3	38	2.87	0.69	3.44	0.55	1.97	85	82	78	57	49	3.4	1.8	910	112
30	2.9	51	2.39	1.09	3.64	0.72	2.61	118	112	107	79	65	4.0	2.4	1,365	168
40	3.4	63	2.39	1.33	3.33	0.88	3.18	141	134	129	95	79	4.3	2.7	1,820	224
50	3.8	75	1.91	1.94	3.87	1.03	3.70	177	169	161	119	92	5.2	3.5	2,275	280
60	4.2	86	1.91	2.20	3.67	1.17	4.20	199	190	181	134	105	5.5	3.9	2,730	336
70	4.6	97	1.91	2.45	3.51	1.30	4.69	220	210	201	148	117	5.9	4.2	3,185	392
80	4.9	107	1.91	2.69	3.36	1.42	5.14	239	228	218	160	128	6.2	4.5	3,640	448
90	5.2	117	1.91	2.91	3.24	1.55	5.57	257	245	235	173	139	6.5	4.8	4,095	504

Mature does (Dairy) Late gestation (Twin kids; BW = 2.6 to 4.8 kg)

20	2.1	66	2.87	0.84	4.20	0.67	2.41	111	106	101	75	60	5.2	2.6	910	112
30	2.6	85	2.87	1.09	3.63	0.87	3.13	141	134	128	95	78	5.5	2.9	1,365	168
40	3	106	2.39	1.59	3.96	1.05	3.79	177	169	161	119	95	6.2	3.6	1,820	224
50	3.4	125	2.39	1.85	3.70	1.23	4.42	203	194	186	137	110	6.6	4.0	2,275	280
60	3.8	143	2.39	2.10	3.50	1.39	5.02	229	219	209	154	125	6.9	4.3	2,730	336
70	4.1	161	2.39	2.33	3.33	1.55	5.57	251	240	229	169	139	7.2	4.6	3,185	392
80	4.5	178	2.39	2.57	3.21	1.70	6.15	276	264	252	186	153	7.6	4.9	3,640	448
90	4.8	194	1.91	3.48	3.87	1.85	6.66	325	310	297	219	166	8.8	6.2	4,095	504

Mature does (Dairy) Late gestation (Three or more kids; BW = 2.6 to 4.1 kg)

30	1.8	79	2.87	1.20	4.00	0.95	3.44	158	151	144	106	66	7.0	3.6	1,365	168
40	2.2	109	2.87	1.47	3.67	1.17	4.21	189	181	173	127	86	7.4	4.0	1,820	224

TABLE 15-4 continued

Class/Age/Other	Body Weight[a] kg	Birth Weight or Milk Yield[b] kg	Body Weight Gain[c] g/d	Energy Concentration in Diet[d] kcal/kg	Daily Dry Matter Intake[e] kg	Daily Dry Matter Intake[e] % BW	Energy Requirements[f] TDN kg/d	Energy Requirements[f] ME Mcal/d	Protein Requirements[g] CP @20% UIP g/d	Protein Requirements[g] CP @40% UIP g/d	Protein Requirements[g] CP @60% UIP g/d	Protein Requirements[g] MP g/d	Protein Requirements[g] DIP g/d	Mineral Requirements[h] Ca g/d	Mineral Requirements[h] P g/d	Vitamin Requirements[i] A RE/d	Vitamin Requirements[i] E IU/d
	50	2.6	137	2.87	1.70	3.41	1.36	4.89	215	205	196	145	105	7.7	4.3	2,275	280
	60	2.9	163	2.39	2.31	3.86	1.53	5.53	256	244	233	172	122	8.6	5.1	2,730	336
	70	3.2	186	2.39	2.58	3.68	1.71	6.16	282	269	258	190	138	8.9	5.5	3,185	392
	80	3.5	209	2.39	2.83	3.54	1.88	6.77	308	294	282	207	154	9.3	5.8	3,640	448
	90	3.8	231	2.39	3.08	3.42	2.04	7.37	334	319	305	225	169	9.6	6.2	4,095	504
Mature does (Nondairy) Early gestation (Single kid; BW = 2.3 to 5.2 kg)																	
	20	2.3	9	1.91	0.64	3.20	0.34	1.22	59	57	54	40	31	3.4	1.7	628	106
	30	2.9	13	1.91	0.86	2.86	0.45	1.64	78	74	71	52	41	3.7	2.0	942	159
	40	3.4	16	1.91	1.05	2.63	0.56	2.01	94	90	86	63	50	3.9	2.3	1,256	212
	50	3.8	19	1.91	1.23	2.47	0.65	2.36	109	104	100	73	59	4.2	2.5	1,570	265
	60	4.2	21	1.91	1.40	2.34	0.74	2.68	124	118	113	83	67	4.4	2.8	1,884	318
	70	4.6	24	1.91	1.57	2.24	0.83	3.00	137	131	125	92	75	4.7	3.0	2,198	371
	80	4.9	27	1.91	1.73	2.16	0.92	3.30	150	143	137	101	82	4.9	3.2	2,512	424
	90	5.2	29	1.91	1.88	2.09	1.00	3.59	162	155	148	109	90	5.1	3.4	2,826	477
Mature does (Nondairy) Early gestation (Twin kids; BW = 2.1 to 4.8 kg)																	
	20	2.1	16	1.91	0.72	3.60	0.38	1.38	71	68	65	48	34	5.0	2.4	628	106
	30	2.6	21	1.91	0.95	3.18	0.51	1.82	92	88	84	62	45	5.3	2.8	942	159
	40	3	26	1.91	1.16	2.91	0.62	2.22	110	105	101	74	56	5.6	3.0	1,256	212
	50	3.4	31	1.91	1.36	2.73	0.72	2.61	128	122	117	86	65	5.9	3.3	1,570	265
	60	3.8	36	1.91	1.56	2.59	0.83	2.98	145	138	132	97	74	6.2	3.6	1,884	318
	70	4.1	40	1.91	1.73	2.48	0.92	3.31	160	153	146	108	83	6.4	3.8	2,198	371
	80	4.5	44	1.91	1.91	2.39	1.01	3.65	176	168	161	118	91	6.7	4.0	2,512	424
	90	4.8	49	1.91	2.08	2.31	1.10	3.98	191	182	174	128	99	6.9	4.3	2,826	477
Mature does (Nondairy) Early gestation (Three or more kids; BW = 1.8 to 4.1 kg)																	
	30	2.2	28	1.91	1.02	3.39	0.54	1.94	100	96	92	67	49	6.8	3.4	942	159
	40	2.6	34	1.91	1.24	3.11	0.66	2.38	121	116	111	81	59	7.1	3.7	1,256	212
	50	2.9	41	1.91	1.45	2.90	0.77	2.78	139	133	127	94	69	7.4	3.9	1,570	265
	60	3.2	47	1.91	1.65	2.75	0.88	3.16	157	150	143	105	79	7.7	4.2	1,884	318
	70	3.5	52	1.91	1.84	2.63	0.98	3.52	174	166	159	117	88	7.9	4.5	2,198	371
	80	3.8	58	1.91	2.03	2.53	1.07	3.88	191	182	174	128	97	8.2	4.7	2,512	424
	90	4.1	63	1.91	2.21	2.45	1.17	4.22	207	197	189	139	105	8.4	5.0	2,826	477
Mature does (Nondairy) Late gestation (Single kid; BW = 2.3 to 5.2 kg)																	
	20	2.3	38	2.39	0.75	3.76	0.50	1.80	88	84	80	59	45	3.5	1.9	910	112
	30	2.9	51	2.39	0.99	3.30	0.66	2.37	114	108	104	76	59	3.9	2.2	1,365	168
	40	3.4	63	2.39	1.21	3.01	0.80	2.88	136	130	124	91	72	4.1	2.5	1,820	224
	50	3.8	75	1.91	1.75	3.51	0.93	3.35	169	162	155	114	84	4.9	3.2	2,275	280
	60	4.2	86	1.91	1.99	3.31	1.05	3.80	190	182	174	128	95	5.2	3.6	2,730	336
	70	4.6	97	1.91	2.22	3.17	1.17	4.24	211	201	192	142	106	5.5	3.9	3,185	392
	80	4.9	107	1.91	2.42	3.03	1.29	4.63	228	218	209	153	116	5.8	4.2	3,640	448
	90	5.2	117	1.91	2.63	2.92	1.39	5.02	246	235	224	165	125	6.1	4.4	4,095	504

Mature does (Nondairy) Late gestation (Twin kids; BW = 2.1 to 4.8 kg)																	
	20	2.1	66	2.87	0.78	3.89	0.62	2.23	108	104	99	73	56	5.1	2.5	910	112
	30	2.6	85	2.87	1.01	3.35	0.80	2.89	137	131	125	92	72	5.4	2.8	1,365	168
	40	3	106	2.39	1.46	3.65	0.97	3.49	172	164	157	115	87	6.0	3.4	1,820	224
	50	3.4	125	2.39	1.70	3.40	1.13	4.06	197	189	180	133	101	6.4	3.8	2,275	280
	60	3.8	143	2.39	1.93	3.22	1.28	4.62	223	212	203	150	115	6.7	4.1	2,730	336
	70	4.1	161	2.39	2.14	3.06	1.42	5.12	244	233	223	164	128	7.0	4.4	3,185	392
	80	4.5	178	1.91	2.95	3.69	1.56	5.64	291	278	266	196	141	8.1	5.5	3,640	448
	90	4.8	194	1.91	3.20	3.55	1.70	6.11	314	300	287	211	153	8.4	5.8	4,095	504
Mature does (Nondairy) Late gestation (Three or more kids; BW = 1.8 to 4.1 kg)																	
	30	2.2	109	2.87	1.12	3.72	0.89	3.20	154	147	141	104	80	6.9	3.5	1,365	168
	40	2.6	137	2.87	1.36	3.41	1.08	3.91	185	177	169	124	98	7.3	3.8	1,820	224
	50	2.9	163	2.87	1.58	3.16	1.26	4.53	210	201	192	141	113	7.6	4.1	2,275	280
	60	3.2	186	2.39	2.14	3.57	1.42	5.12	249	238	227	167	128	8.3	4.9	2,730	336
	70	3.5	209	2.39	2.39	3.41	1.58	5.70	275	262	251	185	142	8.7	5.2	3,185	392
	80	3.8	231	2.39	2.62	3.28	1.74	6.26	300	286	274	202	156	9.0	5.5	3,640	448
	90	4.1	253	2.39	2.85	3.17	1.89	6.82	325	310	297	218	170	9.3	5.8	4,095	504
Mature does (Dairy) Early lactation (Single kid; milk yield = 0.88 to 1.61 kg/d)																	
	30	0.88	−19	1.91	1.38	4.59	0.73	2.64	77	73	70	52	66	5.5	3.5	1,605	168
Milk Fat = 4%	40	1.03	−21	1.91	1.67	4.17	0.89	3.19	93	89	85	63	80	5.9	3.9	2,140	224
	50	1.16	−23	1.91	1.94	3.87	1.03	3.70	109	104	99	73	92	6.3	4.3	2,675	280
	50	1.29	−24	1.91	2.19	3.66	1.16	4.20	124	118	113	83	105	6.7	4.6	3,210	336
	70	1.40	−25	1.91	2.43	3.47	1.29	4.65	138	131	126	92	116	7.0	5.0	3,745	392
	80	1.51	−26	1.91	2.66	3.33	1.41	5.09	151	144	138	101	127	7.3	5.3	4,280	448
	90	1.61	−27	1.91	2.88	3.20	1.53	5.51	164	156	150	110	138	7.6	5.6	4,815	504
Mature does (Dairy) Early lactation (Twin kids; milk yield = 2.06 to 3.22 g/d)																	
	40	2.06	−42	1.91	2.34	5.86	1.24	4.48	120	115	110	81	112	10.0	6.4	2,140	224
	50	2.33	−45	1.91	2.70	5.40	1.43	5.17	139	133	127	94	129	10.5	6.9	2,675	280
	60	2.57	−48	1.91	3.03	5.05	1.61	5.80	157	150	143	105	145	10.9	7.3	3,210	336
	70	2.80	−50	1.91	3.35	4.78	1.77	6.40	174	166	159	117	160	11.4	7.7	3,745	392
	80	3.01	−52	1.91	3.64	4.55	1.93	6.97	190	181	173	128	174	11.8	8.1	4,280	448
	90	3.22	−54	1.91	3.94	4.37	2.09	7.53	206	196	188	138	188	12.2	8.5	4,815	504
Mature does (Dairy) Early lactation (Three or more kids; milk yield = 3.49 to 4.82 kg/d)																	
	50	3.49	−68	2.39	2.77	5.54	1.83	6.61	142	136	130	96	165	13.7	8.5	2,675	280
	60	3.86	−72	2.39	3.10	5.17	2.05	7.41	160	153	146	108	185	14.1	8.9	3,210	336
	70	4.20	−75	2.39	3.41	4.87	2.26	8.15	177	169	162	119	203	14.6	9.4	3,745	392
	80	4.52	−78	1.91	4.63	5.79	2.46	8.85	229	219	209	154	221	16.3	11.0	4,280	448
	90	4.82	−81	1.91	4.98	5.54	2.64	9.53	247	236	226	166	238	16.7	11.5	4,815	504
Mature does (Dairy) Early lactation (Parlor production; milk yield = 4.65 to 6.43 kg/d)																	
	50	4.65	−90	2.87	2.81	5.62	2.24	8.06	144	138	132	97	201	16.8	10.1	2,675	280
	60	5.14	−95	2.87	3.14	5.23	2.50	9.01	162	155	148	109	225	17.3	10.5	3,210	336
	70	5.60	−100	2.39	4.14	5.92	2.74	9.90	206	197	188	139	247	18.7	11.9	3,745	392
	80	6.03	−104	2.39	4.49	5.62	2.98	10.74	224	214	205	151	268	19.2	12.4	4,280	448
	90	6.43	−108	2.39	4.83	5.36	3.20	11.54	242	231	221	163	288	19.6	12.8	4,815	504

TABLE 15-4 continued

Class/Age/Other	Body Weight[a] kg	Birth Weight or Milk Yield[b] kg	Body Weight Gain[c] g/d	Energy Concentration in Diet[d] kcal/kg	Daily Dry Matter Intake[e] kg	Daily Dry Matter Intake[e] % BW	Energy Requirements[f] TDN kg/d	Energy Requirements[f] ME Mcal/d	Protein Requirements[g] CP @20% UIP g/d	Protein Requirements[g] CP @40% UIP g/d	Protein Requirements[g] CP @60% UIP g/d	Protein Requirements[g] MP g/d	Protein Requirements[g] DIP g/d	Mineral Requirements[h] Ca g/d	Mineral Requirements[h] P g/d	Vitamin Requirements[i] A RE/d	Vitamin Requirements[i] E IU/d
Mature does (Dairy) Early lactation (Parlor production; milk yield = 5.82 to 8.04 kg/d)																	
	50	5.82	−113	2.87	3.32	6.64	2.64	9.53	165	157	150	111	238	20.7	12.3	2,675	280
	60	6.43	−119	2.87	3.70	6.17	2.94	10.62	184	176	168	124	265	21.2	12.8	3,210	336
	70	7.00	−125	2.87	4.06	5.80	3.23	11.65	203	194	185	137	291	21.7	13.3	3,745	392
	80	7.53	−130	2.87	4.40	5.50	3.50	12.62	221	211	202	148	315	22.2	13.8	4,280	448
	90	8.04	−135	2.87	4.72	5.25	3.76	13.55	238	227	217	160	338	22.6	14.2	4,815	504
Mature does (Dairy) Early lactation (Parlor production; milk yield = 6.98 to 9.65 kg/d)																	
	50	6.98	−135	2.87	3.83	7.65	3.04	10.98	185	176	169	124	274	24.5	14.5	2,675	280
	60	7.72	−143	2.87	4.26	7.11	3.39	12.23	207	198	189	139	305	25.1	15.1	3,210	336
	70	8.40	−150	2.87	4.67	6.67	3.72	13.40	228	217	208	153	334	25.6	15.7	3,745	392
	80	9.04	−156	2.87	5.06	6.32	4.02	14.50	247	236	226	166	362	26.2	16.2	4,280	448
	90	9.65	−162	2.87	5.43	6.03	4.32	15.56	266	254	243	179	388	26.7	16.7	4,815	504
Mature does (Dairy) Mid-lactation (Single kid; milk yield = 0.63 to 1.15 kg/d)																	
	30	0.63	0	1.91	1.22	4.05	0.64	2.32	70	67	64	47	58	5.3	3.3	1,605	168
	40	0.74	0	1.91	1.48	3.70	0.78	2.83	86	82	78	58	71	5.7	3.7	2,140	224
	50	0.83	0	1.91	1.72	3.44	0.91	3.29	100	96	92	67	82	6.0	4.0	2,675	280
	60	0.92	0	1.91	1.95	3.25	1.04	3.73	114	109	104	77	93	6.3	4.3	3,210	336
	70	1.00	0	1.91	2.17	3.10	1.15	4.15	127	121	116	85	104	6.6	4.6	3,745	392
	80	1.08	0	1.91	2.38	2.98	1.26	4.56	140	133	128	94	114	6.9	4.9	4,280	448
	90	1.15	0	1.91	2.58	2.87	1.37	4.94	152	145	139	102	123	7.2	5.2	4,815	504
Mature does (Dairy) Mid-lactation (Twin kids; milk yield = 1.47 to 2.30 kg/d)																	
	40	1.47	0	1.91	1.96	4.89	1.04	3.74	105	100	96	71	93	9.4	5.9	2,140	224
	50	1.66	0	1.91	2.26	4.53	1.20	4.33	122	116	111	82	108	9.9	6.3	2,675	280
	60	1.84	0	1.91	2.55	4.26	1.35	4.88	138	132	126	93	122	10.3	6.7	3,210	336
	70	2.00	0	1.91	2.82	4.03	1.50	5.40	153	146	140	103	135	10.6	7.0	3,745	392
	80	2.15	0	1.91	3.08	3.85	1.63	5.89	168	160	153	113	147	11.0	7.4	4,280	448
	90	2.30	0	1.91	3.33	3.71	1.77	6.38	182	174	166	122	159	11.3	7.7	4,815	504
Mature does (Dairy) Mid-lactation (Three or more kids; milk yield = 2.49 to 3.44 kg/d)																	
	50	2.49	0	1.91	2.81	5.61	1.49	5.37	143	137	131	96	134	13.7	8.5	2,675	280
	60	2.76	0	1.91	3.16	5.26	1.67	6.03	162	155	148	109	151	14.2	9.0	3,210	336
	70	3.00	0	1.91	3.48	4.97	1.84	6.65	179	171	164	120	166	14.7	9.4	3,745	392
	80	3.23	0	1.91	3.79	4.73	2.01	7.24	196	187	179	131	181	15.1	9.9	4,280	448
	90	3.44	0	1.91	4.08	4.53	2.16	7.80	211	202	193	142	195	15.5	10.3	4,815	504
Mature does (Dairy) Mid-lactation (Parlor production; milk yield = 3.32 to 4.59 kg/d)																	
	50	3.32	0	2.39	2.68	5.36	1.78	6.40	139	133	127	93	160	16.7	9.9	2,675	280
	60	3.67	0	2.39	3.00	5.00	1.99	7.17	156	149	143	105	179	17.1	10.3	3,210	336
	70	4.00	0	1.91	4.13	5.90	2.19	7.90	205	196	187	138	197	18.7	11.9	3,745	392
	80	4.3	0	1.91	4.49	5.61	2.38	8.58	223	213	204	150	214	19.2	12.4	4,280	448
	90	4.59	0	1.91	4.83	5.37	2.56	9.24	241	230	220	162	231	19.6	12.8	4,815	504

Mature does (Dairy) Mid-lactation (Parlor production; milk yield = 4.16 to 5.74 kg/d)															
50	4.16	0	2.87	2.60	5.20	2.07	7.45	136	130	124	91	186	19.7	11.3	2,675	280
60	4.59	0	2.39	3.48	5.80	2.31	8.32	175	167	160	118	208	20.9	12.5	3,210	336
70	5.00	0	2.39	3.83	5.47	2.54	9.15	194	185	177	130	228	21.4	13.0	3,745	392
80	5.38	0	2.39	4.15	5.19	2.75	9.93	211	201	193	142	248	21.8	13.4	4,280	448
90	5.74	0	2.39	4.47	4.96	2.96	10.68	227	217	208	153	266	22.2	13.9	4,815	504
Mature does (Dairy) Mid-lactation (Parlor production; milk yield = 4.99 to 6.89 kg/d)																
50	4.99	0	2.87	2.96	5.92	2.35	8.49	150	143	137	101	212	23.3	13.4	2,675	280
60	5.51	0	2.87	3.30	5.50	2.63	9.47	168	161	154	113	236	23.7	13.8	3,210	336
70	6.00	0	2.87	3.63	5.18	2.88	10.40	186	177	170	125	260	24.2	14.3	3,745	392
80	6.46	0	2.39	4.72	5.90	3.13	11.28	234	223	213	157	282	25.7	15.7	4,280	448
90	6.89	0	2.39	5.07	5.63	3.36	12.11	252	240	230	169	302	26.2	16.2	4,815	504
Mature does (Dairy) Late lactation (Single kid; milk yield = 0.38 to 0.69 kg/d)																
30	0.38	13	1.91	1.05	3.51	0.56	2.01	64	61	58	43	50	5.1	3.1	1,605	168
40	0.44	15	1.91	1.28	3.21	0.68	2.46	78	75	71	53	61	5.4	3.4	2,140	224
50	0.50	17	1.91	1.51	3.01	0.80	2.88	92	88	84	62	72	5.7	3.7	2,675	280
60	0.55	18	1.91	1.71	2.85	0.91	3.27	105	100	95	70	82	6.0	4.0	3,210	336
70	0.60	20	1.91	1.91	2.73	1.01	3.65	117	111	107	78	91	6.3	4.2	3,745	392
80	0.65	22	1.91	2.10	2.63	1.11	4.02	129	123	117	86	100	6.5	4.5	4,280	448
90	0.69	23	1.91	2.28	2.54	1.21	4.36	140	134	128	94	109	6.8	4.8	4,815	504
Mature does (Dairy) Late lactation (Twin kids; milk yield = 0.88 to 1.38 kg/d)																
40	0.88	29	1.91	1.57	3.93	0.83	3.01	90	86	82	60	75	8.9	5.3	2,140	224
50	1.00	33	1.91	1.83	3.66	0.97	3.50	105	100	96	70	87	9.3	5.7	2,675	280
60	1.10	37	1.91	2.07	3.45	1.10	3.96	119	113	108	80	99	9.6	6.0	3,210	336
70	1.20	40	1.91	2.30	3.29	1.22	4.40	132	126	121	89	110	9.9	6.3	3,745	392
80	1.29	43	1.91	2.52	3.15	1.34	4.82	145	139	133	98	120	10.2	6.6	4,280	448
90	1.38	46	1.91	2.73	3.04	1.45	5.23	158	151	144	106	130	10.5	6.9	4,815	504
Mature does (Dairy) Late lactation (Three or more kids; milk yield = 1.50 to 2.07 kg/d)																
50	1.50	50	1.91	2.16	4.32	1.14	4.13	118	112	108	79	103	12.8	7.7	2,675	280
60	1.65	55	1.91	2.43	4.05	1.29	4.65	133	127	122	89	116	13.2	8.0	3,210	336
70	1.80	60	1.91	2.69	3.85	1.43	5.15	148	141	135	99	129	13.6	8.4	3,745	392
80	1.94	65	1.91	2.94	3.68	1.56	5.63	162	155	148	109	141	13.9	8.7	4,280	448
90	2.07	69	1.91	3.18	3.54	1.69	6.09	176	168	161	118	152	14.2	9.1	4,815	504
Mature does (Dairy) Late lactation (Parlor production; milk yield = 1.99 to 2.76 kg/d)																
50	1.99	66	1.91	2.48	4.96	1.31	4.74	130	125	119	88	118	16.4	9.6	2,675	280
60	2.20	73	1.91	2.79	4.65	1.48	5.33	147	141	135	99	133	16.8	10.1	3,210	336
70	2.40	80	1.91	3.09	4.41	1.64	5.90	164	156	149	110	147	17.2	10.5	3,745	392
80	2.58	86	1.91	3.36	4.20	1.78	6.43	179	171	163	120	160	17.6	10.8	4,280	448
90	2.76	92	1.91	3.64	4.04	1.93	6.95	194	185	177	130	173	18.0	11.2	4,815	504
Mature does (Dairy) Late lactation (Parlor production; milk yield = 2.49 to 3.44 kg/d)																
50	2.49	83	1.91	2.81	5.61	1.49	5.37	143	137	131	96	134	16.8	10.1	2,675	280
60	2.76	92	1.91	3.16	5.26	1.67	6.03	162	155	148	109	151	17.3	10.6	3,210	336
70	3.00	100	1.91	3.48	4.97	1.84	6.65	179	171	164	120	166	17.8	11.0	3,745	392
80	3.23	108	1.91	3.79	4.74	2.01	7.24	196	187	179	132	181	18.2	11.4	4,280	448
90	3.44	115	1.91	4.08	4.53	2.16	7.80	211	202	193	142	195	18.6	11.8	4,815	504

TABLE 15-4 continued

Class/Age/Other	Body Weight[a] kg	Birth Weight or Milk Yield[b] kg	Body Weight Gain[c] g/d	Energy Concentration in Diet[d] kcal/kg	Daily Dry Matter Intake[e] kg	Daily Dry Matter Intake[e] % BW	Energy Requirements[f] TDN kg/d	Energy Requirements[f] ME Mcal/d	Protein Requirements[g] CP @20% UIP g/d	CP @40% UIP g/d	CP @60% UIP g/d	MP g/d	DIP g/d	Mineral Requirements[h] Ca g/d	P g/d	Vitamin Requirements[i] A RE/d	E IU/d
Mature does (Dairy) Late lactation (Parlor production; milk yield = 2.99 to 4.13 kg/d)																	
	50	2.99	100	2.39	2.51	5.01	1.66	5.99	132	126	120	89	150	16.4	9.7	2,675	280
	60	3.31	110	1.91	3.52	5.86	1.86	6.72	176	168	161	118	168	17.8	11.0	3,210	336
	70	3.60	120	1.91	3.87	5.53	2.05	7.40	195	186	178	131	185	18.3	11.5	3,745	392
	80	3.87	129	1.91	4.21	5.26	2.23	8.04	212	203	194	143	201	18.8	12.0	4,280	448
	90	4.13	138	1.91	4.53	5.04	2.40	8.66	229	219	209	154	216	19.2	12.4	4,815	504
Mature does (Nondairy) Early lactation (Single kid; milk yield = 0.55 to 1.25 kg/d)																	
	20	0.55	–15	1.91	0.86	4.30	0.46	1.64	50	48	46	34	41	4.8	2.8	1,070	112
	30	0.68	–19	1.91	1.12	3.74	0.59	2.14	67	64	61	45	54	5.2	3.2	1,605	168
	40	0.80	–22	1.91	1.36	3.41	0.72	2.61	81	78	74	55	65	5.5	3.5	2,140	224
	50	0.90	–25	1.91	1.58	3.16	0.84	3.02	95	91	87	64	75	5.8	3.8	2,675	280
	60	1.00	–28	1.91	1.79	2.99	0.95	3.43	108	103	98	72	86	6.1	4.1	3,210	336
	70	1.09	–30	1.91	1.99	2.84	1.06	3.81	120	115	110	81	95	6.4	4.4	3,745	392
	80	1.17	–32	1.91	2.18	2.72	1.15	4.16	132	126	120	89	104	6.6	4.6	4,280	448
	90	1.25	–35	1.91	2.36	2.62	1.25	4.51	143	137	131	96	113	6.9	4.9	4,815	504
Mature does (Nondairy) Early lactation (Twin kids; milk yield = 0.91 to 2.08 kg/d)																	
	20	0.91	–30	2.39	0.88	4.38	0.58	2.09	51	49	47	34	52	7.9	4.4	1,070	112
	30	1.14	–38	1.91	1.42	4.74	0.75	2.72	78	75	72	53	68	8.7	5.1	1,605	168
	40	1.33	–44	1.91	1.71	4.27	0.91	3.27	95	91	87	64	82	9.1	5.5	2,140	224
	50	1.51	–50	1.91	1.98	3.96	1.05	3.79	111	106	101	74	95	9.5	5.9	2,675	280
	60	1.67	–55	1.91	2.23	3.72	1.18	4.27	125	119	114	84	106	9.8	6.2	3,210	336
	70	1.81	–60	1.91	2.46	3.52	1.31	4.71	139	132	127	93	117	10.1	6.5	3,745	392
	80	1.95	–65	1.91	2.69	3.36	1.43	5.14	152	145	139	102	128	10.5	6.8	4,280	448
	90	2.08	–69	1.91	2.90	3.23	1.54	5.55	165	157	150	111	139	10.7	7.1	4,815	504
Mature does (Nondairy) Early lactation (Three or more kids; milk yield = 1.18 to 2.71 kg/d)																	
	30	1.48	–57	2.39	1.32	4.39	0.87	3.14	74	71	68	50	78	11.7	6.5	1,605	168
	40	1.73	–66	1.91	1.97	4.93	1.05	3.77	105	101	96	71	94	12.6	7.4	2,140	224
	50	1.96	–75	1.91	2.27	4.55	1.21	4.35	122	117	112	82	109	13.0	7.8	2,675	280
	60	2.17	–83	1.91	2.56	4.26	1.36	4.89	138	132	126	93	122	13.4	8.2	3,210	336
	70	2.36	–90	1.91	2.82	4.03	1.50	5.39	153	146	140	103	135	13.7	8.6	3,745	392
	80	2.54	–97	1.91	3.07	3.84	1.63	5.88	167	160	153	112	147	14.1	8.9	4,280	448
	90	2.71	–104	1.91	3.32	3.68	1.76	6.34	181	173	165	122	158	14.4	9.2	4,815	504
Mature does (Nondairy) Mid-lactation (Single kid; milk yield = 0.37 to 0.84 kg/d)																	
	20	0.37	0	1.91	0.74	3.71	0.39	1.42	46	44	42	31	35	4.6	2.7	1,070	112
	30	0.37	0	1.91	0.92	3.06	0.49	1.76	58	56	53	39	44	4.9	2.9	1,605	168
	40	0.54	0	1.91	1.19	2.98	0.63	2.28	75	71	68	50	57	5.3	3.3	2,140	224
	50	0.61	0	1.91	1.39	2.78	0.74	2.66	87	83	80	59	66	5.5	3.5	2,675	280
	60	0.67	0	1.91	1.58	2.63	0.84	3.02	99	95	91	67	75	5.8	3.8	3,210	336
	70	0.73	0	1.91	1.76	2.51	0.93	3.36	111	106	101	74	84	6.0	4.0	3,745	392
	80	0.78	0	1.91	1.92	2.40	1.02	3.68	122	116	111	82	92	6.3	4.3	4,280	448
	90	0.84	0	1.91	2.09	2.33	1.11	4.00	132	126	121	89	100	6.5	4.5	4,815	504

Mature does (Nondairy) Mid-lactation (Twin kids; milk yield = 0.61 to 1.40 kg/d)																	
	20	0.61	0	1.91	0.90	4.49	0.48	1.72	52	50	47	35	43	8.0	4.4	1,070	112
	30	0.76	0	1.91	1.17	3.91	0.62	2.25	69	65	63	46	56	8.4	4.8	1,605	168
	40	0.89	0	1.91	1.42	3.56	0.75	2.72	84	80	76	56	68	8.7	5.1	2,140	224
	50	1.01	0	1.91	1.65	3.31	0.88	3.16	98	93	89	66	79	9.0	5.4	2,675	280
	60	1.12	0	1.91	1.87	3.12	0.99	3.58	111	106	101	75	89	9.3	5.7	3,210	336
	70	1.22	0	1.91	2.08	2.97	1.10	3.97	123	118	113	83	99	9.6	6.0	3,745	392
	80	1.31	0	1.91	2.27	2.84	1.20	4.34	135	129	124	91	108	9.9	6.3	4,280	448
	90	1.40	0	1.91	2.46	2.73	1.30	4.70	147	140	134	99	117	10.1	6.5	4,815	504
Mature does (Nondairy) Mid-lactation (Three or more kids; milk yield = 0.79 to 1.81 kg/d)																	
	30	0.99	0	1.91	1.32	4.42	0.70	2.53	75	71	68	50	63	11.7	6.5	1,605	168
	40	1.16	0	1.91	1.60	4.00	0.85	3.06	91	87	83	61	76	12.1	6.9	2,140	224
	50	1.31	0	1.91	1.85	3.70	0.98	3.54	105	101	96	71	88	12.4	7.2	2,675	280
	60	1.45	0	1.91	2.09	3.48	1.11	3.99	119	114	109	80	100	12.7	7.6	3,210	336
	70	1.58	0	1.91	2.31	3.30	1.23	4.42	133	127	121	89	110	13.0	7.9	3,745	392
	80	1.70	0	1.91	2.52	3.16	1.34	4.83	145	139	133	98	120	13.3	8.2	4,280	448
	90	1.81	0	1.91	2.73	3.03	1.45	5.21	158	150	144	106	130	13.6	8.4	4,815	504
Mature does (Nondairy) Late lactation (Single kid; milk yield = 0.18 to 0.41 kg/d)																	
	20	0.18	12	1.91	0.62	3.09	0.33	1.18	41	39	37	27	29	4.5	2.5	1,070	112
	30	0.23	15	1.91	0.83	2.76	0.44	1.58	55	52	50	37	39	4.8	2.8	1,605	168
	40	0.26	18	1.91	1.01	2.53	0.54	1.93	67	64	61	45	48	5.0	3.0	2,140	224
	50	0.30	20	1.91	1.19	2.38	0.63	2.27	79	76	72	53	57	5.3	3.3	2,675	280
	60	0.33	22	1.91	1.35	2.26	0.72	2.59	90	86	83	61	65	5.5	3.5	3,210	336
	70	0.36	24	1.91	1.51	2.16	0.80	2.90	101	97	92	68	72	5.7	3.7	3,745	392
	80	0.39	26	1.91	1.67	2.09	0.88	3.19	111	106	102	75	80	5.9	3.9	4,280	448
	90	0.41	28	1.91	1.81	2.01	0.96	3.46	121	116	111	81	86	6.1	4.1	4,815	504
Mature does (Nondairy) Late lactation (Twin kids; milk yield = 0.30 to 0.69 kg/d)																	
	20	0.30	24	1.91	0.70	3.48	0.37	1.33	44	42	40	30	33	7.7	4.1	1,070	112
	30	0.38	30	1.91	0.93	3.09	0.49	1.77	59	56	54	39	44	8.0	4.5	1,605	168
	40	0.44	35	1.91	1.13	2.82	0.60	2.16	72	69	66	48	54	8.3	4.7	2,140	224
	50	0.50	40	1.91	1.32	2.64	0.70	2.52	84	81	77	57	63	8.6	5.0	2,675	280
	60	0.55	44	1.91	1.50	2.50	0.79	2.87	96	92	88	65	72	8.8	5.2	3,210	336
	70	0.60	48	1.91	1.67	2.39	0.89	3.20	107	102	98	72	80	9.0	5.5	3,745	392
	80	0.64	52	1.91	1.83	2.29	0.97	3.50	118	113	108	79	87	9.3	5.7	4,280	448
	90	0.69	55	1.91	2.00	2.22	1.06	3.81	129	123	117	86	95	9.5	5.9	4,815	504
Mature does (Nondairy) Late lactation (Three or more kids; milk yield = 0.39 to 0.89 kg/d)																	
	30	0.49	45	1.91	1.00	3.33	0.53	1.91	62	59	56	41	48	11.2	6.1	1,605	168
	40	0.57	53	1.91	1.21	3.03	0.64	2.32	75	72	69	51	58	11.5	6.4	2,140	224
	50	0.65	60	1.91	1.42	2.84	0.75	2.71	88	84	81	59	68	11.8	6.7	2,675	280
	60	0.71	66	1.91	1.60	2.67	0.85	3.07	100	96	92	67	77	12.1	6.9	3,210	336
	70	0.78	72	1.91	1.79	2.56	0.95	3.42	112	107	102	75	85	12.3	7.2	3,745	392
	80	0.84	78	1.91	1.96	2.45	1.04	3.75	123	118	112	83	94	12.6	7.4	4,280	448
	90	0.89	83	1.91	2.13	2.36	1.13	4.07	134	128	122	90	101	12.8	7.6	4,815	504
Mature bucks (Dairy)																	
Maintenance	50			1.91	1.36	2.71	0.72	2.59	86	82	78	58	65	2.4	2.0	1,570	265
	75			1.91	1.84	2.45	0.97	3.51	116	111	106	78	88	3.0	2.6	2,355	398

TABLE 15-4 continued

Class/Age/Other	Body Weight[a] kg	Birth Weight or Milk Yield[b] kg	Body Weight Gain[c] g/d	Energy Concentration in Diet[d] kcal/kg	Daily Dry Matter Intake[e] kg	Daily Dry Matter Intake[e] % BW	Energy Requirements[f] TDN kg/d	Energy Requirements[f] ME Mcal/d	Protein Requirements[g] CP @20% UIP g/d	CP @40% UIP g/d	CP @60% UIP g/d	MP g/d	DIP g/d	Mineral Requirements[h] Ca g/d	Mineral Requirements[h] P g/d	Vitamin Requirements[i] A RE/d	Vitamin Requirements[i] E IU/d
	100			1.91	2.28	2.28	1.21	4.36	144	137	131	97	109	3.7	3.2	3,140	530
	125			1.91	2.69	2.16	1.43	5.15	170	162	155	114	129	4.2	3.8	3,925	663
	150			1.91	3.09	2.06	1.64	5.91	195	186	178	131	147	4.8	4.3	4,710	795
Prebreeding	50			1.91	1.49	2.98	0.79	2.85	94	90	86	63	71	2.6	2.1	2,275	280
	75			1.91	2.02	2.69	1.07	3.86	128	122	117	86	96	3.3	2.9	3,413	420
	100			1.91	2.51	2.51	1.33	4.79	158	151	144	106	120	4.0	3.5	4,550	560
	125			1.91	2.96	2.37	1.57	5.67	187	178	171	126	141	4.6	4.1	5,688	700
	150			1.91	3.40	2.27	1.80	6.50	214	204	195	144	162	5.2	4.7	6,825	840
Mature bucks (Nondairy)																	
Maintenance	50			1.91	1.14	2.29	0.61	2.18	77	74	71	52	55	2.1	1.7	1,570	265
	75			1.91	1.55	2.06	0.82	2.96	105	100	96	70	74	2.7	2.2	2,355	398
	100			1.91	1.92	1.92	1.02	3.67	130	124	118	87	92	3.2	2.7	3,140	530
	125			1.91	2.27	1.82	1.20	4.34	153	146	140	103	108	3.7	3.2	3,925	663
	150			1.91	2.60	1.74	1.38	4.98	175	167	160	118	124	4.1	3.7	4,710	795
Prebreeding	50			1.91	1.26	2.51	0.67	2.40	85	81	78	57	60	2.2	1.8	2,275	280
	75			1.91	1.70	2.27	0.90	3.26	115	110	105	77	81	2.9	2.4	3,413	420
	100			1.91	2.11	2.11	1.12	4.04	143	136	130	96	101	3.4	3.0	4,550	560
	125			1.91	2.50	2.00	1.32	4.78	168	161	154	113	119	4.0	3.5	5,688	700
	150			1.91	2.86	1.91	1.52	5.48	193	184	176	130	137	4.5	4.0	6,825	840

[a]Body weight used in estimating requirements is the determined or estimated weight in kilograms (kg) average for the period during which these requirements will be applied.
[b]Birth weight (kg) of single and average of multiple kids or liquid milk yield (kg/d).
[c]Average change in body weight over a 24-hour period.
[d]Three hypothetical diets with increasing energy concentrations (1.91, 2.34, and 2.87 kcal/kg) were used in the calculations of intake and nutrient requirements. For each line entry, a diet was selected to represent the level of energy concentration that approximates that needed by the animal to achieve adequate intake to satisfy its energy requirement.
[e]The daily dry matter intake, expressed as kg or as percentage of body weight, of a diet having the indicated energy concentration (previous column) that is required to meet energy requirements. These energy concentrations should be viewed only as examples. In some cases, diets having greater or lesser concentrations of energy would be more appropriate.
[f]Energy requirements expressed as total digestible nutrients (TDN) in kg/d and metabolizable energy (ME) as kcal/d.
[g]Protein requirements expressed as crude protein (CP), metabolizable protein (MP), and degradable intake protein (DIP). The CP requirement differs with the proportion of undegradable intake protein (UIP) because of the required minimal DIP.
[h]Two macro minerals, calcium (Ca) and phosphorus (P), commonly considered in balancing diets are included. Often, the balance (ratio) of the two minerals also is of concern.
[i]Two fat-soluble vitamins, A and E, that often are deficient in animal diets are expressed as retinol equivalents (RE) and international units (IU) for vitamins A and E, respectively. RE = 1.0 μg of all-trans retinol, 5.0 μg of all-trans betacarotene, and 7.6 μg of other carotenoids.

TABLE 15-5 Nutrient Requirements of Goats (growing kids)

Class/Age/Other	Body Weight[a] kg	Body Weight Gain[b] g/d	Energy Concentration in Diet[c] kcal/kg	Daily Dry Matter Intake[d] kg	Daily Dry Matter Intake[d] % BW	Energy Requirements[e] TDN kg/d	Energy Requirements[e] ME Mcal/d	Protein Requirements[f] CP @ 20% UIP g/d	Protein Requirements[f] CP @ 40% UIP g/d	Protein Requirements[f] CP @ 60% UIP g/d	Protein Requirements[f] MP g/d	Protein Requirements[f] DIP g/d	Mineral Requirements[g] Ca g/d	Mineral Requirements[g] P g/d	Vitamin Requirements[h] A RE/d	Vitamin Requirements[h] E IU/d
Growing Kids (Doelings and male castrates)																
Dairy	10	0	2.39	0.30	2.97	0.20	0.72	26	25	23	17	18	0.9	0.5	1,000	100
	10	25	2.39	0.35	3.55	0.24	0.86	36	35	33	25	21	1.6	0.8	1,000	100
	10	100	2.87	0.40	4.02	0.35	1.27	69	66	63	46	32	3.5	1.6	1,000	100
	10	150	2.87	0.48	4.81	0.43	1.55	90	86	83	61	39	4.8	2.2	1,000	100
	10	200	2.87	0.56	5.57	0.51	1.82	112	107	102	75	46	6.2	2.7	1,000	100
	15	0	1.91	0.54	3.63	0.27	0.98	35	33	32	23	24	1.3	0.9	1,500	150
	15	25	2.39	0.46	3.07	0.31	1.11	46	44	42	31	28	1.8	1.0	1,500	150
	15	100	2.87	0.49	3.25	0.42	1.53	78	74	71	52	38	3.6	1.7	1,500	150
	15	150	2.87	0.57	3.79	0.50	1.80	100	95	91	67	45	5.0	2.3	1,500	150
	15	200	2.87	0.65	4.3[illegible]	0.58	2.08	121	116	111	81	52	6.3	2.8	1,500	150
	20	0	1.91	0.68	3.38	0.34	1.21	43	41	39	29	30	1.4	1.0	2,000	200
	20	25	1.91	0.76	3.79	0.37	1.35	54	52	49	36	34	2.2	1.4	2,000	200
	20	100	2.39	0.73	3.65	0.49	1.76	86	82	79	58	44	4.0	2.0	2,000	200
	20	150	2.87	0.65	3.24	0.57	2.04	108	103	99	73	51	5.1	2.4	2,000	200
	20	200	2.87	0.73	3.64	0.64	2.31	130	124	118	87	58	6.4	3.0	2,000	200
	20	250	2.87	0.81	4.03	0.72	2.59	151	144	138	102	65	7.7	3.5	2,000	200
	25	0	1.91	0.80	3.20	0.40	1.43	51	49	47	34	36	1.6	1.2	2,500	250
	25	25	1.91	0.88	3.53	0.44	1.57	62	59	56	42	39	2.3	1.5	2,500	250
	25	100	2.39	0.82	3.29	0.55	1.98	94	90	86	63	49	4.1	2.2	2,500	250
	25	150	2.39	0.94	3.75	0.63	2.26	116	111	106	78	56	5.5	2.8	2,500	250
	25	200	2.87	0.80	3.21	0.70	2.54	137	131	125	92	63	6.5	3.1	2,500	250
	25	250	2.87	0.88	3.53	0.78	2.81	159	152	145	107	70	7.8	3.6	2,500	250
	30	0	1.91	0.92	3.05	0.46	1.64	59	56	53	39	41	1.8	1.4	3,000	300
	30	25	1.91	1.00	3.33	0.49	1.78	69	66	63	47	44	2.5	1.7	3,000	300
	30	100	2.39	0.91	3.03	0.61	2.19	102	97	93	68	55	4.2	2.3	3,000	300
	30	150	2.39	1.02	3.41	0.68	2.47	123	118	113	83	62	5.6	2.9	3,000	300
	30	200	2.39	1.14	3.80	0.76	2.74	145	138	132	97	69	7.0	3.5	3,000	300
	30	250	2.87	0.95	3.17	0.84	3.02	166	159	152	112	75	7.9	3.7	3,000	300
	30	300	2.87	1.03	3.44	0.91	3.30	188	179	172	126	82	9.3	4.3	3,000	300
	35	0	1.91	1.03	2.94	0.51	1.84	66	63	60	44	46	1.9	1.5	3,500	350
	35	25	1.91	1.11	3.17	0.55	1.98	77	73	70	51	49	2.7	1.9	3,500	350
	35	100	1.91	1.36	3.89	0.66	2.39	109	104	99	73	60	4.8	2.9	3,500	350
	35	150	2.39	1.11	3.[illegible]6	0.74	2.67	130	125	119	88	67	5.7	3.0	3,500	350
	35	200	2.39	1.22	3.49	0.82	2.95	152	145	139	102	74	7.1	3.6	3,500	350
	35	250	2.39	1.34	3.83	0.89	3.22	174	166	159	117	80	8.5	4.2	3,500	350
	35	300	2.87	1.10	3.[illegible]4	0.97	3.50	195	186	178	131	87	9.4	4.4	3,500	350

TABLE 15-5 continued

Class/Age/Other	Body Weight[a] kg	Body Weight Gain[b] g/d	Energy Concentration in Diet[c] Mcal/kg	Daily Dry Matter Intake[d] kg	Daily Dry Matter Intake[d] % BW	Energy Requirements[e] TDN kg/d	Energy Requirements[e] ME Mcal/d	Protein Requirements[f] CP @ 20% UIP g/d	CP @ 40% UIP g/d	CP @ 60% UIP g/d	MP g/d	DIP g/d	Mineral Requirements[g] Ca g/d	Mineral Requirements[g] P g/d	Vitamin Requirements[h] A RE/d	Vitamin Requirements[h] E IU/d
	40	0	1.91	1.14	2.84	0.56	2.04	73	69	66	49	51	2.1	1.7	4,000	400
	40	25	1.91	1.22	3.05	0.60	2.17	83	80	76	56	54	2.8	2.0	4,000	400
	40	100	1.91	1.47	3.67	0.72	2.59	116	111	106	78	65	5.0	3.0	4,000	400
	40	150	2.39	1.19	2.97	0.79	2.86	137	131	125	92	71	5.8	3.1	4,000	400
	40	200	2.39	1.30	3.26	0.87	3.14	159	152	145	107	78	7.2	3.7	4,000	400
	40	250	2.39	1.42	3.55	0.95	3.42	181	172	165	121	85	8.6	4.4	4,000	400
	40	300	2.39	1.54	3.84	1.02	3.69	202	193	185	136	92	10.0	5.0	4,000	400
Boer	10	0	1.91	0.34	3.39	0.17	0.61	26	25	23	17	15	1.0	0.6	1,000	100
	10	25	2.39	0.31	3.08	0.21	0.75	41	39	37	27	19	1.5	0.8	1,000	100
	10	100	2.87	0.36	3.64	0.32	1.16	86	82	78	58	29	3.5	1.5	1,000	100
	10	150	2.87	0.44	4.42	0.40	1.44	116	111	106	78	36	4.8	2.1	1,000	100
	10	200	2.87	0.52	5.15	0.47	1.71	146	139	133	98	43	6.1	2.7	1,000	100
	15	0	1.91	0.46	3.07	0.23	0.82	35	33	32	23	21	1.1	0.7	1,500	150
	15	25	1.91	0.54	3.61	0.27	0.96	50	48	46	34	24	1.9	1.1	1,500	150
	15	100	2.39	0.57	3.81	0.38	1.38	95	91	87	64	34	3.7	1.8	1,500	150
	15	150	2.87	0.52	3.44	0.46	1.65	125	119	114	84	41	4.9	2.2	1,500	150
	15	200	2.87	0.59	3.96	0.53	1.93	155	148	142	104	48	6.2	2.8	1,500	150
	20	0	1.91	0.57	2.85	0.28	1.02	43	41	39	29	25	1.3	0.9	2,000	200
	20	25	1.91	0.65	3.26	0.32	1.16	58	56	53	39	29	2.0	1.2	2,000	200
	20	100	2.39	0.65	3.26	0.44	1.57	103	99	94	69	39	3.9	1.9	2,000	200
	20	150	2.39	0.77	3.85	0.51	1.85	133	127	122	90	46	5.2	2.6	2,000	200
	20	200	2.87	0.66	3.31	0.59	2.13	163	156	149	110	53	6.3	2.9	2,000	200
	20	250	2.87	0.74	3.70	0.67	2.40	194	185	177	130	60	7.6	3.4	2,000	200
	25	0	1.91	0.67	2.70	0.33	1.21	51	49	47	34	30	1.4	1.0	2,500	250
	25	25	1.91	0.76	3.03	0.37	1.35	66	63	60	44	34	2.2	1.4	2,500	250
	25	100	2.39	0.73	2.92	0.49	1.76	111	106	102	75	44	4.0	2.0	2,500	250
	25	150	2.39	0.85	3.38	0.56	2.04	141	135	129	95	51	5.3	2.7	2,500	250
	25	200	2.39	0.96	3.85	0.64	2.31	171	164	156	115	58	6.7	3.3	2,500	250
	25	250	2.37	0.80	3.22	0.72	2.59	201	192	184	135	65	7.7	3.5	2,500	250
	30	0	1.91	0.77	2.58	0.38	1.38	59	56	53	39	35	1.6	1.2	3,000	300
	30	25	1.91	0.86	2.85	0.42	1.52	74	70	67	49	38	2.3	1.5	3,000	300
	30	100	1.91	1.11	3.69	0.54	1.94	119	113	108	80	48	4.5	2.5	3,000	300
	30	150	2.39	0.92	3.06	0.61	2.21	149	142	136	100	55	5.4	2.8	3,000	300
	30	200	2.39	1.04	3.45	0.69	2.49	179	171	163	120	62	6.8	3.4	3,000	300
	30	250	2.39	1.15	3.84	0.77	2.76	209	199	191	140	69	8.2	4.0	3,000	300
	30	300	2.87	0.94	3.14	0.84	3.04	239	228	218	161	76	9.1	4.2	3,000	300

	35	0	1.91	0.87	2.48	0.43	1.55	66	63	60	44	39	1.7	1.3	3,500	350
	35	25	1.91	0.95	2.71	0.47	1.69	81	77	74	54	42	2.4	1.6	3,500	350
	35	100	1.91	1.20	3.43	0.58	2.11	126	120	115	85	53	4.6	2.7	3,500	350
	35	150	1.91	1.37	3.92	0.66	2.38	156	149	142	105	59	6.1	3.4	3,500	350
	35	200	2.39	1.10	3.16	0.74	2.66	186	178	170	125	66	6.9	3.5	3,500	350
	35	250	2.39	1.22	3.49	0.81	2.93	216	206	197	145	73	8.3	4.1	3,500	350
	35	300	2.39	1.34	3.83	0.89	3.21	246	235	225	165	80	9.7	4.7	3,500	350
	40	0	1.91	0.96	2.40	0.48	1.72	73	69	66	49	43	1.8	1.4	4,000	400
	40	25	1.91	1.04	2.60	0.51	1.86	88	84	80	59	46	2.6	1.8	4,000	400
	40	100	1.91	1.29	3.23	0.63	2.27	133	127	121	89	57	4.7	2.8	4,000	400
	40	150	1.91	1.46	3.65	0.71	2.55	163	155	149	109	64	6.2	3.5	4,000	400
	40	200	2.39	1.17	2.93	0.78	2.82	193	184	176	130	70	7.0	3.6	4,000	400
	40	250	2.39	1.29	3.22	0.86	3.10	223	213	204	150	77	8.4	4.2	4,000	400
	40	300	2.39	1.41	3.51	0.94	3.37	253	242	231	170	84	9.8	4.8	4,000	400
Indigenous Local	10	0	1.91	0.34	3.39	0.17	0.61	26	25	23	17	15	1.0	0.6	1,000	100
	10	25	2.39	0.30	3.00	0.20	0.73	36	35	33	25	18	1.5	0.8	1,000	100
	10	50	2.87	0.34	3.42	0.30	1.08	69	66	63	46	27	2.2	1.0	1,000	100
	10	150	2.87	0.41	4.09	0.37	1.32	90	86	83	61	33	4.7	2.1	1,000	100
	10	200	2.87	0.47	4.74	0.43	1.55	112	107	102	75	39	6.1	2.6	1,000	100
	15	0	1.91	0.46	3.07	0.23	0.82	35	33	32	23	21	1.1	0.7	1,500	150
	15	25	1.91	0.53	3.53	0.26	0.94	46	44	42	31	23	1.9	1.1	1,500	150
	15	100	2.39	0.54	3.59	0.36	1.30	78	74	71	52	32	3.7	1.8	1,500	150
	15	150	2.87	0.48	3.22	0.43	1.53	100	95	91	67	38	4.8	2.2	1,500	150
	15	200	2.87	0.55	3.67	0.49	1.77	121	116	111	81	44	6.2	2.7	1,500	150
	20	0	1.91	0.57	2.85	0.28	1.02	43	41	39	29	25	1.3	0.9	2,000	200
	20	25	1.91	0.64	3.20	0.32	1.14	54	52	49	36	28	2.0	1.2	2,000	200
	20	100	2.39	0.62	3.10	0.41	1.49	86	82	79	58	37	3.8	1.9	2,000	200
	20	150	2.39	0.72	3.60	0.48	1.73	108	103	99	73	43	5.2	2.5	2,000	200
	20	200	2.87	0.62	3.09	0.55	1.97	130	124	118	87	49	6.3	2.8	2,000	200
	20	250	2.87	0.68	3.42	0.61	2.20	151	144	138	102	55	7.6	3.4	2,000	200
	25	0	1.91	0.67	2.70	0.33	1.21	51	49	47	34	30	1.4	1.0	2,500	250
	25	25	1.91	0.74	2.98	0.37	1.33	62	59	56	42	33	2.1	1.4	2,500	250
	25	100	1.91	0.96	3.34	0.47	1.68	94	90	86	63	42	4.3	2.3	2,500	250
	25	150	2.39	0.80	3.18	0.53	1.92	116	111	106	78	48	5.3	2.6	2,500	250
	25	200	2.39	0.90	3.58	0.60	2.15	137	131	125	92	54	6.6	3.2	2,500	250
	25	250	2.39	1.00	3.98	0.66	2.39	159	152	145	107	60	8.0	3.8	2,500	250
	30	0	1.91	0.77	2.58	0.38	1.38	59	56	53	39	35	1.6	1.2	3,000	300
	30	25	1.91	0.84	2.81	0.42	1.50	69	66	63	47	38	2.3	1.5	3,000	300
	30	100	1.91	1.06	3.53	0.52	1.86	102	97	93	68	46	4.4	2.5	3,000	300
	30	150	2.39	0.87	2.89	0.58	2.09	123	118	113	83	52	5.4	2.7	3,000	300
	30	200	2.39	0.97	3.23	0.65	2.33	145	138	132	97	58	6.7	3.3	3,000	300
	30	250	2.39	1.07	3.56	0.71	2.57	166	159	152	112	64	8.1	3.9	3,000	300
	30	300	2.39	1.17	3.90	0.78	2.80	188	179	172	126	70	9.5	4.5	3,000	300

TABLE 15-5 continued

Class/Age/Other	Body Weight[a] kg	Body Weight Gain[b] g/d	Energy Concentration in Diet[c] kcal/kg	Daily Dry Matter Intake[d] kg	Daily Dry Matter Intake[d] % BW	Energy Requirements[e] TDN kg/d	Energy Requirements[e] ME Mcal/d	Protein Requirements[f] CP @ 20% UIP g/d	CP @ 40% UIP g/d	CP @ 60% UIP g/d	MP g/d	DIP g/d	Mineral Requirements[g] Ca g/d	P g/d	Vitamin Requirements[h] A RE/d	E IU/d
	35	0	1.91	0.87	2.48	0.43	1.55	66	63	60	44	39	1.7	1.3	3,500	350
	35	25	1.91	0.94	2.68	0.46	1.67	77	73	70	51	42	2.4	1.6	3,500	350
	35	100	1.91	1.15	3.29	0.56	2.03	109	104	99	73	51	4.5	2.6	3,500	350
	35	150	1.91	1.30	3.71	0.63	2.26	130	125	119	88	56	6.0	3.3	3,500	350
	35	200	2.39	1.04	2.97	0.69	2.50	152	145	139	102	62	6.8	3.4	3,500	350
	35	250	2.39	1.14	3.25	0.76	2.74	174	166	159	117	68	8.2	4.0	3,500	350
	35	300	2.39	1.24	3.54	0.82	2.97	195	186	178	131	74	9.6	4.6	3,500	350
	40	0	1.91	0.96	2.40	0.48	1.72	73	69	66	49	43	1.8	1.4	4,000	400
	40	25	1.91	1.03	2.57	0.51	1.84	83	80	76	56	46	2.5	1.7	4,000	400
	40	100	1.91	1.24	3.11	0.61	2.19	116	111	106	78	55	4.7	2.7	4,000	400
	40	150	1.91	1.39	3.47	0.67	2.43	137	131	125	92	61	6.1	3.4	4,000	400
	40	200	1.91	1.53	3.84	0.74	2.66	159	152	145	107	66	7.5	4.0	4,000	400
	40	250	2.39	1.21	3.01	0.80	2.90	181	172	165	121	72	8.3	4.1	4,000	400
	40	300	2.39	1.31	3.26	0.87	3.14	202	193	185	136	78	9.6	4.7	4,000	400
Growing Kids (Intact males)																
Dairy	10	0	2.39	0.35	3.46	0.23	0.84	26	25	23	17	21	1.0	0.6	1,000	100
	10	25	2.87	0.32	3.17	0.27	0.98	36	35	33	25	24	1.6	0.8	1,000	100
	10	100	2.87	0.44	4.42	0.39	1.39	69	66	63	46	35	3.6	1.6	1,000	100
	10	150	2.87	0.52	5.22	0.46	1.67	90	86	83	61	42	4.9	2.2	1,000	100
	10	200	2.87	0.60	5.99	0.54	1.94	112	107	102	75	48	6.2	2.8	1,000	100
	15	0	2.39	0.47	3.12	0.31	1.14	35	33	32	23	28	1.2	0.8	1,500	150
	15	25	2.39	0.53	3.51	0.35	1.27	46	44	42	31	32	1.8	1.1	1,500	150
	15	100	2.87	0.54	3.61	0.47	1.69	78	74	71	52	42	3.7	1.8	1,500	150
	15	150	2.87	0.62	4.15	0.54	1.96	100	95	91	67	49	5.0	2.4	1,500	150
	15	200	2.87	0.70	4.68	0.62	2.24	121	116	111	81	56	6.4	2.9	1,500	150
	20	0	1.91	0.79	3.94	0.39	1.41	43	41	39	29	35	1.6	1.2	2,000	200
	20	25	2.39	0.64	3.20	0.43	1.55	54	52	49	36	39	2.0	1.2	2,000	200
	20	100	2.87	0.63	3.16	0.54	1.96	86	82	79	58	49	3.8	1.9	2,000	200
	20	150	2.87	0.71	3.57	0.62	2.24	108	103	99	73	56	5.2	2.5	2,000	200
	20	200	2.87	0.79	3.97	0.70	2.51	130	124	118	87	63	6.5	3.0	2,000	200
	20	250	2.87	0.87	4.37	0.77	2.79	151	144	138	102	70	7.8	3.6	2,000	200
	25	0	1.91	0.93	3.72	0.46	1.67	51	49	47	34	42	1.8	1.4	2,500	250
	25	25	2.39	0.74	2.98	0.50	1.80	62	59	56	42	45	2.1	1.4	2,500	250
	25	100	2.39	0.92	3.67	0.62	2.22	94	90	86	63	55	4.2	2.3	2,500	250
	25	150	2.87	0.80	3.19	0.69	2.49	116	111	106	78	62	5.3	2.6	2,500	250
	25	200	2.87	0.88	3.52	0.77	2.77	137	131	125	92	69	6.6	3.2	2,500	250
	25	250	2.87	0.96	3.84	0.84	3.05	159	152	145	107	76	7.9	3.7	2,500	250

	30	0	1.91	1.07	3.56	0.53	1.91	59	56	53	39	48	2.0	1.6	3,000	300
	30	25	1.91	1.15	3.83	0.57	2.05	69	66	63	47	51	2.7	1.9	3,000	300
	30	100	2.39	1.02	3.40	0.68	2.46	102	97	93	68	61	4.4	2.4	3,000	300
	30	150	2.39	1.13	3.78	0.76	2.74	123	118	113	83	68	5.7	3.0	3,000	300
	30	200	2.87	0.96	3.21	0.84	3.01	145	138	132	97	75	6.7	3.3	3,000	300
	30	250	2.87	1.04	3.48	0.91	3.29	166	159	152	112	82	8.1	3.8	3,000	300
	30	300	2.87	1.12	3.74	0.99	3.57	188	179	172	126	89	9.4	4.4	3,000	300
	35	0	1.91	1.20	3.42	0.59	2.14	66	63	60	44	54	2.2	1.7	3,500	350
	35	25	1.91	1.28	3.66	0.63	2.28	77	73	70	51	57	2.9	2.1	3,500	350
	35	100	2.39	1.12	3.19	0.75	2.70	109	104	99	73	67	4.5	2.6	3,500	350
	35	150	2.39	1.23	3.52	0.82	2.97	130	125	119	88	74	5.9	3.2	3,500	350
	35	200	2.39	1.35	3.85	0.90	3.25	152	145	139	102	81	7.3	3.8	3,500	350
	35	250	2.87	1.12	3.20	0.98	3.52	174	166	159	117	88	8.2	4.0	3,500	350
	35	300	2.87	1.20	3.43	1.05	3.80	195	186	178	131	95	9.5	4.5	3,500	350
	40	0	1.91	1.32	3.31	0.66	2.37	73	69	66	49	59	2.3	1.9	4,000	400
	40	25	1.91	1.41	3.51	0.70	2.51	83	80	76	56	63	3.1	2.3	4,000	400
	40	100	2.39	1.21	3.02	0.81	2.92	116	111	106	78	73	4.6	2.7	4,000	400
	40	150	2.39	1.32	3.31	0.89	3.20	137	131	125	92	80	6.0	3.3	4,000	400
	40	200	2.39	1.44	3.60	0.96	3.47	159	152	145	107	87	7.4	3.9	4,000	400
	40	250	2.39	1.56	3.89	1.04	3.75	181	172	165	121	94	8.8	4.5	4,000	400
	40	300	2.87	1.28	3.19	1.12	4.03	202	193	185	136	100	9.6	4.6	4,000	400
Boer	10	0	1.91	0.40	3.96	0.20	0.71	26	25	23	17	18	1.1	0.7	1,000	100
	10	25	2.39	0.35	3.50	0.23	0.85	41	39	37	27	21	1.6	0.8	1,000	100
	10	100	2.87	0.40	3.99	0.35	1.26	86	82	78	58	31	3.5	1.6	1,000	100
	10	150	2.87	0.48	4.77	0.43	1.54	116	111	106	78	38	4.8	2.2	1,000	100
	10	200	2.87	0.55	5.53	0.50	1.81	146	139	133	98	45	6.2	2.7	1,000	100
	15	0	1.91	0.54	3.58	0.27	0.96	35	33	32	23	24	1.2	0.9	1,500	150
	15	25	2.39	0.45	3.03	0.30	1.10	50	48	46	34	27	1.7	1.0	1,500	150
	15	100	2.87	0.48	3.22	0.42	1.51	95	91	87	64	38	3.6	1.7	1,500	150
	15	150	2.87	0.56	3.75	0.50	1.79	125	119	114	84	45	5.0	2.3	1,500	150
	15	200	2.87	0.64	4.28	0.57	2.06	155	148	142	104	52	6.3	2.8	1,500	150
	20	0	1.91	0.67	3.33	0.33	1.19	43	41	39	29	30	1.4	1.0	2,000	200
	20	25	1.91	0.75	3.74	0.37	1.33	58	56	53	39	33	2.2	1.4	2,000	200
	20	100	2.39	0.72	3.61	0.48	1.74	103	99	94	69	44	4.0	2.0	2,000	200
	20	150	2.87	0.64	3.21	0.56	2.02	133	127	122	90	50	5.1	2.4	2,000	200
	20	200	2.87	0.72	3.60	0.64	2.30	163	156	149	110	57	6.4	2.9	2,000	200
	20	250	2.87	0.80	4.00	0.71	2.57	194	185	177	130	64	7.7	3.5	2,000	200
	25	0	1.91	0.79	3.15	0.39	1.41	51	49	47	34	35	1.6	1.2	2,500	250
	25	25	1.91	0.87	3.48	0.43	1.55	66	63	60	44	39	2.3	1.5	2,500	250
	25	100	2.39	0.81	3.25	0.54	1.96	111	106	102	75	49	4.1	2.1	2,500	250
	25	150	2.39	0.93	3.71	0.62	2.24	141	135	129	95	56	5.5	2.8	2,500	250
	25	200	2.87	0.79	3.18	0.70	2.51	171	164	156	115	63	6.5	3.0	2,500	250
	25	250	2.87	0.87	3.49	0.77	2.79	201	192	184	135	70	7.8	3.6	2,500	250

TABLE 15-5 continued

Class/Age/Other	Body Weight[a] kg	Body Weight Gain[b] g/d	Energy Concentration in Diet[c] kcal/kg	Daily Dry Matter Intake[d] kg	Daily Dry Matter Intake[d] % BW	Energy Requirements[e] TDN kg/d	Energy Requirements[e] ME Mcal/d	Protein Requirements[f] CP @ 20% UIP g/d	CP @ 40% UIP g/d	CP @ 60% UIP g/d	MP g/d	DIP g/d	Mineral Requirements[g] Ca g/d	P g/d	Vitamin Requirements[h] A RE/d	E IU/d
	30	0	1.91	0.90	3.01	0.45	1.62	59	56	53	39	40	1.8	1.3	3,000	300
	30	25	1.91	0.98	3.28	0.49	1.75	74	70	67	49	44	2.5	1.7	3,000	300
	30	100	2.39	0.90	2.99	0.60	2.17	119	113	108	80	54	4.2	2.3	3,000	300
	30	150	2.39	1.01	3.38	0.68	2.44	149	142	136	100	61	5.6	2.9	3,000	300
	30	200	2.39	1.13	3.77	0.75	2.72	179	171	163	120	68	7.0	3.5	3,000	300
	30	250	2.87	0.94	3.15	0.83	3.00	209	199	191	140	75	7.9	3.7	3,000	300
	30	300	2.87	1.02	3.41	0.91	3.27	239	228	218	161	82	9.3	4.3	3,000	300
	35	0	1.91	1.01	2.89	0.50	1.81	66	63	60	44	45	1.9	1.5	3,500	350
	35	25	1.91	1.09	3.13	0.54	1.95	81	77	74	54	49	2.6	1.8	3,500	350
	35	100	1.91	1.34	3.84	0.66	2.37	126	120	115	85	59	4.8	2.9	3,500	350
	35	150	2.39	1.09	3.13	0.73	2.64	156	149	142	105	66	5.7	3.0	3,500	350
	35	200	2.39	1.21	3.46	0.81	2.92	186	178	170	125	73	7.1	3.6	3,500	350
	35	250	2.39	1.33	3.79	0.89	3.19	216	206	197	145	80	8.5	4.2	3,500	350
	35	300	2.87	1.09	3.11	0.96	3.47	246	235	225	165	87	9.3	4.4	3,500	350
	40	0	1.91	1.12	2.80	0.56	2.00	73	69	66	49	50	2.1	1.6	4,000	400
	40	25	1.91	1.20	3.00	0.59	2.14	88	84	80	59	53	2.8	2.0	4,000	400
	40	100	1.91	1.45	3.63	0.71	2.56	133	127	121	89	64	5.0	3.0	4,000	400
	40	150	2.39	1.17	2.93	0.79	2.83	163	155	149	109	71	5.8	3.1	4,000	400
	40	200	2.39	1.29	3.22	0.86	3.11	193	184	176	130	78	7.2	3.7	4,000	400
	40	250	2.39	1.41	3.52	0.94	3.38	223	213	204	150	84	8.6	4.3	4,000	400
	40	300	2.39	1.52	3.81	1.01	3.66	253	242	231	170	91	9.9	5.0	4,000	400
Indigenous Local	10	0	1.91	0.40	3.96	0.20	0.71	26	25	23	17	18	1.1	0.7	1,000	100
	10	25	2.39	0.34	3.42	0.23	0.83	36	35	33	25	21	1.6	0.8	1,000	100
	10	50	2.87	0.38	3.76	0.33	1.18	69	66	63	46	29	2.2	1.1	1,000	100
	10	150	2.87	0.44	4.44	0.39	1.42	90	86	83	61	35	4.8	2.1	1,000	100
	10	200	2.87	0.51	5.10	0.46	1.65	112	107	102	75	41	6.1	2.7	1,000	100
	15	0	1.91	0.54	3.58	0.27	0.96	35	33	32	23	24	1.2	0.9	1,500	150
	15	25	2.39	0.45	2.97	0.30	1.08	46	44	42	31	27	1.7	1.0	1,500	150
	15	100	2.39	0.59	3.96	0.40	1.43	78	74	71	52	36	3.8	1.9	1,500	150
	15	150	2.87	0.53	3.53	0.46	1.67	100	95	91	67	42	4.9	2.2	1,500	150
	15	200	2.87	0.60	3.98	0.53	1.91	121	116	111	81	48	6.2	2.8	1,500	150
	20	0	1.91	0.67	3.33	0.33	1.19	43	41	39	29	30	1.4	1.0	2,000	200
	20	25	1.91	0.74	3.68	0.36	1.31	54	52	49	36	33	2.1	1.4	2,000	200
	20	100	2.39	0.69	3.45	0.46	1.66	86	82	79	58	42	3.9	2.0	2,000	200
	20	150	2.39	0.79	3.95	0.53	1.90	108	103	99	73	47	5.3	2.6	2,000	200
	20	200	2.87	0.68	3.38	0.59	2.14	130	124	118	87	53	6.3	2.9	2,000	200
	20	250	2.87	0.74	3.72	0.66	2.37	151	144	138	102	59	7.6	3.4	2,000	200

25	0	1.91	0.79	3.15	0.39	1.41	51	49	47	34	35	1.6	1.2	2,500	250
25	25	1.91	0.86	3.43	0.42	1.53	62	59	56	42	38	2.3	1.5	2,500	250
25	100	2.39	0.78	3.12	0.52	1.88	94	90	86	63	47	4.0	2.1	2,500	250
25	150	2.39	0.88	3.51	0.59	2.12	116	111	106	78	53	5.4	2.7	2,500	250
25	200	2.39	0.98	3.91	0.65	2.35	137	131	125	92	59	6.7	3.3	2,500	250
25	250	2.87	0.82	3.27	0.72	2.59	159	152	145	107	65	7.7	3.5	2,500	250
30	0	1.91	0.90	3.01	0.45	1.62	59	56	53	39	40	1.8	1.3	3,000	300
30	25	1.91	0.97	3.24	0.48	1.73	69	66	63	47	43	2.5	1.7	3,000	300
30	100	1.91	1.19	3.95	0.58	2.09	102	97	93	68	52	4.6	2.7	3,000	300
30	150	2.39	0.96	3.21	0.64	2.32	123	118	113	83	58	5.5	2.8	3,000	300
30	200	2.39	1.06	3.54	0.71	2.56	145	138	132	97	64	6.9	3.4	3,000	300
30	250	2.39	1.16	3.88	0.78	2.80	166	159	152	112	70	8.2	4.0	3,000	300
30	300	2.87	0.96	3.18	0.84	3.03	188	179	172	126	76	9.2	4.2	3,000	300
35	0	1.91	1.01	2.89	0.50	1.81	66	63	60	44	45	1.9	1.5	3,500	350
35	25	1.91	1.08	3.09	0.54	1.93	77	73	70	51	48	2.6	1.8	3,500	350
35	100	1.91	1.30	3.70	0.63	2.29	109	104	99	73	57	4.7	2.8	3,500	350
35	150	2.39	1.05	2.99	0.70	2.52	130	125	119	88	63	5.6	2.9	3,500	350
35	200	2.39	1.14	3.27	0.77	2.76	152	145	139	102	69	7.0	3.5	3,500	350
35	250	2.39	1.24	3.55	0.83	3.00	174	166	159	117	75	8.3	4.1	3,500	350
35	300	2.39	1.34	3.84	0.90	3.23	195	186	178	131	81	9.7	4.7	3,500	350
40	0	1.91	1.12	2.80	0.56	2.00	73	69	66	49	50	2.1	1.6	4,000	400
40	25	1.91	1.19	2.97	0.59	2.12	83	80	76	56	53	2.8	2.0	4,000	400
40	100	1.91	1.40	3.51	0.69	2.48	116	111	106	78	62	4.9	2.9	4,000	400
40	150	1.91	1.55	3.87	0.75	2.71	137	131	125	92	68	6.3	3.6	4,000	400
40	200	2.39	1.22	3.06	0.82	2.95	159	152	145	107	74	7.1	3.6	4,000	400
40	250	2.39	1.32	3.31	0.88	3.19	181	172	165	121	80	8.4	4.2	4,000	400
40	300	2.39	1.42	3.56	0.95	3.42	202	193	185	136	85	9.8	4.8	4,000	400

[a]Body weight used in estimating requirements is the determined or estimated weight in kilograms (kg) average for the period during which these requirements will be applied.

[b]Average change in body weight over a 24-hour period.

[c]Three hypothetical diets with increasing energy concentrations (1.91, 2.34, and 2.87 kcal/kg) were used in the calculations of intake and nutrient requirements. For each line entry, a diet was selected to represent the level of energy concentration that approximates that needed by the animal to achieve adequate intake to satisfy its energy requirement.

[d]The daily dry matter intake, expressed as kg or as percentage of body weight, of a diet having the indicated energy concentration (previous column) that is required to meet energy requirements. These energy concentrations should be viewed only as examples. In some cases, diets having greater or lesser concentrations of energy would be more appropriate.

[e]Energy requirements expressed as total digestible nutrients (TDN) in kg/d and metabolizable energy (ME) as kcal/d.

[f]Protein requirements expressed as crude protein (CP), metabolizable protein (MP), and degradable intake protein (DIP). The CP requirement differs with the proportion of undegradable intake protein (UIP) because of the required minimal DIP.

[g]Two macro minerals, calcium (Ca) and phosphorus (P), commonly considered in balancing diets are included. Often, the balance (ratio) of the two minerals also is of concern.

[h]Two fat-soluble vitamins, A and E, that often are deficient in animal diets are expressed as retinol equivalents (RE) and international units (IU) for vitamins A and E, respectively. RE = 1.0 μg of all-trans retinol, 5.0 μg of all-trans betacarotene, and 7.6 μg of other carotenoids

TABLE 15-6 Nutrient Requirements of Goats (Angora)

Class/Age/Other	Body Weight[a] kg	Birth Weight or Milk Yield[b] kg	Daily Gain[c] g/d	Mohair Fiber Growth[d] g/d	Energy Concentration in Diet[e] kcal/kg	Daily Dry Matter Intake[f] kg	Daily Dry Matter Intake[f] % BW	Energy Requirements[g] TDN kg/d	Energy Requirements[g] ME Mcal/d	Protein Requirements[h] CP @20% UIP g/d	Protein Requirements[h] CP @40% UIP g/d	Protein Requirements[h] CP @60% UIP g/d	Protein Requirements[h] MP g/d	Protein Requirements[h] DIP g/d	Mineral Requirements[i] Ca g/d	Mineral Requirements[i] P g/d	Vitamin Requirements[j] A RE/d	Vitamin Requirements[j] E IU/d
Growing Angora Kids																		
Female kids																		
	10		0	4	2.39	0.32	3.21	0.21	0.77	38	36	35	25	19	1.0	0.6	1,000	100
	10		0	8	2.39	0.38	3.84	0.25	0.92	48	46	44	32	23	1.0	0.6	1,000	100
	10		20	4	2.39	0.40	3.96	0.26	0.95	46	44	42	31	24	1.5	0.8	1,000	100
	10		20	8	2.87	0.39	3.87	0.30	1.10	56	53	51	38	27	1.5	0.8	1,000	100
	10		40	4	2.87	0.36	3.57	0.31	1.12	55	52	50	37	28	2.0	1.0	1,000	100
	10		40	8	2.87	0.42	4.20	0.35	1.27	64	61	59	43	32	2.1	1.1	1,000	100
	20		0	4	1.91	0.66	3.28	0.33	1.19	57	54	52	38	30	1.4	1.0	2,000	200
	20		0	8	1.91	0.74	3.69	0.37	1.34	67	64	61	45	33	1.5	1.1	2,000	200
	20		20	4	1.91	0.76	3.80	0.38	1.37	65	62	60	44	34	2.0	1.3	2,000	200
	20		20	8	1.91	0.79	3.97	0.42	1.52	75	72	69	51	38	2.1	1.4	2,000	200
	20		40	4	2.39	0.65	3.24	0.43	1.55	74	70	67	50	39	2.4	1.4	2,000	200
	20		40	8	2.39	0.71	3.55	0.47	1.70	84	80	76	56	42	2.5	1.5	2,000	200
	30		0	4	1.91	1.05	3.50	0.53	1.90	89	85	81	60	47	2.0	1.5	3,000	300
	30		0	8	1.91	1.13	3.77	0.57	2.05	99	94	90	66	51	2.1	1.7	3,000	300
	30		0	12	2.39	0.92	3.06	0.61	2.20	109	104	99	73	55	1.8	1.4	3,000	300
	30		20	4	1.91	1.15	3.84	0.58	2.08	97	93	89	66	52	2.6	1.9	3,000	300
	30		20	8	1.91	1.18	3.94	0.62	2.23	107	102	98	72	56	2.6	1.9	3,000	300
	30		20	12	1.91	1.19	3.97	0.66	2.38	117	112	107	79	59	2.6	1.9	3,000	300
	30		40	4	2.39	0.95	3.15	0.63	2.26	106	101	97	71	56	2.8	1.8	3,000	300
	30		40	8	2.39	1.01	3.35	0.67	2.41	116	110	106	78	60	2.9	1.9	3,000	300
	30		40	12	2.39	1.06	3.55	0.71	2.56	125	120	115	84	64	3.0	1.9	3,000	300
Male kids																		
	10		0	4	2.39	0.36	3.63	0.24	0.87	38	36	35	25	22	1.0	0.6	1,000	100
	10		0	8	2.87	0.34	3.39	0.28	1.02	48	46	44	32	25	1.0	0.6	1,000	100
	10		20	4	2.87	0.35	3.45	0.29	1.05	46	44	42	31	26	1.5	0.8	1,000	100
	10		20	8	2.87	0.42	4.20	0.33	1.20	56	53	51	38	30	1.6	0.9	1,000	100
	10		40	4	2.87	0.39	3.90	0.34	1.23	55	52	50	37	31	2.0	1.0	1,000	100
	10		40	8	2.87	0.45	4.53	0.38	1.38	64	61	59	43	34	2.1	1.1	1,000	100
	20		0	4	1.91	0.75	3.75	0.38	1.36	57	54	52	38	34	1.5	1.1	2,000	200
	20		0	8	2.39	0.63	3.16	0.42	1.51	67	64	61	45	38	1.4	1.0	2,000	200
	20		20	4	2.39	0.64	3.22	0.43	1.54	65	62	60	44	38	1.9	1.2	2,000	200
	20		20	8	2.39	0.70	3.51	0.47	1.69	75	72	69	51	42	2.0	1.3	2,000	200
	20		40	4	2.39	0.72	3.60	0.48	1.72	74	70	67	50	43	2.5	1.5	2,000	200
	20		40	8	2.39	0.78	3.90	0.52	1.87	84	80	76	56	47	2.6	1.6	2,000	200
	30		0	4	2.39	0.91	3.05	0.61	2.19	89	85	81	60	55	1.8	1.4	3,000	300
	30		0	8	2.39	0.98	3.25	0.65	2.34	99	94	90	66	58	1.9	1.4	3,000	300
	30		0	12	2.39	1.04	3.46	0.69	2.49	109	104	99	73	62	1.9	1.5	3,000	300
	30		20	4	2.39	0.99	3.29	0.66	2.36	97	93	89	66	59	2.4	1.6	3,000	300
	30		20	8	2.39	1.05	3.49	0.70	2.51	107	102	98	72	63	2.4	1.7	3,000	300
	30		20	12	2.39	1.10	3.68	0.74	2.66	117	112	107	79	66	2.5	1.8	3,000	300
	30		40	4	2.39	1.07	3.55	0.70	2.54	106	101	97	71	63	3.0	1.9	3,000	3000

30	40	8	2.39	1.13	3.75	0.75	2.69	116	110	106	78	67	3.0	2.0	3,000	300
30	40	12	2.39	1.18	3.95	0.79	2.84	125	120	115	84	71	3.1	2.1	3,000	300
Mature Angora Males																
Maintenance only																
30	0	5	1.91	1.02	3.41	0.51	1.85	76	73	70	51	46	1.9	1.5	942	159
30	0	10	1.91	1.12	3.75	0.57	2.04	88	84	81	59	51	2.1	1.6	942	159
30	0	15	2.39	0.93	3.10	0.62	2.23	101	96	92	68	56	1.8	1.4	942	159
40	0	5	1.91	1.24	3.11	0.63	2.26	92	87	84	62	56	2.2	1.8	1,256	212
40	0	10	1.91	1.35	3.37	0.68	2.44	104	99	95	70	61	2.4	1.9	1,256	212
40	0	15	1.91	1.45	3.62	0.73	2.63	116	111	106	78	66	2.5	2.1	1,256	212
50	0	10	1.91	1.56	3.11	0.78	2.82	118	113	108	79	70	2.7	2.2	1,570	265
50	0	15	1.91	1.66	3.31	0.83	3.01	131	125	119	88	75	2.8	2.4	1,570	265
50	0	20	1.91	1.76	3.52	0.89	3.19	143	136	130	96	80	2.9	2.5	1,570	265
60	0	10	1.91	1.75	2.92	0.88	3.18	132	126	121	89	79	2.9	2.5	1,884	318
60	0	15	1.91	1.85	3.09	0.93	3.37	144	138	132	97	84	3.1	2.6	1,884	318
60	0	20	1.91	1.96	3.26	0.99	3.55	157	149	143	105	89	3.2	2.8	1,884	318
Breeding																
30		5	1.91	1.12	3.75	0.57	2.04	84	80	77	56	51	2.1	1.6	1,365	168
30		10	2.39	0.94	3.13	0.62	2.25	97	93	89	65	56	1.8	1.4	1,365	168
30		15	2.39	1.02	3.41	0.68	2.45	111	106	101	74	61	1.9	1.5	1,365	168
40		5	1.91	1.37	3.42	0.69	2.48	101	96	92	68	62	2.4	2.0	1,820	224
40		10	1.91	1.48	3.70	0.75	2.69	114	109	104	77	67	2.6	2.1	1,820	224
40		15	1.91	1.59	3.98	0.80	2.89	128	122	117	86	72	2.7	2.3	1,820	224
50		10	1.91	1.71	3.42	0.86	3.10	130	124	119	87	77	2.9	2.4	2,275	280
50		15	1.91	1.82	3.64	0.92	3.31	144	137	131	97	83	3.0	2.6	2,275	280
50		20	1.91	1.93	3.86	0.97	3.51	157	150	143	106	88	3.2	2.7	2,275	280
60		10	1.91	1.93	3.21	0.97	3.50	145	139	133	98	87	3.2	2.7	2,730	336
60		15	1.91	2.04	3.39	1.03	3.70	159	152	145	107	92	3.3	2.9	2,730	336
60		20	1.91	2.15	3.58	1.08	3.91	172	164	157	116	98	3.5	3.0	2,730	336
Mature Angora Females																
Maintenance only																
30	0	5	1.91	0.90	3.01	0.45	1.64	76	73	70	51	41	1.8	1.3	942	159
30	0	10	1.91	1.00	3.35	0.51	1.82	88	84	81	59	46	1.9	1.5	942	159
30	0	15	1.91	1.11	3.69	0.56	2.01	101	96	92	68	50	2.0	1.6	942	159
40	0	5	1.91	1.10	2.74	0.55	1.98	92	87	84	62	50	2.0	1.6	1,256	212
40	0	10	1.91	1.20	2.99	0.60	2.17	104	99	95	70	54	2.2	1.7	1,256	212
40	0	15	1.91	1.30	3.25	0.65	2.36	116	111	106	78	59	2.3	1.9	1,256	212
50	0	10	1.91	1.38	2.76	0.69	2.50	118	113	108	79	62	2.4	2.0	1,570	265
50	0	15	1.91	1.48	2.96	0.75	2.69	131	125	119	88	67	2.6	2.1	1,570	265
50	0	20	1.91	1.58	3.16	0.80	2.87	143	136	130	96	72	2.7	2.3	1,570	265
60	0	10	1.91	1.55	2.58	0.78	2.81	132	126	121	89	70	2.7	2.2	1,884	318
60	0	15	1.91	1.65	2.75	0.83	3.00	144	138	132	97	75	2.8	2.4	1,884	318
60	0	20	1.91	1.75	2.92	0.88	3.19	157	149	143	105	80	2.9	2.5	1,884	318
Mature Angora Females																
Breeding																
30		5	1.91	0.99	3.30	0.50	1.80	84	80	77	56	45	1.9	1.5	942	159
30		10	1.91	1.10	3.68	0.56	2.01	97	93	89	65	50	2.0	1.6	942	159

TABLE 15-6 continued

Class/Age/Other	Body Weight[a] kg	Birth Weight or Milk Yield[b] kg	Daily Gain[c] g/d	Mohair Fiber Growth[d] g/d	Energy Concentration in Diet[e] kcal/kg	Daily Dry Matter Intake[f] kg	Daily Dry Matter Intake[f] % BW	Energy Requirements[g] TDN kg/d	Energy Requirements[g] ME Mcal/d	Protein Requirements[h] CP @20% UIP g/d	Protein Requirements[h] CP @40% UIP g/d	Protein Requirements[h] CP @60% UIP g/d	Protein Requirements[h] MP g/d	Protein Requirements[h] DIP g/d	Mineral Requirements[i] Ca g/d	Mineral Requirements[i] P g/d	Vitamin Requirements[j] A RE/d	Vitamin Requirements[j] E IU/d
	30			15	2.39	0.92	3.08	0.61	2.21	111	106	101	74	55	1.8	1.4	942	159
	40			5	1.91	1.20	3.01	0.61	2.18	101	96	92	68	54	2.2	1.8	1,256	212
	40			10	1.91	1.31	3.29	0.66	2.39	114	109	104	77	60	2.3	1.9	1,256	212
	40			15	1.91	1.43	3.57	0.72	2.60	128	122	117	86	65	2.5	2.1	1,256	212
	50			10	1.91	1.51	3.03	0.76	2.75	130	124	119	87	69	2.6	2.2	1,570	265
	50			15	1.91	1.63	3.25	0.82	2.96	144	137	131	97	74	2.8	2.3	1,570	265
	50			20	1.91	1.74	3.47	0.88	3.16	157	150	143	106	79	2.9	2.5	1,570	265
	60			10	1.91	1.70	2.84	0.86	3.09	145	139	133	98	77	2.9	2.4	1,884	318
	60			15	1.91	1.81	3.02	0.91	3.30	159	152	145	107	82	3.0	2.6	1,884	318
	60			20	1.91	1.93	3.21	0.97	3.50	172	164	157	116	87	3.2	2.7	1,884	318
Early gestation (Single kid; BW = 2.9 to 4.2 kg)																		
	30	2.9	13	5	1.91	1.04	3.47	0.52	1.89	98	94	90	66	47	3.9	2.3	942	159
	30	2.9	13	10	1.91	1.14	3.81	0.58	2.08	110	105	101	74	52	4.1	2.4	942	159
	30	2.9	13	15	2.39	0.95	3.15	0.63	2.27	123	117	112	82	57	3.8	2.2	942	159
	40	3.4	16	5	1.91	1.26	3.14	0.63	2.28	117	112	107	79	57	4.2	2.6	1,256	212
	40	3.4	16	10	1.91	1.36	3.39	0.68	2.47	129	123	118	87	62	4.4	2.7	1,256	212
	40	3.4	16	15	1.91	1.46	3.64	0.74	2.65	142	135	129	95	66	4.5	2.8	1,256	212
	50	3.8	19	10	1.91	1.56	3.11	0.78	2.83	147	140	134	99	71	4.6	3.0	1,570	265
	50	3.8	19	15	1.91	1.66	3.31	0.84	3.01	159	152	145	107	75	4.8	3.1	1,570	265
	50	3.8	19	20	1.91	1.76	3.52	0.89	3.20	171	163	156	115	80	4.9	3.3	1,570	265
	60	4.2	21	10	1.91	1.75	2.91	0.88	3.17	163	156	149	110	79	4.9	3.2	1,884	318
	60	4.2	21	15	1.91	1.85	3.08	0.93	3.36	176	168	160	118	84	5.0	3.4	1,884	318
	60	4.2	21	20	1.91	1.95	3.25	0.98	3.55	188	179	171	126	89	5.2	3.5	1,884	318
Early gestation (Twin kids; BW = 2.6 to 3.8 kg)																		
	30	2.6	21	5	1.91	1.11	3.70	0.56	2.02	108	104	99	73	50	5.6	3.0	942	159
	30	2.6	21	10	2.39	0.92	3.07	0.61	2.21	121	115	110	81	55	5.3	2.7	942	159
	30	2.6	21	15	2.39	1.00	3.33	0.66	2.39	133	127	121	89	60	5.4	2.8	942	159
	40	3.0	26	5	1.91	1.33	3.33	0.67	2.43	129	123	117	86	61	5.9	3.3	1,256	212
	40	3.0	26	10	1.91	1.44	3.59	0.72	2.61	141	134	129	95	65	6.0	3.4	1,256	212
	40	3.0	26	15	1.91	1.54	3.84	0.78	2.80	153	146	140	103	70	6.1	3.5	1,256	212
	50	3.4	31	10	1.91	1.65	3.29	0.83	3.00	160	153	146	108	75	6.3	3.7	1,570	265
	50	3.4	31	15	1.91	1.75	3.50	0.88	3.18	172	165	157	116	79	6.4	3.8	1,570	265
	50	3.4	31	20	1.91	1.85	3.70	0.93	3.37	185	176	169	124	84	6.6	4.0	1,570	265
	60	3.8	36	10	1.91	1.85	3.08	0.93	3.36	179	171	163	120	84	6.6	4.0	1,884	318
	60	3.8	36	15	1.91	1.95	3.25	0.98	3.55	191	182	174	128	89	6.7	4.1	1,884	318
	60	3.8	36	20	1.91	2.05	3.42	1.04	3.74	203	194	186	137	93	6.9	4.2	1,884	318
Late gestation (Single kid; BW = 2.9 to 4.2 kg)																		
	30	2.9	51	5	2.39	0.99	3.29	0.65	2.36	128	123	117	86	59	3.8	2.2	1,365	168
	30	2.9	51	10	2.39	1.06	3.55	0.71	2.55	141	134	128	95	64	4.0	2.3	1,365	168
	30	2.9	51	15	2.39	1.14	3.81	0.76	2.74	153	146	140	103	68	4.1	2.4	1,365	168
	40	3.4	63	5	1.91	1.55	3.88	0.78	2.83	152	146	139	102	71	4.6	3.0	1,820	224

40	3.4	63	10	2.39	1.26	3.15	0.84	3.02	165	157	150	111	75	4.2	2.6	1,820	224
40	3.4	63	15	2.39	1.34	3.34	0.89	3.20	177	169	162	119	80	4.3	2.7	1,820	224
50	3.8	75	10	1.91	1.89	3.77	0.95	3.44	186	178	170	125	86	5.1	3.4	2,275	280
50	3.8	75	15	1.91	1.99	3.97	1.01	3.63	198	189	181	133	91	5.2	3.6	2,275	280
50	3.8	75	20	2.39	1.59	3.18	1.06	3.82	211	201	192	142	95	4.7	3.0	2,275	280
60	4.2	86	10	1.91	2.11	3.52	1.07	3.85	207	197	189	139	96	5.4	3.7	2,730	336
60	4.2	86	15	1.91	2.21	3.68	1.12	4.03	219	209	200	147	101	5.5	3.9	2,730	336
60	4.2	86	20	1.91	2.31	3.85	1.17	4.22	231	221	211	155	105	5.7	4.0	2,730	336
Late gestation (Twin kids; BW = 2.6 to 3.8 kg)																	
30	2.6	85	5	2.39	1.11	3.68	0.73	2.65	152	145	138	102	66	5.5	3.0	1,365	168
30	2.6	85	10	2.39	1.18	3.94	0.79	2.84	164	156	150	110	71	5.7	3.1	1,365	168
30	2.6	85	15	2.87	1.01	3.38	0.84	3.02	176	168	161	118	75	5.4	2.8	1,365	168
40	3.0	106	5	2.39	1.31	3.28	0.87	3.15	178	170	163	120	79	5.8	3.2	1,820	224
40	3.0	106	10	2.39	1.39	3.48	0.92	3.34	191	182	174	128	83	5.9	3.3	1,820	224
40	3.0	106	15	2.39	1.47	3.67	0.98	3.52	203	194	185	136	88	6.1	3.5	1,820	224
50	3.4	125	10	2.39	1.59	3.18	1.06	3.81	216	206	197	145	95	6.2	3.6	2,275	280
50	3.4	125	15	2.39	1.67	3.34	1.11	4.00	229	218	209	154	100	6.3	3.7	2,275	280
50	3.4	125	20	2.39	1.75	3.49	1.16	4.19	241	230	220	162	105	6.4	3.8	2,275	280
60	3.8	143	10	1.91	2.34	3.90	1.19	4.28	241	230	220	162	107	7.3	4.6	2,730	336
60	3.8	143	15	2.39	1.86	3.10	1.24	4.46	254	242	232	170	111	6.6	4.0	2,730	336
60	3.8	143	20	2.39	1.94	3.23	1.29	4.65	266	254	243	179	116	6.7	4.1	2,730	336
Early lactation (Single kid; milk yield = 0.57 to 0.83 kg/d)																	
30	0.57	−19	5	2.39	1.02	3.40	0.68	2.44	125	120	114	84	61	3.5	2.3	1,605	168
30	0.57	−19	10	2.39	1.10	3.67	0.73	2.63	138	131	126	92	66	3.6	2.4	1,605	168
30	0.57	−19	15	2.39	1.18	3.93	0.78	2.82	150	143	137	101	70	3.7	2.5	1,605	168
40	0.66	−22	5	1.91	1.53	3.81	0.81	2.92	149	142	136	100	73	4.2	3.0	2,140	224
40	0.66	−22	10	2.39	1.30	3.25	0.86	3.10	161	153	147	108	77	3.9	2.7	2,140	224
40	0.66	−22	15	2.39	1.38	3.44	0.91	3.29	173	165	158	116	82	4.0	2.8	2,140	224
50	0.75	−25	10	1.91	1.86	3.72	0.99	3.56	183	175	167	123	89	4.6	3.4	2,675	280
50	0.75	−25	15	1.91	1.96	3.92	1.04	3.75	195	186	178	131	94	4.8	3.5	2,675	280
50	0.75	−25	20	2.39	1.65	3.29	1.09	3.93	208	198	190	139	98	4.3	3.1	2,675	280
60	0.83	−28	10	1.91	2.08	3.47	1.10	3.98	204	194	186	137	99	4.9	3.7	3,210	336
60	0.83	−28	15	1.91	2.18	3.64	1.16	4.17	216	206	197	145	104	5.1	3.8	3,210	336
60	0.83	−28	20	1.91	2.28	3.80	1.21	4.36	228	218	208	153	109	5.2	4.0	3,210	336
Early lactation (Twin kids; milk yield = 0.94 to 1.38 kg/d)																	
30	0.94	−38	5	2.87	1.03	3.44	0.82	2.96	157	150	144	106	74	5.0	3.1	1,605	168
30	0.94	−38	10	2.87	1.10	3.66	0.87	3.15	170	162	155	114	79	5.1	3.2	1,605	168
30	0.94	−38	15	2.87	1.16	3.88	0.93	3.34	182	174	166	122	83	5.2	3.2	1,605	168
40	1.11	−44	5	2.39	1.49	3.72	0.99	3.55	187	179	171	126	89	5.7	3.7	2,140	224
40	1.11	−44	10	2.39	1.56	3.91	1.04	3.74	200	191	182	134	93	5.8	3.8	2,140	224
40	1.11	−44	15	2.87	1.37	3.42	1.09	3.93	212	202	193	142	98	5.5	3.5	2,140	224
50	1.25	−50	10	2.39	1.78	3.57	1.18	4.27	226	216	206	152	106	6.1	4.1	2,675	280
50	1.25	−50	15	2.39	1.86	3.73	1.23	4.45	238	228	218	160	111	6.2	4.2	2,675	280
50	1.25	−50	20	2.39	1.94	3.88	1.29	4.64	251	239	229	168	116	6.3	4.3	2,675	280
60	1.38	−55	10	2.39	1.99	3.32	1.32	4.76	251	240	229	169	119	6.4	4.4	3,210	336
60	1.38	−55	15	2.39	2.07	3.45	1.37	4.95	263	251	240	177	123	6.5	4.5	3,210	336
60	1.38	−55	20	2.39	2.15	3.58	1.42	5.13	276	263	252	185	128	6.6	4.6	3,210	336

TABLE 15-6 continued

Class/Age/Other	Body Weight[a] kg	Birth Weight or Milk Yield[b] kg	Daily Gain[c] g/d	Mohair Fiber Growth[d] g/d	Energy Concentration in Diet[e] kcal/kg	Daily Dry Matter Intake[f] kg	Daily Dry Matter Intake[f] % BW	Energy Requirements[g] TDN kg/d	Energy Requirements[g] ME Mcal/d	Protein Requirements[h] CP @20% UIP g/d	CP @40% UIP g/d	CP @60% UIP g/d	MP g/d	DIP g/d	Mineral Requirements[i] Ca g/d	P g/d	Vitamin Requirements[j] A RE/d	E IU/d
Late lactation (Single kid; milk yield = 0.28 to 0.41 kg/d)																		
	30	0.28	15	5	1.91	1.06	3.54	0.56	2.03	100	96	92	67	51	3.5	2.3	1,605	168
	30	0.28	15	10	1.91	1.16	3.87	0.62	2.22	113	108	103	76	55	3.7	2.5	1,605	168
	30	0.28	15	15	2.39	1.01	3.36	0.67	2.41	125	119	114	84	60	3.5	2.3	1,605	168
	40	0.33	18	5	1.91	1.28	3.21	0.68	2.45	120	115	110	81	61	3.8	2.6	2,140	224
	40	0.33	18	10	1.91	1.38	3.45	0.73	2.64	132	126	121	89	66	4.0	2.8	2,140	224
	40	0.33	18	15	1.91	1.48	3.70	0.78	2.83	145	138	132	97	71	4.1	2.9	2,140	224
	50	0.38	20	10	1.91	1.59	3.18	0.84	3.04	151	144	138	102	76	4.3	3.0	2,675	280
	50	0.38	20	15	1.91	1.69	3.37	0.89	3.22	163	156	149	110	80	4.4	3.2	2,675	280
	50	0.38	20	20	1.91	1.78	3.57	0.95	3.41	176	168	160	118	85	4.5	3.3	2,675	280
	60	0.41	22	10	1.91	1.77	2.96	0.94	3.39	167	160	153	113	85	4.5	3.3	3,210	336
	60	0.41	22	15	1.91	1.87	3.12	0.99	3.58	180	172	164	121	89	4.7	3.4	3,210	336
	60	0.41	22	20	1.91	1.97	3.28	1.04	3.77	192	183	175	129	94	4.8	3.6	3,210	336
Late lactation (Twin kids; milk yield = 0.47 to 0.69 kg/d)																		
	30	0.47	30	5	2.39	0.96	3.21	0.64	2.30	117	111	107	78	57	5.0	3.0	1,605	168
	30	0.47	30	10	2.39	1.04	3.47	0.69	2.49	129	123	118	87	62	5.1	3.1	1,605	168
	30	0.47	30	15	2.39	1.12	3.73	0.74	2.68	141	135	129	95	67	5.2	3.2	1,605	168
	40	0.55	35	5	1.91	1.44	3.61	0.77	2.76	139	133	127	93	69	5.6	3.6	2,140	224
	40	0.55	35	10	1.91	1.54	3.86	0.82	2.95	151	144	138	102	74	5.8	3.8	2,140	224
	40	0.55	35	15	2.39	1.31	3.28	0.87	3.14	164	156	149	110	78	5.4	3.4	2,140	224
	50	0.63	40	10	1.91	1.77	3.55	0.94	3.39	173	165	158	116	85	6.1	4.1	2,675	280
	50	0.63	40	15	1.91	1.87	3.74	0.99	3.58	185	177	169	124	89	6.2	4.2	2,675	280
	50	0.63	40	20	1.91	1.97	3.94	1.04	3.77	197	188	180	133	94	6.3	4.3	2,675	280
	60	0.69	44	10	1.91	1.98	3.30	1.05	3.79	192	183	175	129	94	6.4	4.3	3,210	336
	60	0.69	44	15	1.91	2.08	3.46	1.10	3.97	204	195	186	137	99	6.5	4.5	3,210	336
	60	0.69	44	20	1.91	2.18	3.63	1.15	4.16	216	206	197	145	104	6.6	4.6	3,210	336

[a]Body weight used in estimating requirements is the determined or estimated weight in kilograms (kg) average for the period during which these requirements will be applied.
[b]Birth weight (kg) of single and average of multiple lambs or liquid milk yield (kg/d).
[c]Average change in body weight over a 24-hour period.
[d]Weight of mohair growth over a 24-hour period.
[e]Three hypothetical diets with increasing energy concentrations (1.91, 2.34, and 2.87 kcal/kg) were used in the calculations of intake and nutrient requirements. For each line entry, a diet was selected to represent the level of energy concentration that approximates that needed by the animal to achieve adequate intake to satisfy its energy requirement.
[f]The daily dry matter intake, expressed as kg or as percentage of body weight, of a diet having the indicated energy concentration (previous column) that is required to meet energy requirements. These energy concentrations should be viewed only as examples. In some cases, diets having greater or lesser concentrations of energy would be more appropriate.
[g]Energy requirements expressed as total digestible nutrients (TDN) in kg/d and metabolizable energy (ME) as kcal/d.
[h]Protein requirements expressed as crude protein (CP), metabolizable protein (MP), and degradable intake protein (DIP). The CP requirement differs with the proportion of undegradable intake protein (UIP) because of the required minimal DIP.
[i]Two macro minerals, calcium (Ca) and phosphorus (P), commonly considered in balancing diets are included. Often, the balance (ratio) of the two minerals also is of concern.
[j]Two fat-soluble vitamins, A and E, that often are deficient in animal diets are expressed as retinol equivalents (RE) and international units (IU) for vitamins A and E, respectively. RE = 1.0 μg of all-trans retinol, 5.0 μg of all-trans betacarotene, and 7.6 μg of other carotenoids.

TABLE 15-7 Mineral Requirements of Meat and Milk Goats[a]

Class/Stage/Other	Body Weight[b] kg	Body Weight Gain[c] g/d	Dry Matter Intake[d] kg/d	Mineral Requirements											
				Na g/d	Cl g/d	K g/d	Mg g/d	S g/d	Co mg/d	Cu mg/d	I mg/d	Fe mg/d	Mn mg/d	Se mg/d	Zn mg/d
Growing Kids (Females, males, and male castrates)															
	10	0	0.35	0.19	0.28	1.6	0.18	0.9	0.04	9	0.18	1	3	0.29	2
	10	25	0.33	0.24	0.31	1.6	0.23	0.9	0.04	8	0.16	9	4	0.33	4
	10	100	0.39	0.39	0.40	1.9	0.38	1.0	0.04	10	0.19	33	9	0.46	10
	15	0	0.50	0.28	0.41	2.3	0.26	1.3	0.06	13	0.25	2	4	0.30	2
	15	25	0.49	0.33	0.44	2.3	0.31	1.3	0.05	12	0.25	10	6	0.34	4
	15	100	0.54	0.48	0.54	2.6	0.46	1.4	0.06	13	0.27	34	10	0.47	11
	20	0	0.66	0.38	0.55	3.0	0.35	1.7	0.07	16	0.33	3	5	0.31	3
	20	25	0.70	0.43	0.58	3.2	0.40	1.8	0.08	17	0.35	11	7	0.35	5
	20	100	0.67	0.58	0.68	3.3	0.55	1.8	0.07	17	0.34	34	12	0.48	11
	20	150	0.71	0.68	0.74	3.6	0.65	1.9	0.08	18	0.36	50	15	0.56	16
	25	0	0.78	0.47	0.69	3.6	0.44	2.0	0.09	19	0.39	4	7	0.32	4
	25	25	0.81	0.52	0.72	3.8	0.49	2.1	0.09	20	0.40	11	8	0.36	6
	25	100	0.84	0.67	0.81	4.1	0.64	2.2	0.09	21	0.42	35	13	0.49	12
	25	150	0.86	0.77	0.88	4.3	0.74	2.2	0.10	22	0.43	51	16	0.57	16
	30	0	0.89	0.56	0.83	4.2	0.53	2.3	0.10	22	0.44	4	8	0.32	5
	30	25	0.97	0.61	0.86	4.5	0.58	2.5	0.11	24	0.48	12	10	0.37	7
	30	100	1.03	0.76	0.95	4.9	0.73	2.7	0.11	26	0.51	36	14	0.49	13
	30	150	0.99	0.86	1.01	4.9	0.83	2.6	0.11	25	0.49	52	17	0.58	17
	30	200	1.05	0.96	1.08	5.2	0.93	2.7	0.12	26	0.52	67	21	0.66	21
	35	0	1.00	0.66	0.96	4.8	0.61	2.6	0.11	25	0.50	5	9	0.33	5
	35	25	1.08	0.71	0.99	5.1	0.66	2.8	0.12	27	0.54	13	11	0.37	7
	35	100	1.24	0.86	1.09	5.8	0.81	3.2	0.14	31	0.62	36	16	0.51	14
	35	150	1.19	0.96	1.15	5.8	0.91	3.1	0.13	30	0.60	52	19	0.59	18
	35	200	1.18	1.06	1.21	5.9	1.01	3.1	0.13	29	0.59	68	22	0.67	22
	35	250	1.23	1.16	1.28	6.2	1.11	3.2	0.14	31	0.62	84	25	0.75	26
	40	0	1.10	0.75	1.10	5.4	0.70	2.9	0.12	28	0.55	6	11	0.33	6
	40	25	1.18	0.80	1.13	5.7	0.75	3.1	0.13	30	0.59	13	12	0.38	8
	40	100	1.34	0.95	1.23	6.4	0.90	3.5	0.15	34	0.67	37	17	0.51	14
	40	150	1.35	1.05	1.29	6.5	1.00	3.5	0.15	34	0.67	53	20	0.59	19
	40	200	1.33	1.15	1.35	6.6	1.10	3.5	0.15	33	0.66	69	23	0.68	23
	40	250	1.37	1.25	1.41	6.8	1.20	3.6	0.15	34	0.68	85	26	0.76	27
	40	300	1.41	1.35	1.48	7.1	1.30	3.7	0.16	35	0.71	100	29	0.85	31
Mature does (Maintenance only)															
	20		0.55	0.38	0.55	2.7	0.35	1.2	0.06	11	0.27	3	5	0.15	6
	30		0.74	0.56	0.83	3.8	0.53	1.6	0.08	15	0.37	4	8	0.16	9
	40		0.92	0.75	1.10	4.9	0.70	2.0	0.10	18	0.46	6	11	0.16	12
	50		1.09	0.94	1.38	5.9	0.88	2.4	0.12	22	0.54	7	13	0.17	15
	60		1.25	1.13	1.65	6.9	1.05	2.7	0.14	25	0.62	8	16	0.17	18
	70		1.40	1.31	1.93	7.9	1.23	3.1	0.15	28	0.70	10	19	0.17	21
	80		1.54	1.50	2.20	8.9	1.40	3.4	0.17	31	0.77	11	21	0.18	24
	90		1.69	1.69	2.48	9.9	1.58	3.7	0.19	34	0.84	13	24	0.18	27
Mature does (Breeding)															
	20		0.60	0.38	0.55	2.8	0.35	1.3	0.07	12	0.30	3	5	0.15	6
	30		0.81	0.56	0.83	4.0	0.53	1.8	0.09	16	0.41	4	8	0.16	9
	40		1.01	0.75	1.10	5.1	0.70	2.2	0.11	20	0.51	6	11	0.16	12
	50		1.19	0.94	1.38	6.2	0.88	2.6	0.13	24	0.60	7	13	0.17	15
	60		1.37	1.13	1.65	7.3	1.05	3.0	0.15	27	0.68	8	16	0.17	18
	70		1.54	1.31	1.93	8.3	1.23	3.4	0.17	31	0.77	10	19	0.18	21
	80		1.70	1.50	2.20	9.4	1.40	3.7	0.19	34	0.85	11	21	0.18	24
	90		1.86	1.69	2.48	10.4	1.58	4.1	0.20	37	0.93	13	24	0.18	27

TABLE 15-7 continued

Class/Stage/Other	Body Weight[b] kg	Body Weight Gain[c] g/d	Dry Matter Intake[d] kg/d	Mineral Requirements Na g/d	Cl g/d	K g/d	Mg g/d	S g/d	Co mg/d	Cu mg/d	I mg/d	Fe mg/d	Mn mg/d	Se mg/d	Zn mg/d
Mature does during early gestation (Single kid)															
	20		0.69	0.40	0.57	3.1	0.39	1.5	0.08	10	0.34	17	8	0.16	9
	30		0.92	0.59	0.85	4.4	0.57	2.0	0.10	14	0.46	22	11	0.17	14
	40		1.13	0.79	1.13	5.5	0.76	2.5	0.12	17	0.56	27	15	0.18	18
	50		1.32	0.98	1.40	6.6	0.94	2.9	0.15	20	0.66	31	18	0.19	21
	60		1.51	1.17	1.68	7.7	1.12	3.3	0.17	23	0.75	35	21	0.20	25
	70		1.69	1.36	1.96	8.8	1.31	3.7	0.19	25	0.84	39	24	0.20	29
	80		1.86	1.55	2.24	9.9	1.49	4.1	0.20	28	0.93	42	27	0.21	33
	90		2.02	1.74	2.51	10.9	1.67	4.4	0.22	30	1.01	45	30	0.22	36
Mature does during early gestation (Twin kids)															
	20		0.69	0.42	0.58	3.1	0.41	1.5	0.08	10	0.34	29	10	0.17	12
	30		1.02	0.62	0.86	4.7	0.61	2.2	0.11	15	0.51	37	14	0.19	17
	40		1.24	0.81	1.15	5.9	0.80	2.7	0.14	19	0.62	43	17	0.20	21
	50		1.46	1.01	1.43	7.1	0.99	3.2	0.16	22	0.73	50	21	0.21	26
	60		1.66	1.21	1.71	8.2	1.18	3.7	0.18	25	0.83	56	25	0.22	30
	70		1.85	1.40	1.99	9.3	1.37	4.1	0.20	28	0.93	61	28	0.23	35
	80		2.04	1.60	2.27	10.4	1.56	4.5	0.22	31	1.02	67	32	0.23	39
	90		2.22	1.79	2.55	11.5	1.75	4.9	0.24	33	1.11	73	35	0.24	43
Mature does during early gestation (Three or more kids)															
	30		1.08	0.63	0.87	4.9	0.63	2.4	0.12	16	0.54	45	15	0.19	19
	40		1.32	0.83	1.16	6.1	0.83	2.9	0.15	20	0.66	54	19	0.21	24
	50		1.54	1.03	1.44	7.3	1.02	3.4	0.17	23	0.77	61	23	0.22	29
	60		1.76	1.23	1.72	8.5	1.22	3.9	0.19	26	0.88	68	27	0.23	34
	70		1.96	1.42	2.00	9.7	1.41	4.3	0.22	29	0.98	75	31	0.24	38
	80		2.16	1.62	2.29	10.8	1.60	4.7	0.24	32	1.08	82	34	0.25	43
	90		2.35	1.82	2.57	11.9	1.79	5.2	0.26	35	1.18	89	38	0.26	48
Mature does during late gestation (Single kid)															
	20		0.72	0.47	0.62	3.3	0.50	1.6	0.08	11	0.36	26	15	0.20	20
	30		1.04	0.69	0.91	4.8	0.71	2.3	0.11	16	0.52	33	21	0.22	27
	40		1.27	0.89	1.20	6.0	0.93	2.8	0.14	19	0.63	40	26	0.23	34
	50		1.84	1.10	1.49	8.3	1.14	4.1	0.20	28	0.92	45	31	0.26	40
	60		2.09	1.30	1.78	9.6	1.35	4.6	0.23	31	1.05	50	35	0.28	46
	70		2.33	1.51	2.06	10.8	1.56	5.1	0.26	35	1.17	56	40	0.29	53
	80		2.56	1.71	2.35	12.1	1.76	5.6	0.28	38	1.28	60	44	0.31	58
	90		2.77	1.91	2.63	13.2	1.97	6.1	0.30	42	1.39	65	49	0.32	64
Mature does during late gestation (Twin kids)															
	20		0.81	0.55	0.68	3.6	0.61	1.8	0.09	12	0.40	45	23	0.23	31
	30		1.05	0.78	0.98	4.9	0.85	2.3	0.12	16	0.52	56	31	0.25	41
	40		1.52	1.01	1.28	6.9	1.09	3.4	0.17	23	0.76	66	37	0.29	50
	50		1.77	1.23	1.58	8.2	1.33	3.9	0.20	27	0.89	75	44	0.31	59
	60		2.02	1.45	1.88	9.5	1.56	4.4	0.22	30	1.01	84	50	0.33	67
	70		2.24	1.66	2.17	10.7	1.79	4.9	0.25	34	1.12	92	56	0.36	75
	80		2.76	1.88	2.47	12.8	2.03	6.1	0.30	41	1.38	101	62	0.39	84
	90		3.34	2.10	2.76	15.1	2.25	7.4	0.37	50	1.67	109	68	0.42	91
Mature does during late gestation (Three or more kids)															
	30		1.16	0.82	1.01	5.3	0.89	2.5	0.13	17	0.58	64	34	0.27	45
	40		1.42	1.06	1.32	6.6	1.16	3.1	0.16	21	0.71	78	42	0.30	57
	50		1.64	1.29	1.62	7.9	1.42	3.6	0.18	25	0.82	90	50	0.33	68
	60		2.23	1.51	1.92	10.2	1.67	4.9	0.25	33	1.11	100	57	0.37	78
	70		2.48	1.74	2.23	11.5	1.92	5.5	0.27	37	1.24	110	65	0.40	87
	80		2.73	1.97	2.53	12.8	2.17	6.0	0.30	41	1.36	121	72	0.43	97
	90		2.97	2.19	2.83	14.1	2.41	6.5	0.33	45	1.48	131	79	0.46	107
Mature does during early lactation (Single kid)															
	20	−14	0.96	0.69	1.42	5.3	0.78	2.5	0.11	14	0.76	9	10	0.27	29
	30	−19	1.25	0.95	1.90	7.0	1.05	3.3	0.14	19	1.00	12	14	0.30	38

TABLE 15-7 continued

Class/Stage/Other	Body Weight[b] kg	Body Weight Gain[c] g/d	Dry Matter Intake[d] kg/d	Mineral Requirements Na g/d	Cl g/d	K g/d	Mg g/d	S g/d	Co mg/d	Cu mg/d	I mg/d	Fe mg/d	Mn mg/d	Se mg/d	Zn mg/d
	40	–22	1.52	1.21	2.36	8.6	1.32	3.9	0.17	23	1.21	15	17	0.33	46
	50	–24	1.76	1.45	2.79	10.1	1.57	4.6	0.19	26	1.41	17	21	0.35	53
	60	–26	1.99	1.70	3.22	11.6	1.82	5.2	0.22	30	1.59	20	24	0.38	60
	70	–28	2.21	1.94	3.64	13.0	2.07	5.7	0.24	33	1.77	22	28	0.40	67
	80	–29	2.42	2.17	4.04	14.4	2.31	6.3	0.27	36	1.94	25	31	0.42	73
	90	–31	2.62	2.40	4.44	15.8	2.54	6.8	0.29	39	2.10	27	34	0.44	79
Mature does during early lactation (Twin kids)															
	20	–28	1.03	0.95	2.14	6.7	1.13	2.7	0.11	15	0.83	14	13	0.35	46
	30	–35	1.68	1.29	2.82	9.7	1.50	4.4	0.18	25	1.34	19	18	0.41	60
	40	–43	2.03	1.60	3.43	11.8	1.84	5.3	0.22	30	1.62	23	22	0.45	71
	50	–48	2.34	1.90	4.02	13.8	2.17	6.1	0.26	35	1.87	26	26	0.50	82
	60	–52	2.63	2.19	4.57	15.6	2.48	6.8	0.29	39	2.10	30	30	0.54	92
	70	–55	2.90	2.47	5.09	17.4	2.78	7.6	0.32	44	2.32	33	34	0.57	101
	80	–59	3.17	2.74	5.61	19.1	3.07	8.2	0.35	47	2.53	36	38	0.61	111
	90	–62	3.42	3.01	6.12	20.8	3.36	8.9	0.38	51	2.74	39	42	0.64	120
Mature does during early lactation (Three or more kids)															
	30	–52	1.54	1.59	3.65	10.7	1.91	4.0	0.17	23	1.23	25	22	0.50	32
	40	–60	2.31	1.95	4.41	14.2	2.32	6.0	0.25	35	1.85	30	27	0.57	38
	50	–72	2.52	2.30	5.12	16.1	2.71	6.6	0.28	38	2.02	34	31	0.63	109
	60	–78	2.83	2.63	5.80	18.2	3.08	7.4	0.31	42	2.26	39	36	0.68	123
	70	–83	3.12	2.95	6.44	20.2	3.43	8.1	0.34	47	2.49	43	40	0.73	135
	80	–88	3.85	3.27	7.05	23.4	3.77	10.0	0.42	58	3.08	47	45	0.79	147
	90	–93	4.15	3.57	7.65	25.4	4.11	10.8	0.46	62	3.32	50	49	0.84	158
Mature does (Dairy) Early lactation (Parlor production; milk yield = 4.65 to 6.43 kg/d)															
	50	–90	2.81	3.26	7.77	21.2	4.13	7.3	0.31	42	2.25	54	42	0.91	171
	60	–95	3.14	3.70	8.72	23.8	4.65	8.2	0.35	47	2.51	60	48	0.99	191
	70	–100	4.14	4.11	9.63	28.3	5.15	10.8	0.46	62	3.31	66	53	1.09	210
	80	–104	4.49	4.52	10.49	30.8	5.62	11.7	0.49	67	3.60	72	59	1.17	228
	90	–108	4.83	4.90	11.32	33.2	6.08	12.6	0.53	72	3.86	77	64	1.24	245
Mature does (Dairy) Early lactation (Parlor production; milk yield = 5.82 to 8.04 kg/d)															
	50	–113	3.32	3.85	9.38	25.3	4.95	8.6	0.37	50	2.66	65	49	1.10	210
	60	–119	3.70	4.34	10.49	28.3	5.55	9.6	0.41	56	2.96	73	56	1.20	234
	70	–125	4.06	4.81	11.55	31.2	6.13	10.6	0.45	61	3.25	80	62	1.30	257
	80	–130	4.40	5.27	12.55	33.9	6.67	11.4	0.48	66	3.52	87	68	1.39	278
	90	–135	4.72	5.71	13.53	36.5	7.20	12.3	0.52	71	3.78	93	75	1.48	299
Mature does (Dairy) Early lactation (Parlor production; milk yield = 6.98 to 9.65 kg/d)															
	50	–135	3.83	4.43	10.97	29.3	5.76	10.0	0.42	57	3.06	77	65	1.40	271
	60	–143	4.26	4.99	12.27	32.8	6.45	11.1	0.47	64	3.41	86	73	1.53	301
	70	–150	4.67	5.51	13.48	36.1	7.11	12.1	0.51	70	3.74	94	80	1.66	329
	80	–156	5.06	6.02	14.63	39.1	7.73	13.1	0.56	76	4.05	102	88	1.77	355
	90	–162	5.43	6.51	15.74	42.1	8.33	14.1	0.60	81	4.34	109	95	1.88	381
Mature does during late lactation (Single kid)															
	20	11	0.70	0.50	0.88	3.7	0.54	1.8	0.08	10	0.56	9	8	0.20	16
	30	14	0.94	0.72	1.24	5.1	0.77	2.4	0.10	14	0.75	12	11	0.22	23
	40	17	1.15	0.93	1.58	6.3	0.98	3.0	0.13	17	0.92	14	14	0.24	28
	50	19	1.35	1.14	1.93	7.6	1.19	3.5	0.15	20	1.08	17	17	0.25	33
	60	20	1.53	1.35	2.26	8.7	1.40	4.0	0.17	23	1.23	19	20	0.27	37
	70	22	1.71	1.55	2.59	9.9	1.61	4.4	0.19	26	1.37	22	24	0.28	42
	80	24	1.88	1.76	2.92	11.0	1.81	4.9	0.21	28	1.51	24	27	0.29	47
	90	26	2.05	1.96	3.23	12.1	2.01	5.3	0.23	31	1.64	26	30	0.30	51
Mature does during late lactation (Twin kids)															
	20	22	0.83	0.60	1.17	4.5	0.71	2.2	0.09	12	0.66	14	10	0.25	26
	30	27	1.10	0.85	1.61	6.1	0.98	2.9	0.12	17	0.88	19	14	0.28	35
	40	32	1.35	1.08	2.01	7.6	1.23	3.5	0.15	20	1.08	22	18	0.31	42

TABLE 15-7 continued

Class/Stage/Other	Body Weight[b] kg	Body Weight Gain[c] g/d	Dry Matter Intake[d] kg/d	Mineral Requirements Na g/d	Cl g/d	K g/d	Mg g/d	S g/d	Co mg/d	Cu mg/d	I mg/d	Fe mg/d	Mn mg/d	Se mg/d	Zn mg/d
	50	37	1.58	1.31	2.41	9.0	1.47	4.1	0.17	24	1.26	26	21	0.33	49
	60	41	1.78	1.54	2.78	10.3	1.71	4.6	0.20	27	1.43	29	25	0.35	55
	70	44	1.99	1.76	3.16	11.6	1.94	5.2	0.22	30	1.59	33	28	0.37	61
	80	48	2.18	1.98	3.53	12.9	2.17	5.7	0.24	33	1.74	36	31	0.39	67
	90	51	2.36	2.21	3.90	14.1	2.40	6.1	0.26	35	1.89	39	35	0.41	73
Mature does during late lactation (Three or more kids)															
	30	41	1.25	0.97	1.94	7.1	1.18	3.3	0.14	19	1.00	25	17	0.34	46
	40	49	1.52	1.22	2.40	8.7	1.46	4.0	0.17	23	1.22	30	21	0.37	55
	50	55	1.79	1.48	2.85	10.3	1.74	4.7	0.20	27	1.43	35	25	0.41	64
	60	61	2.02	1.72	3.27	11.8	2.00	5.2	0.22	30	1.61	39	28	0.44	71
	70	66	2.24	1.96	3.70	13.2	2.26	5.8	0.25	34	1.79	44	32	0.46	79
	80	72	2.45	2.20	4.11	14.6	2.52	6.4	0.27	37	1.96	48	36	0.49	87
	90	76	2.66	2.43	4.51	16.0	2.76	6.9	0.29	40	2.12	51	40	0.51	94
Mature does (Dairy) Late lactation (Parlor production; milk yield = 1.99 to 2.76 kg/d)															
	50	66	2.48	1.93	4.11	14.4	2.40	6.4	0.27	37	1.98	48	32	0.59	99
	60	73	2.79	2.23	4.68	16.3	2.74	7.3	0.31	42	2.23	53	37	0.64	111
	70	80	3.09	2.51	5.23	18.1	3.07	8.0	0.34	46	2.47	59	41	0.68	122
	80	86	3.36	2.79	5.75	19.9	3.38	8.7	0.37	50	2.69	64	46	0.72	133
	90	92	3.64	3.07	6.27	21.6	3.69	9.5	0.40	55	2.91	69	50	0.77	144
Mature does (Dairy) Late lactation (Parlor production; milk yield = 2.49 to 3.44 kg/d)															
	50	83	2.81	2.18	4.80	16.4	2.78	7.3	0.31	42	2.25	58	37	0.69	120
	60	92	3.16	2.51	5.45	18.6	3.17	8.2	0.35	47	2.52	65	42	0.75	135
	70	100	3.48	2.81	6.05	20.6	3.53	9.0	0.38	52	2.78	71	47	0.81	148
	80	108	3.79	3.12	6.64	22.6	3.88	9.8	0.42	57	3.03	78	52	0.86	160
	90	115	4.08	3.41	7.21	24.4	4.21	10.6	0.45	61	3.26	83	56	0.91	172
Mature does (Dairy) Late lactation (Parlor production; milk yield = 2.99 to 4.13 kg/d)															
	50	100	2.51	2.43	5.49	16.7	3.17	6.5	0.28	38	2.01	68	42	0.78	141
	60	110	3.52	2.78	6.20	20.8	3.59	9.1	0.39	53	2.81	76	47	0.87	158
	70	120	3.87	3.11	6.88	23.1	3.99	10.1	0.43	58	3.10	84	53	0.94	173
	80	129	4.21	3.44	7.52	25.2	4.37	10.9	0.46	63	3.37	91	58	1.00	187
	90	138	4.53	3.75	8.15	27.3	4.74	11.8	0.50	68	3.63	97	63	1.05	201
Mature bucks															
	50	0	1.31	0.94	1.38	6.6	0.88	2.9	0.14	26	0.66	7	13	0.17	15
	75	0	1.78	1.41	2.06	9.3	1.31	3.9	0.20	36	0.89	11	20	0.18	23
	100	0	2.21	1.88	2.75	11.9	1.75	4.9	0.24	44	1.10	14	27	0.19	30
	125	0	2.61	2.34	3.44	14.5	2.19	5.7	0.29	52	1.30	18	33	0.20	38
	150	0	2.99	2.81	4.13	17.0	2.63	6.6	0.33	60	1.49	21	40	0.21	45

[a]Calcium and phosphorus requirements for goats are listed in Tables 15-4, 15-5, and 15-6.

[b]Body weight used in estimating requirements is the determined or estimated weight in kilograms (kg) average for the period during which these requirements will be applied.

[c]Average change in body weight over a 24-hour period.

[d]Estimate of dry matter intake of a feed of appropriate energy density to meet energy requirements.

TABLE 15-8 Mineral Requirements of Goats (Angora)[a]

Class/Stage/Other	Body Weight[b] kg	Daily Gain[c] g/d	Mohair Fiber Growth[d] g/d	Dry Matter Intake[e] kg/d	Mineral Requirements[f] Na g/d	Cl g/d	K g/d	Mg g/d	S g/d	Co mg/d	Cu mg/d	I mg/d	Fe mg/d	Mn mg/d	Se mg/d	Zn mg/d
Growing Angora Kids																
	10	20	4	0.37	0.23	0.30	1.7	0.22	1.0	0.04	9	0.19	9	6	0.33	5
	10	20	8	0.40	0.23	0.30	1.8	0.22	1.0	0.04	10	0.20	10	7	0.34	6
	10	40	4	0.37	0.27	0.33	1.7	0.26	1.0	0.04	9	0.19	15	8	0.37	6
	10	40	8	0.44	0.27	0.33	1.9	0.26	1.1	0.05	11	0.22	16	9	0.38	8
	20	20	4	0.70	0.42	0.58	3.2	0.39	1.8	0.08	18	0.35	10	9	0.35	6
	20	20	8	0.75	0.42	0.58	3.3	0.39	1.9	0.08	19	0.37	12	10	0.36	8
	20	40	4	0.68	0.46	0.60	3.2	0.43	1.8	0.08	17	0.34	17	10	0.38	8
	20	40	8	0.74	0.46	0.60	3.4	0.43	1.9	0.08	19	0.37	18	12	0.39	9
	30	0	4	0.98	0.56	0.83	4.5	0.53	2.6	0.11	25	0.49	5	9	0.33	6
	30	0	8	1.05	0.56	0.83	4.7	0.53	2.7	0.12	26	0.53	7	11	0.34	8
	30	0	12	0.98	0.56	0.83	4.5	0.53	2.5	0.11	24	0.49	8	12	0.34	9
	30	20	4	1.07	0.60	0.85	4.8	0.57	2.8	0.12	27	0.54	12	11	0.37	8
	30	20	8	1.11	0.60	0.85	4.9	0.57	2.9	0.12	28	0.56	13	13	0.38	9
	30	20	12	1.15	0.60	0.85	5.0	0.57	3.0	0.13	29	0.57	14	14	0.38	11
	30	40	4	1.01	0.64	0.88	4.7	0.61	2.6	0.11	25	0.50	18	13	0.40	9
	30	40	8	1.07	0.64	0.88	4.9	0.61	2.8	0.12	27	0.53	19	14	0.41	11
	30	40	12	1.12	0.64	0.88	5.0	0.61	2.9	0.12	28	0.56	20	16	0.41	12
Mature Angora Males																
Maintenance only																
	40	0	10	1.35	0.75	1.10	6.1	0.70	3.5	0.15	27	0.67	9	14	0.36	20
	40	0	15	1.45	0.75	1.10	6.4	0.70	3.8	0.16	29	0.72	10	16	0.37	24
	50	0	15	1.66	0.94	1.38	7.6	0.88	4.3	0.18	33	0.83	12	18	0.38	27
	50	0	20	1.76	0.94	1.38	7.9	0.88	4.6	0.19	35	0.88	13	20	0.39	30
	60	0	15	1.85	1.13	1.65	8.7	1.05	4.8	0.20	37	0.93	13	21	0.39	30
	60	0	20	1.96	1.13	1.65	9.0	1.05	5.1	0.22	39	0.98	14	23	0.40	33
Breeding																
	40	0	10	1.48	0.75	1.10	6.5	0.70	3.8	0.16	30	0.74	9	14	0.36	20
	40	0	15	1.59	0.75	1.10	6.8	0.70	4.1	0.17	32	0.80	10	16	0.38	24
	50	0	15	1.82	0.94	1.38	8.0	0.88	4.7	0.20	36	0.91	12	18	0.39	27
	50	0	20	1.93	0.94	1.38	8.4	0.88	5.0	0.21	39	0.97	13	20	0.40	30
	60	0	15	2.04	1.13	1.65	9.2	1.05	5.3	0.22	41	1.02	13	21	0.40	30
	60	0	20	2.15	1.13	1.65	9.5	1.05	5.6	0.24	43	1.07	14	23	0.41	33
Mature Angora Females																
Maintenance only																
	30	0	5	0.90	0.56	0.83	4.3	0.53	2.3	0.10	18	0.45	6	10	0.33	13
	30	0	10	1.00	0.56	0.83	4.6	0.53	2.6	0.11	20	0.50	7	11	0.34	17
	40	0	10	1.20	0.75	1.10	5.7	0.70	3.1	0.13	24	0.60	9	14	0.35	20
	40	0	15	1.30	0.75	1.10	6.0	0.70	3.4	0.14	26	0.65	10	16	0.36	24
	50	0	10	1.38	0.94	1.38	6.8	0.88	3.6	0.15	28	0.69	10	17	0.36	23
	50	0	15	1.48	0.94	1.38	7.1	0.88	3.8	0.16	30	0.74	12	18	0.37	27
	60	0	15	1.65	1.13	1.65	8.1	1.05	4.3	0.18	33	0.83	13	21	0.38	30
	60	0	20	1.75	1.13	1.65	8.4	1.05	4.6	0.19	35	0.88	14	23	0.39	33
Breeding																
	30	30	5	0.99	0.56	0.83	4.5	0.53	2.6	0.11	20	0.50	6	10	0.33	13
	30	30	10	1.10	0.56	0.83	4.9	0.53	2.9	0.12	22	0.55	7	11	0.34	17
	40	40	10	1.31	0.75	1.10	6.0	0.70	3.4	0.14	26	0.66	9	14	0.36	20
	40	40	15	1.43	0.75	1.10	6.3	0.70	3.7	0.16	29	0.71	10	16	0.37	24
	50	50	10	1.51	0.94	1.38	7.2	0.88	3.9	0.17	30	0.76	10	17	0.37	23
	50	50	15	1.63	0.94	1.38	7.5	0.88	4.2	0.18	33	0.81	12	18	0.38	27
	60	60	15	1.81	1.13	1.65	8.6	1.05	4.7	0.20	36	0.91	13	21	0.39	30
	60	60	20	1.93	1.13	1.65	8.9	1.05	5.0	0.21	39	0.96	14	23	0.40	33
Early Gestation (Single kid)																
	30	13	5	1.04	0.59	1.22	4.7	0.57	2.7	0.11	16	0.52	13	13	0.36	17
	30	13	10	1.14	0.59	1.22	5.0	0.57	3.0	0.13	17	0.57	15	15	0.37	21

TABLE 15-8 continued

Class/Stage/Other	Body Weight[b] kg	Daily Gain[c] g/d	Mohair Fiber Growth[d] g/d	Dry Matter Intake[e] kg/d	Mineral Requirements[f]											
					Na g/d	Cl g/d	K g/d	Mg g/d	S g/d	Co mg/d	Cu mg/d	I mg/d	Fe mg/d	Mn mg/d	Se mg/d	Zn mg/d
	40	16	10	1.36	0.79	1.58	6.2	0.76	3.5	0.15	20	0.68	18	18	0.39	25
	40	16	15	1.46	0.79	1.58	6.5	0.76	3.8	0.16	22	0.73	19	20	0.40	29
	50	19	10	1.56	0.98	1.95	7.4	0.94	4.0	0.17	23	0.78	21	22	0.41	29
	50	19	15	1.66	0.98	1.95	7.7	0.94	4.3	0.18	25	0.83	22	23	0.42	33
	60	21	15	1.85	1.17	2.28	8.8	1.12	4.8	0.20	28	0.92	25	26	0.43	37
	60	21	20	1.95	1.17	2.28	9.1	1.12	5.1	0.21	29	0.97	26	28	0.44	40
Early Gestation (Twin kids)																
	30	21	5	1.11	0.62	1.46	5.0	0.61	2.9	0.12	17	0.56	19	16	0.38	21
	30	21	10	0.92	0.62	1.46	4.4	0.61	2.4	0.10	14	0.46	20	18	0.38	25
	40	26	10	1.44	0.81	1.88	6.5	0.80	3.7	0.16	22	0.72	24	21	0.41	29
	40	26	15	1.54	0.81	1.88	6.8	0.80	4.0	0.17	23	0.77	26	23	0.43	33
	50	31	10	1.65	1.01	2.31	7.7	0.99	4.3	0.18	25	0.82	28	25	0.44	34
	50	31	15	1.75	1.01	2.31	8.0	0.99	4.5	0.19	26	0.87	30	27	0.45	37
	60	36	15	1.95	1.21	2.73	9.2	1.18	5.1	0.21	29	0.98	34	31	0.47	42
	60	36	20	2.05	1.21	2.73	9.4	1.18	5.3	0.23	31	1.03	35	32	0.48	46
Late Gestation (Single kid)																
	30	51	5	0.99	0.69	2.36	4.8	0.71	2.6	0.11	15	0.49	36	24	0.44	31
	30	51	10	1.06	0.69	2.36	5.0	0.71	2.8	0.12	16	0.53	38	26	0.45	35
	40	63	10	1.26	0.89	2.99	6.2	0.93	3.3	0.14	19	0.63	45	31	0.48	42
	40	63	15	1.34	0.89	2.99	6.4	0.93	3.5	0.15	20	0.67	47	33	0.49	45
	50	75	10	1.89	1.10	3.63	8.6	1.14	4.9	0.21	28	0.94	53	36	0.54	48
	50	75	15	1.99	1.10	3.63	8.9	1.14	5.2	0.22	30	0.99	54	38	0.55	52
	60	86	15	2.21	1.30	4.23	10.1	1.35	5.7	0.24	33	1.11	61	43	0.58	58
	60	86	20	2.31	1.30	4.23	10.4	1.35	6.0	0.25	35	1.16	63	45	0.59	62
Late Gestation (Twin kids)																
	30	85	5	1.11	0.78	3.38	5.3	0.85	2.9	0.12	17	0.55	59	35	0.52	44
	30	85	10	1.18	0.78	3.38	5.6	0.85	3.1	0.13	18	0.59	60	37	0.53	48
	40	106	10	1.39	1.01	4.28	6.8	1.09	3.6	0.15	21	0.70	72	44	0.58	57
	40	106	15	1.47	1.01	4.28	7.0	1.09	3.8	0.16	22	0.73	74	46	0.59	61
	50	125	10	1.59	1.23	5.13	8.0	1.33	4.1	0.18	24	0.80	83	51	0.62	66
	50	125	15	1.67	1.23	5.13	8.3	1.33	4.3	0.18	25	0.83	85	53	0.64	70
	60	143	15	1.86	1.45	5.94	9.4	1.56	4.8	0.20	28	0.93	96	60	0.68	79
	60	143	20	1.94	1.45	5.94	9.7	1.56	5.0	0.21	29	0.97	98	61	0.69	83
Early Lactation (Single kid)																
	30	–19	5	1.02	0.85	0.83	5.9	0.92	2.7	0.11	15	0.82	11	12	0.52	34
	30	–19	10	1.10	0.85	0.83	6.1	0.92	2.9	0.12	16	0.88	12	14	0.53	38
	40	–22	10	1.30	1.08	1.10	7.4	1.16	3.4	0.14	19	1.04	15	17	0.57	44
	40	–22	15	1.38	1.08	1.10	7.7	1.16	3.6	0.15	21	1.10	16	18	0.58	48
	50	–25	10	1.86	1.31	1.38	9.8	1.40	4.8	0.20	28	1.49	17	20	0.63	50
	50	–25	15	1.96	1.31	1.38	10.1	1.40	5.1	0.22	29	1.57	18	21	0.64	54
	60	–28	15	2.18	1.54	1.65	11.5	1.63	5.7	0.24	33	1.75	20	24	0.68	60
	60	–28	20	2.28	1.54	1.65	11.8	1.63	5.9	0.25	34	1.82	22	26	0.69	64
Early Lactation (Twin kids)																
	30	–38	5	1.03	1.03	0.83	6.7	1.18	2.7	0.11	15	0.83	14	13	0.65	47
	30	–38	10	1.10	1.03	0.83	6.9	1.18	2.9	0.12	16	0.88	16	15	0.66	51
	40	–44	10	1.56	1.31	1.10	9.2	1.48	4.1	0.17	23	1.25	19	18	0.74	60
	40	–44	15	1.37	1.31	1.10	8.6	1.48	3.6	0.15	21	1.10	20	20	0.73	64
	50	–50	10	1.78	1.56	1.38	10.7	1.75	4.6	0.20	27	1.43	21	22	0.80	69
	50	–50	15	1.86	1.56	1.38	10.9	1.75	4.8	0.20	28	1.49	23	23	0.81	72
	60	–55	15	2.07	1.82	1.65	12.4	2.02	5.4	0.23	31	1.66	25	27	0.86	80
	60	–55	20	2.15	1.82	1.65	12.6	2.02	5.6	0.24	32	1.72	27	28	0.87	84
Late Lactation (Single kid)																
	30	15	5	1.06	0.70	21.45	5.4	0.75	2.8	0.12	16	0.85	13	12	0.45	26
	30	15	10	1.16	0.70	21.45	5.7	0.75	3.0	0.13	17	0.93	14	14	0.47	29

TABLE 15-8 continued

Class/Stage/Other	Body Weight[b] kg	Daily Gain[c] g/d	Mohair Fiber Growth[d] g/d	Dry Matter Intake[e] kg/d	Mineral Requirements[f] Na g/d	Cl g/d	K g/d	Mg g/d	S g/d	Co mg/d	Cu mg/d	I mg/d	Fe mg/d	Mn mg/d	Se mg/d	Zn mg/d
	40	18	10	1.38	0.92	25.85	7.0	0.97	3.6	0.15	21	1.10	17	17	0.50	35
	40	18	15	1.48	0.92	25.85	7.3	0.97	3.8	0.16	22	1.18	19	19	0.51	39
	50	20	10	1.59	1.13	28.88	8.3	1.18	4.1	0.17	24	1.27	20	20	0.53	40
	50	20	15	1.69	1.13	28.88	8.5	1.18	4.4	0.19	25	1.35	21	22	0.54	44
	60	22	15	1.87	1.33	31.90	9.7	1.38	4.9	0.21	28	1.50	24	25	0.56	48
	60	22	20	1.97	1.33	31.90	10.0	1.38	5.1	0.22	30	1.58	25	26	0.57	52
Late Lactation (Twin kids)																
	30	30	5	0.96	0.80	42.08	5.6	0.91	2.5	0.11	14	0.77	19	14	0.54	35
	30	30	10	1.04	0.80	42.08	5.8	0.91	2.7	0.11	16	0.83	21	16	0.55	39
	40	35	10	1.54	1.03	49.23	8.0	1.16	4.0	0.17	23	1.23	25	19	0.61	46
	40	35	15	1.31	1.03	49.23	7.3	1.16	3.4	0.14	20	1.05	26	21	0.60	50
	50	40	10	1.77	1.25	56.38	9.4	1.40	4.6	0.20	27	1.42	28	23	0.65	52
	50	40	15	1.87	1.25	56.38	9.7	1.40	4.9	0.21	28	1.50	30	25	0.67	56
	60	44	15	2.08	1.47	62.15	11.0	1.62	5.4	0.23	31	1.66	33	28	0.70	62
	60	44	20	2.18	1.47	62.15	11.3	1.62	5.7	0.24	33	1.74	35	30	0.71	66

[a]Calcium and phosphorus requirements are listed in Table 15-6.
[b]Body weight used in estimating requirements is the determined or estimated weight in kilograms (kg) average for the period during which these requirements will be applied.
[c]Average change in body weight over a 24-hour period.
[d]Weight of mohair growth over a 24-hour period.
[e]The required daily dry matter intake of a diet having appropriate energy density for providing the required energy.
[f]The concentrations in the diet for satisfying mineral requirements can be calculated by dividing the daily requirement by the estimated dry matter intake.

NUTRIENT REQUIREMENTS OF CERVIDS TABLE

Nutrient requirements were determined by the factorial method for white-tailed deer (*Odocoileus virginianus*), reindeer/caribou (*Rangifer tarandus*), red deer (*Cervus elaphus*), and wapiti (*Cervus elaphus*) and when data were adequate or assumptions were deemed reasonable. Maintenance requirements for energy, protein, calcium, phosphorus, and vitamins A and E were estimated for body weights from 10 to 320 kg during winter and summer seasons to apply for all cervid species addressed. Winter (W) and summer (S) are used liberally to refer to the 6-month periods of shortest and longest days, respectively. Coefficients used as multipliers with interspecies metabolic body weights ($kg^{0.75}$) were 0.125 (wt = 20 to 60 kg) and 0.135 (wt = > 60 kg) (W)/0.173 (S) and 3.17 (W)/4.34 (S) for energy (Mcal/d ME) and protein (g/d MP), respectively. Requirements for growth for reindeer/caribou including antler growth were estimated for animals weighing 10 to 100 kg and gaining 50 to 300 g/d, with BWs to 300 kg and 820 g/d for wapiti, by summing requirements for maintenance, for growth (ME_g = 0.00533 [wt = 10 to 20 kg] or 0.00473 [wt > 20 kg] Mcal/g ADG; MP_g = 0.35 g/g ADG), and energy for antler growth ($ME_a = 0.0042 \times Wt^{0.75}$). Summer maintenance requirements included that for hair-coat growth.

Separate listings of requirements for production were included for the different species. The first period of the annual production cycle for the species includes prebreeding (following weaning of offspring), breeding, and early gestation that occurs during mid-summer through mid-winter. Contributing to the total nutrient requirements during this period are demands for maintenance, compensatory growth to recover body reserves used during previous periods, initiation of reproductive processes, and fetal demands for early pregnancy. Average daily gains indicated in Table 15-9 for this period include compensatory growth (ME_g = 0.010 Mcal/g ADG, MP_g = 0.38 g/g ADG), fetal growth, and accumulated growth of maternal reproductive tissue. The second period begins at mid- to late pregnancy when demands for fetal growth increase dramatically. This period is referred to in Table 15-9 as "Late pregnancy" and occurs during late winter and early summer. Equations by Robbins and Moen (1975) were used to calculate requirements for ME_p and MP_p. Lactation begins at parturition and continues approximately 4 months depending on species and conditions. Energy requirements for lactation (ME_l) are scaled to 0.75 power of body weight ($0.104 \times Wt^{0.75}$) using a mean efficiency (0.73) considering equally diet (0.64) and metabolic (0.82) sources of energy. An estimate of energy required for antler growth during lactation ($ME_a = 0.0042 \times Wt^{0.75}$) was included for reindeer/caribou. For MP_l, requirements were calculated with equations of Oftedal (1984), then scaled to body weights by a constant multiplier with ME_l. Assumptions related to the four species (white-tailed deer, reindeer/caribou, red deer, and wapiti) included for gestation period (205, 225, 233, and 260 days); birth weight scaled to body weights below and above averages (4.0 and 3.6 for single and twins, 8, 5, and 15 kg); and day of gestation representing prebreeding, breeding, and early gestation (days 50, 60, 60, 65). The final section in Table 15-9 gives estimates for nutrient requirements of mature males that may lose up to 30 percent of their normal weight during and surrounding the breeding season and may require large weight gains during the late winter to mid-summer period. Requirements for maintenance (ME_m and MP_m) were added to those for growth (ME_g = 0.010 Mcal/g and MP_g = 0.29 g/g ADG) and antler growth ($ME_a = 0.021 \times Wt^{0.75}$ and $MP_a = 0.54 \times Wt^{0.75}$) to calculate energy and protein requirements for adult males. Requirements for Ca, P, vitamin A, and vitamin E for all classes were extrapolated from sheep data.

The values in Table 15-9 are accurate to the extent that data are available to substantiate them. In some areas in which data are scarce, the values may only approximate the true but yet not understood relationships between the animals, their diet, and productivity. The range of conditions that occur in the wild could not be adequately addressed in this publication. Therefore, users are encouraged to modify, interpolate, and be creative in using these guidelines in the nutritional management of these wildlife species. More research is needed in order that future editions of this publication provide improved accuracy and precision in estimating the nutrient requirements and predicting responses.

REFERENCES

Oftedal, O.T. 1984. Milk composition, milk yield and energy output at peak lactation: A comparative review. Symp. Zool. Soc. Lond. 51:33–85.

Robbins, C. T., and A. N. Moen. 1975. Uterine composition and growth in pregnant white-tailed deer. J. Wildl. Manage. 39:684–691.

TABLE 15-9 Nutrient Requirements of Cervid Species (White-tailed Deer, Reindeer/Caribou, Red Deer and Elk/Wapiti)

Class/Age/Other	Body Weight[a] kg	Body Weight Gain[b] g/d	Energy Concentration in Diet[c] kcal/kg	Daily Dry Matter Intake[d] kg	Daily Dry Matter Intake[d] % BW	Energy Requirements[e] TDN kg/d	Energy Requirements[e] ME Mcal/d	Protein Requirements[f] CP g/d	Protein Requirements[f] CP % of Diet	Protein Requirements[f] MP g/d	Mineral Requirements[g] Ca g/d	Mineral Requirements[g] P g/d	Vitamin Requirements[h] A RE/d	Vitamin Requirements[h] E IU/d
Young to Mature														
Maintenance only														
Winter	10		2.4	0.3	2.9	0.2	0.7	25	9	18	1.0	0.4	314	53
	20		2.4	0.5	2.5	0.3	1.2	43	9	30	1.3	0.8	628	106
	30		2.4	0.7	2.2	0.4	1.6	58	9	41	1.6	1.1	942	159
	40		2.4	0.8	2.1	0.6	2.0	72	9	50	1.9	1.4	1256	212
	50		2.4	1.0	2.0	0.7	2.4	85	9	60	2.1	1.7	1570	265
	60		2.4	1.1	1.9	0.7	2.7	98	9	68	2.3	1.9	1884	318
	80		2.4	1.5	1.9	1.0	3.6	121	8	85	2.9	2.6	2512	424
	100		2.4	1.8	1.8	1.2	4.3	143	8	100	3.4	3.1	3140	530
	120		2.4	2.0	1.7	1.4	4.9	164	8	115	3.8	3.6	3768	636
	140		2.4	2.3	1.6	1.5	5.5	184	8	129	4.2	4.1	4396	742
	160		2.4	2.5	1.6	1.7	6.1	204	8	143	4.5	4.5	5024	848
	180		2.4	2.8	1.5	1.8	6.6	223	8	156	4.9	5.0	5652	954
	200		2.4	3.0	1.5	2.0	7.2	241	8	169	5.2	5.4	6280	1060
	220		1.9	4.0	1.8	2.1	7.7	259	6	181	6.9	7.3	6908	1166
	240		1.9	4.3	1.8	2.3	8.2	276	6	193	7.3	7.8	7536	1272
	260		1.9	4.6	1.8	2.4	8.7	293	6	205	7.7	8.3	8164	1378
	280		1.9	4.8	1.7	2.6	9.2	310	6	217	8.1	8.8	8792	1484
	300		1.9	5.1	1.7	2.7	9.7	326	6	229	8.5	9.3	9420	1590
	320		1.9	5.3	1.7	2.8	10.2	343	6	240	8.9	9.7	10048	1696
	340		1.9	5.6	1.6	3.0	10.7	359	6	251	9.3	10.2	10676	1802
	360		1.9	5.8	1.6	3.1	11.2	374	6	262	9.7	10.6	11304	1908
	380		1.9	6.1	1.6	3.2	11.6	390	6	273	10.0	11.1	11932	2014
	400		1.9	6.3	1.6	3.3	12.1	405	6	284	10.4	11.5	12560	2120
Summer	10		2.9	0.3	3.4	0.3	1.0	35	10	24	1.1	0.5	314	53
	20		2.9	0.6	2.9	0.5	1.6	59	10	41	1.5	0.9	628	106
	30		2.9	0.8	2.6	0.6	2.2	79	10	56	1.8	1.3	942	159
	40		2.9	1.0	2.4	0.8	2.8	99	10	69	2.1	1.6	1256	212
	50		2.9	1.1	2.3	0.9	3.3	117	10	82	2.3	1.9	1570	265
	60		2.9	1.3	2.2	1.0	3.7	134	10	94	2.6	2.2	1884	318
	80		2.9	1.6	2.0	1.3	4.6	166	10	116	3.1	2.8	2512	424
	100		2.9	1.9	1.9	1.5	5.5	196	10	137	3.5	3.4	3140	530
	120		2.4	2.6	2.2	1.7	6.3	225	9	157	4.7	4.7	3768	636
	140		2.4	2.9	2.1	2.0	7.0	252	9	177	5.2	5.3	4396	742
	160		2.4	3.3	2.0	2.2	7.8	279	9	195	5.6	5.9	5024	848
	180		2.4	3.6	2.0	2.4	8.5	305	9	213	6.1	6.4	5652	954
	200		2.4	3.8	1.9	2.6	9.2	330	9	231	6.6	7.0	6280	1060
	220		2.4	4.1	1.9	2.7	9.9	354	9	248	7.0	7.5	6908	1166

TABLE 15-9 continued

Class/Age/Other	Body Weight[a] kg	Body Weight Gain[b] g/d	Energy Concentration in Diet[c] kcal/kg	Daily Dry Matter Intake[d] kg	% BW	Energy Requirements[e] TDN kg/d	ME Mcal/d	Protein Requirements[f] CP g/d	CP % of Diet	MP g/d	Mineral Requirements[g] Ca g/d	P g/d	Vitamin Requirements[h] A RE/d	E IU/d
	240		2.4	4.4	1.8	2.9	10.5	378	9	265	7.4	8.0	7536	1272
	260		2.4	4.7	1.8	3.1	11.2	401	9	281	7.9	8.5	8164	1378
	280		2.4	5.0	1.8	3.3	11.8	424	9	297	8.3	9.0	8792	1484
	300		1.9	6.5	2.2	3.5	12.5	447	7	313	10.7	11.9	9420	1590
	320		1.9	6.9	2.1	3.6	13.1	469	7	328	11.2	12.5	10048	1696
	340		1.9	7.2	2.1	3.8	13.7	491	7	344	11.7	13.1	10676	1802
	360		1.9	7.5	2.1	4.0	14.3	512	7	359	12.2	13.7	11304	1908
	380		1.9	7.8	2.1	4.1	14.9	534	7	374	12.7	14.2	11932	2014
	400		1.9	8.1	2.0	4.3	15.5	555	7	388	13.2	14.8	12560	2120
Young-Growing Reindeer/Caribou														
Maintenance and gain	10	50	2.9	0.4	4.4	0.4	1.3	60	14	42	1.4	0.8	1000	100
		100	2.9	0.5	5.3	0.4	1.5	85	16	59	2.2	1.4	1000	100
(Includes allowance for		200	2.9	0.7	7.2	0.6	2.1	135	19	94	3.8	2.6	1000	100
antler growth)	20	50	1.9	1.0	5.1	0.5	1.9	84	8	59	2.0	1.4	2000	200
		100	2.4	0.9	4.6	0.6	2.2	109	12	76	2.6	1.8	2000	200
		200	2.9	1.0	4.8	0.8	2.7	159	17	111	4.0	2.8	2000	200
		300	2.9	1.1	5.7	0.9	3.3	209	18	146	5.6	4.0	2000	200
	30	50	1.9	1.3	4.4	0.7	2.5	104	8	73	2.2	1.7	3000	300
		100	2.4	1.1	3.8	0.8	2.7	129	11	91	2.8	2.0	3000	300
		200	2.4	1.3	4.5	0.9	3.2	179	13	126	4.3	3.2	3000	300
		300	2.9	1.3	4.3	1.0	3.7	229	18	161	5.7	4.2	3000	300
	40	50	1.9	1.3	3.3	0.7	2.5	124	9	87	2.2	1.7	4000	400
		100	1.9	1.4	3.6	0.8	2.8	149	10	104	3.0	2.3	4000	400
		200	2.4	1.4	3.4	0.9	3.2	199	15	139	4.4	3.2	4000	400
		300	2.4	1.5	3.9	1.0	3.7	249	16	174	5.9	4.4	4000	400
		400	2.4	1.7	4.4	1.2	4.2	299	17	209	7.5	5.6	4000	400
	50	50	1.9	1.6	3.2	0.9	3.1	142	9	99	2.5	2.0	5000	500
		100	1.9	1.7	3.5	0.9	3.3	167	10	117	3.3	2.6	5000	500
		200	1.9	2.0	4.0	1.0	3.8	217	11	152	4.9	3.8	5000	500
		300	2.4	1.8	3.6	1.2	4.2	267	15	187	6.1	4.6	5000	500
		400	2.4	2.0	4.0	1.3	4.7	317	16	222	7.7	5.8	5000	500
	60	50	1.9	1.9	3.1	1.0	3.6	159	8	111	2.7	2.2	6000	600
		100	1.9	2.0	3.3	1.1	3.8	184	9	129	3.6	2.8	6000	600
		200	1.9	2.2	3.7	1.2	4.3	234	10	164	5.2	4.1	6000	600
		300	2.4	2.0	3.3	1.3	4.8	284	14	199	6.3	4.8	6000	600
		400	2.4	2.2	3.7	1.5	5.2	334	15	234	7.9	6.0	6000	600

	70	50	1.9	2.4	3.4	1.3	4.5	175	7	123	3.2	2.7	7000	700
		100	1.9	2.5	3.6	1.3	4.8	200	8	140	4.0	3.3	7000	700
		200	1.9	2.7	3.9	1.5	5.2	250	9	175	5.6	4.6	7000	700
		300	2.4	2.4	3.4	1.6	5.7	300	13	210	6.7	5.2	7000	700
		400	2.4	2.6	3.7	1.7	6.2	350	14	245	8.3	6.4	7000	700
	80	50	1.9	2.1	2.7	1.1	4.1	191	9	134	3.0	2.5	8000	800
		100	1.9	2.3	2.8	1.2	4.3	216	10	151	3.8	3.1	8000	800
		200	1.9	2.5	3.1	1.3	4.8	266	11	186	5.4	4.3	8000	800
		300	2.4	2.2	2.8	1.5	5.3	316	14	221	6.5	5.1	8000	800
		400	2.4	2.4	3.0	1.6	5.7	366	15	256	8.1	6.2	8000	800
	90	50	1.9	2.8	3.1	1.5	5.4	206	7	144	3.6	3.1	9000	900
		100	1.9	3.0	3.3	1.6	5.7	231	8	162	4.4	3.8	9000	900
		200	1.9	3.2	3.6	1.7	6.1	281	9	197	6.1	5.0	9000	900
		300	1.9	3.5	3.8	1.8	6.6	331	10	232	7.7	6.3	9000	900
		400	2.4	3.0	3.3	2.0	7.1	381	13	267	8.6	6.8	9000	900
	100	50	1.9	3.1	3.1	1.6	5.8	221	7	155	3.8	3.4	10000	1000
		100	1.9	3.2	3.2	1.7	6.1	246	8	172	4.6	4.0	10000	1000
		200	1.9	3.4	3.4	1.8	6.5	296	9	207	6.3	5.2	10000	1000
		300	1.9	3.7	3.7	1.9	7.0	346	9	242	7.9	6.5	10000	1000
		400	2.4	3.1	3.1	2.1	7.5	396	13	277	8.8	7.0	10000	1000
White-Tailed Deer														
Prebreeding, breeding, and early pregnancy														
Single fetus	40	20	2.4	0.9	2.2	0.6	2.1	93	11	65	3.7	2.4	1256	212
	50	25	2.4	1.0	2.1	0.7	2.5	110	11	77	3.9	2.7	1570	265
	60	30	2.4	1.2	2.0	0.8	2.9	127	11	89	4.1	3.0	1884	318
	80	39	2.4	1.6	2.0	1.1	3.8	160	10	112	4.6	3.7	2512	424
	100	47	2.4	1.9	1.9	1.3	4.5	190	10	133	5.0	4.3	3140	530
	120	56	2.4	2.2	1.8	1.4	5.2	219	10	154	5.3	4.8	3768	636
	140	65	2.4	2.5	1.8	1.6	5.9	248	10	173	5.7	5.3	4396	742
Twin fetuses	40	22	2.4	0.9	2.3	0.6	2.2	100	11	70	5.4	3.2	1256	212
	50	27	2.4	1.1	2.1	0.7	2.6	119	11	84	5.6	3.5	1570	265
	60	32	2.4	1.2	2.1	0.8	2.9	138	11	96	5.8	3.8	1884	318
	80	42	2.4	1.6	2.1	1.1	3.9	173	11	121	6.4	4.6	2512	424
	100	52	2.4	2.0	2.0	1.3	4.7	207	11	145	6.7	5.1	3140	530
	120	62	2.4	2.3	1.9	1.5	5.4	239	11	167	7.1	5.7	3768	636
	140	72	2.4	2.5	1.8	1.7	6.1	270	11	189	7.5	6.2	4396	742
Late pregnancy														
Single fetus	40	48	2.4	1.2	3.0	0.8	2.9	191	16	134	5.3	3.2	1820	224
	50	58	2.4	1.4	2.9	0.9	3.4	214	15	150	5.5	3.6	2275	280
	60	68	2.4	1.6	2.7	1.1	3.9	236	14	165	5.8	4.0	2730	336
	80	87	2.4	2.2	2.8	1.5	5.3	278	13	195	6.5	5.1	3640	448
	100	106	2.4	2.6	2.6	1.7	6.2	319	12	223	7.0	5.8	4550	560
	120	124	2.4	3.0	2.5	2.0	7.1	359	12	251	7.5	6.5	5460	672
	140	142	2.4	3.4	2.4	2.2	8.0	398	12	279	7.9	7.2	6370	784

TABLE 15-9 continued

Class/Age/Other	Body Weight[a] kg	Body Weight Gain[b] g/d	Energy Concentration in Diet[c] kcal/kg	Daily Dry Matter Intake[d] kg	Daily Dry Matter Intake[d] % BW	Energy Requirements[e] TDN kg/d	Energy Requirements[e] ME Mcal/d	Protein Requirements[f] CP g/d	Protein Requirements[f] CP % of Diet	Protein Requirements[f] MP g/d	Mineral Requirements[g] Ca g/d	Mineral Requirements[g] P g/d	Vitamin Requirements[h] A RE/d	Vitamin Requirements[h] E IU/d
Twin fetuses	40	35	2.9	1.3	3.3	1.0	3.8	227	17	159	8.0	4.3	1820	224
	50	43	2.9	1.5	3.1	1.2	4.4	253	16	177	8.3	4.8	2275	280
	60	50	2.9	1.8	3.0	1.4	5.1	278	16	194	8.6	5.2	2730	336
	80	65	2.9	2.4	3.0	1.9	6.8	326	14	228	9.3	6.3	3640	448
	100	79	2.9	2.8	2.8	2.2	8.1	373	13	261	9.9	7.1	4550	560
	120	93	2.9	3.2	2.7	2.6	9.3	419	13	293	10.4	7.9	5460	672
	140	107	2.9	3.6	2.6	2.9	10.4	464	13	325	10.9	8.6	6370	784
Lactation														
Single fawns	40	–30	2.9	1.6	4.1	1.3	4.7	207	13	145	7.3	6.1	2140	224
	50	–35	2.9	1.9	3.9	1.5	5.6	250	13	175	7.7	6.7	2675	280
	60	–40	2.9	2.2	3.7	1.8	6.4	292	13	204	8.0	7.2	3210	336
	80	–50	2.9	2.8	3.5	2.2	7.9	371	13	260	8.7	8.2	4280	448
	100	–59	2.9	3.3	3.3	2.6	9.4	446	14	312	9.3	9.1	5350	560
	120	–68	2.9	3.8	3.1	3.0	10.8	518	14	363	9.9	10.0	6420	672
	140	–76	2.9	4.2	3.0	3.3	12.1	588	14	411	10.5	10.9	7490	784
Twin fawns	40	–45	2.9	2.0	5.0	1.6	5.8	266	13	186	7.8	6.8	2140	224
	50	–53	2.9	2.4	4.8	1.9	6.8	322	14	226	8.2	7.5	2675	280
	60	–60	2.9	2.7	4.6	2.2	7.9	377	14	264	8.7	8.1	3210	336
	80	–75	2.9	3.4	4.2	2.7	9.7	481	14	337	9.5	9.4	4280	448
	100	–89	2.9	4.0	4.0	3.2	11.5	581	14	406	10.3	10.5	5350	560
	120	–102	2.9	4.6	3.8	3.7	13.2	676	15	473	11.0	11.6	6420	672
	140	–114	2.9	5.2	3.7	4.1	14.8	768	15	538	11.7	12.6	7490	784
Reindeer/caribou														
Prebreeding, breeding, and early pregnancy	60	28	2.4	1.2	2.0	0.8	2.9	108	9	76	4.1	3.0	1884	318
	80	36	2.4	1.6	2.0	1.1	3.8	135	8	95	4.6	3.7	2512	424
	100	45	2.4	1.9	1.9	1.3	4.5	161	8	113	5.0	4.3	3140	530
	120	53	2.4	2.2	1.8	1.4	5.2	185	9	130	5.3	4.8	3768	636
	140	61	2.4	2.5	1.8	1.6	5.9	209	9	146	5.7	5.3	4396	742
	160	70	2.4	2.7	1.7	1.8	6.5	232	9	162	6.0	5.8	5024	848
Late pregnancy	60	61	2.9	1.4	2.3	1.1	3.9	236	17	165	5.5	3.5	2730	336
	80	78	2.9	1.8	2.3	1.5	5.3	278	15	195	6.0	4.4	3640	448
	100	95	2.9	2.2	2.2	1.7	6.2	319	15	223	6.5	5.0	4550	560
	120	111	2.9	2.5	2.1	2.0	7.1	359	14	251	6.9	5.6	5460	672
	140	127	2.9	2.8	2.0	2.2	8.0	398	14	279	7.2	6.2	6370	784
	160	143	2.9	3.1	1.9	2.5	8.9	436	14	305	7.6	6.7	7280	896

Lactation	60	–59	2.9	2.2	3.7	1.7	6.3	292	13	204	8.0	7.1	3210	336
	80	–74	2.9	2.7	3.4	2.2	7.8	371	14	260	8.7	8.1	4280	448
(Includes allowance for	100	–87	2.9	3.2	3.2	2.6	9.2	446	14	312	9.3	9.0	5350	560
antler growth)	120	–100	2.9	3.7	3.1	2.9	10.6	518	14	363	9.9	9.9	6420	672
	140	–112	2.9	4.1	3.0	3.3	11.9	588	14	411	10.4	10.7	7490	784
	160	–124	2.9	4.6	2.9	3.6	13.1	655	14	459	11.0	11.6	8560	896
Red deer														
Prebreeding, breeding, and early pregnancy	80	36	2.4	1.6	2.0	1.1	3.8	158	10	110	4.6	3.7	2512	424
	100	44	2.4	1.9	1.9	1.3	4.5	182	10	127	5.0	4.3	3140	530
	120	52	2.4	2.2	1.8	1.4	5.2	206	9	144	5.3	4.8	3768	636
	140	60	2.4	2.5	1.8	1.6	5.9	228	9	160	5.7	5.3	4396	742
	160	68	2.4	2.7	1.7	1.8	6.5	251	9	175	6.0	5.8	5024	848
Late pregnancy	80	74	2.9	1.8	2.3	1.5	5.3	278	15	195	6.0	4.4	3640	448
	100	89	2.9	2.2	2.2	1.7	6.2	319	15	223	6.5	5.0	4550	560
	120	105	2.9	2.5	2.1	2.0	7.1	359	14	251	6.9	5.6	5460	672
	140	120	2.9	2.8	2.0	2.2	8.0	398	14	279	7.2	6.2	6370	784
	160	135	2.9	3.1	1.9	2.5	8.9	436	14	305	7.6	6.7	7280	896
Lactation	80	–111	2.9	2.6	3.2	2.0	7.3	371	15	260	8.4	7.8	4280	448
	100	–131	2.9	3.0	3.0	2.4	8.7	446	15	312	9.0	8.7	5350	560
	120	–150	2.9	3.5	2.9	2.8	9.9	518	15	363	9.6	9.5	6420	672
	140	–168	2.9	3.9	2.8	3.1	11.2	588	15	411	10.1	10.3	7490	784
	160	–186	2.9	4.3	2.7	3.4	12.3	655	15	459	10.6	11.0	8560	896
Wapiti (American Elk)														
Prebreeding, breeding, and early pregnancy	180	74	2.4	3.0	1.7	2.0	7.1	273	9	191	6.3	6.3	5652	954
	200	82	2.4	3.2	1.6	2.1	7.7	295	9	206	6.6	6.7	6280	1060
	220	90	2.4	3.5	1.6	2.3	8.3	315	9	221	6.9	7.2	6908	1166
	240	98	2.4	3.7	1.5	2.5	8.9	336	9	235	7.2	7.6	7536	1272
	260	105	2.4	3.9	1.5	2.6	9.4	356	9	249	7.5	8.0	8164	1378
	280	113	2.4	4.2	1.5	2.8	10.0	376	9	263	7.8	8.5	8792	1484
	300	121	2.4	4.4	1.5	2.9	10.5	396	9	277	8.1	8.9	9420	1590
Late pregnancy	180	142	2.9	3.4	1.9	2.7	9.7	474	14	332	8.0	7.2	8190	1008
	200	156	2.9	3.7	1.8	2.9	10.5	511	14	358	8.3	7.8	9100	1120
	220	169	2.9	3.9	1.8	3.1	11.3	548	14	384	8.7	8.3	10010	1232
	240	183	2.9	4.2	1.8	3.3	12.1	584	14	409	9.0	8.8	10920	1344
	260	196	2.9	4.5	1.7	3.6	12.8	620	14	434	9.3	9.3	11830	1456
	280	209	2.9	4.7	1.7	3.8	13.6	656	14	459	9.6	9.7	12740	1568
	300	223	2.9	5.0	1.7	4.0	14.3	691	14	484	10.0	10.2	13650	1680

TABLE 15-9 continued

Class/Age/Other	Body Weight[a] kg	Body Weight Gain[b] g/d	Energy Concentration in Diet[c] kcal/kg	Daily Dry Matter Intake[d] kg	Daily Dry Matter Intake[d] % BW	Energy Requirements[e] TDN kg/d	Energy Requirements[e] ME Mcal/d	Protein Requirements[f] CP g/d	Protein Requirements[f] CP % of Diet	Protein Requirements[f] MP g/d	Mineral Requirements[g] Ca g/d	Mineral Requirements[g] P g/d	Vitamin Requirements[h] A RE/d	Vitamin Requirements[h] E IU/d
Lactation	180	–121	2.9	4.7	2.6	3.8	13.5	746	16	522	11.1	11.8	9630	1008
	200	–131	2.9	5.1	2.6	4.1	14.6	810	16	567	11.6	12.5	10700	1120
	220	–141	2.9	5.5	2.5	4.4	15.7	872	16	611	12.1	13.2	11770	1232
	240	–150	2.9	5.9	2.4	4.7	16.8	934	16	653	12.5	13.9	12840	1344
	260	–159	2.9	6.2	2.4	4.9	17.8	994	16	696	13.0	14.6	13910	1456
	280	–168	2.9	6.6	2.3	5.2	18.8	1053	16	737	13.4	15.2	14980	1568
	300	–177	2.9	6.9	2.3	5.5	19.8	1111	16	778	13.9	15.9	16050	1680
All Cervids														
Adult males	60	45	2.4	1.9	3.2	1.3	4.6	169	9	118	2.7	2.2	6000	600
(Includes allowance for		90	2.4	2.1	3.5	1.4	5.1	188	9	131	3.5	2.9	6000	600
antler growth)	80	60	2.4	2.4	3.0	1.6	5.8	211	9	148	3.4	2.9	8000	800
		120	2.4	2.7	3.3	1.8	6.4	236	9	165	4.5	3.7	8000	800
	100	75	2.4	2.9	2.9	1.9	6.9	252	9	176	4.0	3.4	10000	1000
		150	2.4	3.2	3.2	2.1	7.6	283	9	198	5.3	4.5	10000	1000
	120	90	2.4	3.3	2.8	2.2	7.9	290	9	203	4.6	4.0	12000	1200
		180	2.4	3.7	3.1	2.4	8.8	327	9	229	6.2	5.3	12000	1200
	140	105	2.4	3.7	2.7	2.5	8.9	327	9	229	5.2	4.6	14000	1400
		210	2.4	4.2	3.0	2.8	10.0	371	9	260	7.1	6.1	14000	1400
	160	120	2.4	4.2	2.6	2.8	9.9	363	9	254	5.8	5.1	16000	1600
		240	2.4	4.7	2.9	3.1	11.1	413	9	289	7.9	6.8	16000	1600
	180	135	2.4	4.6	2.5	3.0	10.9	399	9	279	6.4	5.7	18000	1800
		270	2.4	5.1	2.8	3.4	12.2	454	9	318	8.8	7.6	18000	1800
	200	150	2.4	4.9	2.5	3.3	11.8	433	9	303	7.0	6.2	20000	2000
		300	2.4	5.6	2.8	3.7	13.3	495	9	347	9.6	8.3	20000	2000
	220	165	2.4	5.3	2.4	3.5	12.7	467	9	327	7.5	6.7	22000	2200
		330	2.4	6.0	2.7	4.0	14.4	535	9	374	10.4	9.0	22000	2200
	240	180	2.4	5.7	2.4	3.8	13.6	500	9	350	8.1	7.2	24000	2400
		360	2.4	6.5	2.7	4.3	15.4	574	9	402	11.3	9.7	24000	2400
	260	195	2.4	6.1	2.3	4.0	14.5	532	9	373	8.6	7.7	26000	2600
		390	2.4	6.9	2.6	4.6	16.5	613	9	429	12.1	10.5	26000	2600
	280	210	2.4	6.4	2.3	4.3	15.4	564	9	395	9.2	8.2	28000	2800
		420	2.4	7.3	2.6	4.8	17.5	651	9	456	12.9	11.2	28000	2800
	300	225	2.4	6.8	2.3	4.5	16.2	596	9	417	9.7	8.7	30000	3000
		450	2.4	7.7	2.6	5.1	18.5	689	9	482	13.7	11.9	30000	3000
	320	240	2.4	7.1	2.2	4.7	17.1	627	9	439	10.2	9.2	32000	3200

	480	2.4	8.1	2.5	5.4	19.5	726	9	508	14.5	12.6	32000	3200
340	255	2.4	7.5	2.2	5.0	17.9	658	9	460	10.7	9.7	34000	3400
	510	2.4	8.6	2.5	5.7	20.5	763	9	534	15.3	13.3	34000	3400
360	270	2.4	7.8	2.2	5.2	18.7	688	9	482	11.3	10.2	36000	3600
	540	2.4	9.0	2.5	5.9	21.4	800	9	560	16.1	14.0	36000	3600

[a]Body weight used in estimating requirements is the determined or estimated weight in kilograms (kg) average for the period during which these requirements will be applied.
[b]Average change in body weight over a 24-hour period.
[c]Three hypothetical diets with increasing energy concentrations (1.91, 2.34 and 2.87 kcal/kg) were used in the calculations of intake and nutrient requirements. For each line entry, a diet was selected to represent the level of energy concentration that approximates that needed by the animal to achieve adequate intake to satisfy its energy requirement.
[d]The daily dry matter intake, expressed as kg or as percentage of body weight, of a diet having the indicated energy concentration (previous column) that is required to meet energy requirements. These energy concentrations should be viewed only as examples. In some cases, diets having greater or lesser concentrations of energy would be more appropriate.
[e]Energy requirements expressed as total digestible nutrients (TDN) in kg/d and metabolizable energy (ME) as kcal/d.
[f]Protein requirements expressed as crude protein (CP), metabolizable protein (MP), and degradable intake protein (DIP). The CP requirement differs with the proportion of undegradable intake protein (UIP) because of the required minimal DIP.
[g]Two macro minerals, calcium (Ca) and phosphorus (P), commonly considered in balancing diets are included. Often, the balance (ratio) of the two minerals also is of concern. Estimated requirements for calcium and phosphorus were extrapolated from sheep data.
[h]Two fat-soluble vitamins, A and E, that often are deficient in animal diets are expressed as retinol equivalents (RE) and international units (IU) for vitamins A and E, respectively. RE = 1.0 μg of all-trans retinol, 5.0 μg of all-trans betacarotene, and 7.6 μg of other carotenoids. Estimated requirements for calcium, phosphorus, vitamin A, and vitamin E were extrapolated from sheep data.

NUTRIENT REQUIREMENTS OF NEW WORLD CAMELIDS TABLE

Nutrient requirements in Table 15-10 are listed for new world camelids (NWC; llamas and alpacas) for body weights (BW) between 60 and 160 kg. For growing animals, average daily gains range from 50 to 400 g/d. Pregnancy requirements are given for 8, 9, and 10 months of gestation and with birth weight being 8, 10, or 12 percent of mature female BW. Requirements for lactating animals are for daily milk yield of 0.5, 1.5, and 2.5 kg, with assumed milk energy and protein concentrations of 700 kcal/kg and 3.4 percent, respectively. Fiber growth was based on an annual fleece weight of 3 percent BW. Dry matter intake (DMI) values are to supply needed energy with dietary ME concentrations of either 1.91, 2.39, or 2.87 Mcal/kg DM. Dry matter intake estimates greater than 1.8 and 2.2 percent BW for nonlactating and lactating camelids, respectively, were deemed unachievable and omitted. These requirements do not include an activity energy cost and, thus, can only be directly applied to confined animals in pens, stalls, or small lots. To include an activity energy cost for grazing or working animals, a fractional multiplier can be used. The ME_m value multiplied by an assumed activity cost as a fraction of the maintenance requirement (e.g., 0.25, 0.50, or 0.75) can be added to the sum of the other requirements to derive the total ME need. Estimates of requirements by NWC for Ca and P and vitamins A and E are included in Table 15-10. Much of the bases of these estimates were gleaned from data from other species, mostly sheep. Requirements and maximum tolerances for other minerals and vitamins are discussed in Chapters 7 and 8, respectively.

TABLE 15-10 Nutrient Requirements of New World Camelids (NWC)

Class/Age/Other	Body Weight[a]	Body Weight Gain[b]	Energy Concentration in Diet[c]	Daily Dry Matter Intake[d]		Energy Requirements[e]		Protein[f]	Minerals[g]		Vitamins[h]	
						TDN	ME	CP	Ca	P	A	E
	kg	g/d	kcal/kg	kg	% BW	kg/d	Mcal/d	g/d	g/d	g/d	RE/d	IU/d
Mature												
Maintenance												
	60		1.91	0.82	1.37	0.44	1.57	75	1.6	1.2	1,884	318
	80		1.91	1.02	1.27	0.54	1.95	94	1.9	1.5	2,512	424
	100		1.91	1.21	1.21	0.64	2.30	111	2.2	1.8	3,140	530
	120		1.91	1.38	1.15	0.73	2.64	127	2.4	2.0	3,768	636
	140		1.91	1.55	1.11	0.82	2.97	143	2.7	2.2	4,396	742
	160		1.91	1.71	1.07	0.91	3.28	158	2.9	2.4	5,024	848
Gestation												
At 8-month gestation												
Birth weight = 8% of mature weight												
	60		1.91	0.97	1.61	0.51	1.85	96	3.8	2.2	2,730	336
	80		1.91	1.22	1.53	0.65	2.33	119	4.2	2.5	3,640	448
	100		1.91	1.46	1.46	0.77	2.79	141	4.5	2.9	4,550	560
	120		1.91	1.69	1.41	0.90	3.24	161	4.8	3.2	5,460	672
	140		1.91	1.92	1.37	1.02	3.66	181	5.1	3.5	6,370	784
	160		1.91	2.13	1.33	1.13	4.08	200	5.4	3.8	7,280	896
Birth weight = 10% of mature weight												
	60		1.91	1.01	1.68	0.53	1.93	96	3.9	2.2	2,730	336
	80		1.91	1.28	1.59	0.68	2.44	119	4.2	2.6	3,640	448
	100		1.91	1.53	1.53	0.81	2.92	141	4.6	2.9	4,550	560
	120		1.91	1.77	1.48	0.94	3.39	161	4.9	3.3	5,460	672
	140		1.91	2.01	1.44	1.07	3.85	181	5.3	3.6	6,370	784
	160		1.91	2.24	1.40	1.19	4.29	200	5.6	3.9	7,280	896
Birth weight = 12% of mature weight												
	60		1.91	1.05	1.75	0.56	2.01	96	3.9	2.3	2,730	336
	80		1.91	1.33	1.66	0.71	2.54	119	4.3	2.7	3,640	448
	100		1.91	1.60	1.60	0.85	3.05	141	4.7	3.0	4,550	560
	120		1.91	1.86	1.55	0.98	3.55	161	5.0	3.4	5,460	672
	140		1.91	2.11	1.51	1.12	4.03	181	5.	3.7	6,370	784
	160		1.91	2.35	1.47	1.25	4.50	200	5.7	4.1	7,280	896
At 9-month gestation												
Birth weight = 8% of mature weight												
	60		2.39	0.91	1.51	0.60	2.16	117	3.7	2.1	2,730	336
	80		2.39	1.15	1.44	0.76	2.75	146	4.1	2.4	3,640	448
	100		1.91	1.74	1.74	0.92	3.32	172	4.9	3.2	4,550	560
	120		1.91	2.02	1.68	1.07	3.87	197	5.3	3.6	5,460	672
	140		1.91	2.30	1.64	1.22	4.40	221	5.7	4.0	6,370	784
	160		1.91	2.58	1.61	1.37	4.92	245	6.0	4.4	7,280	896
Birth weight = 10% of mature weight												
	60		2.39	0.97	1.62	0.64	2.32	117	3.8	2.2	2,730	336
	80		2.39	1.24	1.55	0.82	2.96	146	4.2	2.6	3,640	448
	100		2.39	1.50	1.50	0.99	3.58	172	4.6	2.9	4,550	560
	120		2.39	1.75	1.46	1.16	4.18	197	4.9	3.2	5,460	672
	140		1.91	2.49	1.78	1.32	4.77	221	5.9	4.3	6,370	784
	160		1.91	2.80	1.75	1.48	5.34	245	6.4	4.7	7,280	896
Birth weight = 12% of mature weight												
	60		2.39	1.04	1.73	0.69	2.48	117	3.9	2.3	2,730	336
	80		2.39	1.33	1.66	0.88	3.17	146	4.3	2.7	3,640	448
	100		2.39	1.61	1.61	1.07	3.84	172	4.7	3.1	4,550	560
	120		2.39	1.88	1.57	1.25	4.50	197	5.1	3.4	5,460	672
	140		2.39	2.15	1.54	1.42	5.14	221	5.5	3.8	6,370	784
	160		2.39	2.41	1.51	1.60	5.77	245	5.8	4.1	7,280	896

TABLE 15-10 continued

Class/Age/Other	Body Weight[a] kg	Body Weight Gain[b] g/d	Energy Concentration in Diet[c] kcal/kg	Daily Dry Matter Intake[d] kg	Daily Dry Matter Intake[d] % BW	Energy Requirements[e] TDN kg/d	Energy Requirements[e] ME Mcal/d	Protein[f] CP g/d	Minerals[g] Ca g/d	Minerals[g] P g/d	Vitamins[h] A RE/d	Vitamins[h] E IU/d
At 10-month gestation												
Birth weight = 8% of mature weight												
	60		2.87	0.92	1.53	0.73	2.63	145	3.8	2.1	2,730	336
	80		2.39	1.40	1.75	0.93	3.34	180	4.4	2.8	3,640	448
	100		2.39	1.68	1.68	1.11	4.02	213	4.8	3.2	4,550	560
	120		2.39	1.96	1.63	1.30	4.68	244	5.2	3.5	5,460	672
	140		2.39	2.23	1.59	1.48	5.33	274	5.6	3.9	6,370	784
	160		2.39	2.50	1.56	1.66	5.97	303	5.9	4.3	7,280	896
Birth weight = 10% of mature weight												
	60		2.87	1.00	1.67	0.80	2.88	145	3.9	2.2	2,730	336
	80		2.87	1.28	1.60	1.02	3.66	180	4.2	2.6	3,640	448
	100		2.87	1.54	1.54	1.23	4.43	213	4.6	3.0	4,550	560
	120		2.39	2.16	1.80	1.43	5.17	244	5.5	3.8	5,460	672
	140		2.39	2.47	1.76	1.64	5.90	274	5.9	4.2	6,370	784
	160		2.39	2.77	1.73	1.84	6.62	303	6.3	4.6	7,280	896
Birth weight = 12% of mature weight												
	60		2.87	1.09	1.81	0.87	3.12	145	4.0	2.3	2,730	336
	80		2.87	1.39	1.74	1.11	3.99	180	4.4	2.8	3,640	448
	100		2.87	1.68	1.68	1.34	4.83	213	4.8	3.2	4,550	560
	120		2.87	1.97	1.64	1.57	5.66	244	5.2	3.5	5,460	672
	140		2.87	2.26	1.61	1.79	6.47	274	5.6	3.9	6,370	784
	160		2.87	2.54	1.58	2.02	7.27	303	6.0	4.3	7,280	896
Lactation												
Milk yield = 0.5 kg/d	50		1.91	1.07	2.14	0.57	2.04	106	3.5	2.3	2,675	280
	80		1.91	1.27	1.58	0.67	2.42	124	3.8	2.6	4,280	448
	100		1.91	1.45	1.45	0.77	2.78	141	4.1	2.9	5,350	560
	120		1.91	1.63	1.36	0.86	3.11	157	4.3	3.1	6,420	672
	140		1.91	1.80	1.28	0.95	3.44	173	4.6	3.3	7,490	784
	160		1.91	1.96	1.23	1.04	3.75	188	4.8	3.5	8,560	896
Milk yield = 1.5 kg/d	50		2.87	1.04	2.09	0.83	2.99	166	6.6	3.8	2,675	280
	80		1.91	1.76	2.20	0.93	3.37	185	7.6	4.8	4,280	448
	100		1.91	1.95	1.95	1.03	3.72	202	7.9	5.1	5,350	560
	120		1.91	2.12	1.77	1.13	4.06	218	8.1	5.3	6,420	672
	140		1.91	2.29	1.64	1.22	4.38	233	8.3	5.5	7,490	784
	160		1.91	2.46	1.54	1.30	4.70	248	8.6	5.8	8,560	896
Milk yield = 2.5 kg/d	50		2.87	1.36	2.72	1.09	3.91	210	10.2	5.8	2,675	280
	80		2.87	1.50	1.88	1.20	4.31	245	10.4	6.0	4,280	448
	100		2.39	1.95	1.95	1.29	4.67	262	11.0	6.6	5,350	560
	120		1.91	2.62	2.18	1.39	5.01	278	11.9	7.5	6,420	672
	140		1.91	2.79	1.99	1.48	5.33	294	12.1	7.7	7,490	784
	160		1.91	2.95	1.84	1.56	5.64	309	12.4	8.0	8,560	896
Growing												
	40	50	2.39	0.64	1.59	0.42	1.52	70	2.6	1.4	4000	400
		100	2.87	0.66	1.64	0.52	1.88	84	3.9	1.9	4000	400
	60	50	1.91	1.01	1.69	0.54	1.93	90	3.1	2.0	6000	600
		100	2.39	0.96	1.60	0.64	2.30	104	4.3	2.3	6000	600
		200	2.87	1.05	1.76	0.84	3.02	132	6.9	3.4	6000	600
	80	50	1.91	1.21	1.51	0.64	2.31	108	3.4	2.2	8000	800
		100	1.91	1.40	1.75	0.74	2.67	122	4.9	2.9	8000	800
		200	2.39	1.42	1.78	0.94	3.40	150	7.4	3.9	8000	800
		300	2.87	1.44	1.80	1.14	4.12	179	9.8	4.8	8000	800
	100	50	1.91	1.39	1.39	0.74	2.67	125	3.7	2.5	10000	1000
		100	1.91	1.58	1.58	0.84	3.03	139	5.1	3.2	10000	1000

TABLE 15-10 continued

Class/Age/Other	Body Weight[a] kg	Body Weight Gain[b] g/d	Energy Concentration in Diet[c] kcal/kg	Daily Dry Matter Intake[d] kg	Daily Dry Matter Intake[d] % BW	Energy Requirements[e] TDN kg/d	Energy Requirements[e] ME Mcal/d	Protein[f] CP g/d	Minerals[g] Ca g/d	Minerals[g] P g/d	Vitamins[h] A RE/d	Vitamins[h] E IU/d
		200	2.39	1.57	1.57	1.04	3.75	168	7.6	4.1	10000	1000
		300	2.87	1.56	1.56	1.24	4.48	196	10.0	5.0	10000	1000
	120	50	1.91	1.57	1.31	0.83	3.00	141	3.9	2.7	12000	1200
		100	1.91	1.76	1.47	0.93	3.37	155	5.4	3.4	12000	1200
		200	1.91	2.14	1.78	1.13	4.09	184	8.4	4.9	12000	1200
		300	2.39	2.02	1.68	1.34	4.82	212	10.6	5.6	12000	1200
		400	2.87	1.93	1.61	1.54	5.54	241	13.0	6.4	12000	1200
	140	50	1.91	1.74	1.24	0.92	3.33	157	4.1	2.9	14000	1400
		100	1.91	1.93	1.38	1.02	3.69	171	5.6	3.7	14000	1400
		200	1.91	2.31	1.65	1.22	4.42	199	8.6	5.1	14000	1400
		300	2.39	2.15	1.54	1.43	5.14	228	10.8	5.8	14000	1400
		400	2.39	2.45	1.75	1.63	5.87	256	13.7	7.1	14000	1400

[a]Body weight used in estimating requirements is the determined or estimated weight in kilograms (kg) average for the period during which these requirements will be applied.

[b]Average change in body weight over a 24-hour period.

[c]Three hypothetical diets with increasing energy concentrations (1.91, 2.34, and 2.87 kcal/kg) were used in the calculations of intake and nutrient requirements. For each line entry, a diet was selected to represent the level of energy concentration that approximates that needed by the animal to achieve adequate intake to satisfy its energy requirement.

[d]The daily dry matter intake, expressed as kg or as percentage of body weight, of a diet having the indicated energy concentration (previous column) that is required to meet energy requirements. These energy concentrations should be viewed only as examples. In some cases, diets having greater or lesser concentrations of energy would be more appropriate.

[e]Energy requirements expressed as total digestible nutrients (TDN) in kg/d and metabolizable energy (ME) as kcal/d.

[f]Protein requirements expressed as crude protein (CP).

[g]Two macro minerals, calcium (Ca) and phosphorus (P), commonly considered in balancing diets are included. Often, the balance (ratio) of the two minerals also is of concern.

[h]Two fat-soluble vitamins, A and E, that often are deficient in animal diets are expressed as retinol equivalents (RE) and international units (IU) for vitamins A and E, respectively. RE = 1 μg of all-trans retinol, 5.0 μg of all-trans betacarotene, and 7.6 μg of other carotenoids

TABLE 15-11 Composition of Common Feedstuffs[a,b,c]

Feedstuff	DM	Energy[d]						Protein[e]			
		TDN	DE	ME	NE_m	NE_g	NE_l	CP	DP	MP	UIP
	%	%	Mcal/kg					%			
Alfalfa Cubes	91	57	2.5	2.1	1.3	0.6	1.3	18.0	13.2	12.6	5.4
Alfalfa Dehydrated 17% CP	92	61	2.7	2.2	1.4	0.7	1.3	19.0	14.1	13.3	11.4
Alfalfa Fresh	24	61	2.7	2.2	1.4	0.7	1.3	19.0	14.1	13.3	3.4
Alfalfa Hay Early Bloom	90	59	2.6	2.1	1.3	0.6	1.3	19.0	14.1	13.3	3.8
Alfalfa Hay Midbloom	89	58	2.6	2.1	1.3	0.6	1.3	17.0	12.3	11.9	3.9
Alfalfa Hay Full Bloom	88	54	2.4	2.0	1.2	0.4	1.2	16.0	11.4	11.2	4.0
Alfalfa Hay Mature	88	50	2.2	1.8	1.1	0.3	1.1	13.0	8.7	9.1	3.9
Alfalfa Seed Screenings	91	84	3.7	3.0	2.0	1.3	1.9	34.0	27.6	23.8	—
Alfalfa Silage	30	55	2.4	2.0	1.2	0.5	1.2	18.0	13.2	12.6	3.4
Alfalfa Silage Wilted	39	58	2.6	2.1	1.3	0.6	1.3	18.0	13.2	12.6	4.0
Alfalfa Leaf Meal	89	69	3.0	2.5	1.6	0.9	1.5	28.0	22.2	19.6	4.2
Alfalfa Stems	89	47	2.1	1.7	1.0	0.2	1.0	11.0	6.9	7.7	4.8
Almond Hulls	89	59	2.6	2.1	1.3	0.6	1.3	5.0	1.5	3.5	3.0
Ammonium Chloride	99	0	0.0	0.0	0.0	0.0	0.0	163.0	143.7	114.1	0.0
Ammonium Sulfate	99	0	0.0	0.0	0.0	0.0	0.0	132.0	115.8	92.4	0.0
Apple Pomace Wet	20	68	3.0	2.5	1.5	0.9	1.5	6.0	2.4	4.2	0.6
Apple Pomace Dried	89	65	2.9	2.4	1.5	0.8	1.5	5.0	1.5	3.5	0.8
Artichoke Tops (Jerusalem)	27	61	2.7	2.2	1.4	0.7	1.3	6.0	2.4	4.2	—
Avocado Seed Meal	91	52	2.3	1.9	1.1	0.4	1.1	20.0	15.0	14.0	—
Bahiagrass Hay	90	51	2.2	1.8	1.1	0.3	1.1	8.0	4.2	5.6	3.0
Bakery Product Dried	90	90	4.0	3.3	2.2	1.5	2.1	12.0	7.8	8.4	3.6
Barley Hay	90	57	2.5	2.1	1.3	0.6	1.3	9.0	5.1	6.3	—
Barley Silage	35	59	2.6	2.1	1.3	0.6	1.3	12.0	7.8	8.4	2.6
Barley Silage Mature	35	58	2.6	2.1	1.3	0.6	1.3	12.0	7.8	8.4	3.0
Barley Straw	90	43	1.9	1.6	1.0	0.0	0.9	4.0	0.6	2.8	2.8
Barley Grain	89	84	3.7	3.0	2.0	1.3	1.9	12.0	7.8	8.4	3.4
Barley Grain Steam Flaked	85	90	4.0	3.3	2.2	1.5	2.2	12.0	7.8	8.4	4.7
Barley Grain Steam Rolled	86	84	3.7	3.0	2.0	1.3	1.9	12.0	7.8	8.4	4.6
Barley Grain 2-row	87	84	3.7	3.0	2.0	1.3	1.9	12.0	7.8	8.4	—
Barley Grain 6-row	87	84	3.7	3.0	2.0	1.3	1.9	11.0	6.9	7.7	—
Barley Grain Lt.Wt. (42–44 lb/bu)	88	78	3.4	2.8	1.8	1.2	1.8	13.0	8.7	9.1	3.9
Barley Feed Pearl Byproduct	90	73	3.2	2.6	1.7	1.1	1.7	15.0	10.5	10.5	—
Barley Grain Screenings	89	77	3.4	2.8	1.8	1.2	1.7	12.0	7.8	8.4	—
Beans Navy Cull	90	84	3.7	3.0	2.0	1.3	1.9	24.0	18.6	16.8	6.0
Beet Pulp Wet	17	76	3.4	2.7	1.8	1.1	1.7	11.0	6.9	7.7	3.9
Beet Pulp Dried	91	75	3.3	2.7	1.7	1.1	1.7	11.0	6.9	7.7	4.8
Beet Pulp Wet with Molasses	24	77	3.4	2.8	1.8	1.2	1.7	11.0	6.9	7.7	2.8
Beet Pulp Dried with Molasses	92	76	3.4	2.7	1.8	1.1	1.7	11.0	6.9	7.7	3.7
Beet Tops (Sugar)	20	58	2.6	2.1	1.3	0.6	1.3	14.0	9.6	9.8	—
Beet Top Silage	25	52	2.3	1.9	1.1	0.4	1.1	12.0	7.8	8.4	—
Bermudagrass Coastal Dehydrated	90	62	2.7	2.2	1.4	0.7	1.4	16.0	11.4	11.2	6.4
Bermudagrass Coastal Hay	89	56	2.5	2.0	1.2	0.5	1.2	10.0	6.0	7.0	2.0
Bermudagrass Hay	89	53	2.3	1.9	1.2	0.4	1.2	10.0	6.0	7.0	1.8
Bermudagrass Silage	26	50	2.2	1.8	1.1	0.3	1.1	10.0	6.0	7.0	1.5
Birdsfoot Trefoil Fresh	22	66	2.9	2.4	1.5	0.8	1.5	21.0	15.9	14.7	4.2
Birdsfoot Trefoil Hay	89	57	2.5	2.1	1.3	0.6	1.3	16.0	11.4	11.2	3.5
Biuret	99	0	0.0	0.0	0.0	0.0	0.0	248.0	220.2	173.6	0.0
Blood Meal, Swine/Poultry	91	66	2.9	2.4	1.5	0.8	1.5	92.0	79.8	64.4	73.6
Bluegrass KY Fresh Early Bloom	36	69	3.0	2.5	1.6	0.9	1.5	15.0	10.5	10.5	3.0
Bluegrass Straw	93	45	2.0	1.6	1.0	0.1	1.0	6.0	2.4	4.2	—
Bluestem Fresh Mature	61	50	2.2	1.8	1.1	0.3	1.1	6.0	2.4	4.2	—
Bone Meal Steamed, Swine/Poultry	95	16	0.7	0.6	0.6	0.0	0.2	13.0	8.7	9.1	—
Bread Byproduct	68	91	4.0	3.3	2.2	1.5	2.1	14.0	9.6	9.8	3.4
Brewers Grains Wet	23	85	3.7	3.1	2.1	1.4	1.9	27.0	21.3	18.9	14.0
Brewers Grains Dried	92	84	3.7	3.0	2.0	1.3	1.9	25.0	19.5	17.5	13.5
Brewers Yeast Dried	94	79	3.5	2.9	1.9	1.2	1.8	48.0	40.2	33.6	—
Bromegrass Fresh Immature	30	64	2.8	2.3	1.4	0.8	1.4	15.0	10.5	10.5	3.3
Bromegrass Hay	89	55	2.4	2.0	1.2	0.5	1.2	10.0	6.0	7.0	3.3
Bromegrass Haylage	35	57	2.5	2.1	1.3	0.6	1.3	11.0	6.9	7.7	2.9
Buckwheat Grain	88	77	3.4	2.8	1.8	1.2	1.7	12.0	7.8	8.4	—
Buttermilk Dried	92	88	3.9	3.2	2.2	1.4	2.0	34.0	27.6	23.8	0.0

Fiber[f]						Mineral Elements						Vitamins[h,i]	
CF	ADF	NDF	eNDF	EE[g]	ASH	Ca	P	K	Cl	S	Zn	A	E
%				%	%	%	%	%	%	%	ppm	RE/kg	ppm
29.0	36.0	46.0	40.0	2.0	11.0	1.30	0.23	1.9	0.37	0.33	20.0	–	—
26.0	34.0	45.0	6.0	3.0	11.0	1.42	0.25	2.5	0.45	0.28	21.0	26,200	121.0
27.0	35.0	46.0	41.0	3.0	9.0	1.35	0.27	2.6	0.40	0.29	18.0	37,000	—
28.0	35.0	45.0	92.0	2.5	8.0	1.41	0.26	2.5	0.38	0.28	22.0	28,000	26.0
30.0	36.0	47.0	92.0	2.3	9.0	1.40	0.24	2.0	0.38	0.27	24.0	—	—
34.0	40.0	52.0	92.0	2.0	8.0	1.20	0.23	1.7	0.37	0.25	23.0	13,000	—
38.0	45.0	59.0	92.0	1.3	8.0	1.18	0.19	1.5	0.35	0.21	23.0	2,400	—
13.0	15.0	—	—	10.5	6.0	0.30	0.67	—	—	—	—	—	—
28.0	37.0	49.0	82.0	3.0	9.0	1.40	0.29	2.6	0.41	0.29	26.0	19,800	—
28.0	37.0	49.0	82.0	3.0	9.0	1.40	0.29	2.6	0.41	0.29	26.0	12,000	—
15.0	25.0	34.0	35.0	2.7	15.0	2.88	0.34	2.2	—	0.32	39.0	17,600	—
44.0	51.0	68.0	100.0	1.3	6.0	0.90	0.18	2.5	—	—	—	—	—
16.0	27.0	35.0	100.0	3.3	7.0	0.25	0.10	2.0	0.03	0.07	20.0	—	—
0.0	0.0	0.0	0.0	0.0	0.0	0.00	0.00	0.0	66.00	0.00	0.0	—	—
0.0	0.0	0.0	0.0	0.0	0.0	—	—	—	—	24.15	—	—	—
17.0	34.0	40.0	34.0	5.6	4.0	0.14	0.14	0.6	—	0.06	11.0	—	—
19.0	35.0	45.0	34.0	5.2	4.0	0.13	0.12	0.5	—	0.02	—	—	—
18.0	30.0	41.0	40.0	1.1	10.0	1.62	0.11	1.4	—	—	—	—	—
19.0	24.0	—	—	1.2	16.0	—	—	—	—	—	—	—	—
32.0	41.0	72.0	98.0	1.9	8.0	0.48	0.20	1.4	—	0.21	—	36,600	—
4.0	6.0	14.0	0.0	11.0	4.0	0.18	0.28	0.3	2.25	0.15	33.0	3,100	45.0
28.0	37.0	65.0	98.0	2.1	8.0	0.30	0.28	1.6	—	0.19	25.0	10,600	—
34.0	37.0	58.0	61.0	3.0	9.0	0.46	0.30	2.4	—	0.22	28.0	—	—
30.0	34.0	50.0	61.0	3.5	9.0	0.30	0.20	1.5	—	0.15	25.0	—	—
42.0	52.0	78.0	100.0	1.9	7.0	0.33	0.08	2.1	0.67	0.16	7.0	400.0	—
5.0	7.0	20.0	34.0	2.1	3.0	0.06	0.38	0.6	0.18	0.16	23.0	263.2	25.0
5.0	7.0	20.0	30.0	2.1	3.0	0.06	0.35	0.6	0.18	0.16	23.00	—	—
5.0	7.0	20.0	27.0	2.1	3.0	0.06	0.41	0.6	0.18	0.17	30.0	—	—
6.0	8.0	24.0	34.0	2.3	2.0	0.05	0.31	0.6	0.18	0.17	—	—	—
6.0	8.0	24.0	34.0	2.2	3.0	0.05	0.36	0.6	0.18	0.15	—	—	—
9.0	12.0	30.0	34.0	2.3	4.0	—	—	—	—	—	—	—	—
12.0	15.0	—	—	3.9	5.0	0.05	0.45	0.7	—	0.06	—	—	—
9.0	11.0	—	—	2.6	4.0	0.30	0.33	0.7	—	0.15	—	—	—
5.0	8.0	20.0	0.0	1.4	5.0	0.15	0.59	1.4	0.06	0.26	45.0	—	—
20.0	23.0	48.0	33.0	0.7	6.0	0.68	0.08	1.4	0.40	0.21	20.0	—	—
21.0	21.0	41.0	33.0	0.7	6.0	0.65	0.08	1.4	0.40	0.22	22.0	—	—
16.0	21.0	39.0	33.0	0.6	6.0	0.60	0.10	1.8	—	0.42	11.0	—	—
17.0	22.0	40.0	33.0	0.6	6.0	0.60	0.10	1.8	—	0.42	11.0	—	—
10.0	14.0	25.0	41.0	1.5	24.0	1.20	0.23	5.1	0.20	0.45	20.0	—	—
12.0	—	—	—	2.0	32.0	1.38	0.22	5.7	—	0.57	20.0	—	—
26.0	29.0	40.0	10.0	3.8	7.0	0.40	0.25	1.8	—	0.23	18	—	—
30.0	36.0	73.0	98.0	2.1	6.0	0.47	0.21	1.5	—	0.22	16.0	21,000	—
30.0	39.0	78.0	98.0	1.9	8.0	0.46	0.20	1.5	—	0.25	33.0	11,600	—
30.0	37.0	77.0	48.0	1.9	8.0	0.46	0.20	1.5	—	0.25	33.0	—	—
21.0	31.0	47.0	41.0	4.4	9.0	1.78	0.25	2.6	—	0.25	31.0	—	—
31.0	38.0	50.0	92.0	2.2	8.0	1.73	0.24	1.8	—	0.25	28.0	—	—
0.0	0.0	0.0	0.0	0.0	0.0	0.00	0.00	0.0	0.00	0.00	0.0	—	—
1.0	2.0	10.0	0.0	1.4	3.0	0.32	0.28	0.2	0.30	0.70	22.0	—	—
27.0	32.0	60.0	41.0	3.9	7.0	0.37	0.30	1.9	0.42	0.19	25.0	43,800	—
40.0	50.0	78.0	90.0	1.1	6.0	0.20	0.10	—	—	—	—	—	—
34.0	—	—	—	2.5	5.0	0.40	0.12	0.8	—	0.05	28.0	—	—
1.0	0.0	0.0	0.0	11.6	77.0	27.00	12.74	0.2	—	2.50	290.0	—	—
1.0	2.0	3.0	0.0	3.2	3.0	0.09	0.18	0.2	0.76	0.15	40.0	—	—
13.0	21.0	45.0	18.0	7.6	4.0	0.29	0.61	0.1	0.15	0.32	78.0	—	—
14.0	24.0	49.0	18.0	8.2	4.0	0.29	0.60	0.1	0.15	0.32	78.0	—	29.0
3.0	—	—	—	1.0	7.0	0.10	1.56	1.8	—	0.41	41.0	—	—
28.0	33.0	54.0	40.0	4.1	10.0	0.45	0.34	2.3	—	0.21	20.0	38,400	—
35.0	41.0	66.0	98.0	2.3	9.0	0.40	0.23	1.9	0.40	0.19	19.0	6,800	—
36.0	44.0	69.0	61.0	2.5	8.0	0.38	0.30	2.0	—	0.20	19.0	—	—
12.0	17.0	—	—	2.8	2.0	0.11	0.36	0.5	0.05	0.16	10.0	—	—
5.0	0.0	0.0	0.0	5.0	10.0	1.44	1.00	0.9	—	0.09	44.0	—	7.0

TABLE 15-11 Continued

Feedstuff	DM	TDN	DE	ME	NE_m	NE_g	NE_l	CP	DP	MP	UIP
			Energy[d]					Protein[e]			
	%	%	Mcal/kg					%			
Cactus	26	63	2.8	2.3	1.4	0.7	1.4	5.0	1.5	3.5	—
Calcium Carbonate	99	0	0.0	0.0	0.0	0.0	0.0	0.0	–3.0	0.0	—
Canarygrass Hay	91	53	2.3	1.9	1.2	0.4	1.2	9.0	5.1	6.3	2.3
Canola Meal Solvent	90	71	3.1	2.6	1.6	1.0	1.6	40.0	33.0	28.0	12.0
Carrot Pulp	14	62	2.7	2.2	1.4	0.7	1.4	6.0	2.4	4.2	—
Carrot Root Fresh	12	83	3.7	3.0	2.0	1.3	1.9	10.0	6.0	7.0	—
Carrot Tops	16	73	3.2	2.6	1.7	1.1	1.7	13.0	8.7	9.1	—
Cattle Manure Dried	92	38	1.7	1.4	0.9	0.0	0.8	17.0	12.3	11.9	—
Cheatgrass Fresh Immature	21	68	3.0	2.5	1.5	0.9	1.5	16.0	11.4	11.2	—
Citrus Pulp Dried	90	79	3.5	2.9	1.9	1.2	1.8	7.0	3.3	4.9	2.7
Clover Ladino Fresh	19	69	3.0	2.5	1.6	0.9	1.5	25.0	19.5	17.5	5.0
Clover Ladino Hay	90	61	2.7	2.2	1.4	0.7	1.3	21.0	15.9	14.7	5.3
Clover Red Fresh	24	64	2.8	2.3	1.4	0.8	1.4	18.0	13.2	12.6	3.8
Clover Red Hay	88	55	2.4	2.0	1.2	0.5	1.2	15.0	10.5	10.5	4.2
Clover Sweet Hay	91	53	2.3	1.9	1.2	0.4	1.2	16.0	11.4	11.2	4.8
Coconut Meal	92	71	3.1	2.6	1.6	1.0	1.6	21.0	15.9	14.7	11.8
Coffee Grounds	88	20	0.9	0.7	0.8	0.0	0.4	13.0	8.7	9.1	—
Corn Whole Plant Pelleted	91	63	2.8	2.3	1.4	0.7	1.4	9.0	5.1	6.3	4.1
Corn Fodder	80	67	3.0	2.4	1.5	0.9	1.5	9.0	5.1	6.3	4.1
Corn Stover Mature (Stalks)	80	59	2.6	2.1	1.3	0.6	1.3	5.0	1.5	3.5	1.5
Corn Silage Milk Stage	26	65	2.9	2.4	1.5	0.8	1.5	8.0	4.2	5.6	1.4
Corn Silage Mature Well Eared	34	72	3.2	2.6	1.7	1.0	1.6	8.0	4.2	5.6	2.2
Corn Silage Sweet Corn	24	65	2.9	2.4	1.5	0.8	1.5	11.0	6.9	7.7	—
Corn Grain Whole	88	88	3.9	3.2	2.2	1.4	2.0	9.0	5.1	6.3	5.2
Corn Grain Rolled	88	88	3.9	3.2	2.2	1.4	2.0	9.0	5.1	6.3	4.9
Corn Grain Steam Flaked	85	93	4.1	3.4	2.3	1.6	2.1	9.0	5.1	6.3	5.3
Corn Grain High Moisture	74	93	4.1	3.4	2.3	1.6	2.1	10.0	6.0	7.0	4.2
Corn Grain High Oil	88	91	4.0	3.3	2.2	1.5	2.1	8.0	4.2	5.6	4.3
Corn Grain Hi-Lysine	92	87	3.8	3.1	2.1	1.4	2.0	12.0	7.8	8.4	7.0
Corn and Cob Meal	87	82	3.6	3.0	2.0	1.3	1.9	9.0	5.1	6.3	4.7
Corn Cobs	90	48	2.1	1.7	1.1	0.2	1.0	3.0	–0.3	2.1	1.5
Corn Screenings	86	91	4.0	3.3	2.2	1.5	2.1	10.0	6.0	7.0	5.2
Corn Bran	91	76	3.4	2.7	1.8	1.1	1.7	11.0	6.9	7.7	—
Corn Gluten Feed	90	80	3.5	2.9	1.9	1.2	1.8	22.0	16.8	15.4	5.5
Corn Gluten Meal 41% CP	91	85	3.7	3.1	2.1	1.4	1.9	46.0	38.4	32.2	26.7
Corn Gluten Meal 60% CP	91	89	3.9	3.2	2.2	1.5	2.1	67.0	57.3	46.9	40.2
Corn Cannery Waste	29	68	3.0	2.5	1.5	0.9	1.5	8.0	4.2	5.6	1.2
Cottonseed Whole	91	95	4.2	3.4	2.4	1.6	2.2	23.0	17.7	16.1	8.7
Cottonseed, Whole, Extruded	92	87	3.8	3.1	2.2	1.5	2.0	26.0	20.4	18.2	13.0
Cottonseed, Whole, Delinted	90	95	4.2	3.4	2.4	1.6	2.2	24.0	18.6	16.8	9.4
Cotton Gin Trash (Burrs)	91	42	1.9	1.5	0.9	0.0	0.9	10.0	6.0	7.0	—
Cottonseed Hulls	90	45	2.0	1.6	1.0	0.1	1.0	5.0	1.5	3.5	2.3
Cottonseed Meal Mech. 41% CP	92	80	3.5	2.9	1.9	1.2	1.8	46.0	38.4	32.2	23.0
Cottonseed Meal Solvent 41% CP	90	77	3.4	2.8	1.8	1.2	1.7	48.0	40.2	33.6	20.2
Crab Waste Meal	91	29	1.3	1.0	0.8	0.0	0.7	32.0	25.8	22.4	20.8
Crambe Meal Solvent	91	81	3.6	2.9	1.9	1.3	1.9	31.0	24.9	21.7	14.0
Crambe Meal Mech.	92	88	3.9	3.2	2.2	1.4	2.0	28.0	22.2	19.6	14.0
Cranberry Pulp Meal	88	49	2.2	1.8	1.1	0.2	1.1	7.0	3.3	4.9	—
Crawfish Waste Meal	94	25	1.1	0.9	0.8	0.0	0.6	35.0	28.5	24.5	25.9
Curacao Phosphate	99	0	0.0	0.0	0.0	0.0	0.0	0.0	–3.0	0.0	—
Defluorinated Phosphate	99	0	0.0	0.0	0.0	0.0	0.0	0.0	–3.0	0.0	—
Diammonium Phosphate	98	0	0.0	0.0	0.0	0.0	0.0	115.0	100.5	80.5	0.0
Dicalcium Phosphate	96	0	0.0	0.0	0.0	0.0	0.0	0.0	–3.0	0.0	—
Distillers Grains Wet	25	90	4.0	3.3	2.2	1.5	2.1	28.0	22.2	19.6	14.6
Distillers Grain Barley	90	77	3.4	2.8	1.8	1.2	1.7	30.0	24.0	21.0	16.8
Distillers Grain, Corn, Dry	91	92	4.1	3.3	2.3	1.5	2.1	29.0	23.1	20.3	17.4
Distillers Grain, Corn, Wet	36	98	4.3	3.5	2.4	1.6	2.2	29.0	23.1	20.3	16.0
Distillers Grain Corn with Solubles	90	92	4.1	3.3	2.3	1.5	2.1	29.0	23.1	20.3	14.5
Distillers Corn Stillage	7	92	4.1	3.3	2.3	1.5	2.1	22.0	16.8	15.4	12.1
Distillers Grain, Sorghum, Dry	91	85	3.7	3.1	2.1	1.4	1.9	32.0	25.8	22.4	19.8

Fiber[f]						Mineral Elements						Vitamins[h,i]	
CF	ADF	NDF	eNDF	EE[g]	ASH	Ca	P	K	Cl	S	Zn	A	E
	%			%	%	%	%	%	%	%	ppm	RE/kg	ppm
18.0	23.0	29.0	—	2.1	17.0	3.50	0.10	1.7	—	0.20	—	—	—
0.0	0.0	0.0	0.0	0.0	99.0	38.50	0.04	0.1	—	0.00	0.0	—	—
32.0	34.0	67.0	98.0	2.7	8.0	0.38	0.25	2.7	—	0.14	18.0	5,200	—
12.0	20.0	29.0	23.0	4.0	8.0	0.75	1.16	1.3	0.07	0.78	68.0	—	—
19.0	23.0	40.0	0.0	7.8	9.0	—	—	—	—	—	—	—	—
9.0	11.0	20.0	0.0	1.4	10.0	0.60	0.30	2.4	0.50	0.17	—	135,600	60.0
18.0	23.0	45.0	41.0	3.8	15.0	1.94	0.19	1.9	—	—	—	—	—
34.0	37.0	55.0	0.0	2.6	14.0	1.35	1.00	0.6	—	1.78	240.0	—	—
23.0	—	—	—	2.7	10.0	0.60	0.28	—	—	—	—	—	—
13.0	18.0	21.0	33.0	2.2	7.0	1.81	0.12	0.8	0.04	0.08	14.0	0.0	—
14.0	33.0	35.0	41.0	4.8	11.0	1.27	0.38	2.4	—	0.20	20.0	70,600	—
22.0	32.0	36.0	92.0	2.0	9.0	1.35	0.32	2.4	0.30	0.20	17.0	16,600	—
24.0	33.0	44.0	41.0	4.0	9.0	1.70	0.30	2.0	0.60	0.17	23.0	40,400	—
30.0	39.0	51.0	92.0	2.5	8.0	1.50	0.25	1.7	0.32	0.17	17.0	4,000	—
30.0	38.0	50.0	92.0	2.4	9.0	1.27	0.25	1.8	0.37	0.46	—	19,800	—
12.0	22.0	56.0	23.0	6.7	7.0	0.63	0.21	0.6	0.33	0.04	—	—	—
41.0	68.0	77.0	10.0	15.0	2.0	0.10	0.08	—	—	—	—	—	—
21.0	24.0	40.0	6.0	2.4	6.0	0.50	0.24	0.9	—	0.14	—	—	—
25.0	29.0	48.0	100.0	2.4	7.0	0.50	0.25	0.9	0.20	0.14	—	526.4	—
35.0	44.0	70.0	100.0	1.3	7.0	0.35	0.19	1.1	0.30	0.14	22.0	—	—
26.0	32.0	54.0	60.0	2.8	6.0	0.40	0.27	1.6	—	0.11	20.0	—	—
21.0	27.0	46.0	70.0	3.1	5.0	0.28	0.23	1.1	0.20	0.12	22.0	5,922	—
20.0	32.0	57.0	60.0	5.0	5.0	0.24	0.26	1.2	0.17	0.16	39.0	1,711	—
2.0	3.0	9.0	60.0	4.3	2.0	0.02	0.30	0.4	0.05	0.12	18.0	394.8	25.0
2.0	3.0	9.0	34.0	4.3	2.0	0.02	0.30	0.4	0.05	0.12	18.0	—	—
2.0	3.0	9.0	40.0	4.1	2.0	0.02	0.27	0.4	0.05	0.12	18.0	—	—
2.0	3.0	9.0	0.0	4.0	2.0	0.02	0.30	0.4	0.06	0.13	20.0	—	—
2.0	3.0	8.0	60.0	6.9	2.0	0.01	0.30	0.3	0.05	0.13	18.0	—	—
4.0	4.0	11.0	60.0	4.4	2.0	0.03	0.24	0.4	0.05	0.11	18.0	658.0	—
9.0	10.0	26.0	56.0	3.7	2.0	0.06	0.28	0.5	0.05	0.13	16.0	526.4	20.0
36.0	39.0	88.0	56.0	0.5	2.0	0.12	0.04	0.8	—	0.40	5.0	131.6	—
3.0	4.0	9.0	20.0	4.3	2.0	0.04	0.27	0.4	0.05	0.12	16.0	—	—
10.0	17.0	51.0	0.0	6.3	3.0	0.04	0.15	0.1	0.13	0.08	18.0	—	—
9.0	12.0	38.0	36.0	3.2	7.0	0.12	0.85	1.3	0.25	0.33	84.0	921.2	14.0
5.0	9.0	32.0	23.0	3.2	3.0	0.13	0.55	0.2	0.07	0.55	35.0	2,369	34.0
4.0	6.0	11.0	23.0	2.6	3.0	0.06	0.54	0.2	0.10	0.82	40.0	4,474	26.0
28.0	36.0	59.0	0.0	3.0	5.0	0.10	0.29	1.0	—	0.13	25.0	—	—
29.0	39.0	47.0	100.0	17.8	4.0	0.14	0.64	1.1	0.06	0.24	34.0	—	—
32.0	44.0	53.0	33.0	9.5	5.0	0.17	0.68	1.3	—	0.24	38.0	—	—
20.0	29.0	40.0	100.0	22.2	4.0	0.13	0.55	1.2	—	0.24	36.0	—	—
34.0	51.0	70.0	100.0	2.0	14.0	1.70	0.25	1.9	—	0.14	25.0	—	—
48.0	68.0	87.0	100.0	1.9	3.0	0.15	0.08	1.1	0.02	0.05	10.0	—	—
13.0	18.0	31.0	23.0	5.0	7.0	0.21	1.19	1.7	0.05	0.42	64.0	0.0	—
13.0	17.0	25.0	23.0	1.8	7.0	0.22	1.25	1.7	0.05	0.44	66.0	—	—
11.0	13.0	—	—	3.0	43.0	15.00	1.88	0.5	1.63	0.27	107.0	—	—
25.0	35.0	47.0	23.0	1.4	8.0	1.27	0.86	1.1	0.70	1.26	44.0	—	—
24.0	33.0	42.0	25.0	17.0	7.0	1.22	0.78	1.0	0.65	1.18	41.0	—	—
26.0	47.0	54.0	33.0	15.7	2.0	—	—	—	—	—	—	—	—
—	15.0	—	—		42.0	13.10	0.85	—	—	—	—	—	—
0.0	0.0	0.0	0.0	0.0	95.0	34.00	15.00	—	—	—	—	—	—
0.0	0.0	0.0	0.0	0.0	95.0	32.60	18.07	1.0	—	—	100.0	—	—
0.0	0.0	0.0	0.0	0.0	35.0	0.52	20.41	0.0	—	2.16	—	—	—
0.0	0.0	0.0	0.0	0.0	94.0	22.00	18.65	0.1	—	1.00	70.0	—	—
8.0	18.0	40.0	4.0	9.6	6.0	0.28	0.78	1.2	0.28	0.40	95.0	—	—
18.0	22.0	45.0	4.0	3.7	4.0	0.15	0.67	1.0	0.18	0.43	50.0	—	—
8.0	21.0	42.0	4.0	10.5	4.0	0.15	0.78	0.9	0.14	0.45	65.0	394.8	—
8.0	21.0	41.0	4.0	10.5	4.0	0.15	0.78	0.9	0.14	0.45	65.0	—	—
9.0	17.0	43.0	4.0	10.6	6.0	0.28	0.79	1.0	0.18	0.39	80.0	394.8	43.0
8.0	10.0	21.0	0.0	8.1	5.0	0.14	0.72	0.2	—	0.60	60.0	—	—
13.0	22.0	44.0	4.0	10.0	3.0	0.22	0.63	0.3	—	0.45	50.0	—	—

TABLE 15-11 Continued

Feedstuff	DM	TDN	DE	ME	NE_m	NE_g	NE_l	CP	DP	MP	UIP
			Energy[d]					Protein[e]			
	%	%	Mcal/kg					%			
Distillers Grain, Sorghum, Wet	35	89	3.9	3.2	2.2	1.5	2.1	32.0	25.8	22.4	17.6
Distillers Grain Sorghum with Solubles	92	85	3.7	3.1	2.1	1.4	1.9	31.0	24.9	21.7	16.4
Distillers Dried Solubles	93	88	3.9	3.2	2.2	1.4	2.0	29.0	23.1	20.3	0.0
Elephant (Napier) Grass Hay/Chopped	92	55	2.4	2.0	1.2	0.5	1.2	9.0	5.1	6.3	—
Fat, Animal, Poultry, Vegetable	99	195	8.6	7.1	6.3	5.1	6.3	0.0	–3.0	0.0	—
Feather Meal Hydrolyzed	92	69	3.0	2.5	1.6	0.9	1.5	86.0	74.4	60.2	62.8
Fescue KY 31 Fresh	29	64	2.8	2.3	1.4	0.8	1.4	15.0	10.5	10.5	3.0
Fescue KY 31 Hay Early Bloom	88	65	2.9	2.4	1.5	0.8	1.5	18.0	13.2	12.6	4.0
Fescue KY 31 Hay Mature	88	52	2.3	1.9	1.1	0.4	1.1	11.0	6.9	7.7	3.3
Fescue (Red) Straw	94	43	1.9	1.6	1.0	0.0	0.9	4.0	0.6	2.8	—
Fish Meal	90	74	3.3	2.7	1.7	1.1	1.7	66.0	56.4	46.2	39.6
Garbage Municipal Cooked	23	80	3.5	2.9	1.9	1.2	1.8	16.0	11.4	11.2	—
Grain Screenings	90	65	2.9	2.4	1.5	0.8	1.5	14.0	9.6	9.8	—
Grain Dust	92	73	3.2	2.6	1.7	1.1	1.7	10.0	6.0	7.0	—
Grape Pomace Stemless	91	30	1.3	1.1	0.8	0.0	0.6	12.0	7.8	8.4	5.4
Grass Hay	88	58	2.6	2.1	1.3	0.6	1.3	10.0	6.0	7.0	3.0
Grass Silage	30	61	2.7	2.2	1.4	0.7	1.3	11.0	6.9	7.7	2.6
Guar Meal	90	72	3.2	2.6	1.7	1.0	1.6	39.0	32.1	27.3	13.3
Hominy Feed	90	89	3.9	3.2	2.2	1.5	2.1	11.0	6.9	7.7	5.3
Hop Leaves	37	49	2.2	1.8	1.1	0.2	1.1	15.0	10.5	10.5	—
Hop Vine Silage	30	53	2.3	1.9	1.2	0.4	1.2	15.0	10.5	10.5	—
Hops Spent	89	37	1.6	1.3	0.9	0.0	0.8	23.0	17.7	16.1	—
Kelp Dried	91	32	1.4	1.2	0.8	0.0	0.6	7.0	3.3	4.9	—
Kenaf Hay	92	48	2.1	1.7	1.1	0.2	1.0	10.0	6.0	7.0	—
Kochia Fresh	29	55	2.4	2.0	1.2	0.5	1.2	16.0	11.4	11.2	—
Kochia Hay	90	53	2.3	1.9	1.2	0.4	1.2	14.0	9.6	9.8	—
Kudzu Hay	90	54	2.4	2.0	1.2	0.4	1.2	16.0	11.4	11.2	—
Lespedeza Fresh Early Bloom	25	60	2.6	2.2	1.3	0.7	1.3	16.0	11.4	11.2	8.0
Lespedeza Hay	92	54	2.4	2.0	1.2	0.4	1.2	14.0	9.6	9.8	8.4
Limestone Ground	98	0	0.0	0.0	0.0	0.0	0.0	0.0	–3.0	0.0	0.0
Limestone Dolomitic Ground	99	0	0.0	0.0	0.0	0.0	0.0	0.0	–3.0	0.0	0.0
Linseed Meal Solvent	91	76	3.4	2.7	1.8	1.1	1.7	39.0	32.1	27.3	14.0
Meadow Hay	90	50	2.2	1.8	1.1	0.3	1.1	7.0	3.3	4.9	1.6
Meat Meal, Swine/Poultry	93	71	3.1	2.6	1.6	1.0	1.6	56.0	47.4	39.2	35.8
Meat and Bone Meal, Swine/Poultry	93	72	3.2	2.6	1.7	1.0	1.6	56.0	47.4	39.2	13.4
Milk, Dry, Skim	94	87	3.8	3.1	2.1	1.4	2.0	36.0	29.4	25.2	0.0
Mint Slug Silage	27	55	2.4	2.0	1.2	0.5	1.2	14.0	9.6	9.8	—
Molasses Beet	77	75	3.3	2.7	1.7	1.1	1.7	9.0	5.1	6.3	0.0
Molasses Cane	76	75	3.3	2.7	1.7	1.1	1.7	6.0	2.4	4.2	0.0
Molasses Cane Dried	94	74	3.3	2.7	1.7	1.1	1.7	9.0	5.1	6.3	0.0
Molasses Cond. Fermentation Solubles	46	0	0.0	0.0	0.0	0.0	0.0	80.0	69.0	56.0	—
Molasses Citrus	65	77	3.4	2.8	1.8	1.2	1.7	10.0	6.0	7.0	0.0
Molasses Wood Hemicellulose	61	76	3.4	2.7	1.8	1.1	1.7	1.0	–2.1	0.7	0.0
Monoammonium Phosphate	98	0	0.0	0.0	0.0	0.0	0.0	70.0	60.0	49.0	0.0
Mono-Dicalcium Phosphate	97	0	0.0	0.0	0.0	0.0	0.0	0.0	–3.0	0.0	—
Oat Hay	90	54	2.4	2.0	1.2	0.4	1.2	10.0	6.0	7.0	2.5
Oat Silage	35	60	2.6	2.2	1.3	0.7	1.3	12.0	7.8	8.4	2.5
Oat Straw	91	48	2.1	1.7	1.1	0.2	1.0	4.0	0.6	2.8	1.6
Oat Grain	89	76	3.4	2.7	1.8	1.1	1.7	13.0	8.7	9.1	2.3
Oat Grain Steam Flaked	84	88	3.9	3.2	2.2	1.4	2.0	13.0	8.7	9.1	3.4
Oat Groats	91	91	4.0	3.3	2.2	1.5	2.1	18.0	13.2	12.6	2.7
Oat Middlings	90	90	4.0	3.3	2.2	1.5	2.1	17.0	12.3	11.9	3.4
Oat Mill Byproduct	89	33	1.5	1.2	0.8	0.0	0.7	8.0	4.2	5.6	—
Oat Hulls	93	40	1.8	1.4	0.9	0.0	0.8	4.0	0.6	2.8	1.0
Orange Pulp Dried	89	80	3.5	2.9	1.9	1.2	1.8	9.0	5.1	6.3	—

Fiber[f]						Mineral Elements						Vitamins[h,i]	
CF	ADF	NDF	eNDF	EE[g]	ASH	Ca	P	K	Cl	S	Zn	A	E
%				%	%	%	%	%	%	%	ppm	RE/kg	ppm
13.0	22.0	44.0	4.0	10.0	3.0	0.22	0.63	0.3	—	0.45	50.0	—	—
13.0	19.0	47.0	4.0	10.0	3.0	0.25	0.65	0.5	—	0.40	55.0	—	—
4.0	7.0	22.0	4.0	9.2	7.0	0.33	1.38	1.8	0.28	0.40	91.0	—	—
24.0	46.0	63.0	85.0	2.0	10.0	0.35	0.30	1.3	0.10	—	—	—	55.0
0.0	0.0	0.0	0.0	99.0	0.0	0.00	0.00	0.0	—	—	—	—	—
2.0	16.0	44.0	23.0	6.5	4.0	0.60	0.62	0.2	0.30	1.85	95.0	—	—
25.0	32.0	64.0	40.0	5.5	9.0	0.48	0.37	2.5	—	0.18	22.0	—	—
25.0	31.0	64.0	98.0	6.6	8.0	0.45	0.37	2.7	—	0.24	24.0	—	—
30.0	42.0	73.0	98.0	5.0	6.0	0.45	0.26	1.7	—	0.14	22.0	—	—
41.0	—	—	—	1.1	6.0	0.00	0.06	—	—	—	—	—	—
1.0	2.0	12.0	10.0	8.0	20.0	5.50	3.15	0.7	0.76	0.80	130.0	—	13.0
9.0	50.0	59.0	30.0	20.0	10.0	1.20	0.43	0.6	0.67	—	—	—	—
14.0	—	—	—	5.5	9.0	0.25	0.34	—	—	—	30.0	—	—
11.0	—	—	—	2.2	10.0	0.30	0.18	—	—	—	42.0	—	—
32.0	48.0	53.0	34.0	7.5	9.0	0.50	0.08	0.5	0.01	—	24.0	—	—
33.0	41.0	63.0	98.0	3.0	6.0	0.60	0.21	2.0	—	0.20	28.0	—	—
32.0	39.0	60.0	61.0	3.4	8.0	0.70	0.24	2.1	—	0.22	29.0	—	—
16.0			3.9	5.0	—	—	—	—	—	—	—	—	75.0
5.0	7.0	21.0	9.0	6.1	3.0	0.04	0.54	0.6	0.06	0.10	32.0	1,316	—
15.0	—	—	—	3.6	35.0	2.80	0.64	—	—	—	—	—	—
21.0	24.0	—	—	3.1	20.0	3.30	0.37	1.8	—	0.22	44.0	—	—
26.0	30.0	—	—	4.5	7.0	1.60	0.60	—	—	—	—	—	—
7.0	10.0	—	—	0.5	39.0	2.72	0.31	—	—	—	—	—	—
31.0	44.0	56.0	98.0	2.9	12.0	—	—	—	—	—	—	—	—
23.0	—	—	—	1.2	18.0	1.10	0.30	—	—	—	—	—	—
27.0	—	—	—	1.7	14.0	1.00	0.20	—	—	—	—	—	—
33.0	—	—	—	2.6	7.0	3.00	0.23	—	—	—	—	—	—
32.0	—	—	—	2.0	10.0	1.20	0.24	1.1	—	0.21	—	—	—
30.0	—	—	—	3.0	7.0	1.10	0.22	1.0	—	0.19	29.0	8,000	—
0.0	0.0	0.0	0.0	0.0	98.0	34.00	0.02	—	—	0.03	—	—	—
0.0	0.0	0.0	0.0	0.0	98.0	22.30	0.04	0.4	—	—	—	—	—
10.0	18.0	25.0	23.0	1.9	6.0	0.43	0.93	1.5	0.04	0.47	60.0	—	15.0
33.0	44.0	70.0	98.0	2.5	9.0	0.61	0.18	1.6	—	0.17	24	—	—
2.0	7.0	48.0	0.0	10.5	24.0	9.00	4.42	0.5	1.27	0.48	190.0	—	—
1.0	5.0	34.0	0.0	10.0	29.0	13.50	6.50	—	—	—	—	—	—
0.0	0.0	0.0	0.0	1.0	8.4	1.36	1.09	1.7	0.96	0.34	41	3,690	—
24.0	—	—	—	1.8	16.0	1.10	0.57	—	—	—	—	—	—
0.0	0.0	0.0	0.0	0.2	12.0	0.12	0.03	6.0	1.64	0.60	18.0	—	5.0
0.0	0.0	0.0	0.0	0.8	12.0	0.97	0.10	3.7	2.50	0.53	25.0	—	7.0
2.0	3.0	7.0	0.0	0.3	14.0	1.10	0.15	3.6	3.00	—	30.0	—	—
—	—	—	—		16.0		0.25	—	—	12.60	—	—	—
0.0	0.0	0.0	0.0	0.3	8.0	1.90	0.17	0.2	0.11	0.23	137.0	—	—
1.0	2.0	4.0	0.0	0.7	9.0	1.30	0.09	0.1	—	0.05	—	—	—
0.0	0.0	0.0	0.0	0.0	24.0	0.30	24.70	0.0	—	1.42	81.0	—	—
0.0	0.0	0.0	0.0	0.0	94.0	16.70	21.10	0.1	—	1.20	70.0	—	—
31.0	39.0	63.0	98.0	2.3	8.0	0.40	0.27	1.6	0.42	0.21	28.0	5,600	—
31.0	39.0	59.0	61.0	3.2	10.0	0.34	0.30	2.4	0.50	0.25	27.0	9,000	—
41.0	48.0	73.0	98.0	2.3	8.0	0.24	0.07	2.4	0.78	0.22	6.0	800	—
11.0	15.0	28.0	34.0	5.0	4.0	0.05	0.41	0.5	0.11	0.20	40.0	—	15.0
11.0	15.0	30.0	32.0	4.9	4.0	0.05	0.37	0.5	0.11	0.20	40.00	—	—
3.0	—	—	—	6.6	2.0	0.08	0.47	0.4	0.10	0.20	—	—	16.0
3.0	4.0	—	—	6.0	3.0	0.06	0.48	0.5	—	0.23	—	—	—
25.0	37.0	—	—	2.6	6.0	0.12	0.23	0.6	—	0.24	—	—	—
32.0	40.0	75.0	90.0	1.5	7.0	0.16	0.15	0.6	0.08	0.14	31.0	—	—
9.0	16.0	20.0	33.0	1.8	4.0	0.71	0.11	0.6	—	0.05	—	—	—

TABLE 15-11 Continued

Feedstuff	DM	TDN	DE	ME	NE_m	NE_g	NE_l	CP	DP	MP	UIP
		Energy[d]						Protein[e]			
	%	%	Mcal/kg					%			
Orchardgrass Fresh Early Bloom	24	65	2.9	2.4	1.5	0.8	1.5	14.0	9.6	9.8	3.2
Orchardgrass Hay	88	59	2.6	2.1	1.3	0.6	1.3	10.0	6.0	7.0	2.7
Pea Vine Hay	89	60	2.6	2.2	1.3	0.7	1.3	10.0	6.0	7.0	—
Pea Vine Silage	25	58	2.6	2.1	1.3	0.6	1.3	16.0	11.4	11.2	—
Pea Straw	89	50	2.2	1.8	1.1	0.3	1.1	7.0	3.3	4.9	—
Peas Cull	89	86	3.8	3.1	2.1	1.4	2.0	25.0	19.5	17.5	5.5
Peanut Hulls	91	22	1.0	0.8	0.8	0.0	0.4	7.0	3.3	4.9	—
Peanut Meal Solvent	91	77	3.4	2.8	1.8	1.2	1.7	50.0	42.0	35.0	13.5
Peanut Skins	92	0	0.0	0.0	0.0	0.0	0.0	17.0	12.3	11.9	—
Pearl Millet Grain	87	82	3.6	3.0	2.0	1.3	1.9	13.0	8.7	9.1	—
Pineapple Greenchop	17	45	2.0	1.6	1.0	0.1	1.0	8.0	4.2	5.6	—
Pineapple Bran	89	71	3.1	2.6	1.6	1.0	1.6	5.0	1.5	3.5	—
Pineapple Presscake	21	72	3.2	2.6	1.7	1.0	1.6	5.0	1.5	3.5	—
Potato Vine Silage	15	59	2.6	2.1	1.3	0.6	1.3	15.0	10.5	10.5	—
Potatoes Cull	21	80	3.5	2.9	1.9	1.2	1.8	10.0	6.0	7.0	0.0
Potato Waste Wet	14	82	3.6	3.0	2.0	1.3	1.9	7.0	3.3	4.9	0.0
Potato Waste Dried	89	85	3.7	3.1	2.1	1.4	1.9	8.0	4.2	5.6	0.0
Potato Waste Wet with Lime	17	80	3.5	2.9	1.9	1.2	1.8	5.0	1.5	3.5	0.0
Potato Waste Filter Cake	14	77	3.4	2.8	1.8	1.2	1.7	5.0	1.5	3.5	0.0
Poultry Byproduct Meal	93	79	3.5	2.9	1.9	1.2	1.8	62.0	52.8	43.4	30.4
Poultry Manure Dried	89	38	1.7	1.4	0.9	0.0	0.8	28.0	22.2	19.6	6.2
Prairie Hay	91	50	2.2	1.8	1.1	0.3	1.1	7.0	3.3	4.9	2.6
Pumpkins Cull	10	85	3.7	3.1	2.1	1.4	1.9	16.0	11.4	11.2	0.0
Rice Straw	91	40	1.8	1.4	0.9	0.0	0.8	4.0	0.6	2.8	—
Rice Straw Ammoniated	87	45	2.0	1.6	1.0	0.1	1.0	9.0	5.1	6.3	—
Rice Grain	89	79	3.5	2.9	1.9	1.2	1.8	8.0	4.2	5.6	2.4
Rice Polishings	90	90	4.0	3.3	2.2	1.5	2.1	14.0	9.6	9.8	—
Rice Bran	91	72	3.2	2.6	1.7	1.0	1.6	14.0	9.6	9.8	4.2
Rice Hulls	92	13	0.6	0.5	0.8	0.0	0.2	3.0	–0.3	2.1	1.4
Rice Mill Byproduct	91	42	1.9	1.5	0.9	0.0	0.9	7.0	3.3	4.9	—
Rye Grass Hay	90	58	2.6	2.1	1.3	0.6	1.3	10.0	6.0	7.0	3.0
Rye Grass Silage	32	59	2.6	2.1	1.3	0.6	1.3	14.0	9.6	9.8	3.5
Rye Straw	89	44	1.9	1.6	1.0	0.0	0.9	4.0	0.6	2.8	—
Rye Grain	89	82	3.6	3.0	2.0	1.3	1.9	12.0	7.8	8.4	2.4
Safflower Meal Solvent	91	55	2.4	2.0	1.2	0.5	1.2	24.0	18.6	16.8	—
Safflower Meal Dehulled Solvent	91	76	3.4	2.7	1.8	1.1	1.7	48.0	40.2	33.6	—
Sagebrush Fresh	50	50	2.2	1.8	1.1	0.3	1.1	13.0	8.7	9.1	—
Sanfoin Hay	88	61	2.7	2.2	1.4	0.7	1.4	14.0	9.6	9.8	8.4
Shrimp Waste Meal	90	48	2.1	1.7	1.1	0.2	1.0	50.0	42.0	35.0	30.0
Sodium Tripolyphosphate	96	0	0.0	0.0	0.0	0.0	0.0	0.0	–3.0	0.0	0.0
Sorghum Stover	87	55	2.4	2.0	1.2	0.5	1.2	5.0	1.5	3.5	—
Sorghum Silage	32	59	2.6	2.1	1.3	0.6	1.3	9.0	5.1	6.3	2.7
Sorghum Grain (Milo) Ground	89	82	3.6	3.0	2.0	1.3	1.9	11.0	6.9	7.7	6.1
Sorhum Grain (Milo) Flaked	82	90	4.0	3.3	2.2	1.5	2.1	11.0	6.9	7.7	6.8
Soybean Hay	89	52	2.3	1.9	1.1	0.4	1.1	15.0	10.5	10.5	—
Soybean Straw	88	42	1.9	1.5	0.9	0.0	0.9	5.0	1.5	3.5	—
Soybeans Whole	88	93	4.1	3.4	2.3	1.6	2.1	40.0	33.0	28.0	11.2
Soybeans Whole, Extruded	88	93	4.1	3.4	2.3	1.6	2.1	40.0	33.0	28.0	14.0
Soybeans Whole, Roasted	88	93	4.1	3.4	2.3	1.6	2.1	40.0	33.0	28.0	19.2
Soybean Hulls	90	77	3.4	2.8	1.8	1.1	1.7	13.0	8.7	9.1	3.6
Soybean Meal Solvent 44% CP	91	84	3.7	3.0	2.0	1.3	1.9	49.0	41.1	34.3	17.2
Soybean Meal Solvent 49% CP	91	87	3.8	3.1	2.1	1.4	2.0	54.0	45.6	37.8	19.4
Soybean Mill Feed	90	51	2.2	1.8	1.1	0.3	1.1	15.0	10.5	10.5	—
Spelt Grain	88	75	3.3	2.7	1.7	1.1	1.7	13.0	8.7	9.1	3.5
Sudangrass Fresh Immature	18	70	3.1	2.5	1.6	1.0	1.6	17.0	12.3	11.9	—
Sudangrass Hay	88	57	2.5	2.1	1.3	0.6	1.3	9.0	5.1	6.3	2.7
Sudangrass Silage	31	58	2.6	2.1	1.3	0.6	1.3	10.0	6.0	7.0	2.8

Fiber[f]						Mineral Elements						Vitamins[h,i]	
CF	ADF	NDF	eNDF	EE[g]	ASH	Ca	P	K	Cl	S	Zn	A	E
%				%	%	%	%	%	%	%	ppm	RE/kg	ppm
30.0	32.0	54.0	41.0	4.0	9.0	0.33	0.39	2.7	0.08	0.20	21.0	60,400	436.0
34.0	40.0	67.0	98.0	3.3	8.0	0.32	0.30	2.6	0.41	0.20	26.0	4,400	191.0
32.0	52.0	62.0	92.0	1.8	7.0	1.20	0.21	1.2	—	0.20	20.0	—	—
29.0	44.0	55.0	61.0	3.3	8.0	1.25	0.28	1.6	—	0.29	32.0	37,800	—
42.0	49.0	72.0	98.0	1.3	7.0	0.60	0.15	1.1	—	0.15	—	—	—
7.0	9.0	15.0	0.0	1.5	4.0	0.15	0.45	1.1	0.06	0.26	30.0	200.0	3.0
63.0	65.0	74.0	98.0	1.5	5.0	0.20	0.07	0.9	—	—	—	—	—
8.0	15.0	27.0	23.0	3.6	6.0	0.24	0.58	1.0	0.03	0.30	38.0	—	—
13.0	20.0	28.0	0.0	22.0	3.0	0.19	0.20	—	—	—	—	—	—
2.0	6.0	18.0	34.0	4.5	3.0	0.03	0.36	0.5	—	—	—	—	—
23.0	35.0	64.0	41.0	2.6	7.0	0.28	0.08	—	—	—	—	—	—
19.0	31.0	66.0	20.0	1.5	3.0	0.26	0.12	—	—	—	—	—	—
23.0	35.0	69.0	20.0	0.9	3.0	0.24	0.10	—	—	—	—	—	—
26.0	—	—	—	3.7	19.0	2.10	0.29	4.0	—	0.37	—	—	—
2.0	3.0	4.0	0.0	0.4	5.0	0.03	0.24	2.2	0.30	0.09	—	—	—
9.0	11.0	18.0	0.0	1.5	3.0	0.16	0.25	1.2	0.36	0.11	12.0	—	—
7.0	9.0	15.0	0.0	0.5	5.0	0.16	0.25	1.2	0.39	0.11	12.0	—	—
10.0	12.0	16.0	0.0	0.3	9.0	4.20	0.18	—	—	—	—	—	—
2.0	—	—	—	7.7	3.0	0.10	0.19	0.2	—	—	—	—	—
2.0	—	—	—	14.5	17.0	4.00	2.25	0.5	0.58	0.56	129.0	—	—
13.0	15.0	35.0	0.0	2.1	33.0	10.20	2.80	2.3	1.05	0.20	520.0	—	—
34.0	47.0	67.0	98.0	2.0	8.0	0.40	0.15	1.1	0.06	0.06	34.0	4,800	—
14.0	18.0	25.0	0.0	8.9	9.0	0.24	0.43	3.3	—	—	—	—	—
40.0	55.0	72.0	100.0	1.4	12.0	0.25	0.08	1.1	—	0.11	—	—	—
39.0	53.0	68.0	100.0	1.3	12.0	0.25	0.08	1.1	—	0.11	—	—	—
10.0	12.0	16.0	34.0	1.9	5.0	0.07	0.32	0.4	0.09	0.05	17.0	—	—
4.0	5.0	—	—	14.0	9.0	0.05	1.36	1.2	0.12	0.19	28.0	—	—
13.0	18.0	24.0	0.0	17.0	11.0	0.07	1.70	1.8	0.09	0.19	40.0	—	—
44.0	70.0	81.0	90.0	0.9	20.0	0.14	0.07	0.5	0.08	0.08	24.0	—	—
32.0	48.0	60.0	0.0	5.7		0.40	0.31	2.2	—	0.30	31.0	—	—
33.0	38.0	65.0	98.0	3.3	8.0	0.45	0.30	2.2	—	0.18	27.0	24,000	211.0
22.0	37.0	59.0	61.0	3.3	8.0	0.43	0.38	2.9	0.73	0.23	29.0	11,600	—
44.0	55.0	71.0	100.0	1.5	6.0	0.24	0.09	1.0	0.24	0.11	—	—	—
2.0	9.0	19.0	34.0	1.7	2.0	0.07	0.39	0.5	0.03	0.17	33.0	0.0	17.0
33.0	41.0	57.0	36.0	1.2	6.0	0.35	0.78	1.0	0.21	0.23	65.0	—	—
9.0	—	—	—	0.6	7.0	0.38	1.60	1.2	0.18	0.22	36.0	—	—
25.0	28.0	36.0	—	9.2	10.0	1.00	0.25	—	—	0.22	—	3,200	—
24.0	—	—	—	3.1	9.0	—	—	—	—	—	—	—	—
11.0	—	—	—	5.5	25.0	8.50	1.75	—	1.15	—	—	—	—
0.0	0.0	0.0	0.0	0.0	96.0	0.00	25.98	0.0	—	0.00	—	—	—
33.0	41.0	65.0	100.0	1.9	10.0	0.49	0.12	1.2	—	—	—	—	—
27.0	38.0	59.0	70.0	2.7	6.0	0.48	0.21	1.7	0.45	0.11	30.0	3,000	662.0
3.0	6.0	15.0	5.0	3.1	2.0	0.04	0.32	0.4	0.10	0.14	18.0	131.6	12.0
3.0	6.0	15.0	38.0	3.1	2.0	0.04	0.28	0.4	0.10	0.14	18.0	—	—
35.0	40.0	55.0	92.0	2.2	8.0	1.29	0.30	1.1	0.15	0.24	24.0	9,000	30.0
44.0	54.0	70.0	100.0	1.4	6.0	1.59	0.06	0.6	—	0.26	—	—	—
9.0	11.0	15.0	100.0	18.8	5.0	0.27	0.64	2.0	0.03	0.34	56.0	200.0	37.0
9.0	11.0	15.0	100.0	18.8	5.0	0.27	0.64	2.0	0.03	0.34	56.0	0.0	7.0
9.0	11.0	15.0	100.0	18.8	5.0	0.27	0.64	2.0	0.03	0.34	56.0	—	—
38.0	46.0	62.0	28.0	2.6	5.0	0.55	0.17	1.4	0.02	0.12	38.0	—	—
6.0	10.0	15.0	23.0	1.6	7.0	0.38	0.71	2.3	0.07	0.45	62.0	0.0	3.0
3.0	6.0	9.0	23.0	1.2	6.0	0.28	0.71	2.2	0.08	0.49	61.0	—	3.0
36.0	46.0	—	—	2.0	6.0	0.49	0.18	1.7	—	0.07	—	—	—
10.0	17.0	21.0	34.0	2.1	4.0	0.04	0.40	0.4	—	0.15	47.0	—	—
23.0	29.0	55.0	41.0	3.9	9.0	0.46	0.36	2.0	—	0.11	24	39,600	—
36.0	43.0	67.0	98.0	1.8	10.0	0.50	0.22	2.2	0.80	0.12	26.0	11,800	—
30.0	42.0	64.0	61.0	3.1	10.0	0.58	0.27	2.4	0.52	0.14	29.0	21,000	—

TABLE 15-11 Continued

Feedstuff	DM	TDN	DE	ME	NE_m	NE_g	NE_l	CP	DP	MP	UIP
				Energy[d]					Protein[e]		
	%	%		Mcal/kg					%		
Sunflower Seed Meal Solvent	92	65	2.9	2.4	1.5	0.8	1.5	38.0	31.2	26.6	10.3
Sunflower Seed Meal with Hulls	91	57	2.5	2.1	1.3	0.6	1.3	31.0	24.9	21.7	10.9
Sunflower Seed Hulls	90	40	1.8	1.4	0.9	0.0	0.8	4.0	0.6	2.8	2.6
Sugar Cane Bagasse	91	36	1.6	1.3	0.9	0.0	0.7	1.0	–2.1	0.7	—
Tapioca Meal	89	83	3.7	3.0	2.0	1.3	1.9	2.0	–1.2	1.4	—
Timothy Fresh Pre-bloom	26	64	2.8	2.3	1.4	0.8	1.4	11.0	6.9	7.7	2.2
Timothy Hay Early Bloom	88	59	2.6	2.1	1.3	0.6	1.3	11.0	6.9	7.7	2.4
Timothy Hay Full Bloom	88	57	2.5	2.1	1.3	0.6	1.3	8.0	4.2	5.6	2.4
Timothy Silage	34	59	2.6	2.1	1.3	0.6	1.3	10.0	6.0	7.0	2.5
Tomato Pomace Dried	92	64	2.8	2.3	1.4	0.8	1.4	23.0	17.7	16.1	—
Triticale Hay	90	56	2.5	2.0	1.2	0.5	1.2	10.0	6.0	7.0	—
Triticale Silage	34	58	2.6	2.1	1.3	0.6	1.3	14.0	9.6	9.8	—
Triticale Grain	89	85	3.7	3.1	2.1	1.4	1.9	14.0	9.6	9.8	3.5
Turnip Tops (Purple)	18	69	3.0	2.5	1.6	0.9	1.5	16.0	11.4	11.2	—
Turnip Roots	9	86	3.8	3.1	2.1	1.4	2.0	12.0	7.8	8.4	0.0
Urea 46%N	99	0	0.0	0.0	0.0	0.0	0.0	288.0	256.2	201.6	0.0
Vetch Hay	89	58	2.6	2.1	1.3	0.6	1.3	18.0	13.2	12.6	2.5
Wheat Fresh Pasture	21	71	3.1	2.6	1.6	1.0	1.6	20.0	15.0	14.0	3.2
Wheat Hay	90	57	2.5	2.1	1.3	0.6	1.3	9.0	5.1	6.3	2.3
Wheat Silage	33	59	2.6	2.1	1.3	0.6	1.3	12.0	7.8	8.4	2.5
Wheat Straw	91	42	1.9	1.5	0.9	0.0	0.9	3.0	–0.3	2.1	1.8
Wheat Straw Ammoniated	85	50	2.2	1.8	1.1	0.3	1.1	9.0	5.1	6.3	2.3
Wheat Grain	89	88	3.9	3.2	2.2	1.4	2.0	14.0	9.6	9.8	3.2
Wheat Grain Hard	89	88	3.9	3.2	2.2	1.4	2.0	14.0	9.6	9.8	3.9
Wheat Grain Soft	89	88	3.9	3.2	2.2	1.4	2.0	12.0	7.8	8.4	2.8
Wheat Grain Steam Flaked	85	91	4.0	3.3	2.2	1.5	2.1	14.0	9.6	9.8	4.1
Wheat Grain Sprouted	86	88	3.9	3.2	2.2	1.4	2.0	12.0	7.8	8.4	2.2
Wheat Bran	89	70	3.1	2.5	1.6	1.0	1.6	17.0	12.3	11.9	4.8
Wheat Middlings	89	82	3.6	3.0	2.0	1.3	1.9	19.0	14.1	13.3	4.2
Wheat Mill Run	90	75	3.3	2.7	1.7	1.1	1.7	17.0	12.3	11.9	4.8
Wheat Shorts	89	80	3.5	2.9	1.9	1.2	1.8	20.0	15.0	14.0	5.0
Wheatgrass Crested Fresh Early Bloom	37	60	2.6	2.2	1.3	0.7	1.3	11.0	6.9	7.7	2.8
Wheatgrass Crested Fresh Full Bloom	50	55	2.4	2.0	1.2	0.5	1.2	10.0	6.0	7.0	3.3
Wheatgrass Crested Hay	92	54	2.4	2.0	1.2	0.4	1.2	10.0	6.0	7.0	3.3
Whey Dried	94	82	3.6	3.0	2.0	1.3	1.9	14.0	9.6	9.8	2.1

[a]NRC expresses appreciation to R. L. Preston and Beef Magazine (http://www.beef-mag.com) for allowing the use of *Typical Composition of Feeds for Cattle and Sheep* as the initial basis for this table.

[b]All values except dry matter (DM) are shown on a dry matter basis.

[c]Entry of a dash (—) indicates that there are insufficient data to include a value.

[d]Energy expressions include total digestible nutrients (TDN), digestible energy (DE), metabolizable energy (ME), net energy for maintenance (NE_m), net energy for gain (NE_g), and net energy for lactation (NE_l). TDN expresses an estimate of the extent of digestion of all organic components (DM minus Ash) of the feed plus an extra contribution from digestible fat (2.25 × digestible EE). Approximate conversions between energy expressions are as follows:

1 kg TDN = 4.4 Mcal DE = 3.6 Mcal ME

NE = ME – heat increment. The conversion of ME to NE varies with use of the NE (NE_m, NE_g, or NE_l) and energy density of the feedstuff (see Chapter 4).

[e]Protein expressions include crude protein (CP; nitrogen × 6.25), digestible protein (DP), metabolizable protein (MP), and undegraded intake protein (UIP). Apparent digestible protein (DP) is calculated from CP assuming a true digestibility of 90 percent and a correction of 3 percent for metabolic fecal protein (DP = (CP × 0.9) – 3). Metabolizable protein is calculated as 70 percent of DP (MP = (DP × 0.7)). Undegraded intake protein is an estimate of the amount of CP contained in the feed that is not degraded in the ruminoreticulum (see Chapter 5).

[f]Fiber expressions include crude fiber (CF), acid detergent fiber (ADF), neutral detergent fiber (NDF), and effective neutral detergent fiber (eNDF). See Chapter 10 for details on the significance of each of these fiber components.

[g]Ether extract (EE) includes fatty acids, triglycerides, and other lipid compounds.

[h]Values taken from NRC (1982), where 1.0 retinol equivalent = 1.0 μg of all-*trans* retinol, 5.0 μg of all-*trans* betacarotene, and 7.6 μg of other carotenoids.

[i]Vitamins vary in content in feedstuffs because of differences in maturity, conditions at harvests, and length and conditions of storage. Values entered in the table should be considered as approximations.

Fiber[f]						Mineral Elements						Vitamins[h,i]	
CF	ADF	NDF	eNDF	EE[g]	ASH	Ca	P	K	Cl	S	Zn	A	E
%				%	%	%	%	%	%	%	ppm	RE/kg	ppm
20.0	24.0	36.0	23.0	2.5	8.0	0.44	0.97	1.2	0.15	0.33	55.0	—	12.0
27.0	32.0	44.0	37.0	2.4	7.0	0.40	1.03	1.0	—	0.30	85.0	—	—
52.0	63.0	73.0	90.0	2.2	3.0	0.00	0.11	0.2	—	0.19	200.0	—	—
49.0	59.0	86.0	100.0	0.7	3.0	0.90	0.29	0.5	—	0.10	—	—	—
5.0	8.0	34.0	—	0.8	3.0	0.03	0.05	—	—	—	—	—	—
31.0	36.0	59.0	41.0	3.8	7.0	0.40	0.28	1.9	0.57	0.15	28.0	35,800	111.0
32.0	39.0	63.0	98.0	2.7	6.0	0.58	0.26	1.9	0.51	0.21	30.0	5,600	38.0
34.0	40.0	65.0	98.0	2.6	5.0	0.43	0.20	1.8	0.62	0.13	25.0	—	—
34.0	45.0	70.0	61.0	3.4	7.0	0.50	0.27	1.7	—	0.15	—	18,000	—
26.0	50.0	55.0	34.0	10.6	6.0	0.43	0.59	3.6	—	—	—	—	—
34.0	41.0	69.0	98.0			0.30	0.26	2.3	—	—	25.0	—	—
30.0	39.0	56.0	61.0	3.6		0.58	0.34	2.7	—	0.28	36.0	—	—
4.0	5.0	22.0	34.0	2.4	2.0	0.07	0.39	0.5	—	0.17	37.0	—	—
10.0	13.0	—	—	2.6	13.0	3.20	0.31	3.0	1.80	0.27	—	—	—
11.0	34.0	44.0	40.0	1.5	8.0	0.70	0.34	3.2	0.65	0.43	40.0	—	—
0.0	0.0	0.0	0.0	0.0	0.0	0.00	0.00	0.0	0.00	0.00	0.0	—	—
30.0	33.0	48.0	92.0	1.8	8.0	1.25	0.34	2.4	—	0.13	—	92,200	—
18.0	30.0	50.0	41.0	4.0	13.0	0.35	0.36	3.1	0.67	0.22	—	—	—
29.0	38.0	66.0	98.0	2.0	8.0	0.21	0.22	1.4	0.50	0.19	23.0	17,000	—
28.0	37.0	62.0	61.0	3.2	8.0	0.40	0.28	2.1	0.50	0.21	27.0	29,400	—
43.0	58.0	81.0	98.0	1.8	8.0	0.16	0.05	1.3	0.32	0.17	6.0	400	—
40.0	55.0	76.0	98.0	1.5	9.0	0.15	0.05	1.3	0.30	0.16	6.0	—	—
3.0	4.0	12.0	0.0	2.3	2.0	0.05	0.43	0.4	0.09	0.15	40.0	0.0	17.0
3.0	6.0	14.0	0.0	2.0	2.0	0.05	0.43	0.5	—	0.16	45.0	—	15.0
3.0	4.0	12.0	0.0	2.0	2.0	0.06	0.40	0.4	—	0.15	30.0	—	19.0
3.0	4.0	12.0	0.0	2.3	2.0	0.05	0.39	0.4	—	0.15	40.0	—	—
3.0	4.0	13.0	0.0	2.0	2.0	0.04	0.36	0.4	—	0.17	45.0	—	—
11.0	13.0	46.0	4.0	4.5	7.0	0.13	1.29	1.4	0.05	0.24	96.0	600.0	21.0
8.0	12.0	36.0	2.0	4.6	5.0	0.15	1.02	1.4	0.05	0.20	98.0	—	—
9.0	12.0	37.0	0.0	4.4	5.0	0.12	1.00	1.2	0.07	0.22	90.0	—	—
7.0	7.0	30.0	0.0	5.4	5.0	0.10	0.95	1.1	0.08	0.20	118.0	—	61.0
26.0	28.0	50.0	41.0	1.6	7.0	0.46	0.32	2.4	—	—	—	42,600	—
33.0	36.0	65.0	41.0	1.6	7.0	0.39	0.28	2.1	—	—	—	—	—
33.0	36.0	65.0	98.0	2.4	7.0	0.33	0.20	2.0	—	—	32.0		—
0.0	0.0	0.0	0.0	1.0	9.0	1.00	0.90	1.4	1.20	0.92	10.0	—	—

TABLE 15-12 Composition of Pasture or Range Forage, Browse, and Other Novel Feedstuffs[a]

Major Classifications of Feedstuffs			Contents		Energy Contents[b]	
Common Names	Scientific Names	Anatomical Parts	DM %	Ash %	GE Mcal/kg	TDN %
Forest, Pasture, or Range Forages and Browse						
Acacia	*Acacia catechu*	Leaves, fresh	30			19
Agave, century plant	*Agave* spp.	Browse, fresh	12			61
Alder	*Alnus incana*		40	15	4.6	
American beauty berry	*Callicarpa americana*		39	9		
Artichoke, jeruselum	*Helianthus tuberosus*	Leaves, fresh	22	16		62
Ash	*Fraxinus* spp.	Leaves, sun-cured	85	7	4.4	
Ash, green	*Fraxinus pennsylvanica*		44	10		
Aspen	*Populus* spp.	Leaves, sun-cured	85	9	4.3	
Aspen	*Populus* spp.	Flower buds, spring	38		4.8	
Bamboo	*Aruninaria cannaviera*	Leaves, fresh	45	11	4.4	59
Banana	*Musa* spp.	Leaves, fresh	19			50
Banana	*Musa* spp.	Leaves, young	18	8		69
Banana	*Musa* spp.	Leaves, post harvest	24	10		72
Banana	*Musa* spp.	Leaves, dried	94	9		56
Banyantree	*Ficus benghalensis*	Leaves, fresh	32			51
Bean, Mung	*Phaseolus aureus*	Leaves, post harvest	24	9		60
Bean, purple	*Phaseolus atropurpureus*	Leaves, fresh	15			53
Beech	*Carpinus* spp.		62	8		
Beech, American	*Fagus grandifolia*	Leaves, sun-cured				
Beggars lice	*Desmodium canescans*		42	5		
Birch, Paper	*Betula papyrifera*	Leaves				
Birch, Sweet	*Betula lenta*	Browse, immature, fresh	92	8	4.7	
Blackberry	*Rubus ulmifolius*		49	8		
Blackberry, July	*Rubus ulmifolius*		45			72
Blackberry, September	*Rubus ulmifolius*		44			73
Broom sedge	*Carex scoparia*		77			54
Buckeye	*Aesculus* spp.		43	9		
Cassava	*Manihot esculenta*	Leaves, fresh	25	6		73
Cherokee rose	*Rosa laevigata*		35			84
Chinaberry	*Melia azedarach*	Leaves, fresh	21			67
Cottongrass, tussock	*Eriphorum vaginatum*	Seeds				
Cowpea	*Vigna sinensis*	Fresh	15			64
Cucumber	*Cucumis sativus*		39	10		
Devils walking stick	*Aralia spinosa*		36	9		
Dogwood	*Cornus* spp.		43	14		
Elderberry	*Sambucus canadensis*		37	11		
Elm	*Ulmus* spp.		41	11		
Elm, southern	*Ulmus* spp.		31	12		
Elm, white	*Ulmus americana*		34	12		
Fig, cluster	*Ficus glomerata*	Leaves, fresh	30			54
Grape	*Vitis vinifera*		43	10		
Grape	*Vitis vinifera*	Vine, leaves	35			72
Greenbriar	*Smilax* spp.		38	16		
Greenbriar, early veg.	*Smilax* spp.		29			63
Guinea grass	*Panicum maximum*	Leaves, early growth	15	7		65
Guinea grass	*Panicum maximum*	Leaves, veg.	25	13		62
Gum, black	*Nyssa sylmatica*		47	13		
Hackberry	*Celtis reticulata*	Browse, fresh, mature	56			43
Hackberry	*Celtis reticulata*					
Hairy vetch	*Vicia villosa*		45			51
Hickory	*Carya* spp.		55	15		
Holly	*Ilex* spp.		70	9		
Honeysuckle, bush	*Lonicera albiflora*	Leaves, fresh	33			69
Honeysuckle, September	*Lonicera* spp.		37			62
Huckleberry	*Gaylussacia* spp.		43	10		
Jujube	*Ziziphus jujuba*	Browse, fresh	32			31
Juniper, ashe	*Juniperus ashei*	Leaves, fresh	52			64
Kale	*Brassica oleracea*	Leaves and stems, fresh	16	10	4.3	
Kudzu	*Pueraria* spp.		39	8		

				Protein Contents[c]			Fiber Contents[d]			Minerals		
DE Mcal/kg	ME Mcal/kg	NE_m Mcal/kg	NE_g Mcal/kg	CP %	DP %	MP %	NDF %	ADF %	EE[e] %	Ca %	P %	Sources[f]
0.84	0.69	0.77	0.00	5.0	1.2	0.8						(5)
2.69	2.21	1.33	0.69	6.8	2.9	2.0					0.11	(5)
				7.7			43.7	40.8				(2)
				11.2			62.3	48.8				(2)
	2.24			20.7	16.2	11.3			2.3			(1)
				14.6								(6)
				10.9			51.2	38.4				(2)
				17.2								(6)
				13.5								(6)
	2.13			17.4	13.2	9.2			0.2	1.43	0.23	(1)
2.21	1.81	1.07	0.28	15.7	6.7	4.7					0.70	(5)
	2.48			20.0	15.6	10.9			4.1	0.24	0.21	(1)
	2.60			17.9	13.6	9.5			8.2	1.14	0.19	(1)
	2.01			9.8					1.5			(1)
2.25	1.84	1.10	0.32	9.6	4.1	2.9					0.40	(5)
	2.16			9.9	5.4	3.8			3.0	1.43	0.35	(1)
2.34	1.92	1.14	0.40	23.0	9.2	6.4						(5)
				6.4			51.5	43.8				(2)
							64.7	47.6				(6)
				15.3			42.8	24.3				(2)
							44.7	30.8				(6)
				28.1								(6)
				9.7			54.2	39.7				(2)
				8.6								(3)
				8.2								(3)
				6.0								(3)
				15.9			38.2	25.3				(2)
	2.64			23.2	18.6	13.0			5.0	1.25	0.07	(1)
				12.8		0.0						(3)
2.95	2.42	1.50	0.88	18.7	13.9	9.7						(5)
				15.0			66.8	22.8				(4)
2.82	2.31	1.41	0.78	16.2	11.7	8.2					0.28	(5)
				14.1			51.6	40.1				(2)
				13.4			44.8	33.5				(2)
				7.4			39.6	29.8				(2)
				14.2			49.6	32.5				(2)
				7.8			50.3	33.0				(2)
				7.4			43.4	25.0				(2)
				10.8			53.4	36.2				(2)
2.38	1.95	1.16	0.43	11.2	6.7	4.7					0.71	(5)
				11.0			55.1	48.8				(2)
				9.1								(3)
				8.0			51.3	34.6				(2)
				12.2								(3)
	2.35			20.0	15.6	10.9			2.5	0.59	0.40	(1)
	2.25			9.6	5.9	4.1			1.2	0.52	0.60	(2)
				8.1			49.5	39.7				(6)
1.90	1.56	0.94	0.00	7.8	3.8	2.7					0.08	(5)
												(5)
				14.9								(3)
				10.8			48.0	34.5				(2)
				10.3			45.6	39.9				(2)
3.04	2.50	1.55	0.94	10.0	5.9	4.1	20.0				0.11	(5)
				7.4								(3)
				10.1			69.2	42.8				(5)
1.37	1.12	0.79	0.00	8.6	3.1	2.2						(5)
2.82	2.31	1.41	0.78	6.5	2.6	1.8					0.08	(5)
				21.2			18.2	13.3				(6)
				16.0			54.9	36.0				(2)

TABLE 15-12 continued

Major Classifications of Feedstuffs			Contents		Energy Contents[b]	
Common Names	Scientific Names	Anatomical Parts	DM %	Ash %	GE %	TDN %
Kudzu	*Pueraria lobata*	Aerial part, fresh	26	8	4.2	
Kudzu, July	*Pueraria* spp.		45			58
Kudzu, September	*Pueraria* spp.		44			61
Leadtree, little leaf	*Leucaena retusa*	Browse, fresh, early veg.	27			68
Lespediza	*Sericia lespediza*		36	12		
Lettuce	*Lactuca sativa*	Fresh	5	23	3.6	70
Maple, red	*Acer rubrum*		44	11		
Maple, sugar	*Acer saccharum*	Leaves				
Mesquite, honey	*Prosopis glandulosa.*	Browse, fresh, late veg.	48			45
Mimosa	*Mimosa* spp.	Browse, fresh, early veg.	26			69
Mulberry	*Morus* spp.		35	9		
Mulberry	*Morus* spp.	Browse, fresh	40	15	4.1	71
Mustard	*Brassica oleracea*	Leaves and stems, fresh	9	15	4.0	
Napiergrass	*Pennisetum purpureum*	Leaves, early growth	10	12		64
Napiergrass	*Pennisetum purpureum*	Leaves, veg.	21	8		60
Oak, laurel	*Quercus laurifolia*		52	6		
Oak, live	*Quercus virginiana.*	Browse, fresh, early veg.	36			54
Oak, live	*Quercus virginiana.*	Leaves, fresh	50			46
Oak, red	*Quercus rubra*		48	7		
Oak, shin	*Quercus sinuata breviloba*	Browse, fresh, early veg.	32			72
Oak, white	*Quercus albus*		49	9		
Oak, white	*Quercus albus*		45			61
Pangolagrass	*Digitaria decumbens*	Leaves, early growth	20	8		62
Pangolagrass	*Digitaria decumbens*	Leaves, veg.	26	8		59
Parsley	*Carum petroselinum*	Leaves and stems, fresh	12	12		
Pea	*Pisum* spp.	Vines, late veg.	14			67
Peanut, ground nut	*Arachis hypogaea*	Vines, young	16	8		62
Peanut, ground nut	*Arachis hypogaea*	Vines, post harvest	18	5		59
Peepultree	*Ficus religiosa*	Leaves, fresh	17			36
Persimmon	*Diospyros texana*	Leaves, fresh	48			54
Persimon	*Diospyros* spp.		38	10		
Pigweed	*Amaranthus retroflexus*		19			80
Pine, loblolly	*Pinus taeda*	Needles	41			72
Plum	*Prunus* spp.		43			86
Plum, Java	*Syzygium cumini*	Leaves, fresh	30			43
Plum, white	*Prunus* spp.		37	5		
Poke salad, green	*Phytolacca americana*		15			86
Poke salad, mature	*Phytolacca americana*		42	12		
Poplar, black	*Populus nigra*	Leaves, sun-cured	85	7	4.3	
Poplar, yellow	*Populus deltoides*		27			72
Pricklypear	*Opuntia* spp.	Fruit, fresh, immature	26			34
Pricklypear	*Opuntia* spp.	Leaves, fresh, mature	21			51
Privit hedge, August	*Ligustrum* spp.		37			75
Privit hedge, September	*Ligustrum* spp.		28			65
Ragweed, common	*Ambrosia artemisiifolia*		21			75
Ragweed, tall	*Ambrosia trifida*		22			71
Redberry juniper	*Juniperus pinchotii*	Leaves, fresh	53			60
Redbud	*Cercis canadensis*		44	10		
Sacahuista	*Nolina texana*	Buds, fresh	32			63
Sacahuista	*Nolina texana*	Leaves, fresh	57			47
Sassafras	*Sassafras albidum*		41	10		
Sedge	*Carex planostachys*	Fresh, late veg.	39			50
Sensitivebrier	*Schrankia roemeriana*	Browse, fresh, late veg.	32			73
Sesbania pea	*Sesbania cannabina*	Browse, fresh	19			60
Sotol	*Dasylirion texanum*	Leaves, fresh	57			58
Sour wood	*Oxydendrum arboreum*		38	10		
Sumac	*Rhus* spp.		42	10		
Sumac, July	*Rhus* spp.		42			83
Sumac, scented	*Rhus aromatica*	Browse, fresh, early veg.	40			77
Sumac, September	*Rhus* spp.		19			73

DE Mcal/kg	ME Mcal/kg	NE$_m$ Mcal/kg	NE$_g$ Mcal/kg	Protein Contents[c] CP %	DP %	MP %	Fiber Contents[d] NDF %	ADF %	EE[e] %	Minerals Ca %	P %	Sources[f]
				17.6								(6)
				19.0								(3)
				21.7								(3)
3.00	2.46	1.52	0.91	17.6	13.0	9.1						(5)
				17.2			53.6	41.5				(2)
3.09	2.53	1.58	0.97	22.0	17.0	11.9						(2)
				9.0			58.1	48.1				(2)
							58.9	43.9				(6)
1.98	1.63	0.98	0.06	16.2	11.7	8.2	47.0				0.08	(5)
3.04	2.50	1.55	0.94	20.6	15.8	11.1					0.17	(5)
				13.2			44.4	18.0				(2)
3.13	2.57	1.61	1.00	18.1	13.4	9.4					0.24	(5)
				29.3			19.7	16.8				(6)
	2.31			24.0	19.4	13.6			3.5			(1)
	2.17			10.7	7.0	4.9			2.9	0.41	0.72	(1)
				14.3			57.9	34.8				(2)
2.38	1.95	1.16	0.43	20.3	15.5	10.9	34.0				0.38	(5)
2.03	1.66	0.99	0.10	10.2	6.1	4.3	45.0				0.11	(5)
				9.7			52.1	36.6				(2)
3.17	2.60	1.64	1.03	17.4	12.8	9.0	23.0				0.31	(5)
				11.1			40.2	32.3				(2)
				11.9								(3)
	2.25			17.7	13.5	9.5			2.9			(1)
	2.13			12.9	9.0	6.3			1.7	0.40	0.23	(1)
				24.1			21.1	17.8				(6)
2.95	2.42	1.50	0.88	27.4	22.1	15.5						(5)
	2.25			20.9	15.5	10.9			2.0			(1)
	2.12			15.3	10.3	7.2			2.6	0.98	0.36	(1)
1.59	1.30	0.84	0.00	14.0	7.6	5.3						(5)
2.38	1.95	1.16	0.43	11.8	7.6	5.3					0.11	(5)
				10.7			44.9	39.0				(2)
				22.1								(3)
				6.8								(3)
				13.9								(3)
1.90	1.56	0.94	0.00	7.8	0.1	0.1						(5)
				10.7			33.3	26.6				(2)
				25.3								(3)
				20.5			51.7	27.2				(2)
				18.8								(6)
				13.3								(2)
1.50	1.23	0.82	0.00	6.8	3.5	2.5	52.0				0.13	(5)
2.25	1.84	1.10	0.32	3.1	0.0	0.0	21.0				0.03	(5)
				16.4								(5)
				12.4								(3)
				26.4								(3)
				17.4								(3)
2.65	2.17	1.31	0.65	7.5	3.5	2.5					0.11	(5)
				10.3			38.4	25.9				(2)
2.78	2.28	1.39	0.75	19.4	14.7	10.3	28.0				0.38	(5)
2.07	1.70	1.01	0.15	5.6	1.8	1.3	63.0				0.06	(5)
				10.5			60.2	37.4				(5)
2.21	1.81	1.07	0.28	11.8	7.6	5.3					0.13	(5)
3.22	2.64	1.67	1.06	32.3	26.7	18.7					0.22	(5)
2.65	2.17	1.31	0.65	27.5	22.3	15.6						(5)
2.56	2.10	1.26	0.58	7.1	3.2	2.2					0.08	(5)
				10.2			57.9	51.6				(2)
				10.9			43.3	24.6				(2)
				9.0								(3)
3.40	2.78	1.79	1.17	13.7	9.3	6.5					0.20	(5)
				14.4								(3)

TABLE 15-12 continued

Major Classifications of Feedstuffs			Contents		Energy Contents[b]	
Common Names	Scientific Names	Anatomical Parts	DM %	Ash %	GE %	TDN %
Summer cypress, kocia	*Kocia vestita*	Fresh, mature	65			56
Sunflower	*Helianthus* spp.	Fresh, late veg.	12			64
Sweet potato	*Ipomoea batatas*	Vines	13	13		67
Sweetgum	*Liquidambar styraciflua*		34	9		
Sweetgum	*Liquidambar styraciflua*	Leaves	36			80
Sweetgum	*Liquidambar styraciflua*	Twigs	31			82
Sycamore	*Platanus occidentalis*		32	8		
Sycamore	*Platanus occidentalis*		25			67
Teaweed	*Sida spinosa*		28			66
Texas bluebonnet	*Lupinus texensis*	Fresh, early veg.	18			59
Vetch	*Vicia sativa*	Fresh	20			59
Virginia creeper	*Vitis quinquefolia*		39	7		
Wax myrtle	*Myrica cerifera*		33	11		
Wax myrtle, July	*Myrica cerifera*		43			69
Wax myrtle, September	*Myrica cerifera*		46			70
Wild cherry	*Prunus serotina*		50	12		
Willow	*Salix* spp.	Browse, fresh	41	7	4.2	
Willow	*Salix* spp.		63	10		
Winterfat	*Eurotia lanata*	Fresh, early veg.	30			64
Yucca	*Yucca* spp.	Flowers, fresh	15			70
Yucca	*Yucca* spp.	Leaves, fresh, immature	41			43
Hays, Silages, and Other Roughages						
Alfalfa, lucerne	*Medicago sativa*	Silage, late veg.	21			63
Alfalfa, lucerne	*Medicago sativa*	Silage, full bloom	26			58
Beet	*Beta vulgaris altissima*	Silage, aerial parts	22			51
Napiergrass	*Pennisetum purpureum*	Silage	26			43
Oats	*Avena sativa*	Silage, whole plant	31			62
Pangolagrass	*Digitaria decumbens*	Silage, mature	32			56
Pea	*Pisum* spp.	Silage	24			54
Soybean	*Glycine max*	Silage, wilted	35			55
High-energy Feeds						
Apple	*Malas* spp.	Golden delicious	14	2	4.2	
Apple	*Malas* spp.	Red delicious	13	3		
Apple	*Malas* spp.	Pomace, wet	20			74
Apricot	*Prunus armeniaca*		12	4	4.2	
Banana	*Musa* spp.	Baby	26	4		
Banana	*Musa* spp.	Burro	27	4		
Banana	*Musa* spp.	Green	19	5		
Banana	*Musa* spp.	Ripe	20	4	4.2	
Blackberries	*Rubus* spp.		14	3	4.2	
Blood	*Bovis, Ovis,* etc	Meal, spray dehydrated	93		5.3	91
Blueberries	*Viccinium* spp.		13	1	4.3	
Cabbage	*Brassica oleracea capitata*	Fresh	9	9	4.2	84
Cantaloupe	*Cucumis melo*	Whole	8	8		
Carob beans	*Ceratonia siliqua*	Pods with seeds	88			79
Carrots	*Daucus* spp.	Roots, fresh	12	7	4.0	84
Cassava	*Manihot esculenta*	Peelings, dehydrated	88			86
Cassava	*Manihot esculenta*	Tubers, fresh	37	4	4.8	80
Cassava	*Manihot esculenta*	Fresh	38	2		87
Cassava	*Manihot esculenta*	Peeled, dry	90	0		88
Cassava	*Manihot esculenta*	Meal	87	3		82
Chickpea	*Cicer arietinum*	Seeds, dry	91			76
Citrus	*Citrus* spp.	Pumace or pulp, dried	90			73
Coconut	*Cocos nucifera*	Meats, oil residue	91			75
Coconut	*Cocos nucifera*	Meat, fresh	50	2		
Coconut	*Cocos nucifera*	Meat, dried	93	3		
Figs	*Ficus carica*		65	3	4.1	
Grapefruit	*Citrus paradisi*		15	3	4.2	

				Protein Contents[c]			Fiber Contents[d]			Minerals		
DE Mcal/kg	ME Mcal/kg	NE_m Mcal/kg	NE_g Mcal/kg	CP %	DP %	MP %	NDF %	ADF %	EE[e] %	Ca %	P %	Sources[f]
2.47	2.03	1.21	0.51	9.0	5.0	3.5						(5)
2.82	2.31	1.41	0.78	8.3	4.3	3.0						(2)
	2.40			18.2	14.0	9.8			2.3	1.10	0.68	(1)
				9.6			54.7	50.2				(2)
				11.1								(3)
				9.4								(3)
				9.8			45.9	30.3				(2)
				13.7								(3)
				15.9								(3)
2.60	2.13	1.28	0.62	16.1	11.5	8.1	24.0				0.14	(5)
2.60	2.13	1.28	0.62	18.6	13.9	9.7					0.34	(5)
				13.9			52.8	33.8				(2)
				10.4			40.9	23.0				(2)
				10.5								(2)
				9.0								(2)
				14.9			64.2	39.5				(2)
				9.8								(6)
				9.7			48.1	39.9				(2)
2.82	2.31	1.41	0.78	21.0	16.2	11.3					0.12	(5)
3.09	2.53	1.58	0.97	19.7	14.9	10.4	13.0				0.48	(5)
1.90	1.56	0.94	0.00	7.3	3.4	2.4	69.0				0.10	(5)
												(5)
												(2)
2.78	2.28	1.39	0.75	20.0	14.4	10.1	55.0	47.0				(5)
2.56	2.10	1.26	0.58	17.5	12.1	8.5		38.0				(5)
2.25	1.84	1.10	0.32	13.4	8.4	5.9					0.29	(5)
1.90	1.56	0.94	0.00	4.8	0.5	0.4					0.31	(5)
2.73	2.24	1.36	0.72	9.6	3.8	2.7					0.24	(5)
2.47	2.03	1.21	0.51	8.9	4.3	3.0					0.08	(5)
2.38	1.95	1.16	0.43	25.7	19.6	13.7					0.48	(5)
2.43	1.99	1.19	0.47	18.0	12.5	8.8					0.36	(5)
				2.5			9.8	5.5	5.8			(7)
				3.0			10.2	6.0	5.8			(7)
3.26	2.68	1.74	1.08	5.6	2.4	1.7				0.10	0.10	(5)
				7.3			7.3	4.7	4.9			(7)
				5.5			16.1	5.1	3.0			(7)
				4.4			15.2	4.6	1.7			(7)
				5.4			12.4	4.5	6.2			(7)
				5.7			12.3	2.8	5.3			(7)
				9.8			25.4	18.0	9.3			(7)
4.04	3.29	2.22	1.52	89.0	84.5	59.2				0.52	0.26	(5)
				3.7			13.2	7.1	7.6			(7)
3.70	3.04	2.00	1.35	20.6	16.1	11.3	17.2	10.4		0.64	0.35	(5)
				13.1			22.0	20.4	7.2			(7)
3.48	2.86	1.85	1.22	6.3	3.0	2.1				0.23	0.34	(5)
3.70	3.04	2.00	1.35	9.9	6.3	4.4				0.40	0.35	(5)
3.79	3.11	2.06	1.40	2.0	0.0	0.0						(5)
3.53	2.89	1.88	1.24	3.6	0.5	0.4	11.9	4.3				(5)
	3.14			1.1					0.5			(1)
	3.18			2.7					0.3	0.10	0.08	(1)
	2.98			2.8					0.4			(1)
3.35	2.75	1.76	1.14	21.7	15.2	10.6				0.17	0.37	(5)
3.22	2.64	1.67	1.06	6.9	3.5	2.5				1.98	0.13	(5)
3.31	2.71	1.73	1.11	23.4						0.19	0.66	(5)
				7.4	4.0	2.8			68.0	0.04	0.60	(5)
				7.3	3.9	2.7			68.0			(5)
				4.2			10.0	8.0	2.5			(7)
				4.8			7.2	6.1	4.5			(7)

TABLE 15-12 continued

Major Classifications of Feedstuffs			Contents		Energy Contents[b]	
Common Names	Scientific Names	Anatomical Parts	DM %	Ash %	GE %	TDN %
Grapes	*Vitis* spp.	Black	16	3	4.3	
Grapes	*Vitis* spp.	Green	16	2		
Grapes	*Vitis* spp.	Red	14	2		
Honeydew	*Cucumis melo*	Whole	8	7		
Honeydew	*Cucumis melo*	Without rind	10	6	4.2	
Jerusalem artichoke	*Helianthus tuberosus*	Roots, fresh	17	6		83
Kiwi	*Aclinidai* spp.		13	5	4.2	
Lemon	*Citrus limonia*		11	3		
Lime	*Citrus aurantiifolia*		12	5		
Mango	*Mangifera indica*		19	2	4.2	
Mung beans	*Phaseolus aureus*	Meal	91	3		
Nectarine	*Prunus persica*		13	4	4.3	
Oak	*Quercus* spp.	Fruit (acorns)	64			47
Orange	*Citrus sinensis*	Whole fruit	16	3	4.2	
Papaya	*Carica papaya*		8	9	4.1	
Peanut, groundnut	*Arachis hypogaea*		95			134
Pear	*Pyrus* spp.	Anjou	14	2	4.2	
Pear	*Pyrus* spp.	Bartlett	13	2		
Pear	*Pyrus* spp.	Bosc	12	2		
Peas	*Pisum* spp.	Cowpeas, fresh	12	14		74
Peas	*Pisum* spp.	Cowpeas, dry	93	4		83
Pineapple	*Ananas comosus*		10	3	4.3	
Plantain	*Musa* spp.		30	3	4.1	
Plum	*Prunus* spp.		10	3	4.3	
Potatos	*Solanum tuberosum*	Tubers, fresh	23		4.1	81
Pumpkin	*Cucrbuta pepo*	Melon	20	5		
Raspberries	*Rubus idaeus*		14	3	4.4	
Seaweed, kelp	*Laminariales-fucales (Ord)*	Seaweed, kelp, dried	89			32
Sesame	*Sesamum indicum*	Seeds, dry	94	3	6.9	
Sesame	*Sesamum indicum*	Meal	92	14		
Strawberries	*Fragaria ananassa*		9	5	4.3	
Sugarcane	*Saccharum officinarum*	Molasses, high brix	75		3.8	72
Sweetpotatos	*Ipomoea batatas*	Tubers, fresh	33		4.1	81
Sweetpotatos	*Ipomoea batatas*	Tubers, fresh	27	5		84
Sweetpotatos	*Ipomoea batatas*	Meal	87	3		86
Tomatos	*Lycopersicon esculentum*	Pomace, wet	13			62
Tomatos	*Lycopersicon esculentum*	Pomace, dehydrated	92	8	4.7	58
Turnips	*Brassica rapa rapa*	Roots, fresh	9	9	4.0	86
Watermelon	*Citrullus lanatus*	Whole	7	5		
Watermelon	*Citrullus lanatus*	Without rind	7	4	4.4	
Produce, vegetables						
Atrichoke	*Helianthus tuberosus*		13	7		
Asparagus	*Asparagus officinalis*		7	6	4.4	
Bean sprouts	*Phaseolus* spp.		6	6		
Beans	*Phaseolus* spp.	Green	7	8	4.2	
Broccoli	*Brassica oleracia*		10	8	4.4	
Brussel sprouts	*Brassica oleracia*		17	6	4.2	
Carrots	*Daucus carota*		12	6	4.0	
Cauliflower	*Brassica oleracia*		6	12	4.3	
Celery	*Apium graveoleus*		5	12	3.8	
Chickpeas	*Cicer arietinum*		30	2		
Corn	*Zea mays*	Corn-cob-husk	21	3	4.5	
Cucumber	*Cucumis sativus*		4	11	4.1	
Eggplant	*Solanum melongena*		8	7	4.1	
Mushroom	*Genus* spp.(Varied)		7	9		
Okra	*Abelmoschus esculentus*		13	8	4.1	
Onion	*Allium cepa*	Green	9	9		
Onion	*Allium cepa*	Red	9	5		
Onion	*Allium cepa*	Yellow	10	4		

DE Mcal/kg	ME Mcal/kg	NE_m Mcal/kg	NE_g Mcal/kg	Protein Contents[c] CP %	DP %	MP %	Fiber Contents[d] NDF %	ADF %	EE[e] %	Minerals Ca %	P %	Sources[f]
				4.4			3.3	2.4	2.8			(7)
				3.6			3.1	1.8	2.4			(7)
				2.7			12.7	8.5	4.2			(7)
				8.9			15.0	12.5	5.8			(7)
				9.6			17.4	14.1	12.0			(7)
	3.00			8.3	4.9	3.4			0.6	0.30	0.83	(1)
				8.3			16.2	12.6	5.3			(7)
				11.0			18.2	14.9	14.4			(7)
				9.4			17.9	14.8	12.6			(7)
				3.1			11.5	6.3	4.5			(7)
				25.5					0.7	0.24	0.47	(1)
				4.6			7.3	3.2	3.8			(7)
2.07	1.70	1.01	0.15	4.8	1.7	1.2						(5)
				6.0			11.0	7.1	3.8			(7)
				13.6			13.7	12.2	3.5			(7)
5.91	4.85	3.51	2.54	29.9	24.9	17.4				0.06	0.45	(5)
				3.0			16.4	9.5	4.5			(7)
				3.7			12.7	8.1	5.8			(7)
				1.8			15.6	10.5	6.9			(7)
	2.68			30.8	25.5	17.9			1.7			(1)
	3.01			24.9	20.1	14.1			1.5			(1)
				3.3			15.3	5.8	1.9			(7)
				3.1			8.6	2.3	5.3			(7)
				6.1			6.1	3.6	5.2			(7)
3.57	2.93	1.91	1.27	9.5	5.9	4.1				0.04	0.24	(5)
				7.3			21.7	7.7	7.2			(7)
				9.4			26.8	22.0	10.6			(7)
1.41	1.16	0.80	0.00	9.8	6.2	4.3				1.48	0.18	(5)
				25.7					47.9			(1)
				42.7					8.9	2.44	1.29	(1)
				9.0			11.4	7.5	7.7			(7)
3.17	2.60	1.64	1.03	5.8	2.6	1.8				1.00	0.11	(5)
3.57	2.93	1.91	1.27	5.0	1.9	1.3				0.10	0.15	(5)
	3.03			6.5	3.2	2.2			1.0			(1)
	3.10			3.1					0.8	0.09	0.15	(1)
2.73	2.24	1.36	0.72	21.7								(5)
2.56	2.10	1.26	0.58	23.5			55.0			0.43	0.60	(5)
3.79	3.11	2.06	1.40	11.8	8.1	5.7				0.59	0.26	(5)
				7.8			11.6	9.9	6.4			(7)
				7.5			6.1	5.1	6.7			(7)
												(5)
				17.3			29.4	20.7	3.2			(7)
				19.9			17.9	12.4	4.2			(7)
				39.7			18.0	13.1	3.9			(7)
				26.3			21.8	18.3	5.5			(7)
				31.2			16.6	14.6	4.8			(7)
				27.2			18.1	10.5	4.5			(7)
				5.9			9.7	8.9	3.5			(7)
				26.5			19.1	17.2	3.8			(7)
				17.2			15.7	12.6	3.0			(7)
				20.3			30.1	9.6	4.1			(7)
				10.9			44.2	19.0	3.9			(7)
				16.8			18.6	15.5	4.7			(7)
				15.5			22.0	11.0	6.5			(7)
				31.0			15.8	10.6	5.6			(7)
				17.4			14.2	9.7	4.5			(7)
				20.7			13.8	7.0	6.1			(7)
				15.5			9.4	7.4	5.8			(7)
				9.1			10.2	7.4	4.8			(7)

TABLE 15-12 continued

Major Classifications of Feedstuffs			Contents		Energy Contents[b]	
Common Names	Scientific Names	Anatomical Parts	DM %	Ash %	GE %	TDN %
Peas	*Pisum* spp.	Snow	9	4		
Pepper	*Capsicum annum*	Green	5	8	4.2	
Potato	*Solanum tuberosum*		28	4	4.1	
Radishes	*Raphanus sativus*		6	6	4.4	
Rutabega	*Brassica napus*		11	5	4.1	
Squash	*Cucurbita* spp.	Acorn	12	5	4.0	
Squash	*Cucurbita* spp.	Butternut	8	8	4.0	
Squash	*Cucurbita* spp.	Chayote	6	6		
Squash	*Cucurbita* spp.	Spaghetti	11	8	4.5	
Squash	*Cucurbita* spp.	Yellow	6	7		
Squash	*Cucurbita* spp.	Zucchini	4	13	4.2	
Sweet potato	*Ipomoea batatas*	Raw	24	3		
Sweet potato	*Ipomoea batatas*	Steamed	23	3	4.1	
Tomatillos	*Lycium* spp.		8	6	4.8	
Tomato	*Solanum lycopersiem*		5	10	4.4	
Turnip	*Brassica rapa*		7	11	4.0	
Produce, leafy green vegetables and other items						
Alfalfa sprouts	*Medicago sativa*		5	5		
Banana flower	*Musa* spp.		9	11		
Bok choy	*Brassica rapa*		5	11		
Cabbage	*Brassica oleracea*		5	8		
Collards	*Brassica oleracea*		9	11		
Greens, mustard	*Brassica juncea*		9	13	4.0	
Greens, turnip	*Brassica oleracea*		9	14	3.9	
Kale	*Brassica oleracea*		14	8	4.3	
Lettuce	*Laciuca* spp.	Iceburg	4	7	4.3	
Lettuce	*Laciuca* spp.	Romaine	7	9	4.1	
Napa	*Brassica rapa*		4	10		
Parsley	*Petroselinum crispum*		12	12		
Spinach	*Spinacia oleracea*		9	20	4.0	
Sugarcane	*Saccharum officinarum*		20	1	3.8	

[a]All values except dry matter (DM) are shown on a dry matter basis.

[b]Energy concentrations include gross energy (GE), total digestible nutrients (TDN), digestible energy (DE), metabolizable energy (ME), net energy for maintenance (NE_m), and net energy for gain (NE_g). Values listed in the column labelled "GE" were taken from NRC (2003) and should be considered only approximations of the gross energy content for the particular feedstuffs described. Definitions and conversions of energy expressions are as follows:

GE = Total energy in the feeds including both available and unavailable energy.

1 kg TDN = 4.4 Mcal DE = 3.6 Mcal ME

NE = ME – heat increment. The conversion of ME to NE varies with use of the NE (NE_m or NE_g) and energy density of the feedstuff (see Chapter 4).

[c]Protein expressions include crude protein (CP; nitrogen × 6.25), digestible protein (DP), and metabolizable protein (MP). An estimate of apparent digestible protein (DP) can be calculated from CP assuming a true digestibiltiy of 90 percent and a correction of 3 percent for metabolic fecal protein (DP = (CP × 0.9) – 3). Values in the MP column were calculated assuming the relationship (MP = DP × 0.7). Greater detail on protein expressions are contained in Chapter 5.

[d]Fiber expressions include neutral detergent fiber (NDF) and acid detergent fiber (ADF). See Chapter 10 for details on the significance of each of these fiber fractions.

[e]Ether extract (EE) includes fatty acids, triglycerides, and other lipid compounds.

[f]Sources of the nutrient composition of the feeds.

1. Devendra, C. 1979. Malaysian Feedingstuffs. Malaysian Agricultural Research and Development Institute. Serdang, Selangor, Malaysia.

2. Fagan, G. L., S. G. Solaiman. 1993. Nutritional analysis of forest vegetation during 1991 and 1992 browsing season. Goat Forestry Seminar, Tuskegee University, January 1993, Tuskegee AL.

3. Burton L. N., and A. D. Scarf. 1991. Angora goats in Alabama Woodland. Pp. 78–83 in Using Goats to Manage Forest Vegetation: A Regional Inquiry. S. G. Solaiman and W. A. Hill (eds). Tuskegee, AL, Tuskegee University.

4. Jorgenson, J. C., M. S. Udevitz, N. A. Felix. 2002. Forage quantity and quality. Pages 46–50. in D. C. Douglas, P. E. Reynolds, and E. B. Rhode, ed. Arctic Refuge Coastal Plain Terrestrial Wildlife Research Summaries. U.S. Geological Survey, Biological Resources Division, Biological Science Report USGS/BRD/BSR-2002-0001.

5. NRC. 1981. Nutrient Requirements of Goats. Washington, DC: National Academy Press.

6. NRC. 2003. Nutrient Requirements of Nonhuman Primates, 2nd ed. Washington, DC: National Academy Press.

7. Schmidt, D. A., M. S. Kerley, J. H. Porter, and J. L. Dempsey. 2005. Structural and nonstructural carbohydrate, fat, and protein compostion of commercially available, whole produce. Zoo Biol. 0:1–15.

				Protein Contents[c]			Fiber Contents[d]			Minerals		
DE Mcal/kg	ME Mcal/kg	NE_m Mcal/kg	NE_g Mcal/kg	CP %	DP %	MP %	NDF %	ADF %	EE[e] %	Ca %	P %	Sources[f]
				31.4			16.3	10.9	6.7			(7)
				17.7			19.6	17.0	6.4			(5)
				9.6			7.5	2.5	5.3			(7)
				15.7			15.5	14.1	3.7			(7)
				16.0			14.5	11.0	8.1			(7)
				11.2			19.7	16.6	11.4			(7)
				26.0			17.5	14.7	5.8			(7)
				15.8			16.6	12.1	4.5			(7)
				17.2			30.9	24.2	4.9			(7)
				14.6			13.8	7.3	6.3			(7)
				24.9			15.1	10.2	8.4			(7)
				4.2			20.0	4.9	5.6			(7)
				4.9			11.0	3.6	4.0			(7)
				14.3			26.2	17.8	12.0			(7)
				25.9			16.6	14.2	6.1			(7)
				20.8			19.7	14.6	6.2			(7)
				58.4			27.7	20.8	3.1			(7)
				15.8			41.2	22.6	6.8			(7)
				23.7			13.3	10.3	7.3			(7)
				22.6			17.2	10.4	4.6			(7)
				23.1			19.0	12.6	7.9			(7)
				36.7			19.7	16.8	4.5			(7)
				34.1			20.1	17.5	4.4			(7)
				27.2			18.2	13.1	8.7			(7)
				21.9			16.9	13.1	6.3			(7)
				17.5			16.3	14.1	6.2			(7)
				27.6			17.1	14.0	4.3			(7)
				24.0			21.1	17.8	5.2			(7)
				38.7			20.1	11.7	8.0			(7)
				1.3			32.6	21.2	4.3			(7)

TABLE 15-13 Compositions of Inorganic Mineral Sources on a 100% Dry Matter Basis

Mineral Element Source	International Feed No.[a]	Dry Matter[b]	Crude Protein Equivalent (CPE) = N% × 6.25	Primary Mineral Element Content
Calcium Sources		(DM%)	(CPE%)	Ca (%)
Bone meal, steamed, fg[c]	6–00–400	97	13.2	30.71
Calcium carbonate, $CaCO_3$, fg	6–01–069	100	—[d]	39.39
Calcium chloride anhydrous, $CaCl_2$, cp [e, *]	NA[f]	100	—	36.11
Calcium chloride dihydrate, $CaCl_2$•$2H_2O$, cp [*]	NA	100	—	27.53
Calcium hydroxide, $Ca(OH)_2$, cp	NA	100	—	54.09
Calcium oxide, CaO, cp [*]	NA	100	—	71.47
Calcium phosphate (monobasic), $Ca(H_2PO_4)_2$, from defluorinated phosphoric acid, fg	6–01–082	97	—	16.40
Calcium sulfate dihydrate, $CaSO_4$•$2H_2O$, cp	6–01–089	97	—	23.28
Curacao, phosphate, fg	6–05–586	99	—	34.34
Dicalcium phosphate (dibasic), $CaHPO_4$, from defluorinated phosphoric acid, fg	6–01–080	97	—	22.00
Dolomitic limestone (magnesium), fg	6–02–633	99	—	22.30
Limestone, ground, fg	6–02–632	100	—	34.00
Magnesium oxide, MgO, fg	6–02–756	98	—	3.07
Oystershell, flour (ground), fg	6–03–481	99	—	38.00
Phosphate, defluorinated, fg	6–01–780	100	—	32.00
Phosphate rock, fg	6–03–945	100	—	35.00
Phosphate rock, low-fluorine, fg	6–03–946	100	—	36.00
Soft rock phosphate colloidal clay, fg	6–03–947	100	—	17.00
Phosphorus Sources		(DM%)	(CPE%)	P (%)
Ammonium phosphate (dibasic), $(NH_4)_2HPO_4$, fg	6–00–370	97	115.9	20.60
Ammonium phosphate (monobasic), $(NH_4)H_2PO_4$, fg	6–09–338	97	70.9	24.74
Bone meal, steamed, fg	6–00–400	97	13.2	12.86
Calcium phosphate (monobasic), $Ca(H_2PO_4)_2$, from defluorinated phosphoric acid, fg	6–01–082	97	—	21.60
Curacao, phosphate, fg	6–05–586	99	—	14.14
Dicalcium phosphate (dibasic), $CaHPO_4$, from defluorinated phosphoric acid, fg	6–01–080	97	—	19.30
Phosphate, defluorinated, fg	6–01–780	100	—	18.00
Phosphate rock, fg	6–03–945	100	—	13.00
Phosphate rock, low-fluorine, fg	6–03–946	100	—	14.00
Phosphoric acid, $-H_3PO_4$, fg [*]	6–03–707	75	—	31.60
Sodium phosphate (monobasic) monohydrate, NaH_2PO_4•H_2O, fg	6–04–288	97	—	22.50
Sodium tripolyphosphate (meta- and pyro-phosphate) $Na_5P_3O_{10}$, fg	6–08–076	96	—	25.00
Soft rock phosphate, colloidal clay, fg	6–03–947	100	—	9.00
Sodium Sources		(DM%)	(CPE%)	Na (%)
Bone meal, steamed, fg	6–00–400	97	13.2	5.69
Phosphate, defluorinated, fg	6–01–780	100	—	4.90
Potassium chloride, KCl, fg	6–03–755	100	—	1.00
Sodium bicarbonate, $NaHCO_3$,fg	6–04–272	100	—	27.00
Sodium carbonate monohydrate, Na_2CO_3•H_2O, cp	NA	100	—	37.08
Sodium chloride, NaCl, fg	6–04–152	100	—	39.34
Sodium phosphate (monobasic) monohydrate, NaH_2PO_4•H2O, fg	6–04–288	97	—	16.68
Sodium selenate decahydrate, Na_2SeO_4•$10H_2O$, cp	NA	100	—	12.46
Sodium selenite, Na_2SeO_3, fg	6–26–013	98	—	26.60
Sodium sesquicarbonate dihydrate, Na_2CO_3 + $NaHCO_3$•$2H_2O$, fg	NA	100	—	30.50
Sodium sulfate decahydrate, Na_2SO_4•$10H_2O$, cp	6–04–292	97	—	14.27
Sodium tripolyphosphate(meta- and pyro-phosphate, $Na_5P_3O_{10}$, fg	6–08–076	96	—	31.00
Chloride Sources		(DM%)	(CPE%)	Cl (%)
Ammonium chloride, cp	NA	100	163.63	66.28
Calcium chloride anhydrous, $CaCl_2$, cp[*]	NA	100	—	63.89
Calcium chloride dihydrate, $CaCl_2$•$2H_2O$, cp[*]	NA	100	—	48.23
Cobalt dichloride hexahydrate, $CoCl_2$•$6H_2O$, cp	NA	100	—	29.80
Cupric chloride dihydrate, $CuCl_2$•$2H_2O$, cp	NA	100	—	41.65
Magnesium chloride hexahydrate, $MgCl_2$•$6H_2O$, cp	NA	100	—	34.88
Manganese dichloride, $MnCl_2$, cp	NA	100	—	56.34
Manganese chloride tetrahydrate, $MnCl_2$•$4H_2O$, cp	NA	100	—	35.80

TABLE 15-13 continued

Mineral Element Source	International Feed No.[a]	Dry Matter[b]	Crude Protein Equivalent (CPE) = N% × 6.25	Primary Mineral Element Content
Potassium chloride, KCl, fg	6–03–755	100	—	47.30
Sodium chloride, NaCl, fg	6–04–152	100	—	60.66
Zinc chloride, $ZnCl_2$, cp	NA	100	—	52.03
Potassium Sources		(DM%)	(CPE%)	K (%)
Potassium bicarbonate, $KHCO_3$, cp	6–29–493	99	—	39.05
Potassium carbonate, K_2CO_3, cp	NA	100	—	56.58
Potassium chloride, KCl, fg	6–03–755	100	—	50.00
Potassium iodide, KI, fg	6–03–759	100	—	21.00
Potassium sulfate, K_2SO_4, fg	6–06–098	98	—	41.84
Magnesium Sources		(DM%)	(CPE%)	Mg (%)
Dolomitic limestone (magnesium), fg	6–02–633	99	—	9.99
Limestone, ground, fg	6–02–632	100	—	2.06
Magnesium carbonate, $MgCO_3$, fg	6–02–754	98		30.81
Magnesium chloride hexahydrate, $MgCl_2•6H_2O$, cp	NA	100	—	11.96
Magnesium hydroxide, $Mg(OH)_2$, cp	NA	100	—	41.69
Magnesium oxide, MgO, fg	6–02–756	98	—	56.20
Magnesium sulfate heptahydrate, $MgSO_4•7H_2O$, fg	6–02–758	98	—	9.80
Sulfur Sources		(DM%)	(CPE%)	S (%)
Ammonium phosphate (dibasic), $(NH_4)_2HPO_4$, fg	6–00–370	97	115.9	2.16
Ammonium phosphate (monobasic), $(NH_4)H_2PO_4$, fg	6–09–338	97	70.9	1.46
Ammonium sulfate, $(NH_4)_2SO_4$, fg	6–09–339	100	134.1	24.10
Bone meal, steamed, fg	6–00–400	97	13.2	2.51
Calcium phosphate (monobasic), $Ca(H_2PO_4)_2$, from defluorinated phosphoric acid, fg	6–01–082	97	—	1.22
Calcium sulfate, dihydrate $CaSO_4•2H_2O$, fg	6–01–089	97	—	18.62
Cupric sulfate pentahydrate, $CuSO_4•5H_2O$	6–01–720	100	—	12.84
Dicalcium phosphate (dibasic), $CaHPO_4$, from defluorinated phosphoric acid, fg	6–01–080	97	—	1.14
Ferrous sulfate heptahydrate, $FeSO_4•7H_2O$, fg	6–20–734	98	—	12.35
Magnesium sulfate heptahydrate, $MgSO_4•7H_2O$, fg	NA	98	—	13.31
Manganese sulfate monohydrate, $MnSO_4•H_2O$, cp	NA	100	—	18.97
Manganese sulfate pentahydrate, $MnSO_4•5H_2O$, cp	NA	100	—	13.30
Phosphoric acid, $-H_3PO_4$, fg *	6–03–707	75	—	1.55
Potassium sulfate, K_2SO_4, fg	6–06–098	98	—	17.35
Sodium sulfate decahydrate, $Na_2SO_4•10H_2O$, cp	6–04–292	97	—	9.95
Zinc sulfate monohydrate, $ZnSO_4•H_2O$, fg	6–05–555	99	—	17.68
Cobalt Sources		(DM%)	(CPE%)	Co (mg/kg)
Cobalt carbonate, $CoCO_3$, fg	6–01–566	99	—	460,000
Cobalt carbonate hexahydrate, $CoCO_3•6H_2O$, cp	NA	100	—	259,000
Cobalt dichloride hexahydrate, $CoCl_2•6H_2O$, cp	NA	100	—	247,800
Copper (Cupric) Sources		(DM%)	(CPE%)	Cu (mg/kg)
Cupric chloride dihydrate, $CuCl_2•2H_2O$, cp	NA	100	—	372,000
Cupric oxide, CuO, cp	NA	100	—	798,800
Cupric sulfate pentahydrate, $CuSO_4•5H_2O$, cp	6–01–720	100	—	254,500
Iodine Sources		(DM%)	(CPE%)	I (mg/kg)
Ethylenediaminodihydroiodide (EDDI), fg	6–01–842	98	—	803,400
Potassium iodide, KI, fg	6–03–759	100	—	681,700
Iron Sources		(DM%)	(CPE%)	Fe (mg/kg)
Ammonium phosphate (dibasic), $(NH_4)_2HPO_4$, fg	6–00–370	97	115.9	12,400
Ammonium phosphate (monobasic), $(NH_4)H_2PO_4$, fg	6–09–338	97	70.9	17,400
Bone meal, steamed, fg	6–00–400	97	13.2	26,700
Calcium phosphate (monobasic), $Ca(H_2PO_4)_2$, from defluorinated phosphoric acid, fg	6–01–082	97	—	15,800
Dicalcium phosphate (dibasic), $CaHPO_4$, from defluorinated phosphoric acid, fg	6–01–080	97	—	14,400

TABLE 15-13 continued

Mineral Element Source	International Feed No.[a]	Dry Matter[b]	Crude Protein Equivalent (CPE) = N% × 6.25	Primary Mineral Element Content
Ferrous sulfate heptahydrate, $FeSO_4 \cdot 7H_2O$, fg	6–20–734	98	—	218,400
Phosphate rock, fg	6–03–945	100	—	16,800
Phosphoric acid, $-H_3PO_4$, fg *	6–03–707	75	—	17,500
Soft rock phosphate, colloidal clay, fg	6–03–947	100	—	19,000
Manganese (Manganous) Sources		(DM%)	(CPE%)	Mn (mg/kg)
Manganese carbonate, $MnCO_3$, cp	6–03–036	97	—	478,000
Manganese chloride, $MnCl_2$, cp	NA	100	—	430,000
Manganese chloride tetrahydrate, $MnCl_2 \cdot 4H_2O$, cp	NA	100	—	277,000
Manganese oxide, MnO, cp	6–03–056	99	—	774,500
Manganese sulfate monohydrate, $MnSO_4 \cdot H_2O$, cp	NA	100	—	325,069
Manganese sulfate pentahydrate, $Mn\ SO_4 \cdot 5H_2O$, cp	NA	100	—	227,891
Selenium Sources		(DM%)	(CPE%)	Se(mg/kg)
Sodium selenate decahydrate, $Na_2SeO_4 \cdot 10H_2O$, cp	NA	100	—	213,920
Sodium selenite, Na_2SeO_3, cp	6–26–013	98	—	456,000
Zinc Sources		(DM%)	(CPE%)	Zn (mg/kg)
Zinc carbonate, $ZnCO_3$, cp	NA	100	—	521,400
Zinc chloride, $ZnCl_2$, cp	NA	100	—	479,700
Zinc oxide, ZnO, cp	6–05–533	100	—	780,000
Zinc sulfate monohydrate, $ZnSO_4 \cdot H_2O$, fg	6–05–555	99	—	363,600
Fluorine Sources			(CPE%)	Fl (mg/kg)
Ammonium phosphate (dibasic), $(NH_4)_2HPO_4$, fg	6–00–370	97	115.9	2,100
Ammonium phosphate (monobasic), $(NH_4)H_2PO_4$, fg	6–09–338	97	70.9	2,500
Calcium phosphate (monobasic), $Ca(H_2PO_4)_2$, from defluorinated phosphoric acid, fg	6–01–082	97	—	2,100
Curacao, phosphate, fg	6–05–586	99	—	5,550
Dicalcium phosphate (dibasic), $CaHPO_4$, from defluorinated phosphoric acid, fg	6–01–080	97	—	1,800
Phosphate, defluorinated, fg	6–01–780	100	—	1,800
Phosphate rock, fg	6–03–945	100	—	35,000
Phosphoric acid, H_3PO_4, fg *	6–03–707	75	—	3,100
Soft rock phosphate, colloidal clay, fg	6–03–947	100	—	15,000

NOTE: The compositions of hydrated mineral sources (e.g., $CaSO_4 \cdot 2H_2O$) are shown including the waters of hydration. Mineral element compositions of feed-grade sources vary by source, processing method, site of mining, and manufacturer. Sources should be analyzed or manufacturer's analyses should be used when available. Element composition of a source is listed if specific element concentration is ≥ 1.0 percent for macromineral elements, or ≥ 10,000 mg/kg for micromineral elements, except for fluorine concentrations which are listed because of potential toxicity.

[a]First digit denotes the class of feed: 1, dry forages and roughages; 2, pastured, range plants, and forages fed green; 3, silages; 4, energy feeds; 5, protein supplement; 6, minerals; 7, vitamins; 8, additives. The other five digits identify the individual feed.

[b]Dry matter contents have been estimated for the sources; actual analysis will be more accurate.

[c]fg = Feed-grade source.

[d]None present.

[e]cp = Chemically pure form.

[f]NA = Not available.

*Use caution when handling and mixing, can be extremely hazardous.

TABLE 15-14 Table of Conversion Factors

Units	Multiplied by Equals	Units	Multiplied by Equals	Units
pound (lb)	0.4536	kilogram (kg)	2.205	pound (lb)
ounce (oz)	28.35	gram (g)	0.03527	ounce (oz)
gallon, U.S. liquid (gal)	3.785	liter (L)	0.2642	gallon, U.S. liquid (gal)
gallon, U.K. (gal)	4.546	liter (L)	0.2200	gallon, U.K. (gal)
bushel, U.S. (bu)	35.24	liter (L)	0.02838	bushel, U.S. (bu)
bushel, U.K. (bu)	36.37	liter (L)	0.02750	bushel, U.K. (bu)
calorie (cal)	4.184	joule (J)	0.2390	calorie (cal)
mile (mi)	1.609	kilometer (km)	0.6214	mile (mi)
acre (ac)	0.4047	hectare (ha)	2.471	acre (ac)
hectare (ha)	10,000	square meter (m^2)	0.0001	hectare (ha)
ppm	1	mg/kg	1	ppm
ppm	1	μg/g	1	ppm
ppm	0.0001	%	10,000	ppm

Prefixes for the International System of Units (SI)

Units Greater Than the Standard Unit

Item	Prefix	To convert from standard unit multiply by[a]
G	giga	1,000,000,000
M	mega	1,000,000
k	kilo	1,000

Units Less Than the Standard Unit

Item	Prefix	To convert from standard unit divide by[b]
d	deci	10
c	centi	100
m	milli	1,000
μ	micro	1,000,000
n	nano	1,000,000,000

[a]For example, 1 kg (kilogram) = 1 g multiplied by 1,000 = 1,000 g.
[b]For example, 1 mg (milligram) = 1 g divided by 1,000 = 1/1,000 g.

Fahrenheit to Celsius (Centigrade) Conversions

Fahrenheit	Celsius
110	43.3
105	40.6
100	37.8
95	35.0
90	32.2
85	29.4
80	26.7
75	23.9
70	21.1
65	18.3
60	15.6
55	12.8
50	10.0
45	7.2
40	4.4
35	1.7
30	–1.1
25	–3.9
20	–6.7
15	–9.4
10	–12.2
5	–15.0
0	–17.8
–5	–20.6
–10	–23.3
–15	–26.1
–20	–28.9
–25	–31.7
–30	–34.4
–35	–37.2
–40	–40.0

Appendix A

Committee Statement of Task

The Committee on Animal Nutrition proposes to convene a subcommittee to revise two reports in its series: Nutrient Requirements of Goats (1981) and Nutrient Requirements of Sheep (1985). The two reports will be revised in a single report on nutrient requirements of small ruminants. A thorough review of the scientific literature and data on nutrient requirements of small ruminants will be conducted. All life phases and types of small ruminant animal production will be addressed. Updated recommendations will be made with consideration for the increased performance of different types of sheep and goats, as well as other uses of small ruminants. Effects of the environment, feed additives, and metabolism modifiers on nutrient requirements will be addressed. In addition, quantitative information on rumen and tissue requirements for protein will be incorporated, as well as new information on bioavailability of various nutrients. This revision will provide the user with recommendations for predicting nutrient requirements of small ruminants with consideration of various management situations. New and expanded information will be provided on feed composition. Areas of needed research also will be identified.

Appendix B

Abbreviations and Acronyms

25-(OH)D	25-hydroxyvitamin D
AA	Amino acid
AC	Absorption coefficient
ACT	Grazing activity
ADF	Acid detergent fiber
ADFI	Average daily feed intake
ADG	Average daily gain
ADG_{mbw}	Average daily gain scaled for body weight
ADG_{obs}	Observed average daily gain
ADG_{pred}	Prediction of average daily gain
$ADG_{pred\text{-}en}$	Average daily gain based on energy
ADP	Adenosine diphosphate
AF	Adjustment factor
AF_{act}	Adjustment factor for activity
AFRC	Agriculture and Food Research Council
AGE	Age
AGEM	Age in months
AOAC	Association of Official Analytical Chemists
ARC	Agricultural Research Council
ARS	Agricultural Research Service
ASIA	American Sheep Industry Association
ATP	Adenosine triphosphate
BCS	Body condition score
BCS_{fin}	Final body condition score
BCS_{init}	Initial body condition score
BIRWT	Average birth weight
BL	Body length
BMR	Basal metabolic rate
bST	Bovine somatotrophin
BW	Body weight
CAD	Cation and anion differences
cal	Calorie
CF	Crude fiber
CFW	Clean fleece weight
CHO	Carbohydrate
CLA	Conjugated linoleic acid
CNCPS	Cornell Net Carbohydrate and Protein System
CP	Crude protein
CPI	Crude protein intake
CS	Concentrate selectors
CSF	Cerebrospinal fluid
CSIRO	Commonwealth Scientific and Industrial Research Organisation
CSM	Cottonseed meal
CSREES	Cooperative State Research, Education, and Extension Service
CT	Condensed tannins
CWC	Cell wall constituents
d	Day
DAY	Day of gestation
DE	Digestible energy
DEB	Dietary electrolyte balance
DEE	Daily energy expenditure
DEI	Digestible energy intake
Dig	Digestibility
DIP	Degradable intake protein
DM	Dry matter
DMD	Dry matter digestibility
DMI	Dry matter intake
DMI_g	Dry matter intake required for gain
DMI_m	Dry matter intake required for maintenance
DOH	Deuterated water
DP	Digestible protein
DT	Distance traveled
EAT	Effective ambient temperature
EB	Empty body
EBW_{fin}	Final empty body weight
EBW_{init}	Initial empty body weight
ECF	Extracellular fluid
EDDI	Ethylenediamine dihydroiodate
EDTA	ethylenediaminetetraacetic acid
EE	Ether extract
EI	External insulation

eNDF	Effective neutral detergent fiber
EUCP	Endogenous urinary crude protein loss
EVG	Energy concentration in empty body gain
EWL	Insensible water loss
FAO/WHO	Food and Agriculture Organization/World Health Organization
FAOSTAT	Food and Agriculture Organization of the United Nations, FAO Statistical Databases
$FatFr_{fin}$	Final fraction of fat in the empty body
$FatFr_{init}$	Initial fraction of fat in the empty body
$FatM_{fin}$	Final fat mass
$FatM_{init}$	Initial fat mass
FBW	Full body weight
FBW_{fin}	Final full body weight
FBW_{init}	Initial full or unshrunk body weight
$F\text{-}CP_e$	Metabolic fecal crude protein
FCM	Fat-corrected milk
FDA	Food and Drug Administration
FE	Fecal energy
FHP	Fasting heat production
FmatBW	Estimate of final mature body weight
FWI	Free water intake
FWL	Fecal water loss
GasE	Gaseous energy
GE	Gross energy
GIT	Gastrointestinal tract
GPx	Glutathione peroxidase
GR	Grass/roughage eaters
GRF	Growth hormone releasing factor
GWT	Grazing plus walking time
h	Hour
H	Height
H_e	Minimal evaporative heat loss
HE	Heat energy
HiE	Heat increment
HjE	Activity
I	Intake or Iodine
ICF	Intracellular fluid
IFBW	Ingesta-free body weight
IM	Intermediate types
IN	Total insulation
INRA	Institut National de la Recherche Agronomique
IU	International units
IVDMD	In vitro dry matter digestibility
IW	Inspired water
J	Joule
k_f	Efficiency of metabolizable energy utilization for fiber growth
k_g	Efficiency of metabolizable energy utilization for gain
k_l	Efficiency of metabolizable energy utilization for lactation
k_{lt}	Efficiency of mobilized tissue energy use for lactation
k_m	Efficiency of metabolizable energy utilization for maintenance
k_{mt}	Efficiency of mobilized tissue energy use for maintenance
k_{pf}	Efficiency of metabolizable protein use for fiber growth
k_{pg}	Efficiency of metabolizable protein use for gain
k_{pl}	Efficiency of metabolizable protein use for lactation
k_{p-lt}	Efficiency of use of maternal tissue
k_{pl-t}	Efficiency of mobilized tissue protein for milk production
k_{pm}	Efficiency of metabolizable protein use for maintenance
$k_{p\text{-}preg}$	Efficiency of metabolizable protein use for pregnancy
k_{preg}	Efficiency of metabolizable energy use for pregnancy
LBM	Lean body mass
LBW	Litter birth weight
LCT	Lower critical temperature
LEAD	Livestock, Environment, and Development Initiative
LS	Litter size
LW	Live weight
LWG	Live weight gain
MAFF	UK Ministry of Agriculture, Fisheries and Food
MATRBW	Mature ram body weight
ME	Metabolizable energy
ME_a	Metabolizable energy for antler growth
MEC	Metabolizable energy concentration in the diet
ME_f	Metabolizable energy used for fiber growth
ME_f/ME_g	Proportion of metabolizable energy for gain used for fiber growth
ME_g	Metabolizable energy used for tissue gain
MEI	Metabolizable energy intake
ME_l	Metabolizable energy used for lactation
$ME_{l\text{-}d}$	Dietary metabolizable energy for lactation
$ME_{l\text{-}t}$	Mobilized tissue energy used for lactation when average daily gain is negative
ME_m	Metabolizable energy required for maintenance
ME_{preg}	Metabolizable energy used for pregnancy
ME_{tg}	Metabolizable energy used for nonfiber tissue gain
MFC	Milk fat concentration
MFCP	Metabolic fecal crude protein (or nitrogen)
$MFCP_m$	Metabolic fecal crude protein (or nitrogen) for maintenance

MP	Metabolizable protein or Milk production
MP_{antler}	Metabolizable protein for antlers
MPC	Milk true protein concentration
MP_f	Metabolizable protein for fiber
MP_g	Metabolizable protein available for gain or growth
$MP_{g\text{-}used}$	Metabolizable protein used for gain or mobilized
MP_{gest}	Metabolizable protein for gestation
MPI	Metabolizable protein intake
MP_l	Metabolizable protein used for lactation
$MP_{l\text{-}d}$	Dietary (including microbial) metabolizable protein used or required for lactation
$MP_{l\text{-}t}$	Mobilized tissue protein used for lactation when average daily gain is negative
MP_m	Metabolizable protein required for maintenance
MPI_{mbw}	Metabolizable protein intake scaled for body weight
MP_{preg}	Metabolizable protein used for pregnancy
MPR	Metabolic protein requirement
MP_{req}	Total metabolizable protein requirement
MP-SCURF	Metabolizable protein used for scurf
MTPC	Milk true protein concentration
MUCP	Metabolic urinary crude protein
MW	Mature weight or Metabolic water
MWL	Milk water loss
MY	Milk yield
N	Nitrogen
NAD	Nicotinamide adenine dinucleotide
NADP	Nicotinamide adenine dinucleotide phosphate
NASS	National Agricultural Statistics Service
NDF	Neutral detergent fiber
NDS	Neutral detergent solubles
NDSF	Neutral detergent-soluble fiber
NE	Net energy
NE_f	Net energy for fiber growth
NE_g	Net energy for gain
$NE_{g\text{-}ADG}$	Net energy for gain requirement on an average daily gain basis
NE_l	Net energy for lactation
$NE_{l\text{-}d}$	Dietary net energy for lactation
$NE_{l\text{-}obs}$	Observed milk energy yield
$NE_{l\text{-}pred}$	Predicted milk energy yield
NE_m	Net energy for maintenance
$NE_{m\text{-}SBW}$	Unadjusted energy requirement for fasting metabolism
NE_{preg}	Net energy used for pregnancy
NFC	Non-neutral detergent fiber carbohydrates
NFE	Nitrogen-free extract
NP	Net protein
NP_f	Net protein for fiber
NP_g	Net protein for gain
$NP_{g\text{-}used}$	Net protein gained or replacing maintenance protein with tissue mobilization
NP_l	Net protein for lactation
$NP_{l\text{-}d}$	Net protein for lactation from the diet
$NP_{l\text{-}t}$	Net protein for lactation from the tissue
NPN	Nonprotein nitrogen
NP_{preg}	Net protein used for pregnancy
NRC	National Research Council
NWC	New World camelids
OM	Organic matter
oST	Ovine somatotrophin
P	Maturity index or Protein or Phosphorus
PEG	Polyethylene glycol
$ProFr_{fin}$	Final fraction of protein in the empty body
$ProFr_{init}$	Initial fraction of protein in the empty body
$ProM_{fin}$	Final protein mass in the empty body
$ProM_{init}$	Initial protein mass in the empty body
PRP	Proline-rich proteins
PSM	Plant secondary metabolites
PTH	Parathyroid hormone
PW	Preformed water in or on food
Q	Energy content of milk
RE	Retinol equivalents or Recovered energy
R-R	Rumen-reticulum
RW	Water released from food or tissue
SA	Surface area
SBM	Soybean meal
SBW	Shrunk body weight
SCA	Standing Committee on Agriculture
SCURF	Scurf
SE	Standard error
$SF\text{-}CP_E$	Scurf and fiber crude protein
SFW	Standard fleece weight
SGE	Sheep growth energy
SGP	Sheep growth protein
SLE	Sheep lactation energy
SLMP	Scurf loss metabolizable protein
ST	Somatotrophin
T_3	Triiodothyronine
T_4	Tetraiodothyronine or thyroxin
T_a	Ambient temperature
TAC	True absorption coefficient
TBW	Total body water
TDN	Total digestible nutrients
TE_{fin}	Final tissue energy
TE_{init}	Initial tissue energy
TEC	Energy concentration in tissue accreted or mobilized
TEC_{avg}	Average energy concentration on a full body weight basis during the feeding period
TECFBW	Energy concentration in tissue lost or gained
TEMA	Trace Elements in Man and Animals

TER	Terrain score
TI	Tissue insulation
TNR	Thermoneutral range
TOH	Tritiated water
TPC	Protein concentration in tissue accreted or mobilized
TPFr	Protein concentration in tissue accreted or mobilized on an empty BW basis
$TPFr_{avg}$	Average protein concentration as a fraction on a full body weight basis during the feeding period
T_{lc}	Lower critical temperature
T_{uc}	Upper critical temperature
TWI	Total water intake
TWL	Total water loss
$U\text{-}CP_E$	Endogenous urinary crude protein
UE	Urinary energy
UIP	Undegradable intake protein
UME_m	Unadjusted metabolizable energy requirement for maintenance
UME_{req}	Unadjusted total metabolizable energy requirement
UNE_m	Unadjusted net energy requirement for maintenance
USDA	United States Department of Agriculture
UWL	Urinary water loss
VFA	Volatile fatty acid
VO	Visceral organ tissue energy use
W	Weight
WAAF	Wool age adjustment factor
W_b	Birth weight
WCS	Whole cottonseed
WEI	Water economy index
WI	Water intake
wk	Week
WL	Water loss
WP	Total annual wool production
WR	Water requirement
WSC	Water-soluble carbohydrate
WTR	Water transfer rate
WW	Wet weight

Appendix C

Committee Member Biographies

James E. (Ed) Huston, Ph.D. (Chair) is professor (emeritus) of animal science and range science at the Texas A&M University Research Center, San Angelo. Huston received a B.S. (1963), M.S. (1965), and Ph.D. (1971), all from Texas A&M University. He was a member of the 1981 NRC committee on the *Nutrient Requirements of Goats*. Before his recent retirement, Huston spent more than 30 years researching the nutritional needs of goats, sheep, and wildlife. Most of his research has involved the feeding of livestock on range. He currently serves on the editorial boards of the *Sheep and Goat Research Journal* and *Small Ruminant Research*. He has chaired regional committees on Sheep and Goat Research and Education Programs and on Grazing Behavior and Nutritional Status of Domestic Ruminants.

Robert G. White, Ph.D. (Vice-Chair) is professor (emeritus) and director, Institute of Arctic Biology (emeritus) at the University of Alaska Fairbanks. He received a B.Ag.S. (1962) from the University of Melbourne (Australia), and an M.Rur.S. (1968) and Ph.D. (1974) from the University of New England (Australia). White is a fellow of the American Association for the Advancement of Science, a fellow of the Arctic Institute of North America, and a past president of the Comparative Nutrition Society. He has published research on a wide range of wild and domestic animals, including caribou, reindeer, moose, voles, muskoxen, and sheep. His primary research interests are the nutritional and physiological adaptations of animals to the environment, nutritional and physiological ecology, and modeling physiological and ecological processes.

Brian J. Bequette, Ph.D. is an assistant professor in the Department of Animal and Avian Sciences at the University of Maryland. He received a B.S. (1983) from the University of Illinois, an M.S. (1986) from the Southern Illinois University, and a Ph.D. (1990) from the University of Missouri. The goal of his research program is to reduce the amount of nitrogen that ruminants and other farm animals excrete into the environment by improving an animal's ability to conserve nitrogen. The three ruminant-related areas on which he focuses are urea recycling, digestive metabolism, and modeling limiting amino acids for growth and lactation. Before his current position, Bequette spent 10 years at the Rowett Research Institute in Scotland. He is a member of the editorial board of the *British Journal of Nutrition*. Bequette has published extensively and written book chapters on the amino acid metabolism of sheep, goats, and dairy cattle, especially metabolism by the gastrointestinal tissues and the mammary gland. He is familiar with small ruminant production in both the United States and the United Kingdom.

Hugh Dove, Ph.D. is a chief research scientist at the Commonwealth Scientific and Industrial Research Organisation (CSIRO) in Canberra, Australia. He received a B.Agr.Sci. (1968), Dip.Ed. (1969), and Ph.D. (1976) from the University of Melbourne (Australia). Dove is coeditor of the textbook *Sheep Nutrition*. He is an associate editor of the *Journal of the Science of Food and Agriculture* and a member of the editorial board of the Nutrition Society of Australia. His research has focused on the nutrition and management of ruminants in grazing systems, and on the measurement of herbage, supplement, and milk intakes. He is familiar with sheep production in Australia, New Zealand, and the United Kingdom.

Arthur L. Goetsch, Ph.D. is research leader at the E. (Kika) de la Garza American Institute for Goat Research at Langston University. He received a B.S. (1979) from Illinois State University, an M.S. (1980) from the University of Missouri, and a Ph.D. (1982) from New Mexico State University. He has investigated energy and protein utilization, feed intake, growth and lactation performance, and body composition in both sheep and goats. Goetsch is a past section editor of the *Journal of Animal Science*. He is currently a member of the editorial board of the journal *Small Ruminant*

Research and is on the advisory boards for the *Journal of Applied Animal Research* and *Egyptian Journal of Nutrition and Feeds*. He has extensive experience in the determination of nutrient requirements of goats and in the development of a web-based nutrient requirement calculation system for goats.

Bret W. Hess, Ph.D. is an associate professor in the Department of Animal Science at the University of Wyoming. He received a B.S. (1991) and an M.S. (1993) from the University of Nevada and a Ph.D. (1996) from the University of Missouri. Hess has actively participated as a member of the Western Section of the American Society of Animal Science and in collaborative regional projects on improving ruminant use of forages. He is a past president of the Colorado/Wyoming/Western Nebraska/Western Kansas Area Chapter of the American Registry of Professional Animal Scientists and is an associate editor for the *Journal of Animal Science*. He received the Young Scientist Award from the Western Section of the American Society of Animal Science. He has expertise in energy and lipid nutrition of sheep, especially in western range production systems. His current research is focused on nutritional management to improve livestock production.

Maximino Huerta Bravo, Ph.D. is a professor of animal sciences at the University of Chapingo (Mexico). He received a B.S. (1977) from the University of Chapingo and an M.S. (1980) and Ph.D. (2000) from Washington State University. Huerta Bravo is currently president of the Mexican Society of Animal Science. He has developed software to estimate nutrient requirements of sheep based on U.S., British, and French estimates of requirements. His primary area of research is the mineral nutrition of ruminants. He also has expertise in fiber utilization by ruminants.

David G. Pugh, D.V.M., M.S. is a veterinary consultant for Fort Dodge Animal Health in Waverly, Alabama. He received a B.S. (1976), an M.S. (1978), and a D.V.M. (1981), all from the University of Georgia. Pugh is the author of the textbook *Sheep and Goat Medicine* and the sheep and goat nutrition section of the *Merck Veterinary Manual*. Pugh has published research on the health and nutrition of sheep, goats, alpacas, and llamas. His primary contributions to nutrition knowledge have been in the area of trace mineral nutrition.

Sandra G. Solaiman, Ph.D., PAS, is an associate professor of animal and poultry sciences at Tuskegee University and is an affiliated associate professor in animal sciences at Auburn University. She received a B.S. (1974) from the University of Urmia (Iran), an M.S. (1978) from Oklahoma State University, and a Ph.D. (1984) from the University of Missouri-Columbia. She is also a class 10 graduate (2001) of the U.S. Department of Agriculture Leadership Development Program. Her research contributions for the last 15 years have been in the area of goat nutrition, kinetics of digestion and passage, trace mineral copper, alternative feeds, and forage/pasture utilization. Her major contribution to goat nutrition is her study on copper requirement for goats. Currently she continues her copper work and is involved in sustainable goat production systems research using year-round foraging and comparing different goat production systems in the southern United States. Other areas of interest include the environmental and sustainability aspects of ruminant nutrition.

Appendix D

Board on Agriculture and Natural Resources Publications

Policy and Resources

Agricultural Biotechnology and the Poor: Proceedings of an International Conference (2000)
Agricultural Biotechnology: Strategies for National Competitiveness (1987)
Agriculture and the Undergraduate: Proceedings (1992)
Agriculture's Role in K–12 Education: A Forum on the National Science Education Standards (1998)
Alternative Agriculture (1989)
Animal Biotechnology: Science-Based Concerns (2002)
Brucellosis in the Greater Yellowstone Area (1998)
Colleges of Agriculture at the Land Grant Universities: A Profile (1995)
Colleges of Agriculture at the Land Grant Universities: Public Service and Public Policy (1996)
Designing an Agricultural Genome Program (1998)
Designing Foods: Animal Product Options in the Marketplace (1988)
Ecological Monitoring of Genetically Modified Crops (2001)
Ecologically Based Pest Management: New Solutions for a New Century (1996)
Emerging Animal Diseases—Global Markets, Global Safety: A Workshop Summary (2002)
Ensuring Safe Food: From Production to Consumption (1998)
Exploring Horizons for Domestic Animal Genomics: Workshop Summary (2002)
Forested Landscapes in Perspective: Prospects and Opportunities for Sustainable Management of America's Nonfederal Forests (1997)
Frontiers in Agricultural Research: Food, Health, Environment, and Communities (2002)
Future Role of Pesticides for U.S. Agriculture (2000)
Genetic Engineering of Plants: Agricultural Research Opportunities and Policy Concerns (1984)
Genetically Modified Pest-Protected Plants: Science and Regulation (2000)
Incorporating Science, Economics, and Sociology in Developing Sanitary and Phytosanitary Standards in International Trade: Proceedings of a Conference (2000)
Investing in Research: A Proposal to Strengthen the Agricultural, Food, and Environmental System (1989)
Investing in the National Research Initiative: An Update of the Competitive Grants Program in the U.S. Department of Agriculture (1994)
Managing Global Genetic Resources: Agricultural Crop Issues and Policies (1993)
Managing Global Genetic Resources: Forest Trees (1991)
Managing Global Genetic Resources: Livestock (1993)
Managing Global Genetic Resources: The U.S. National Plant Germplasm System (1991)
National Research Initiative: A Vital Competitive Grants Program in Food, Fiber, and Natural Resources Research (2000)
New Directions for Biosciences Research in Agriculture: High-Reward Opportunities (1985)
Pesticide Resistance: Strategies and Tactics for Management (1986)
Pesticides and Groundwater Quality: Issues and Problems in Four States (1986)
Pesticides in the Diets of Infants and Children (1993)
Precision Agriculture in the 21st Century: Geospatial and Information Technologies in Crop Management (1997)
Professional Societies and Ecologically Based Pest Management (2000)
Rangeland Health: New Methods to Classify, Inventory, and Monitor Rangelands (1994)
Regulating Pesticides in Food: The Delaney Paradox (1987)
Resource Management (1991)

The Role of Chromium in Animal Nutrition (1997)
The Scientific Basis for Estimating Air Emissions from Animal Feeding Operations: Interim Report (2002)
Soil and Water Quality: An Agenda for Agriculture (1993)
Soil Conservation: Assessing the National Resources Inventory, Volume 1 (1986); Volume 2 (1986)
Standards in International Trade (2000)
Sustainable Agriculture and the Environment in the Humid Tropics (1993)
Sustainable Agriculture Research and Education in the Field: A Proceedings (1991)
Understanding Agriculture: New Directions for Education (1988)
The Use of Drugs in Food Animals: Benefits and Risks (1999)
Water Transfers in the West: Efficiency, Equity, and the Environment (1992)
Wood in Our Future: The Role of Life Cycle Analysis (1997)

Nutrient Requirements of Domestic Animals Series and Related Titles

Building a North American Feed Information System (1995) (available from the Board on Agriculture)
Metabolic Modifiers: Effects on the Nutrient Requirements of Food-Producing Animals (1994)
Mineral Tolerance of Animals (2005)
Nutrient Requirements of Beef Cattle, Seventh Revised Edition, Update (2000)
Nutrient Requirements of Dairy Cattle, Seventh Revised Edition (2001)
Nutrient Requirements of Dogs and Cats (2006)
Nutrient Requirements of Fish (1993)
Nutrient Requirements of Horses, Fifth Revised Edition (1989)
Nutrient Requirements of Laboratory Animals, Fourth Revised Edition (1995)
Nutrient Requirements of Nonhuman Primates, Second Revised Edition (2003)
Nutrient Requirements of Poultry, Ninth Revised Edition (1994)
Nutrient Requirements of Swine, Tenth Revised Edition (1998)
Predicting Feed Intake of Food-Producing Animals (1986)
Role of Chromium in Animal Nutrition (1997)
Scientific Advances in Animal Nutrition: Promise for the New Century (2001)
Vitamin Tolerance of Animals (1987)

Further information, additional titles (prior to 1984), and prices are available from the National Academies Press, 2101 Constitution Avenue, NW, Washington, DC 20418, 202-334-3313 (information only). To order any of the titles above, visit the National Academies Press bookstore at *http://www.nap.edu/bookstore.*

Index

C

D

E

F

G

H

I

J

K

L

M

R

S

X

Y

Z